'The *Handbook of Sport Neuroscience and Psychophysiology* is a useful reference source for educators, researchers, students and practitioners in sport psychology and allied fields. If sports provide a microcosm for life's physical and mental struggles and achievements, this book is a great way to learn more about the brain, and how it can be optimized for both performance and recovery. Emphasizing ecological approaches that have gained widespread use in the high-performance training culture, the authors convey how the core principles of neuroscience/social neuroscience, psychophysiology, and biofeedback can help athletes and coaches optimize training, performance, and rehabilitation, each by understanding how the human brain has evolved to optimize skill performance, cope with expected and unexpected challenges, and remain robust to injuries and defeats through biologically-mediated healing and recovery. Understanding these systems will help athletes of all levels learn how to leverage them most effectively, just like honing any performance-related skill. Whether you are seeking an introduction to the neuropsychology of sports or a primer on the brain, this book is a well-written, well-curated new resource for the community.'
– **Justin Baker, MD, PhD**, Scientific Director, Institute for Technology in Psychiatry, McLean Hospital, Harvard Medical School

'The *Handbook of Sport Neuroscience and Psychophysiology* combines the latest theory, research, and practical insights in this rapidly evolving space. The breadth of topics covered by the team of renowned experts, led by Dr. Roland A. Carlstedt and Dr. Michela Balconi, represents a landmark contribution to the field. While not sacrificing scientific rigor, the book is accessible and relevant not only to clinicians and scientists but also students, coaches, and athletes. From the most recent advances utilizing digital technologies to the fundamental theories grounding the field of sport neuroscience and psychophysiology, this book offers unrivaled access and information.'
– **John Torous, MD, MBI,** Director of the Division of Digital Psychiatry, Beth Israel Deaconess Medical Center, Harvard Medical School

'Elegantly written, the *Handbook of Sport Neuroscience and Psychophysiology* takes on a journey through the neural pathways of sport. This book is a clear guide to what is going on in our brains in real time as we engage in physical activity and participate in our favorite past times. Using the advanced technology, including neuroimaging, EEG, bio and neurofeedback, the authors probe deep into our brains and map out our electrophysiological and hemodynamic responses during sport activity and physical exercise. This is a must read for clinicians, researchers, instructors, students, athlete, and coaches. It is a seminal reference for how the brain works in the context of sport and evidence-based, biomarker approaches to assessing and enhancing athletic performance as well as the clinical neuroscience of exercise and brain concussion. Welcome to the present and future of sport neuroscience.'
– **Philippe Douyon, MD,** Assistant Professor of Neurology, Seton Hall-Hackensack Meridian School of Medicine; Founder & CEO of The Inle BrainFit Institute

'Expanding on his own pioneering studies of professional athletes, Dr. Roland A. Carlstedt, together with Dr. Michela Balconi, recruited prominent contemporary researchers and practitioners to produce the first comprehensive handbook offering both applied and theoretical perspectives on the neuroscience and psychophysiology of sport performance—again a pioneering contribution. Underscoring the timeliness of this handbook, there is a growing interest in how best to nurture and monitor both the progress and long-term well-being of athletic talents at any level.'
– **Auke Tellegen, PhD,** Professor Emeritus, Department of Psychology, University of Minnesota

'In this cutting-edge book, Dr. Roland A. Carlstedt has assembled a blue-ribbon collection of international authors to present the state of the art in sport neuroscience and psychophysiology. Did you know that "motor imagery" can now be imaged using creative experimental paradigms and sophisticated brain imaging technology? Or that teams seem to produce a "group mind" that can be quantified using "mind-body" measures or that heart rate deceleration during pre-action phases of competition appears to be a biomarker of being In-the-Zone? These and many other questions are addressed and answered in this comprehensive handbook, making it a must-read for students, clinicians, sport psychologists, coaches and athletes. It is an excellent reference source and the go-to textbook for college courses in sport neuroscience and psychophysiology (that I think will proliferate because of this book).'

– **Stanley Krippner, PhD,** Professor of Psychology, Saybrook University; American Board of Sport Psychology

'The *Handbook of Sport Neuroscience and Psychophysiology* is an invaluable sport psychology resource— in addition to those in the psychology field, it will also be of interest to practitioners in sports medicine as well as coaches and athletes. I will be using the book in my Sports Medicine Fellowship training program. The book is a review of the literature in-of-itself, providing readers with a survey of seminal research in the context of evidence-based, validated approaches to athlete assessment/diagnostics, mental and peak performance training. As a former tennis professional, I appreciate how this book can also benefit competitive athletes by exposing them to advanced procedures, methods and analytics. I will recommend it to my colleagues, trainees, student-athletes, coaches, and patients. All-in-all, this is a landmark book that I think will have a major impact in a number of fields that focus on sports and athletes and beyond.'

– **Clifford Stark, DO,** Clinical Director, Sports Medicine at Chelsea, New York City; Director, Northwell Health Plainview Hospital Sports Medicine Fellowship; Clinical Instructor, New York University Langone Medical Center

Handbook of Sport Neuroscience and Psychophysiology

Out of the broad arena of sport science and sport psychology, Roland A. Carlstedt presents a comprehensive collection on the neuroscience and associated psychophysiology that underlies and drives sport performance. Featuring sections ranging from the basics and foundations (anatomy and physiology) to the applied (assessment during competition, training, and mental training), *Handbook of Sport Neuroscience and Psychophysiology* is the first volume to provide students, researchers, practitioners, and coaches the latest knowledge on the brain, mind-body processes, and psychophysiological responding in the context of sport performance.

Roland A. Carlstedt, PhD, McLean Hospital/Harvard Medical School and American Board of Sport Psychology.

Michela Balconi, PhD, Catholic University of the Sacred Heart - UCSC, Milan, Italy.

Handbook of Sport Neuroscience and Psychophysiology

Edited by Roland A. Carlstedt

ASSOCIATE EDITOR

MICHELA BALCONI

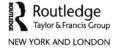

NEW YORK AND LONDON

First published 2019
by Routledge
711 Third Avenue, New York, NY 10017

and by Routledge
2 Park Square, Milton Park, Abingdon, Oxon, OX14 4RN

Routledge is an imprint of the Taylor & Francis Group, an informa business

Library of Congress Cataloging-in-Publication Data
Names: Carlstedt, Roland A., editor. | Balconi, Michela, associate editor.
Title: Handbook of sport neuroscience and psychophysiology /
Edited by Roland Carlstedt; Associate Editor, Michela Balconi.
Description: New York, NY: Routledge, 2019. |
Includes bibliographical references and index.
Identifiers: LCCN 2018021219 | ISBN 9781138852174 (hbk: alk. paper) |
ISBN 9781138852181 (pbk: alk. paper) | ISBN 9781315723693 (ebk)
Subjects: LCSH: Sports—Psychological aspects. |
Sports—Physiological aspects. | Neurosciences.
Classification: LCC GV706.4 .H3714 2019 | DDC 796.01/5—dc23
LC record available at https://lccn.loc.gov/2018021219

ISBN: 978-1-138-85217-4 (hbk)
ISBN: 978-1-138-85218-1 (pbk)
ISBN: 978-1-315-72369-3 (ebk)

Typeset in Bembo
by codeMantra

Contents

Contents

Contributors

Ziba Atak, BA, John F. Kennedy University, American Board of Sport Psychology: Research Fellow

Michela Balconi, PhD, Catholic University of Milan, Italy, Department of Psychology: Professor of Cognitive Neuroscience and Psychophysiology; Research Unit of Affective and Social Neuroscience, Department of Psychology: Director

Eduardo Bellomo, MSc, Institute for the Psychology of Elite Performance (IPEP) School of Sport, Health & Exercise Sciences, Bangor University, UK

Daniel T. Bishop, PhD, CPsychol, Centre for Cognitive Neuroscience, Senior Lecturer and Researcher (Psychology) Program Lead for Sport-Health-and-Exercise-Psychology, Brunel University London

Ambra Bisio, Professor of Human Physiology, Department of Experimental Medicine, Section of Human Physiology, University of Genoa, Italy

Marco Bove, PhD, Associate Professor of Human Physiology, Department of Experimental Medicine, Section of Human Physiology, University of Genoa, Italy

Roland A. Carlstedt, PhD, ABSP, McLean Hospital: Research Associate in Psychology, Developmental Biopsychiatry Research Program/Department of Psychiatry; Harvard Medical School: Research Associate in Psychology, Department of Psychiatry; American Board of Sport Psychology: Chairman & Chief Sport Psychologist

Paola Cesari, PhD, Associate Professor, Department of Neurosciences Biomedicine & Movement Sciences, University of Verona, Italy

Ming-Yang Cheng, PhD Candidate, Bielefeld University, Faculty of Psychology and Sports Science & Cognitive Interaction Technology Center of Excellence (CITEC)

Andrew M. Cooke, PhD, Institute for the Psychology of Elite Performance (IPEP), School of Sport, Health & Exercise Sciences, Bangor University, UK

Davide Crivelli, MPsych, PhD, Catholic University of the Sacred Heart, Department of Psychology, Research Unit in Affective and Social Neuroscience, Milan, Italy: Post-Doc Researcher

Arne Dietrich, PhD, Professor of Psychology, Department of Psychology, American University of Beirut, Beirut, Lebanon

Julien Dirani, Department of Psychology, American University of Beirut, Lebanon

Edson Filho, PhD, Certified Mental Performance Consultant (AASP), United States Olympic Committee - Sport Psychology Registry, University of Central Lancashire, School of Psychology, Director - Social Interaction and Performance Science (SINAPSE) Lab

Germano Gallicchio, MSc, School of Sport, Exercise and Rehabilitation Sciences, University of Birmingham, UK

Jodie R. Gawryluk, PhD, RPsych, Assistant Professor, Department of Psychology, University of Victoria, Canada

Tsung-Min Hung (Ernest), PhD, FNAK, Research Chair Professor, Department of Physical Education, National Taiwan Normal University, Taiwan

Divya Jain, MA, ABSP, Fortis Healthcare, Department of Mental Health and Behavioural Sciences: Head, Psychological Services; American Board of Sport Psychology: Research Fellow and Instructor

Karla A. Kubitz, PhD, FACSM, Associate Professor, Department of Kinesiology, Towson University

Phan Luu, PhD, Brain Electrophysiology Laboratory Company, University of Oregon, Department of Psychology & Neuroinformatics Center

Chantel Mayo, MSc, Department of Psychology, University of Victoria

Valeria Milone, Department of Psychology, Catholic University of the Sacred Heart, Italy

David Moreau, PhD, Cognitive Neuroscientist, Lecturer, The University of Auckland, Centre for Brain Research & School of Psychology

Kyle K. Morgan, MS, University of Oregon, Department of Psychology

Francesca Pala, MPsych, Catholic University of the Sacred Heart, Department of Psychology, Milan, Italy: Research Assistant

Kenneth Perrine, PhD, ABPP-CN, Associate Professor of Neuropsychology in Neurological Surgery, New York-Presbyterian Hospital/Weill Cornell Medical Center, USA

Christopher Ring, PhD, School of Sport, Exercise and Rehabilitation Sciences, University of Birmingham, UK

Philip E. Stieg, MD, PhD, Professor and Chairman, Department of Neurological Surgery, New York-Presbyterian Hospital/Weill Cornell Medical Center, USA

Richard O. Temple, PhD, ABSP American Board of Sport Psychology: Clinical Fellow; Mind For Sports, Austin, Texas

Gershon Tenenbaum, PhD, FAPA, FAASP, FISSP, Benjamin S. Bloom Professor, Director, Graduate Program in Sport Psychology, College of Education, Department of Educational Psychology & Learning Systems, Florida State University

Contributors

Don M. Tucker, PhD, Brain Electrophysiology Laboratory Company, University of Oregon, Department of Psychology & Neuroinformatics Center

Cosimo Urgesi, PhD, University of Udine, Laboratory of Cognitive Neuroscience, Department of Languages and Literatures, Communication, Education and Society: Lecturer, Scientific Institute (IRCCS) Eugenio Medea: Senior Researcher

Sam Vine, PhD, CPsychol, Associate Professor of Psychology, Department of Sport & Health Sciences; College of Life and Environmental Sciences University of Exeter, UK

Mark Wilson, PhD, Department of Sport & Health Sciences; College of Life and Environmental Sciences University of Exeter, UK

Michael J. Wright, PhD, CPsychol, Centre for Cognitive Neuroscience, Brunel University London

Zeead Yaghi, Department of Psychology, American University of Beirut, Lebanon

Suzanne Zuckerman, BA, Research Associate, Department of Neurological Surgery, New York-Presbyterian Hospital/Weill Cornell Medical Center, USA

About the Editors

Roland A. Carlstedt, Editor, PhD, ABSP is a Licensed Clinical Psychologist and Board Certified Sport Psychologist-Diplomate. He chairs the American Board of Sport Psychology and is its Director of Research and Training and Chief Sport Psychologist. Dr. Carlstedt holds academic appointments with McLean Hospital and Harvard Medical School where he is a Research Associate in Psychology in the Department of Psychiatry and Developmental Biopsychiatry Research Program (McLean Hospital). He also is the Clinical and Research Director of Integrative Psychological Services of New York City. An honors graduate of Saybrook University, his doctoral dissertation on cerebral laterality, personality and sport performance was honored with the American Psychological Association's-Division 47, 2001 Dissertation Award and has led to his Theory of Critical Moments and Athlete's Profile models of peak performance. His Master's thesis on Psychologically Mediated Heart Rate Deceleration was published in Biofeedback. Dr. Carlstedt completed a Visiting Fellowship in fMRI and NIH sponsored training program in multi-modal brain imaging in the joint Harvard Medical School-MGH-MIT program and holds post-doctoral certificates in psychiatric neuroscience, applied biostatistics and clinical and translational research from Harvard Medical School Department of Continuing Education and the Harvard Catalyst Clinical and Translational Science Center. Dr. Carlstedt is a pioneer in ambulatory, ecological and biomarker-based athlete assessment and intervention efficiency and efficacy testing, having published and presented on a number of first time investigations of heart rate deceleration/heart rate variability during official competition including a season-long study of heart rate variability/heart rate deceleration biofeedback in youth baseball players and a multi-site replication follow-up investigation. He and his students presented first time findings on heart rate deceleration in baseball, tennis and basketball players and golfers at American Psychological Association and other conferences and are preparing additional publications. Dr. Carlstedt directs the American Board of Sport Psychology Summer Internship and Visiting Fellowship program and has trained over 150 students, faculty, clinicians, sport psychologists and researchers from 14 countries in this New York City based program (now in its 13th year) in applied sport psychology, clinical sport psychology and sport neuroscience and psychophysiology. He has also trained over 50 practitioners in the ABSP certification program including a number of Olympic Sport Psychologists for Team India. Clinically, Dr. Carlstedt's practice and research intersects with sport psychology and sport neuroscience/psychophysiology and vice-versa. At McLean and Harvard Medical School his research centers on Behavioral Medicine/Health Psychology. His Dual Placebo-Pseudo "Effect" and Placebo and Clinical Trial contamination hypotheses are currently being tested with one collaboration in place in the U.K. He is also advancing his Diagnostic Aversion/Clinical Denial hypothesis in conjunction with Dr. Deepak Bhatt, Professor of Medicine (Cardiology) at HMS and Brigham & Women's Hospital. These hypotheses are elucidated in Dr. Carlstedt's clinical book, *Handbook of Integrative Clinical Psychology, Psychiatry and Behavioral Medicine.* He is also advancing a clinical exercise biomarker-guided protocol to quantify angio- and neurogenesis on the basis of

HRV-SDNN, neurocognition and MRI. He is also the author of *Critical Moments During Competition: A Mind-Body Model of Sport Performance When It Counts the Most*, *Evidence-Based Applied Sport Psychology* and *Mentales Tennis* (in German). Dr. Carlstedt has contributed a number of invited and reviewed book chapters including for the forthcoming American Psychological Association's *Handbook of Sport and Exercise Psychology* and in *Handbook of Medical and Psychological Hypnosis*. Dr. Carlstedt is also a former professional tennis player and coach and sport psychology practitioner on the ATP/WTA/ITF tennis tours, a pre-doctoral career that set the stage for a number of his lines of inquiry.

Michela Balconi, Associate Editor, PhD, is Professor of Neuropsychology and Cognitive Neuroscience at the Faculty of Psychology of the Catholic University of the Sacred Heart – UCSC, Milan, Italy. She is also Director and Scientific and Educational Coordinator of the Second-level Master Program in Clinical Neurosciences, as well as of many Advanced Training Courses and Summer Schools supported by UCSC Postgraduate Schools. She is the Head of the Research Unit in Affective and Social Neuroscience, which – thanks to its international, young, and active team – carries out basic and applied research in the fields of neuropsychology and of affective, cognitive and social neurosciences, as well as advanced training activities dedicated to national and international participants. She also founded and is Editor-in-Chief of the international peer-reviewed journal *Neuropsychological Trends* (indexed in the main international scientific databases, such as PsycINFO and Scopus). Prof. Balconi's research interests mainly concern *cognitive and affective neuroscience* and *psychophysiology*. In line with mind-body integration models, she has devised and introduced new methods to explore the relationship between affective communication and cognitive processes and neural-physiological markers. She has also focused on multi-method investigation of psychological phenomena, by integrating optical imaging (fNIRS), electrophysiology (EEG/ERPs), psychophysiological (autonomic indices), and behavioral (eye-tracking, neuropsychological testing) techniques. Furthermore, she has worked on the applications of neuroscience and psychophysiology techniques for neurocognitive rehabilitation and empowerment, with a focus on new technologies for supporting self-enhancement.

Acknowledgements

This is the second multi-author handbook that I have conceptualized, served as the editor for, and contributed chapters to and it never gets easier. I'd like to thank all of the authors who contributed their valuable time and knowledge to producing this book. Prof. Michela Balconi, who helped immensely with the recruiting process, bringing in authors teams from Italian universities to write important chapters, including ones she served as the lead author for, deserves a special *grazie*! I must also commend Georgette Enriquez of Taylor & Francis for her patience and helping see this project through to the end despite a number of missed deadlines, thank you Georgette. Personally, my journey in neuroscience and psychophysiology in both sport and clinical contexts has been enriched by a number of stalwarts in a number of fields and specialties, some who have become colleagues and collaborators and friends. My accomplishments to a certain extent are theirs as well since they have afforded me with opportunities that I never thought would be possible. So, shout-outs of thanks go to Dr. Martin Teicher, my Lab Chief at McLean Hospital/ Harvard Medical School (Developmental Biopsychiatry Research Program), who brought me to McLean/HMS and has been a tremendous source of support. Dr. Frederic Schiffer, also of DBRP, whose research on cerebral laterality has influenced my clinical and sport psychological work must also be thanked along with Dr. Leslie Weiser (McLean/DBRP) a psychologist colleague, collaborator, and friend. Dr. Deepak Bhatt of Brigham & Women's Hospital and HMS, who I cold-contacted in response to a clinical trial that he was the PI of, has become an advisor and collaborator relative to a number of projects we are pursuing, I can't thank him enough for his support. I'd also like to thank a number of Harvard Medical School faculty for supporting the Sport Psychology/Psychiatry in Medical Schools initiative, including Dr. Alvaro Pascaul-Leone a Director of the Football Player's Health Study at Harvard University and professor of Neurology at Beth Israel Deaconess Medical Center/HMS, Dr. William Meehan of Children's Hospital/ HMS and Dr. Ross Zafonte of Spaulding Rehabilitation Hospital/HMS, an initiative that could have important implications for sport neuroscience and psychophysiology. Professors from the past still deserve my thanks, including Dr. Roger Drake of Western State Colorado University, Dr. Stanley Krippner of Saybrook University, and the legendary Dr. Auke Tellegen of the University of Minnesota who served as my doctoral dissertation chairman.

Last but not least, I'd like to thank Dr. James Tabano, Vice-Chair of the American Board of Sport Psychology, for his support of ABSP and myself over the years; Dr. Cliff Stark, my tennis sparring partner and symptom sounding board; and my life-partner Dr. Denise Fortino, a psychologist's psychologist and true humanist.

Applied, Integrative and Ecological Biomarker-Guided Sport Neuroscience and Psychophysiology

Fundamentals, Research, Procedures, Methods and Analytics: An Overview of Chapters

Roland A. Carlstedt

The Handbook of Sport Neuroscience and Psychophysiology was conceptualized about three years ago. Producing an expansive book that covered the broad fields of neuroscience and psychophysiology was both ambitious and challenging, especially in the context of athletes and sport. In the end, I believe we have succeeded in producing a work that has sufficient depth and breadth to satisfy potentially critical peers and colleagues as well as researchers, practitioners/clinicians, instructors and students. While the book is technical, it is also accessible and importantly, it presents critical perspectives that are crucial to the advancement of evidence-based applied sport neuroscience and psychophysiology. In this introduction, synopses of the book's chapters are presented.

The book is divided into four sections: (1) SECTION I, Fundamentals and Research in Sport Neuroscience and Psychophysiology; (2) SECTION II, Applied Sport Neuroscience and Psychophysiology: Intervention and Mental Training; (3) SECTION III, Clinical Sport Neuroscience and Psychophysiology; and (4) SECTION IV, Technology and Products in Sport Neuroscience and Psychophysiology. Section I was designed to introduce readers to the basics, frameworks and conceptual models of sport neuroscience and psychophysiology and the foundational research that is informing researchers, practitioners and students as well as coaches and athletes. Authors were selected on the basis of not only their stature in the field, research and publications, but importantly their commitment to critical analysis of their own research findings and others'. Chapter 2, *The Neural Pathway of Sport Actions: From Seeing and Hearing to Doing: Perception-Action Relationships* by Cesari and Urgesi, and the first chapter in Section I, was a "wish" chapter of mine. I wanted neuroscientists to describe a sport-specific action from the perspective of the brain-mind-body-motor response system (imagine being inside the body in a traveling capsule as in the cult movie of the 70s, the *Fantastic Voyage*) as it happens. What brain areas activate during a sport action? What happens to the mind and body from the beginning to the end of such an action?

This chapter fills the bill in helping illuminate the complex chain of from seeing and hearing to doing.

Chapter 3 by Balconi and Crivelli, *Fundamentals of Electroencephalography and Optical Imaging for Sport and Exercise Science: From the Laboratory to On-the-Playing-Field Acquired Evidence*, focuses on the use of electroencephalography (EEG) and cerebral optical imaging (*functional Near-Infrared Spectroscopy*, [*fNIRS*]) techniques within the domain of sport and exercise sciences. After a brief introduction on brain functioning and how it is mirrored by electrophysiological and hemodynamic responses, examples of research using EEG and fNIRS are presented in the context sport activity and physical exercise, with a focus on both clinical and non-pathological domains. The chapter also presents a technical-methodological primer for the use of EEG and fNIRS.

Chapter 4 is *Sport-Related EEG Activity: What Have We Learned from a Quarter-Century's Worth of Research?* by Kubitz. This survey review of twenty-five years of EEG research in sports asks the following important questions and provides answers to them, including: Based on the afore-mentioned reviews of the sport-related EEG research studies over the past quarter-century, this chapter focuses on eight questions, including: How does EEG activity change across the pre-performance period? How is EEG activity different during good and poor performances? How is EEG activity different in experts and novices? How is EEG activity different in competitive athletes and nonathletes? How is EEG activity different in disabled and nondisabled athletes? How does practice/ learning change EEG activity? Is EEG activity during a sport task different from EEG activity during other tasks (e.g., balancing on a stabilometer)? Is sport-related EEG activity changed by socio-environmental manipulations (e.g., adding competition)?

Chapter 5, *Neuroimaging: Techniques and Applications in Sports* by Mayo and Gawryluk, helps us understand which regions and networks of the brain are involved in the complex set of behaviors required in sports. They also address the following questions: Are the brains of some athletes big-ger than others? Are there differences at a microstructural level? Are different regions recruited during a task given an athlete's training in sport? One of the key methodologies that has been employed to date to address questions like these is magnetic resonance imaging. It compliments Chapter 2, extending on the illumination of brain activation, neural pathways and motor output using action in basketball as an example.

Chapter 6, titled *fMRI in Sport and Performance Research: A Synthesis of Research Findings* by Bishop and Wright, delivers a critical overview of the body of literature that has been devoted to the use of fMRI in attempts to elucidate the neural processes that underpin performance in sport and related areas. Contextual examples include anticipation and prediction tasks, motor prepara-tion, motor imagery, action observation, manipulation of affective state and investigation of brain injury. Limitations of fMRI, potential alternatives or complementary techniques, methodological considerations and future research directions are discussed.

Chapter 7, by the author team Balconi, Pala, Crivelli and Milone and titled *From Investigation to Intervention: Biofeedback and Neurofeedback Biomarkers in Sport*, investigates and discusses psychophys-iological and electrophysiological techniques, including biofeedback and neurofeedback, in sports. They expound on and describe principles and techniques in BF/NF.

Chapter 8. *Understanding Neural Mechanisms of Memory in Rapid Recognition of Football Formations* by Morgan, Tucker and Luu, addresses the neural mechanisms of the cognitive processes that take place when a new quarterback is taught how to analyze defensive formations to make play deci-sions. Through the training process, this information must be consolidated to the point where the athlete is game-ready in the fall. The authors focus on the stages of learning, the brain mechanisms involved in each and the human neuroscience technologies that allow us to study these brain mechanisms. Important challenges, including the effects of stress and the lack of sleep, that must be considered to maximize health and performance are highlighted.

Chapter 9 *Psychologically Mediated Heart Rate Variability During Official Competition: Ecological Investigations of the Heart Rate Deceleration Response with Implications for Quantifying Flow*, by Carlstedt, presents two case-study investigations of heart rate deceleration and HRV on the basis of data derived during official tennis tournament matches. It advances the perspective that HRD is the most revealing and predictive biomarker of psychological performance, especially as pressure increases during competition. A case is made, using a novel analytics, for why HRD is the ideal measure for quantifying "Flow," "Mental Toughness" and psychological performance.

An HRV/HRD primer and literature review of seminal HRD research is presented.

Section II is devoted to neuroscience and psychophysiology guided athlete assessment and intervention (mental training). Novel approaches to ecologically based and biomarker-guided assessment during on-the-playing field training and official competition are presented in this section along with intervention efficiency and efficacy testing. Neurofeedback and biofeedback methods and procedures are also covered in the context of critical perspectives, extant and previous research and future directions.

Chapter 10, *Ecological, Volitional Inducement of Heart Rate Deceleration in Athletes During Competition: A Mental Training Protocol,* a follow-up to Chapter 9, also by Carlstedt, starts the Applied Sport Neuroscience & Psychophysiology section with another HRD/HRV-centric elucidation of an HRD-biofeedback protocol along with an efficiency and efficacy testing case study.

The author contends that the volitional inducement of HRD through sport-specific, pre-action timed inhalation-exhalation cycles that must be established in a training phase is the key to setting off a cascade of performance facilitative brain-heart-mind-body-motor responses mechanistically and eventually subliminally. HRD is also advanced as mental training biomarker efficacy metric that is central to evidence-based mental training efficacy testing.

Chapter 11, *The Use of Gaze Training to Expedite Motor Skill Acquisition* by Wilson and Vine, elucidates an emerging mental training procedure involving the control of eye movements and focus.

The chapter centers primarily on research examining *novice* motor skill acquisition, where consistent findings reveal that gaze training is more effective than traditional instructions focusing on movement control. The premise behind gaze training interventions (e.g., quiet eye training) is that if a performer can learn to optimize the information they receive from their eyes, then they can optimize movement without having to explicitly focus on the control of this movement. As such, by adopting the gaze strategies of experienced performers, novices can "cheat" the learning process where effective sensorimotor mapping must be established. This chapter also outlines the process that is followed in order to develop a practical gaze training program (using examples from laparoscopic surgery, sport and clinical populations) and highlights some of the caveats to consider.

Chapter 12, titled *Cognitive Strategies to Enhance Motor Performance: Examples of Applying Action Observation, Motor Imagery and Psyching-Up Techniques* and written by Bisio and Bove, focuses on different aspects of motor cognition and on the possibility of stimulating the motor system and improving motor performance by acting at the central level (CNS). Studies on healthy subjects, with particular emphasis on athletes and sport science, are presented. Motor resonance and its role in movement planning and execution is discussed along with a motor imagery technique and why it might be considered an "offline operation" of the motor system. The possibility of learning new motor abilities by means of motor resonance, in particular via action observation and motor imagery, is also addressed. Recent findings on the application of these techniques in sport science are reviewed, as well as cognitive strategies, known as psyching-up techniques, and their application in sport domains.

Chapter 13, *Neurofeedback Research in Sport: A Critical Review of the Field* by Cooke Bellomo, Gallicchio and Ring, is one of two chapters on neurofeedback (NF) in the book. It reviews the available evidence and considers some of the reasons why neurofeedback training remains only a minor player in applied sport science. The authors especially focus on exploring some key methodological shortcomings and interpretational caveats that pervade much of the extant neurofeedback research. In doing so, this chapter provides a concise introduction to neurofeedback training, and a critical and balanced view of the current state of knowledge regarding neurofeedback and sport performance. The chapter also offers some guidelines for future research, which the authors hope will stimulate more high-quality neurofeedback experiments to further interrogate and unearth its putative performance-enhancing qualities in the years and decades to come. This is a much needed chapter in light of the eclectic and non-standardized/validated approaches to NF.

Chapter 14, *Neurofeedback in Sport: Theory, Methods, Research and Efficacy* by Hung and Cheng, the second chapter on NF, covers relevant information regarding the application of NF in attempts to enhance sports performance. The aims of this chapter are three-fold: first, to provide both the theoretical and methodological basis of NF in sport performance; and second, to evaluate the quality of studies regarding this line of research, with particular focus on methodological

Roland A. Carlstedt

regarding how to evaluate the effects of NF on sports performance; and finally, the authors conclude with several recommendations for future research.

Chapter 15, *Social Neuroscience: We Think, Therefore We Exist: Team Dynamics, Hyper-brains, and Hyper-minds* by Filho and Tennenbaum, introduces the "notion" of "collective mind" an integral part of many team processes described in the Sport, Exercise and Performance Psychology literature. Most recently, the growth of social neuroscience has ushered new approaches to the study of team dynamics, particularly those focused on capturing the reflective and formative indicators of team processes through peripheral and central psychophysiological methods. The purpose of this chapter is to present the theories and methodologies that lay the foundation for the study of hyper-brains and hyper-minds in interactive motor tasks at large, and the sports domain in particular. The authors advance applied implications stemming from the research conducted thus far, and conclude by discussing future research avenues in this realm.

Section III focuses on Clinical Sport Neuroscience and Psychophysiology. In addition to two chapters relating to sport-induced brain concussions, one on the neuroanatomy and the other the clinical neuropsychology and cellular mechanisms of concussion, emerging explanatory models of exercise-mediated brain mechanisms and cognitive functioning and emotions are presented.

Chapter 16, *Neuroanatomy and Cellular Mechanisms of Sports-Related Concussion and Traumatic Brain Injury* by Perrine, Zuckerman, and Stieg, reviews the latest definitions of concussions and traumatic brain injury, the mechanisms underlying each and how they differ between sports. The discussion incorporates recent research on the gross anatomy and cellular changes that occur in these injuries, how they vary between sports, the controversial syndrome of Chronic Traumatic Encephalopathy, neuroimaging of brain injury, a brief hypothetical case study incorporating each of these subjects and directions for future research.

Chapter 17, *The Neuropsychology of Concussion*, by Temple, extends and compliments Chapter 16.

Chapter 18, *Beyond Physical Exercise: Designing Physical Activities for Cognitive Enhancement* by Moreau, advocates for incorporating additional cognitive tasks/demands within physical training to possibly maximize intervention outcomes. The author reviews research exploring such dual exercise-cognition training and presents an approach that he used within his own line of work – "a blend of physical and cognitive demands integrated within complex environments." The rationale for such along with recent experimental findings are presented. He concludes with prospective trends and recommendations for future research.

Chapter 19, *The Reticular-Activating Hypofrontality (RAH) Model* by Dietrich, Dirani and Yaghi, summarizes the key points of a neurocognitive model of the effects of acute exercise on the brain. This model, which is known as the reticular-activating hypofrontality or RAH model, proposes a set of neural mechanisms for the cognitive and emotional changes that occur during exercise. To make sense of the varied data in the field, any attempt to provide a brain mechanism for the psychological effects of exercise has to make two categorical distinctions: (1) between chronic and acute exercise and (2) between executive functions and all other kinds of cognitive processes. While chronic exercise refers to exercise over long periods of time (e.g., weeks or months), acute exercise refers to exercise that is currently ongoing. As we will see, whether cognitive and emotional processes are facilitated or impaired with exercise depends on both factors, that is, what kind of mental process is measured and at what time point (during or after exercise) it is measured. Because the effects are orthogonal, any global statement about exercise and cognition is likely to be meaningless.

Section IV focuses on technology. Chapter 20, *Technology Product Options in Sport Neuroscience and Psychophysiology* by Jain and Atak, is the final chapter. It presents an overview of select data acquisition and monitoring instrumentation for sport neuroscience and psychophysiology research and practice.

Fundamentals and Research in Sport Neuroscience and Psychophysiology

The Neural Pathway of Sport Actions

From Seeing and Hearing to Doing: Perception-Action Relationships

Paola Cesari and Cosimo Urgesi

The Functional Organization of Perception and Action

Our body is a beautiful machine able to receive different sources of information from the environment and to produce actions that in turn transform the environment. We perceive our body in each instant of the day; the body represents the present through our perceptual and motor experience, the past through the memory of our perceptual and motor experience, and the future through the anticipation of perceptual and motor experience. We perceive the bodies of other people in the same vein. We understand their aims through the movements they perform. As a consequence, we are able to predict their intentions through the movements they perform. Is there a difference between how we perceive our own body and other people's bodies? Even though differences are clearly present, our own body perception and our perception of other people's bodies are closely linked. In this chapter, we will address all these issues taking into consideration different points of view derived from different scientific approaches.

Traditionally, scientists from biomechanics, motor control and robotics were the specialists interested in understanding the body and its movements. More recently, there has been an increased attention on the body from cognitive psychology and neuroscience. More specifically, some neuroscientists became interested in understanding the functioning of bodies that express excellent performance, as shown by elite athletes. The idea is to study these athletes in order to explore the maximum potential the brain is able to achieve. As a consequence, a new field of research was created, known as "Sport Neuroscience".

Before going into the core of recent research in Sport Neuroscience, we need to start by recalling some neurophysiological fundamental concepts which inspired research into the functional organization, combining both perception and action, that underlies the multiple types of information which are organized within the body.

Body and Multimodal Perception

The understanding of the basic processes of brain functioning was initially achieved by observing the anatomical structure of the brain and by delineating its relevant functional connections. As a consequence, we can comprehend with a certain level of detail how visual stimuli are transformed into sensations by the central nervous system and then organized into a neuronal pattern for preplanning voluntary actions. The body produces perceptions that, despite deriving by different sensory modalities, are transformed across modalities, to convey the final idea of an event, which is then perceived as a unitary experience. Despite this, each perceptual modality is defined to give us the idea of different aspects of the physics of the surrounding environment: haptic to discriminate between surfaces made of different materials, vision to localize and recognize objects, sound to recognize the dynamics of objects, such as when they are approaching or receding from our body. Perceptions then, by using analogous mechanisms, decode different information by using different sensorial systems. What makes the very first differentiation between the different types of information are the receptors, located distally within the body, each one sensitive to a specific type of physical energy such as sound light pressure and odor. This sensory information, transformed at the level of receptors, is then transmitted to the cerebral cortex towards regions that are sensory specific.

The multimodality is sustained by the connections that these specific brain regions contain, through their intra-cortical pathways, linked also to the associative and multimodal brain regions. These associative and multimodal regions select and incorporate all the information obtained, which, if coherently organized, give us the impression of a coherent scenario. The ability that the brain has to produce integrated perceptions is due to the structure of the connections between its neuronal cells: they are linked to each other by following a precise and ordered schema that appears quite similar when compared within a normal population. Nevertheless, it has been shown that these connections change under the effect of training and learning, and this has a particular relevance for athletes. We need to notice that we remember a particular event because the structure of the connections has been changed by that event. In this way, "practice" is a key concept, an issue of relevant importance when we deal with motor learning and particularly with extremely sophisticated learning such as that achieved by elite athletes. As we will see, athletes are very efficient in performing actions, but also in recognizing actions performed by others. Indeed, the perceptual information required to perform depends on the interactions between the motor systems and the perceptual systems, coupled with the external environment.

One of the principal roles played by the connection between perceptual and motor functions is organizing actions in advance. What are the parameters that the brain uses to plan an action? We can consider this simple situation: we see a cup on the table and our aim is to drink; we start moving, we reach towards the cup and we drink. Every movement we perform is executed without our conscious control of the details of the action; in other words, to execute a voluntary action it is not necessary to think and consciously control the muscles that we are contracting. This means that at higher levels of sensory-motor interaction, neurons are not coding stimuli characteristics, such as movement force or movement direction (Cesari, Pizzolato, & Fiorio, 2011), but something more general, such as the type of action to be performed and the aim of that action. For instance, since the aim is to drink coffee, a specific neuronal hand configuration will be active which is appropriate for the cup's shape in order for the prehensile to be successful. It has been shown, indeed, that object characteristics (shape, density and mass) are incorporated and decoded under the specification of a pre-organized grip configuration (Cesari & Newell, 1999, 2000a, 2000b; Cesari & Newell, 2002; Newell & Cesari, 1999). Contrary to what was believed to be the case, these brain areas do not contain only motor information, but also relevant cognitive functions.

Where are these neurons located? For action preplanning, these neurons are located in the premotor area of the brain (Figure 2.1). It is important to recall that the neurons involved in movement preparation are clearly differentiated from neurons involved in the actual movements:

a They show a higher level of activity when the actual movement is not present.
b They are particularly active within the time window between the appearance of the target stimuli and movement initiation.

Nevertheless, premotor areas have direct connections with the spinal cord, with the primary motor cortex and the associative areas of the posterior parietal area. The direct connection with the primary motor cortex assures the relationship between action preplanning and action execution, while the direct connection with the associative areas define the visuo-motor circuits that guide the actions under the control of vision. These visuo-motor circuits are thought to contain two main functions: some are dedicated to the processing of the object shape, while others are more involved in processing the object location to program the reaching of the object. For instance, if you want to grasp an object, you need to code for the position of the object with respect to your body and plan an appropriate limb transportation movement. At the same time, you need to perceive the object size, weight and form and pre-shape hands and fingers in an appropriate way. Two different patches of the premotor cortex, which have different types of cells and intra-cortical connections (Rizzolatti & Luppino, 2001), code these two types of visuo-motor transformations. The dorsal premotor cortex (PMd) is interconnected with the primary motor cortex and with medial and lateral intraparietal area, while the ventral premotor cortex (PMv) projects to the hand area of the primary motor cortex, the somatosensory cortex, the anterior intraparietal area and the parietal occipital areas (Stepniewska, Preuss, & Kaas, 2006). These structural differences reflect distinct functional roles in motor control and planning. Indeed, while the PMd is primarily involved in coding information with regards to the direction, amplitude and speed of an occurring limb action, the PMv is primarily involved in preparing and executing visually guided movements for grasping a target. For example, (Fogassi et al., 2001) reversibly inactivated the PMv area of monkeys and tested their performance in a task involving the reaching and grasping of objects. They found that inactivation of the PMv neurons caused a severe deficit in the grasping component of the hand movement, as both the shaping and the posture of the hand were inappropriate for the execution of the grasping task. However, the selective inactivation of the PMv did not affect the limb transport movement. Thus, the PMd, connected with the superior parietal cortex, forms a dorso-dorsal stream that is more involved in the on-line control of movements in space, while the PMv, connected with the inferior parietal cortex, forms a ventro-dorsal stream that is involved in translating the visuospatial information deriving from objects into motor commands that match their physical properties. Both streams, however, are involved in the visuo-motor transformations required for the voluntary control of movements and receive visuo-spatial inputs from the dorsal visual areas that are part of the *vision-for-action* pathway (Milner & Goodale, 2002). Conversely, the visual ventral pathway answers the question "What do I see?" and treats visual information for object recognition (*vision-for-perception* pathway; Milner & Goodale, 2002). More specifically, in the ventral path, the neurons selectively active for specific stimuli, particularly faces and body parts, are located, while the dorsal neurons code information about an object location.

What is the involvement of these two cortical pathways for perceiving and understanding human actions? One supposition is that the dorsal pathway is involved when the perceived action will be executed in the near future; indeed, this path plays a central role in online control of actions. On the other hand, the ventral pathway is involved when perception is simply for action recognition and has not a specific goal (Decety & Grezes, 1999). This distinction might also explain the visual-motor strategies that athletes apply when they observe actions performed by others: action observation may serve to predict the consequences of an action but it might also predict the intention and goal of that particular action. In the next chapter, we will explain the ways sport practice can enhance both these predictive capacities.

Another approach used to understand the neuronal mechanisms underlying action recognition is to design experiments on motor imagery. Results obtained indicate a substantial similarity in the rules and mechanisms underlying execution, observation and imagery of actions, along with a large overlap in their neural substrates (Jeannerod, 2003). Perception for action presents a similar neuronal network to when this action is imagined, and both these networks overlap with the one activated by action execution. Interestingly, as mentioned earlier, these networks are not fixed, but change with body development and with the acquisition of new experience or training. As we will see, studying the ability to observe and imagine an action opens an interesting window for better explaining sport training.

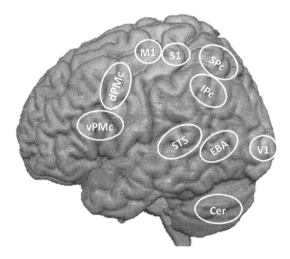

Figure 2.1 Schematic representation of the main brain areas involved in action-perception coupling.
Note: Cer: cerebellum; dPMc: dorsal premotor cortex; EBA: extrastriate body area; IPc: inferior parietal cortex; M1: primary motor cortex; S1: primary somatosensory area; SPc: superior parietal cortex; STS: superior temporal sulcus; V1: primary visual cortex; vPMc, ventral premotor cortex.

Body Representation

We perceive the environment and we move through it: it is reasonable to think that, in order to do this, we need an internal representation of both our body and the surrounding space. The representation of our personal space corresponds to the neural representation of our body surface. This neuronal representation might indicate the presence of a topographic map of the receptors defined by the anatomical organization of the sensitive afferent paths (which goes from the periphery of the body to the brain). To better exemplify this concept, we can think about touching an object. The tactile perception delivers information about the body surface and the object characteristics (its form, weight and density). In the same vein, proprioception delivers information about the body position and movements, such as the hand position and the movement of the fingers. The neuronal path that goes from these receptors (located in the hand) to the brain (the somato-sensitive areas) maintains, from the beginning to the end, the same spatial relationships by preserving along the path the same topographical organization: each piece of information is associated with a specific area of the body. How was this important information obtained? In other words, how were these topological maps defined?

With the application of neuronal registration techniques (the so-called evoked potential), Wade Marshall realized in 1930 that, by touching a specific part of the body of an animal, it was possible to register a related activity in an area at the level of the brain. Later, by using a similar procedure, the neurosurgeon Wilder Penfield delineated the first somatosensory map of the human brain. He defined the map during several brain operations he performed with patients affected by epilepsy and other brain lesions that needed surgery. While under local anesthesia, Penfield stimulated different sites of the primary somatosensory area and asked patients what they felt. Penfield realized that by stimulating specific populations of neurons, the patient perceived tactile perceptions in specific areas of the body and always on the opposite side of the body. In other words, when the stimulated neurons were in the left hemisphere of the brain, the tactile sensations were perceived on the right side of the body. By operating in this way, Penfield was able to delineate a map of the neuronal representation of the entire body at the level of the primary somato-sensory cortex. At the time of Penfield, it was believed that there was just one map for each brain hemisphere and that these maps were relatively stable and fixed. We now know that this is not correct, and that the brain is more dynamic than previously thought, being a system showing a high level of plasticity. As a consequence of Penfield's pioneering work, several maps were found, each representing different aspects of the body. Some maps receive information preferentially from muscles, some from the skin or from the joints. Interestingly, these multiple maps are not fixed but change as the body develops; they also change under the effect of practice or experience and due to learning.

What are the underlying mechanisms at the base of this neuronal modification? This question is particular pertinent in the field of sports since it might provide new knowledge on the ability that the brain has to change under the effect of massive practice or in the presence of an extremely sophisticated skill. What we know up to now about these modifications is that a neuronal connection is facilitated when bursts of neurons are correlated. For instance, when two fingers are tied together in such a way that the two digits are used as one, this provokes a dramatic change in the afferent bursts by increasing the firing correlation of the neuronal activation of the two fingers' paths. This causes, after a while, the disappearance of the discontinuity of the two maps representing the two digits in the brain (Kaas et al., 1981). Moreover, under continuous practice of a particular sequence of finger touching (a few minutes every day for three weeks), performance precision and velocity increased, along with an increase of the involved brain area (Karni et al., 1998). Due to neural plasticity, the brain of an athlete should appear different from the brain of somebody who is not an athlete. To confirm this prediction, the extension of the cortical representation of the hand muscles has been compared between expert and novice badminton players. Experts presented higher motor-evoked potentials and larger motor maps compared to novices, particularly for the hand used toy grasp the racket (Pearce Thickbroom, Byrnes, & Mastaglia, 2000).

Body representation could also be interpreted in a different way and not just, as mentioned earlier, as a representation of the different parts of the body and sensations, but as related to a more complex and dynamical representation that includes the space surrounding the body. In this case, the representation is not necessarily topographic, nor directly linked to receptors. This surrounding space has been denoted as peri-personal space (Previc, 1998) and distinguished from a more external space because events that happen within this space have been shown to provoke a specific neuronal activation. Indeed, when stimuli enter this space, they evoke higher brain activation compared to the same stimuli perceived outside this space (Finisguerra, Canzoneri, Serino, Pozzo, & Bassolino, 2015). The definition of a peri-personal space is the space surrounding the body that is reachable by extending the arms (around one meter) (Rizzolatti, Fadiga, Fogassi, & Gallese, 1997). The neurons that are sensitive to stimuli that reach the peri-personal space are multisensory in nature and are located in the fronto-parietal areas. These neurons, which combine information from somatosensation and spatial position (Graziano, 1999), represent the perfect candidates for action preplanning, especially if the stimuli convey information of an incoming potential threat (Camponogara, Komeilipoor, & Cesari, 2015; Serino, Annella, & Avenanti, 2009).

Moreover, it seems that this space changes under the effect of stimuli semantics and a person's individual experience (Geronazzo, Cesari, in preparation). In summary, it can be said that the body and its surroundings are well represented within the brain. This representation is not fixed but changes constantly under the effect of the meaning conveyed by the stimuli and the experience of the stimuli that each individual develops during his or her life. This underlines once again the existence of a high level of plasticity in the brain and the fact that neuronal connections are not totally preprogrammed genetically, but they are instead highly subject to change under the effect of learning.

Representation of the human body is not only tied to sensori-motor information. Indeed, perceiving one's own and others' body heavily relies on visual information. Along the ventral, vision-for-perception pathway, patches of cortex selectively responding to specific stimuli categories have been described. In particular, social stimuli, namely faces and bodies which convey important information about others' behavior, are selectively represented in the extrastriate visual cortex (Haxby, Hoffman, & Gobbini, 2002). Presentation of human faces triggers the responses of neurons in the lateral occipital cortex, referred to as *occipital face area* (OFA), as well as in the medial temporal cortex, referred to as *fusiform face area* (FFA). The properties of activation of these two areas have been widely explored and reflect the extraordinary ability to detect and recognize human faces among the many stimuli that meet the sensory system. These areas are involved in processing the static features of human faces, allowing for prompt recognition of an individual's physiognomy by considering not only the single details and face parts, but also the relation of each single part in the context of the whole face space. This processing strategy is referred to as *configural processing* and is often used for stimuli highly familiar to the observer, in particular faces and bodies. Dynamic aspects of human faces, such as gaze and emotional expressions, are treated by other areas in the superior temporal sulcus, in the somatosensory cortex and by the amygdala, which is a subcortical structure involved in emotional processing.

A parallel neural network serves the perception of non-facial body parts. Visual presentation of human bodies and body parts triggers the response of neurons in two patches of the extra-striate visual cortex, which are separated from those responding to faces (Peelen & Downing, 2007). Body selective areas have been described in the lateral occipital cortex, the *extrastriate body area* (EBA) and in the medial temporal cortex, the *fusiform body area* (FBA). Analogously to the activation profile of face-selective areas, EBA and FBA seem to be involved in the processing the static aspects of human bodies, allowing for the recognition of the morphology of the bodies that conveys information about gender, age and identity (Moro et al., 2008; Urgesi, Candidi, Ionta, & Aglioti, 2007), along with the aesthetic appearance of others (Cazzato, Mele, & Urgesi, 2016). Importantly, the pattern of activation of these areas is not fixed, but is influenced by the degree of expertise of the observers. For example, observation of domain-specific actions in athletes (i.e., basketball throws in basketball players) recruits activation of EBA to a greater extent than in non-experts (Abreu et al., 2012). This suggests that visual expertise acquired by athletes during sport practice changes the way the body is represented in the visual system, contributing to the superior perceptual abilities of athletes that we will explore below.

Action Recognition and Action Execution

Perception of Biological Motion

How is it that we become aware of things that we observe? An important staring point to understand this complex concept is to think about selective attention. When we observe an event, we just focus our attention on some particular items of the scene, while other items are ignored. Imagine I am concentrating on fixing my bicycle when somebody suddenly enters the room. I will switch my attention from the bike to the person and I will not show any interest in the objects lying on the table in front of me, or in the big window on my right. This selective focalization on one aspect of a scene among the many that are present represents a fundamental characteristic of perceptual elaboration, as pointed out by William James in his book, Principles of Psychology, as early as 1890. Later, it was shown that selective attention increases brain activity in different areas, including the frontal part of the brain involved in action preplanning and the elaboration of movement strategies.

The ability to selectively point our attention toward relevant cues extrapolated from the environment is crucial for understanding action. We know that we have a detailed internal representation of our body parts and sequence of movements, and this is due, as mentioned earlier, to the activation of detailed topographic maps of the receptors and muscles defined by the anatomical organization of the sensitive and motor paths. Does this knowledge also allow us to understand movements when performed by others? To answer this question, a very elegant experiment was designed by Johansson (1973) by testing what he called the observation of "biological motion". Johansson's original idea was to study the information we obtain by observing a pattern of human motion without any interference coming from the form of the body. In order to satisfy these experimental requirements, he used the "point-light figure" which is obtained while recording movement kinematics using a technique known as "motion-capture". This technique uses reflective markers which are attached on the main joints of an actor, who is then asked to walk. Reflective high-speed cameras register the walking and, after an ad-hoc procedure of movement rendering, only the reflective markers moving in a 3D space are visible. When subjects tested as observers were exposed to a single frame (one picture) of the movie, they were unable to identify either that this constellation of markers formed a human figure, or that the human figure was positioned in the typical posture of a walker. However, when the movie started and the lights (markers) started to move, the observers realized that the lights formed a human figure and that that human figure was walking.

By using this paradigm, several experiments were performed using a wide range of different actions and tasks, and results indicated that the observers were able to deliver precise and detailed descriptions of the actions simply by observing the point-light displays. Considering the act of walking for instance, they were able to discriminate whether the walker was a man or a woman (Kozlowski & Cutting, 1977) or whether the walker was a person that they know (Cutting & Kozlowski, 1977). Interestingly, action recognition was impaired when the point-lights figure was shown upside down (Sumi, 1984), a procedure that disrupts our ability to perform configural processing of familiar stimuli.

These experiments suggest important considerations:

1   The visual perception of human movement seems mediated by an implicit knowledge of the production of movements.
2   Movements display specific rules.
3   Rules provide strategies to pick up relevant information for recognizing biological motion.

The type of information captured during action recognition implies that perception and action share a common structural mechanism. Moreover, if, as it was suggested earlier, human movement recognition is mediated by knowledge of the rules related to its production, then we might hypothesize that the more rules we know, the better we are able to recognize an action. We might also anticipate that it is probably the level of action recognition that allows for the ability, shown by animals, to anticipate the forthcoming sequences of an action when observed. This is a promising idea since this is exactly what athletes seem to be able to do when they react to actions performed by their opponents during a sports match. This is what we will present later in more detail and by showing interesting experimental evidence.

Neuronal Underpinning of Action Observation and Execution

A fundamental characteristic of animals' movements is that they express intentionality. Animals are able to initiate their actions voluntarily and their movements continuously change to satisfy the individual's desires and to adapt to different environmental requirements. Reflexes, on the other hand, are different from voluntary actions in that they involve movements which are highly stereotyped and do not change much when repeated. Voluntary actions are generated centrally and central commands are sent in a feed-forward manner from the motor cortex to the distal muscles. Moreover, voluntary actions, while representing manifestations of intentions, give the animal the possibility to choose: an animal can decide whether a stimulus is interesting or not, it might decide to react differently (with different biomechanic actions) to the same stimulus; it may decide whether to approach, to avoid or even to ignore that stimulus. In order to better understand the neuronal mechanisms underlining action intention, experiments on primates were initially performed, preferentially selecting a grasping action as the testing movement.

What is the neuronal mechanism that transforms an object from its sensitive representation to the motor representation that allows for the actual grasp? Sakata, Taira, Murata, & Mine (1995) explored the anterior intra-parietal area of the brain, an area that previously had been identified as the location of neurons active in association with prehension. They recorded single neurons in awake monkeys that had been trained to grasp several objects, while applying different prehensile configurations. The monkeys were also trained to grasp the objects both in daylight and in the dark. With these experiments, Sakata identified three types of neurons: neurons having motor dominance, with comparable response in the dark and in the light; neurons with visual and motor dominance, excited when the monkey was grasping either in daylight or in the dark, but with reduced response in the dark; and neurons with only visual dominance, active during grasping in daylight only. Interestingly, these neurons were active even when the monkey was observing the object without moving. These results suggested the presence of neurons that are active specifically for transforming perceptions into actions, such as transforming perceptual object characteristics into a motor representation of how to shape the grasping hand. Later, Rizzolatti and collaborators (1992) recorded neuronal activity from the monkey's ventral premotor cortex (the area F5) while the animals were performing different tasks. They noticed that a group of neurons (called canonical neurons) were firing in two different conditions: when the monkeys reached towards the object and when they were observing that object without any intention of movement. Importantly, both cases, object observation and object grasping, presented an almost comparable neuronal activity along with the information shared with other brain areas. What was considered particularly interesting was not just that these neurons were firing during the monkey's actions (in fact, these neurons are located in the motor area of the monkey's brain), but rather that these neurons were firing during the observation of the object. Why should these neurons be active in absence of an action? The main interpretation is that they represent the potential to move, indicating the presence of neuronal activity just for the possible planning of an action without the intention of actually performing that action. These potential actions are important in our daily life since they allow us to select whether to react or not to stimuli. For instance, we may choose whether to grasp the object, or just observe it in order to memorize some of its perceptual (i.e., its appearance) or motor (i.e., its usability) characteristics.

An even more interesting discovery made by the same scientific team involved the existence of another group of neurons, located in the same F5 area as the canonical neurons, but delivering a different type of information. These neurons, in contrast to canonical neurons, did not discharge when the monkey observed the objects, but rather while the monkey was performing an action and when the monkey observed another individual (either a human being or another monkey) performing the same action. Because of the dual activation for action execution and observation, they have been called mirror neurons. In other words, the same neuronal pattern is active in two different instances: in forming an internal representation of an action when observing and in performing the same action (di Pellegrino, Fadiga, Fogassi, Gallese, & Rizzolatti, 1992). In the nearly thirty years since the discovery of mirror neurons in the monkey brain, many experiments have been performed and mirror neurons have been found in different areas (including the motor cortex) and have been discovered to be sensitive to different stimuli (Kilner & Lemon, 2013). For instance, some neurons in F5 respond to the sound of an action: the so-called auditory mirror neurons (Koeler et al., 2002).

In humans, mirror neurons are thought to exist within the premotor cortex, a brain area where action preplanning is organized, but they have been also recorded in other medial prefrontal and temporal areas (Mukamel, Ekstrom, Kaplan, Iacoboni, & Fried, 2010). Furthermore, a few fMRI studies performed in humans indicate the existence of a dual activation (action observation and execution) within the same premotor area (Molenberghs, Cunnington, & Mattingley, 2012). Conversely, many studies using Transcranial Magnetic Stimulation (TMS) have found indirect evidence for the existence of mirror neurons in humans by testing several actions and by using several stimuli (vision or sound related). These studies have also been used to test athletes and their superior ability to recognize actions relating to their sporting domain as we will see in more details in the next section.

It is worthwhile to note that, even if mirror neurons are motor neurons in nature, they can also be activated during action observation without the need to send out a motor command for actual action execution. In other words, observing an action triggers within the motor system a simulation of that action even though the perceiver is not obliged to move. Is there an inhibitory mechanism? The answer to this question has not been completely defined, but we do have evidence showing that when the premotor and the motor cortex are damaged, mechanisms controlling movement initiation and movement inhibition are impaired. Furthermore, two types of neurons have been described in the monkey's motor and premotor cortices showing activity modulation during action observation: one type of neurons increases activation when seeing specific actions, while other neurons are inhibited, likely mediating cortico-spinal mechanisms that allow simulating others' actions without necessarily executing them (Kraskov, Dancause, Quallo, Shepherd, & Lemon, 2009; Vigneswaran, Philipp, Lemon, & Kraskov, 2013).

In conclusion, we can say that the discovery of mirror neurons has further reinforced the idea that action execution and action observation are closely related processes. The current hypothesis is that it is through these neurons that we express the ability to understand and interpret actions performed by others, and that in order to understand other people's actions we need the involvement of our motor system and our motor experience.

The Ecological Approach

The idea that perception and action are intimately connected was in principle introduced already in the 70s by JJ Gibson (1979). Gibson's ecological approach to perception and action emphasizes the connection between the organism and the environment in specifying both the information for and the organization of an action (Bertucco & Cesari, 2008, 2010; Cesari, 2005; Cesari, Formenti, & Olivato, 2003; Cesari & Newell, 1999). A central hypothesis of Gibson's theory of direct perception is that there are low dimensional invariants of the organism-environment relationship that specify the goals and organization of movement in action. Animals are thought to visually guide their behavior by perceiving what action possibilities are offered by the environment. Gibson defined the information that emerges from the relationship organism/environment as an "affordance"; thus, if an animal guides its activity by perceiving affordances, then it must be capable of perceiving the relationship between environmental properties and the properties of its own action system. Importantly, in order for the visual guidance of an activity to be successful, the perceiver must be capable of identifying the limits of the action and, then, selecting the most efficient path for the action.

One important implication for this hypothesized relationship between perception and action is that predictions can be made from an analysis of an action to define perception and vice versa. The actor, through training, is then able to perform more efficient actions, but at the same time, through training, she or he becomes more efficient in recognizing that action. Moreover, due to training, individuals learn the limits of actions and then select and recognize the best path for that action among different possibilities available. It is by following these principles that the action-perception relationship becomes relevant not only for action performance but also for action recognition.

We might speculate that the neuronal mechanism for direct perception operates at the level of the dorsal path formed by neurons that present motor and visual dominance. As we have shown earlier, this circuit decodes the different possibilities for action representations offered by the observation of an object. This might be a way to describe how objects and events are "transformed" into potential actions. In real life, however, an object offers more than one possibility of action: a cup might be grasped by the handle for drinking or instead from the cup contour for placing it into a drawer. How can the brain select the best grip configuration? One possibility, suggested by Gibson, is by applying direct perception and using the affordances offered by the object, which are the specific characteristics for performing that specific action. If the intention is to drink, then the handle of the cup offers an affordance.

The question of how actions may be perceived in relation to their potential use raises an important theoretical concept related to the action capabilities of the perceiver. Following on from Gibson's concept of "affordances" (Gibson, 1979), structures and events in the environment, which support or invite different behaviors, do so in relation to the capacity of the perceiver to act successfully upon them. Action-capabilities may be species-specific, developmental, or determined by the relevant skill level of the perceiver-actor. For instance, expert soccer goal-keepers were found to be better than novices at detecting and acting upon the spin that influences the ball flight path in curved free kicks in soccer (Dessing & Craig, 2010). This example suggests that the effect of skill-based action-capabilities on perception may be more effective when perception is coupled to action and when the task requires participants to act inside their domain of expertise (Brault, Bideau, Craig, & Kulpa, 2010; Correia, Araújo, Vilar, & Davids, 2012; Dessing & Craig, 2010).

Several sports, emphasizing different perceptual modalities for action execution and recognition, were tested following this ecological approach. In particular, interceptive movements were considered, such as catching and hitting in sport contexts (Craig, 2013). These movements are particularly attractive because athletes are required to perform fast actions as for instance in baseball where players need to catch balls approaching a speed of 45 m/s. At this velocity, the time window for a) identifying the ball, b) reacting and c) moving and controlling on-line the body's segments in order to be at the right place at the right time is very narrow and the definition of which type of control is required is critical. In this scenario, it appears "expensive" and "unrealistic" to consider the control of movement as performed via indirect perception, given all the codifications that the brain and the body together must elaborate in order to accomplish the task. Instead, the ecological approach proposes direct perception as an alternative and this appears more "economical" and "realistic", given the little time available in these contexts. David Lee was one of the scientists that proposed the parameter of direct perception as used by individuals for interceptive actions (Lee, 1974; Lee, Young, Reddish, Lough, & Clyton, 1983). Lee's idea is that we do not guide our actions through the on-line control of muscle contractions together with their synergies in order to orient the displacement of the body's segments in combination with the displacement of the eyes, instant by instant, toward the direction of the ball. Instead, Lee proposed the use of direct perception via an invariant property that he called tau, which specifies the action-environment relationship. Lee showed that the time to contact (TTC) is optically specified by the ratio of an approaching object size in the optic array to its rate of optical expansion; this is tau (Lee, 1974). The interesting aspect that renders tau a variable in successfully catching a ball is its invariant property. Since tau does not depend on the change of an object's size, it is not required to process an object's changing in size, thus allowing a direct and immediate perception of the ball trajectory. This idea has inspired several authors to apply tau to different sports (Craig, 2013).

Is there a neuronal mechanism that might explain direct perception? One of the possible candidates might be the mirror system. Many scientists interpreted the relationship between action observation and skill experience in terms of the presence of a mirror neuronal network. To test this hypothesis, they performed several experiments having novice and expert players compared while measuring their level of skill and related underlined neuronal activation (Aglioti, Cesari, Romani, & Urgesi, 2008). These experiments were performed to see whether athletes were able to use specific embedded information while observing an action (Aglioti et al., 2008) or while listening to the sound produced by that action (Camponogara, Rodger, Craig & Cesari, 2016). Initially, most of the experiments were run by testing action observation, and only later did the sound produced by an action become a focus of interest. As we will see in more detail later, through the combination of psychophysics and TMS measurements, several sports were tested to identify the behavioral and neural mechanisms underlying the developed sensorimotor abilities of elite athletes in their domain of expertise. The result was that athletes were more accurate and better able to pick up relevant cues for judging observed actions from their domain of expertise, compared either to non-expert individuals or to expert watchers, such as sport journalists or coaches, who were not performers (Aglioti et al., 2008). Moreover, the experiments showed that the higher proficiency of elite athletes parallels an increased excitability of their cortico-spinal system, specifically contingent on observation of actions from their domain of expertise (Aglioti et al., 2008).

As mentioned earlier, the sound of action was also used for testing action perception capability along with the related neuronal underpinning in sport. Does listening to the sound of an action specifically activate the athlete's brain? The answer is yes. An fMRI study, for instance, showed greater activation in the premotor and motor areas of the cortex when expert tennis or basketball players listened to sports sounds from their own sport, compared to sounds from a different sport or non-sporting sounds (Woods, Hernandez, Wagner, & Beilock, 2014). Moreover, several experiments measuring Anticipatory Muscular Adjustments (APA) indicated that the sound of an action contains relevant information about an action-related event that facilitates the reenactment of the listened-to action in a highly sophisticated manner by allowing the extraction of key dynamic kinematic features as supported by direct perception (Camponogara, Rodger, Craig & Cesari, 2016; Cesari, Camponogara, Papetti, Rocchesso, & Fontana, 2014; Young, Rodger, & Craig, 2013; Young, Sherve, Quinn, Craig, & Bronte-Stewart, 2016). For instance, it has been shown that, by listening to the sound of footsteps when walking, humans are able to pick up and use the timing and velocity features of the gait pattern along with the force exerted on the ground to produce strides of different lengths (Camponogara, Turchet, Carner, Marchioni, & Cesari, 2016; Turchet, Camponogara, & Cesari, 2014; Turchet, Serafin, & Cesari, 2013; Young et al., 2013, 2016). These examples highlight the importance of not only assessing what auditory information is picked up and used by the perceiver, but also of how the sound is "brought into use" to regulate action (Dias & Rosenblum, 2016). In other words, these studies highlight the importance of sensory information in the guidance of action, as Lee had proposed (Lee, 1974).

In the following section, we will present in more detail recent evidence in sport settings showing how the extremely sophisticated ability expressed by athletes in recognizing actions from their domain of expertise allows them to exploit one of the most important skills for athletes: action anticipation.

The Neurophysiology of Action Anticipation: Action Anticipation Tasks

Perception Is Predictive

The full sequence of motion is rarely visible during interactions with a dynamic world and missing information needs completion via top-down modulation (Komatsu, 2006; Pessoa, Thompson, & Noë, 1998). Furthermore, perceiving an external stimulus as well as planning the appropriate motor response takes time, inducing an intrinsic delay of brain reactions to external stimuli, which is incompatible with the dynamics of moving stimuli. Thus, to interact optimally with moving objects or creatures, the perceptual system needs to build up an anticipatory representation of the motion sequence in order to predict and anticipate the forthcoming position of moving entities or creatures (Ingvar, 1985). Behavioral studies in humans, for example, have shown that memory for the final position or configuration of a moving object is distorted forward along its path of motion, an effect known as *representational momentum*. In a typical representational momentum experiment, a series of snapshots eliciting the perception of apparent motion is presented. Observers show a tendency to mislocalize the final position of the moving entity further along the anticipated trajectory. This effect has been demonstrated with a variety of stimuli including dot patterns (Finke & Freyd, 1985), common objects (Finke & Shyi, 1988), dynamic facial expressions (Yoshikawa & Sato, 2008) and human figures (Verfaillie & Daems, 2002). It is worth noting that the effect is found even when the actual motion is not present but only implied by static images of moving entities (Freyd, 1983). The anticipatory representation of motion demonstrates the ability of our brain to bridge discontinuities in visual inputs by using internal models of the physical rules that govern object motion in the environment, such as gravity, and thus create a representation of events occurring in the near future by using internal models of the rules that govern the motion of objects in the environment (Hubbard, 2005; Motes, Hubbard, Courtney, & Rypma, 2008; Zago, McIntyre, Senot, & Lacquaniti, 2008).

The internal models use previous experience to complete missing information (Urgesi, Savonitto, Fabbro, & Aglioti, 2012). Visual experience with moving objects or creatures along with auditory experience about the sound produced by moving objects or creatures (Camponogara, Rodger, Craig, & Cesari, 2016; Camponogara, Turchet et al., 2016; Komeilipoor, Rodger, Cesari, & Craig, 2015; Komeilipoor, Rodger, Craig, & Cesari, 2015; Turchet, Camponogara, Nardello, Zamparo, Cesari, 2018; Young, Rodger, & Craig, 2013) may contribute to the creation of predictive models of motion; however, we may additionally use our previous motor experience and knowledge to create an anticipatory representation of human actions (Flach, Knoblich, & Prinz, 2004; Ramnani & Miall, 2004; Verfaillie & Daems, 2002). In fact, accessing the motor representations used during planning and execution of actions might be a deceivingly simple mechanism for the striking ability to create an anticipatory representation of others' actions (Avenanti, Candidi, & Urgesi, 2013; Avenanti & Urgesi, 2011; Gazzola & Keysers, 2009; Perrett, Xiao, Barraclough, Keysers, & Oram, 2009; Schütz-Bosbach & Prinz, 2007; Wilson & Knoblich, 2005).

Action Anticipation in Sports

The ability to create an anticipatory representation of ongoing actions is crucial in sport, where, due to the dramatically fast times required by motor performance, athletes must base their prediction on the initial action cues provided by the opponent players. Indeed, waiting to fully perceive the consequences of their moves would be highly ineffective. Several studies have indeed tested the superior action anticipation abilities of athletes in their specific domain of expertise by using a *temporal occlusion paradigm* (Figure 2.2). In a typical temporal occlusion paradigm, the presentation of sport actions is interrupted at different delays from onset. Domain-specific motor experts

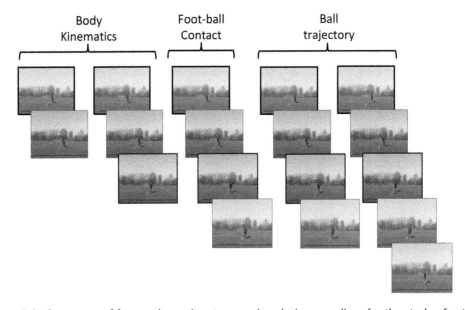

Figure 2.2 Sequences of frames shown in a temporal occlusion paradigm for the study of action prediction in soccer (adapted from Tomeo et al., 2013).

and naïve participants are required to predict the direction or the correctness of the action after viewing only the initial body kinematics of the model player or also the visual consequences of the movements (e.g., ball trajectory). Research in a variety of different sports showed that motor experts are more accurate than expert observers (e.g., coaches) and naïve participants in predicting the fate of the observed actions after viewing the initial body movements. This suggests elite athletes "read" the body kinematics of the observed actions (Abernethy & Zawi, 2007; Smeeton & Huys, 2011).

This temporal occlusion paradigm must be distinguished from one other type of occlusion paradigm (Springer, Parkinson, & Prinz, 2013), referred to as *occluder paradigm*, in which action video presentation is temporarily masked (occluded) for, then reappearing after a variable amount of time, which can be compatible or not with the course of actions during the occlusion period. Observers are asked to judge whether the spatial arrangements of the action kinematics after the occlusion match or do not match those of the action before occlusion. Studies have shown better spatial perception abilities when the temporal dynamics of the action behind the occluder corresponded to the duration of the occlusion. This has been held as suggesting that observers are engaged in mental simulation of the occluded action and present better performance when the state of such simulation process matches the perceived action phase at reappearance. Using this paradigm, basketball and volleyball players and non-experts were presented with short video-clips of free basketball throws that were partially occluded ahead of realization and were asked to judge whether a subsequently presented pose was either taken from the same throw depicted in the occluded video. Results showed that domain-specific experts (i.e., basketball players) outperformed non-experts in detecting whether the test pose matched the spatial characteristics of the action before the occlusion when it was taken from a phase of the action that had occurred some time before the disappearance of the occluder. Thus, action compatibility was better recognized by experts when the pose depicted earlier or synchronous, but not later phases of the movement sequence as compared to the natural course of the action during occlusion (Vicario, Makris, & Urgesi, 2017). Following the logic behind the *occlusion paradigm*, the authors suggested that the experts' mental representation of a domain-specific action is tuned to a slowed-down replica of the action, which may allow them for a better detection of the kinematics and, ultimately, for superior action perception abilities.

In several studies, we investigated in professional pianists (Chen, Pizzolato, & Cesari, 2014) and athletes (Chen & Cesari, 2015; Chen, Pizzolato, & Cesari, 2013; Chen, Verdinelli, & Cesari, 2016) the perception of time, both in sub- and supra-second timescales. We were particularly interested in elite athletes, since they are considered to be individuals with highly developed motor perceptual capabilities and to have a great sense of time, particularly for the extremely short timescales. For this purpose, we asked to elite pole-vaulters to reproduce the exposure times of a familiar image showing a pole-vault jump and non-familiar images, such as a fencing lunge, and scrambled pixels and compared their estimates with controls (Chen et al., 2013). While the time distortion in the supra-second range was similar for athletes and controls independently from the image presented, in the sub-second range of time, athletes were more accurate and less variable than controls. Furthermore, for all the participants, time perception varied according to the image presented: time was perceived as shorter when viewing the pole-vault jump image, followed by the fencing lunge and last the scrambled pixels, providing evidence that action observation distorts individuals' time perception by compressing the perceived passage of time. Remarkably though, pole-vaulters' higher precision and lower variability than controls indicated their ability to compensate for this distortion due to a well-refined internal clock developed through sport training.

Thus, the experts' perception of action is not only characterized by a refined spatial processing of action kinematics, but also by an altered temporal dynamics of the mental representation of the action, implying a motion bias that might subserves their superior perceptual abilities.

Paola Cesari and Cosimo Urgesi

Neurocognitive Mechanism of Action Anticipation

What are the neurocognitive mechanisms underlying experts' superior abilities in perceiving, understanding, predicting and anticipating domain-specific actions? Recent Cognitive Neuroscience studies have addressed this issue, either for the interest of studying motor expertise *per se* or as a model of more general expertise in everyday actions. Two different perspectives exist on the relationship between expert perception and action in sport performance. They claim, respectively, that it is dependent upon perceptual experience or direct motor experience (for a review see Craig, 2013).

Proposers of the role of perceptual experience suggest that expertise is grounded in sensory information and internal representations that are stored in memory, and recalled during action execution to influence choice and performance (Handford, Davids, Bennett, & Button, 1997; Runeson & Frykholm, 1983). In the same vein, during foresight, prediction and anticipation of actions, experts outperform novices in attending to the most relevant source of visual information, verifying it with the information previously stored in memory and making faster and more accurate predictions of the outcome of time-constrained action sequences. For example, a study with French boxers (Ripoll, Kerlirzin, Stein, & Reine, 1995) investigated the specific visual search strategies, information processing and decision-making mechanisms of expert athletes, intermediates and novices. Participants were tested in a virtual environment replicating a boxing field and had to respond to maneuvers of an on-screen opponent in either a simple or a complex environment. The results showed that expert boxers were better at predicting and responding to the maneuvers of the opponent as compared to intermediates and novices, especially in more complex environments. Importantly, it was found that this superiority was reflected in their visual strategies, with expert boxers exhibiting unique characteristics of visual search activity. Similarly, skilled athletes are better at recalling and recognizing patterns of play compared to the less skilled players and show superior ability of controlling eye movements for selecting the most important sources of visual information (Williams, 2000).

Proposers of the role of motor expertise (Hommel, Müsseler, Aschersleben, & Prinz, 2001; Prinz, 1997) endorse a common representation of observed and executed actions and attribute a greater importance to the role of motor expertise in endowing athletes with a heightened perceptual sensitivity to domain-specific actions. Seminal evidence supporting the unique role of motor expertise comes from the comparison of the action anticipation abilities of basketball players not only with those of non-experts, but also with those of expert observers, for example coaches or sports journalists (Aglioti et al., 2008). In a temporal occlusion paradigm, elite basketball athletes, expert observers and novices were presented with videos of basketball free shots whose presentation was interrupted at different time intervals. At these different intervals before action unfolding, the observers were asked to predict the fate of the shots (i.e., whether the ball ended in or out the basket). The behavioral data showed that professional basketball players were better into making accurate predictions at shorter video presentation times, compared to both expert observers (i.e., coaches and sports journalists) and non-experts. Crucially, experts, but not the other groups, were able to reliably predict the outcome of the actions before the ball left the player's hands, thus basing their judgments on the body kinematics without any information from the ball trajectory. This finding pointed to the unique role of motor experience into simulating observed actions and predicting their outcome, which can establish motor model of how to perform the action that are used also during perception of the same actions.

A subsequent study (Urgesi et al., 2012) replicated the aforementioned findings by applying similar experiment paradigms in volleyball. The performance of expert volleyball players was compared to that of expert observers (volleyball team supporters) and novices, in a temporal occlusion paradigm requiring predictions of the fate of volleyball floating services. Crucially, rather than interrupting video presentation at different instants after the beginning of the action, showing videos of increasing length, this study used a modified temporal occlusion paradigm, in which only initial body movements or only ball trajectory of volleyball floating services was shown. This way, this study avoided confounding the presentation of body- vs. ball-related cues, which hints at the experts' ability to read body kinematics, with increasing viewing time and cumulative presentation of more information available on the action, which hint at experts' faster processing speed and need of less information to make a decision. The results showed that both expert players and expert observers were better than novices into making accurate predictions on the basis of the ball trajectory, but only expert players could also base these predictions on body kinematics.

A limit of comparing experts vs. non-experts in cross-sectional studies is that it cannot be established whether superior perceptual abilities of experts reflect sports training or their inherently better sensorimotor skills. Indeed, one can argue that reaching higher levels of sports performance is a consequence of better predispositions to sensorimotor tasks of those who are engaged in sports, which can also explain their superior action perception abilities. To address this issue, Urgesi et al. (2012) used a longitudinal approach to directly test the effects of motor training based on action execution vs. action observation. A group of adolescents were randomly assigned to: (i) a physical practice training that allowed participants to repeatedly execute volleyball floating services after presentation of a model and following a series of instructions; (ii) an observational practice training, in which participants watched videos of floating services and heard the same instructions provided to the execution group; and (iii) a control training showing videos of volleyball defense actions in which the floating services were cut out and giving instructions on the volleyball actions. The adolescents assigned to the volleyball physical practice training improved their perceptual predictions on body kinematics, but not on ball trajectory; importantly, however, the adolescents assigned to the observational practice training improved only in perceiving the ball trajectory. These results suggest that visual and motor experience may play different, complementary roles in action prediction. Visual experience may foster visual representations of actions that are used to describe and to understand the visual dynamics of the actions and of the related contexts (e.g., the ball trajectory). In contrast, motor experience may allow for motor, simulative, body-kinematics-based representations that are used to predict and to anticipate the ongoing actions of other individuals.

Motor Simulation and Action Anticipation

The complementary roles of visual and motor representations of actions were also apparent when the neural bases of experts' perceptual abilities were addressed. As mentioned before, TMS has offered a unique opportunity to study the activity of experts' motor cortex during observation of domain-specific actions. Single pulse TMS is a neurophysiological method that applies single magnetic pulses over the observers' primary motor cortex to record motor-evoked potentials (MEPs) from the targeted muscles (Figures 2.3 & 2.4). This way, it allows assessing the excitability of muscle corticospinal representation during action observation. Many studies have shown that observing others' actions increases the excitability of the onlookers' cortico-spinal motor system (Avenanti, Candidi, et al., 2013; Fadiga, Craighero, & Olivier, 2005), thus inducing motor facilitation that is held as an index of motor simulation processes. Motor facilitation during action is specific for the muscle involved in the observed action and is temporally coupled with the action course (Naish, Houston-Price, Bremner, & Holmes, 2014). Crucially, studies using dynamic (Borroni, Montagna, Cerri, & Baldissera, 2005) or static images of actions (Avenanti, Annella, Candidi, Urgesi, & Aglioti, 2013; Urgesi, Moro, Candidi, & Aglioti, 2006; Urgesi et al., 2010) also indicate that action simulation may be biased toward the future phases of the observed movements, suggesting that the motor system may be involved in the anticipatory simulation of observed actions.

Combining a temporal occlusion paradigm and single-pulse TMS, Aglioti et al. (2008) presented free basket shots with correct, in-basket or erroneous, out-of-basket outcome to athletes, expert observers (i.e., coaches or sport journalists) and non-experts and recorded, at different time intervals from action onset, the corticospinal reactivity of muscles associated with the observed actions. They found two different types of responses that differentiated the three groups. At a first level, they found that observing basketball as compared to soccer actions engendered greater motor responses in both athletes and expert observers but not in non-experts. This suggested that both motor and visual expertise allowed greater recruitment of the motor system during observation of domain-specific actions. Importantly, however, at a second level of analysis, a differential response of the motor cortex of athletes and expert observers was detected when separating corticospinal reactivity to correct or erroneous shots. Indeed, only athletes, but not expert observers or novices, showed fine-tuned modulation of motor facilitation according to the shot outcome. Among the athletes, greater facilitation of the little finger motor representation was obtained during observation of erroneous compared to correct shots. This modulation was only obtained when viewing videos showing the ball leaving the hand, thus, when the model player could exert the last control over the ball trajectory using distal movements of the fingers. This muscle-selective and time-coupled response of the motor cortex of expert players points to a fine-tuned motor simulation mechanism that is established during physical practice and allows for an earlier and more accurate prediction of the future of others' actions. This ultimately supports the roles of motor expertise into predicting the future of observed actions.

Motor simulation, however, is not the only mechanism subserving the superior action perception abilities in athletes. Indeed, the afore mentioned study by Abreu et al. (2012) used functional magnetic resonance imaging (fMRI) to explore the wider neural network whose activity is modulated by domain-specific expertise with the observed actions. In their study, expert basketball players and novices determined the outcome of free shots performed by model players while lying in a fMRI scanner. During the action prediction task, they found comparable activation in basketball experts and novices in areas belonging to the fronto-parietal network that is activated during both action observation and action execution. However, specific activation in the experts' brain was found in, beside the visual EBA (as previously mentioned), the inferior frontal gyrus and the anterior insular cortex when the observers made erroneous predictions in the task. Furthermore, in expert athletes, correct action prediction induced higher activity in the posterior insular cortex, whereas this type of activation in novices was observed in areas of the orbitofrontal cortex. Thus, sports expertise induces functional reorganization of a wide network involving not only motor, fronto-parietal areas, but also visual, body-selective regions as well as of prefrontal areas related to error monitoring and decision-making processes.

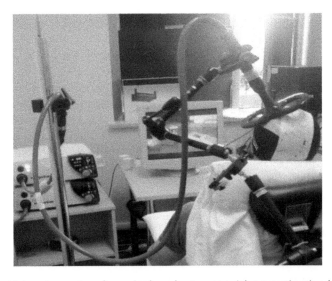

Figure 2.3 Typical laboratory set-up for a single pulse transcranial magnetic stimulation experiment to record motor evoked potentials from limb muscles during observation of action videos.

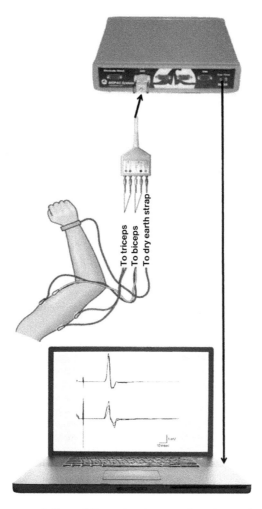

Figure 2.4 Schematic representation of the setup to record motor evoked potentials from hand and forearm muscles.

The Case of the Penalty Kick in Soccer

Novice and Expert Samples

The penalty kick in soccer has been recently used as a model to test the role of action-perception coupling, as well as of higher-level cognitive functions in sports. While kicking to the goal, the player can change the direction of the ball up to about 170 ms before the foot-ball contact (van der Kamp, 2006). This is a big challenge for the goalkeeper, considering humans may take more than 100 ms to initiate a non-discriminative response. Indeed, expert soccer goalkeepers tend to wait more than novice goalkeepers before initiating a response and to respond more on the last part of the kicker's leg kinematics before the foot-ball contact rather than on the initial running phase (Dicks, Davids, & Button, 2010; Savelsbergh, Williams, Van der Kamp, & Ward, 2002). The case of penalty kick in soccer is also relevant for another aspect of sports performance. In sports, as in any competitive social setting, players aim to fool the opponents by attempting to mask their genuine intention (i.e., disguise) or to provide information that leads the observer to make an incorrect prediction (i.e., deceive).

Studies of movement kinematics during fooling actions in sports (Brault et al., 2010) have shown that the players try to reduce the kinematics information that is crucial for performing the intended action (e.g., orientation of the feet during a soccer penalty kick) in order to disguise the opponents and to emphasize those cues that are associated to the movement but are less relevant for action performance (e.g., shaking of the upper limbs) in order to deceive them. Thus, two complementary aspects of fooling actions are the decreasing of the information available and the providing of misleading information that makes the observers more error prone (Jackson, Warren, & Abernethy, 2006).

How does expertise influence the ability to deal with fooling actions? Studies on rugby (Jackson et al., 2006), basketball (Sebanz & Shiffrar, 2009) and handball (Cañal-Bruland & Schmidt, 2009; Cañal-Bruland, van der Kamp, & van Kesteren, 2010) have shown that expert players are better than novices in recognizing when other players are attempting to deceive them. In particular, by using a temporal occlusion paradigm, Jackson et al. (2006) showed that expert players, but not the novice ones, were able to recognize the deceptive intentions of the opponent players by observing their initial body movements. In that study, the player changed the direction of the body by introducing or not a deceptive movement. The observers had to predict the direction of the change and it was found that the experts' responses were less susceptible to the deceptive movement, as compared to the responses made by novices. Indeed, experts were better than novices at predicting the outcome of the direction change in the case of deception trials. Thus, since during deceptive actions players may be able only to approximate the general kinematics of an action but not its full characteristics, experts have acquired the capability to detect the exaggerations of the body kinematics that arise from intended deceptions, suggesting that kinematics offers relevant information about a player's deceptive intentions.

The ability of elite athletes in reading deceptive kinematics seemingly relies on their refined anticipatory simulation abilities, as discussed above. However, since the initial body kinematics of fooling actions is easier to be disguised and more prone to contain deceptive information, anticipatory simulation of the initial kinematics may mislead a correct judgment. Thus, in certain situations, such as reacting to a boxing opponent's stroke (Ripoll et al., 1995) or a goalkeeper's attempt to intercept a penalty kick (Dessing & Craig, 2010), it is crucial that the athletes rely on the visual processing of the last action phases (e.g., consequences on the object motion) rather than on the possibly misleading body kinematics of the opponent player. In these situations, anticipatory simulation may not be the most appropriate mechanism. Expert visual processing of the ball trajectory may be, indeed, much more helpful.

This point was made clear by an elegant study of the ability of novice and expert goalkeepers in detecting deception of a free ball kicks in soccer (Dessing & Craig, 2010). In this study, deception was based on the bending of free kicks and gravitational acceleration of the ball. Importantly, rather than requiring the goalkeepers to make perceptual judgments on the outcome of the observed action, this study used an immersive Virtual-Reality setting to record the hand movement of the goalkeepers in response to a free ball kick. Thus, they recorded an interceptive response, which is more likely to engage the vision-for-action pathway in the brain and to involve implicit perceptuo-motor coupling. Surprisingly, the results showed that the hand movements of the goalkeepers were biased to the direction of the initial ball heading. Therefore, for curved free kicks, the interceptive response of the goalkeepers was in the opposite direction to that required to save the goal. These results indicate that, despite extensive visual and motor experience with defending ball kicks, even expert goalkeepers were frequently bluffed when the ball followed a bending trajectory, as they could not account for the spin-induced visual acceleration of the ball. Thus, detecting deceptive behaviors may be a challenging task even for experts (Dicks, Button, & Davids, 2010; Sebanz & Shiffrar, 2009), who may end up by performing at the same level as novices do (Rowe, Horswill, Kronvall-Parkinson, Poulter, & McKenna, 2009).

24

The Role of Specific Expertise: The Kicker and the Goalkeeper

In the previous paragraph, we have discussed that both motor simulation and perceptual sensitivity are crucial for successful detection of deceptive movements in high-demanding sports. How can these abilities be acquired during sport practice? A prominent role of visual expertise would point to superior abilities in expert observers; a prominent role of motor expertise would point to the prominent role of players. Team field sports, such as handball and soccer, offer an extraordinary setting to investigate the role of perceptual and motor expertise by comparing the performance of field players and goalkeepers. In a seminal study, (Cañal-Bruland et al., 2010) studied deception in handball field players, goalkeepers and novices and found that the two expert groups outperformed novices into predicting the outcome of true or fake shots by a penalty-taker. However, they failed to detect any difference between the two expert groups, even when the actions were seen from the typical goalkeepers' frontal view. This suggested that neither the degree of motor experience nor that of visual familiarity could account for successful recognition of deceptive actions. However, it is possible that the superior perceptual performance of field players and goalkeepers relied on partially different processes. Indeed, field-players may have been more able to detect the deceptive kinematics information of the initial body movements, while the goalkeepers may have based their response on the visual processing of the initial ball trajectory. The complementary contribution given by execution and observation training to learning to predict, respectively, body kinematics and ball trajectory in adolescents learning volleyball (Urgesi et al., 2012) would point to this suggestion.

To directly address this issue, (Tomeo, Cesari, Aglioti, & Urgesi, 2013) investigated how incongruent body kinematics affect judgments for the outcome of soccer penalty kicks in expert goalkeepers, outfield players and novices. Applying a temporal occlusion paradigm, the authors presented video clips of a model player executing a penalty kick. The player was front-viewed as from the goalkeeper's perspective. Half of the movies were congruent kicks, in which the model shot directly to the left or to the right, while the other half were incongruent kicks, in which the initial running phase was incongruent with the foot-ball contact and the initial ball trajectory so that the model seemed to fake to kick to one direction and then kicked to the other. Movie presentation could be interrupted before or after the beginning of the ball trajectory and, at the end of each video, outfield players, goalkeepers and novices were asked to predict the actual outcome of the kick (i.e., ball placed to the left or to the right of the goal). Participants were required to press as fast and accurately as possible one of two keys corresponding to left and right kicks. Results showed that the expert kickers and the goalkeepers outperformed the novices with regards to predicting the outcome of observed congruent penalty kicks after seeing only the initial running phase. On the other hand, when the foot-ball contact was also presented, the results indicated a comparable high-level performance in all expert and novice participants. Thus, while sport experts have superior action-prediction abilities with respect to novices, this perceptual advantage is specific for reading body kinematics. On the other hand, the availability of crucial visual information extracted by scenes, such as the foot-ball contact and the initial ball trajectory, can also give an advantage and increase the performance of novices in predicting the fate of on-going actions.

Importantly, however, the specific role of perceptual and motor expertise became apparent when the outfield players, the goalkeepers and the novices predicted videos containing incongruent information between the initial body kinematics and the foot-ball contact and the initial ball trajectory. In these cases, indeed, the responses of outfield players were still based on the initial body kinematics, even if it could not predict anymore the final outcome of the kick. In contrast, goalkeepers, who were comparably able to predict the final outcome of congruent videos on the basis of the initial body kinematics, were able to update their prediction of the ongoing actions when incongruent foot-ball contact and initial ball trajectory were presented. Thus, outfield players were more susceptible, with respect to goalkeepers and novices, to be fooled by the incongruence between the initial body kinematics and the initial ball trajectory, likely because of their automatic tendency to respond on the basis of the initial running phase. In contrast, goalkeepers were more resistant to fooling body movements, likely as a consequence of their training to respond on the basis of the ball trajectory.

All in all, these findings indicate that outfield players automatically create anticipatory representations of perceived actions based on the observation of initial body kinematics and so they are more prone to be fooled. Goalkeepers are equally able to create such anticipatory representations of the outcome of actions by reading the initial body kinematics, but they can inhibit these inner anticipatory representations and thus update them when incongruent perceptual cues are present. This flexibility may derive from goalkeepers' continuous training to watch the ball, not the player, exerting a regulatory control on automatic simulation of body kinematics (see also below).

Neural Underpinnings of Superior Deception Detection in Sports

What are the neural underpinnings of the superior perceptual abilities of expert athletes in detecting deception in the action of opponent players? Studies of everyday actions have shown that, when we observe an actor lifting a heavy box pretending it is light (and vice versa), the activation of the motor cortex reflects the deceptive intention, allowing us to discriminate between honest and bluffing kinematics and to infer the intention of the actor from the observed kinematics (Tidoni, Borgomaneri, di Pellegrino, & Avenanti, 2013). Importantly, both the deceptive intention of the actor and the kinematic alterations required to attain a deceptive movements are parallel represented in the observer's motor system, likely subserved by different interconnected networks. Indeed, different motor responses have been obtained to the kinematics alterations of actively fooling movements (i.e., increased activity of the motor cortex), when the actor tries to deceive the observer, and of the movements of a fooled actor who has received misleading information about the weight of the to-be-lifted object (i.e., reduced activation of the motor cortex) (Finisguerra, Amoruso, Makris, & Urgesi, 2016).

Using single-pulse TMS, the activity of the motor cortex of outfield players, goalkeepers and novices was recorded during observation of penalty kicks containing, or not, incongruent information between the initial body kinematics and the foot-ball contact and initial ball trajectory (Tomeo et al., 2013). Both expert players (kickers and goalkeepers) and novices presented an increase of cortico-spinal excitability during observation of the kick actions as compared to baseline. However, when facing incongruent videos, the motor reactivity of novices was increased, in keeping with the facilitation of motor activity in response to deceptive movements (Finisguerra et al., 2016; Tidoni et al., 2013). The motor reactivity of goalkeepers was instead reduced when facing with incongruent videos, suggesting that they were able to suppress the motor simulation of the initial body kinematics to favor the visual representation of the foot-ball contact and initial ball trajectory. Conversely, congruent and incongruent actions engendered a comparable facilitation of outfield players' lower-limb motor representation, and their neurophysiological response was correlated with their greater susceptibility to be fooled. Indeed, the greater their motor facilitation during observation of incongruent kicks, the lower their accuracy in predicting the actual outcome of the ball. These data revealed the 'dark side' of motor expertise for action perception, wherein motor experts cannot refrain from representing actions on the basis of simulative processes and by reading body kinematics, even when these last cues are incongruent with upcoming contextual cues. Once again, elite perceptual performance of athletes cannot be explained by the use of motor representations alone, but must be ascribed to the fine-tuning of perceptuo-motor representations.

The complementary contributions of visual and motor representations of others' actions were further revealed by a companion study using repetitive TMS (Makris & Urgesi, 2015). With this technique, the aim is not to probe the activation of the area underlying the coil, as with single-pulse TMS, but to administer a train of magnetic pulses in order interfere with neural activity in the target area during (online repetitive TMS) or just before (offline repetitive TMS) the performance of a perceptual, motor or cognitive task. The rationale behind the technique is that, if neural activity of the target areas is necessary for performing the task, its alteration with repetitive TMS should interfere with behavioral performance, thus providing causative evidence that the area is functionally relevant for the task.

In the study by Makris and Urgesi (2015), the same task used by Tomeo et al. (2013) was employed while expert outfield players, goalkeepers and novices received online repetitive TMS over a premotor area (i.e., dorsal premotor cortex) and over a visual, temporal area (superior temporal sulcus), which are both critical areas involved during action observation. However, while the premotor cortex also responds during action execution, underlying the direct perceptuo-motor coupling, the superior temporal sulcus is specifically involved in the visual representation of actions. The results showed that interferential stimulation over the superior temporal sulcus disrupted performance in both novices and experts, but the effect was greater in those with greater visual expertise (i.e., goalkeepers). Conversely, interferential stimulation over the dorsal premotor cortex impaired performance only in expert players (i.e., outfield players and goalkeepers) who exhibit strong motor expertise in facing domain-specific actions in soccer games. This occurred especially for kicks with incongruent body kinematics, revealing that using motor representations to read the body kinematics of others' movements and predict their outcome is specifically dependent on motor expertise. In sum, while both experts and novices can access visual action representations, only experts are able to use internal motor representations to predict others' behavior. This suggests that we need to embody others' actions in order to anticipate their future behavior, but it also indicates that in some circumstances, for example when facing deceptive intentions, we need to flexibly inhibit such embodied representations to favor a more abstract aspect of social perception based on visual models of others' actions.

The Role of Higher-Level Cognitive Functions in Sports

Detecting deceptive behaviors may require both motor and visual expert abilities. However, deception may disrupt any expertise-related advantage. Expert lie catchers (e.g., police officers) who try to detect deception from non-verbal body cues often end up attributing others' behaviors to genuine rather than to deceptive intentions (Vrij, 2004). Thus, somewhat paradoxically, extensive expertise may, under specific circumstances, produce detrimental results because it does not allow the observer to attribute altered kinematics to deceptive intention. In keeping with this suggestion, a greater susceptibility to opponents' body deceptive movements has been found among expert French boxers, who presented more false alarms in responding to feint actions than intermediate and novice players (Ripoll et al., 1995).

Expertise may change the criterion of responses in detecting deceptive intentions, independently from refined perceptual or motor simulation abilities. A study (Cañal-Bruland & Schmidt, 2009) compared the deception-detection performance of expert handball outfield players, goalkeepers and novices using a signal detection theory (SDT) approach. In SDT, the responses of detecting whether an observed movement is fake or not (e.g., whether a penalty-taker shoots or fakes a shot at the goal) can be separated in those cases in which deception is present and the observer reports it (hits) and those in which the fake is not present and the observer erroneously reports it (false alarms). These complement the cases in which the fake is present and the observer does not report it (misses) and the cases in which the fake is not present and the observer correctly does not report it (correct rejections). The rationale behind this analysis is that the sensitivity of the observer to deception is better caught by the difference between the hits and false alarms, rather than by the number of correct responses. Indeed, if an observer always reports deception, he or she will always detect deception when it is present, in front of tremendously erroneous performance when deception is not present and is nevertheless reported. Thus, optimal sensitivity to deception is revealed when the observer presents a high number of hits, but no false alarms. Any increase of false alarms, as shown by experts in the study of French boxers (Ripoll et al., 1995), reveals a change in response criterion rather than refined perceptual sensitivity. This was the finding of the study by Cañal-Bruland and Schmidt (2009). They found that both expert outfield players and goalkeepers had higher sensitivity to deceptive penalty shots as compared to novices, but the sensitivity of the two expert groups was comparable. However, goalkeepers, as compared to novices and outfield players, were biased to report deceptive movements even for genuine penalty shots.

Saving a penalty kick is a complex decision-making task for goalkeepers; it involves not only perceptual and motor abilities, but also cognitive and affective evaluations. Such complexity may induce specific response biases aimed at optimizing the performance and at inhibiting automatic responses to perceptual cues, which can convey disguising or deceiving information. In the case of soccer penalty kicks, for example, it is crucial for the goalkeeper to wait for longer before deciding where to dive (Dicks, Davids, et al., 2010; Savelsbergh et al., 2002) and to shift from the predictions based on the initial body kinematics to those base on the final movement kinematics and initial ball trajectory. Inhibition of automatic responses and cognitive flexibility are fundamental aspects of executive functions, which have been shown to predict sport performance in both adults (Vestberg, Gustafson, Maurex, Ingvar, & Petrovic, 2012) and adolescents (Vestberg, Reinebo, Maurex, Ingvar, & Petrovic, 2017).

In a recent study, we assessed whether intention can be inferred from the sound an action makes, and whether this information can be used to prospectively guide movement. In two experiments, experienced and novice basketball players had to virtually intercept an attacker by listening to audio recordings of that player's movements. In the first experiment, participants had to move a slider, while, in the second one, they had to move their body in order to block the perceived passage of the attacker as they would do in a real basketball game. Combinations of deceptive and non-deceptive movements were used to see if novice and/or experienced listeners could perceive the attacker's intentions through sound alone. Basketball players were better able to accurately predict the final running direction compared to non-players, particularly when the interceptive action was more basketball specific. Interestingly though, only the basketball players adopted two separated strategies for deceptive and non-deceptive movements. When confronted with a deceptive movement, basketball players waited longer, to pick up more auditory information and to be more fully informed of the attacker's final running direction. Conversely, for the non-deceptive movements, they moved as soon as they heard and understood the attacker's intention (Camponogara & Rodger et al., 2016).

These studies highlight that success in sports does not rely on only superior perceptual and motor abilities, but on a complex pattern of refined perceptuo-motor, cognitive and social skills. The link between sports performance and cognitive development is, however, bidirectional. Indeed, not only is success at sports predicted by the inherent levels of cognitive functioning of an individual, but greater amount of sport practice may lead the development of higher cognitive functions. In particular, while more frequent sport practice is related to better inhibitory control and working memory, longer sports experience is associated with better cognitive flexibility (Ishihara, Sugasawa, Matsuda, & Mizuno, 2017).

Motor Learning and Neuroplasticity

Physical Learning

The repeated execution of a given motor task leads to the reorganization of the cortical and subcortical brain structures involved in its execution. Motor learning triggers neuroplastic changes in the brain, which can be short or long term according to the duration and intensity of the motor learning practice. Thus, sports performance enhances of neurofunctional reorganization of the brain and not only reinforces muscular physiology. The availability of neurofunctional and neuroimaging methods has allowed in the last thirty years to non-invasively document these neuroplastic changes in vivo (Nielsen & Cohen, 2008). What has been detected is that, during optimization of motor performance, the representation of the practiced movement in the primary motor cortex expands and this is accompanied by an increase of the cortico-spinal excitability of the involved body part as measured, for example, with single pulse TMS. With this method, as previously reminded for studies on action observation, the amplitude of MEPs recorded by muscles that are involved vs. non-involved in the practice movements is increased after physical practice, thus pointing to increased cortico-spinal excitability of the underlying motor representation. Furthermore, the optimal scalp position to reliably evoke MEPs from the muscles involved in the practiced movements is larger after training (i.e., MEPs can be evoked, at a fixed intensity, form a wider area of the scalp), pointing to an enlarged cortical representation. These changes outlast the changes of the cortico-motor representation of an active muscle, which decrease after a few minutes and are likely induced by a reduction of intra-cortical inhibition (mediated by GABAergic activity), boosting cortico-spinal excitability. Importantly, similar changes (i.e., expansion of cortical representation and increased cortico-spinal excitability) can last for longer after continuous repetition and optimization of a motor task, leading to a structural reorganization of the motor networks. Such reorganization may have long-lasting functional significance. For example, the repetition of thumb movements in a specific direction biases the contraction of the thumb muscles that are evoked by single-pulse TMS into the practiced direction (Classen, Liepert, Wise, Hallett, & Cohen, 1998), thus suggesting that the motor cortex keeps a memory trace of the learned movement. Indeed, interfering with the primary motor cortex with repetitive TMS alters the motor consolidation process, either at the neural level (i.e., suppressing the expansion and increased excitability of the cortical representation) or at the behavioral level (i.e., reduced improvement of motor performance with learning) (Muellbacher et al., 2002). That these neuroplastic changes reflect the acquisition and consolidation processes was suggested by the finding that the longer-term expansion of the cortical representation was reduced after a motor task had been fully acquired after several weeks of training and motor knowledge became explicit (Pascual-Leone, Grafman, & Hallett, 1994). These changes do not only affect the cortical representation of the practicing limb, but also generalize to the cortical representation of the non-practice hand, reflecting the inter-manual generalization of skill learning (Perez, Wise, Willingham, & Cohen, 2007).

The studies of motor plasticity discussed above used a longitudinal approach to document, within the same individuals, the neuroplastic changes occurring after training as compared to before the training. Due to the intrinsic limitations of longitudinal studies, the follow-up evaluation is only limited to a few weeks/months of training. However, sports expertise requires years of continuous practice. What are the neurofunctional markers of long-term motor expertise? A response (albeit limited) to this question can come from cross-sectional studies comparing the cortical representations of domain-specific actions in experts and non-experts. For example, it has been shown that the cortical representation of the hand used for playing is larger in elite racquet players as compared with novices (Pearce et al., 2000). In a similar vein, the cortico-spinal excitability of elite tennis players was higher, as compared to non-tennis athletes, during imagery of tennis actions but not of golf or table-tennis moves (Fourkas, Bonavolontà, Avenanti, & Aglioti, 2008). All in all, these studies point to long-term neurofunctional reorganization of the motor representation of domain-specific actions in experts.

Observational Learning

The use of motor imagery to reinforce skill learning in sports has been well established in current practice, in spite of limited and contrasting evidence on its efficacy (Holmes & Calmels, 2008;

Murphy, 1994). Its use has frequently invoked the advantage to acquire or boost new motor skills despite the limitations to physical learning caused by injury-related immobilization or physical fatigue. The notion of common representation for executed and observed actions has attracted the interest of scholars interested in sport learning to exploit the possibility to use also action observation (Holmes & Calmels, 2008). Furthermore, in contrast to motor imagery, action observation does not require active effort by the trainee to imagine the movements, and is thus not affected by mental fatigue. Another benefit of action observation compared to motor imagery is that observation can be more easily controlled by the trainer and, as such, is less susceptible to any given individuals' previous knowledge or imagery abilities.

Behavioral studies in the field of motor control have shown that observational practice of movements leads to subsequent improved motor performance (Ashford, Davids, & Bennett, 2007), although the extent of the benefit may be lower as compared to physical practice. Indeed, the neuroplastic changes associated to motor learning (i.e., expansion and increased excitability of cortical representations) can also occur after motor imagery (Facchini, Muellbacher, Battaglia, Boroojerdi, & Focal, 2002) and observational (Stefan, Classen, Celnik, & Cohen, 2008) training even in the absence of actual muscle contraction and perception of sensory feedback. The mechanism of motor memory trace formation induced by physical learning and action observation seems to involve changes of movement representation in the primary motor cortex (Censor & Cohen, 2011). Interference with repetitive TMS over the primary motor cortex disrupts the consolidation of motor memories acquired after both physical (Muellbacher et al., 2002) and observational (Brown, Wilson, & Gribble, 2009) learning. Importantly, not only is the general coordination pattern of movements acquired during observational practice (Gruetzmacher, Panzer, Blandin, Shea, & Charles, 2011), specifying "what" must be performed, but also acquired are the specific parameters, such as timing (Hayes, Elliott, & Bennett, 2010) and force scaling (Cesari, Pizzolato, & Fiorio, 2011; Porro, Facchin, Fusi, Dri, & Fadiga, 2007), which specify "how" to perform the movements. Furthermore, in keeping with the effects of physical training, the observation-related improvements can be transferred to a different motor task (Mattar & Gribble, 2005; Shea, Wright, Wulf, & Whitacre, 2000). Importantly, however, the mechanism of motor skill acquisition during physical and observational practice seems not only quantitatively, but also qualitatively different. Evidence for this can be taken from work showing that their combination results in a greater advantage on transfer tasks (Shea et al., 2000), compared to either kind of training in isolation. Furthermore, the advantages of physical practice transfer to motor tasks with analogous motor coordinates (i.e., using the opposite limb to control the same pattern of muscle contractions and joint angles). In contrast, advantages of observational practice transfer to tasks in which the motor coordinates of the movements are changed, but the visuo-spatial coordinates are maintained (i.e., using the opposite limb to control movements with the same direction in the external space) (Gruetzmacher et al., 2011). In a similar vein, and in contrast to action execution, adapting to the repeated observation of reaching movements in a perturbed environment did not induce any *after-effects*. On the contrary, adaptation to the repeated execution of the same movements induced after-effects, suggesting that observational practice does not allow an update to an internal sensorimotor model of actions (Ong & Hodges, 2010). These studies suggest that observational learning may facilitate the development of a representation of the visuospatial coordinates of a given action but not of its specific motor codes (in terms of joint angles and activation patterns), which require direct motor experience. When the task to be learned, however, is structured, sequential and repetitive, observational learning may help establishing appropriate mental representations of the spatial structure of the task, thus leading to more efficient learning as compared to experiential learning (Foti et al., 2017).

Even if this ability is present since the early infancy (Foti et al., 2017), the extent to which action observation leads to motor skill acquisition may vary across different individuals, and such inter-individual variability at the behavioral level correlates with the extent of functional connectivity between sensory and motor areas, not limited to the primary somatosensory and motor areas, but extending into dorsal premotor cortex and superior parietal lobule, which are critical nodes of the action observation network matching action observation and execution. This might posit limitations to the widespread use of observational training in sports, since different individuals may respond differently to it. Interestingly, recent studies have documented possible genetic determinants of the sensitivity to observational training. In particular, a polymorphism (i.e., a discontinuous genetic variation of a gene in the population) of the brain-derived neurotrophic factor gene (BDNF) is associated with reduced cortical plasticity in the motor cortex during physical practice (Kleim et al., 2006) and to also reduced motor reactivity to action observation (Taschereau-Dumouchel et al., 2016).

Boosting Motor Learning with Brain Stimulation

The use of brain stimulation technique, such as TMS, has opened new possibilities not only for the study of the neural bases of perceptual, motor and cognitive learning, but also for the boosting of neuroplasticity for the rehabilitation of brain damaged patients, as well as for boosting the acquisition of new skills in healthy individuals. In the field of sport, this has led to the issue of "neurodoping" (Davis, 2013), referring to the use of electric or magnetic field applied to the scalp of healthy individuals to enhance physical and mental performance in sports. By varying the frequency of TMS pulse trains, it is possible to facilitate (e.g., 10 Hz) or inhibit (e.g., 1 Hz) cortico-spinal excitability (Pascual-Leone et al., 1999). Indeed, facilitating the excitability of the primary motor cortex can boost motor learning, while inhibiting it slows down learning. Conversely, opposite effects were obtained when the prefrontal cortex was targeted with repetitive TMS, with impaired learning after applying facilitatory stimulation.

In a similar vein, by applying low-intensity, continuous electric current to the scalp for a few minutes (about twenty) it is possible to change the excitability of the underling cortex with transcranial direct current stimulation (tDCS). The applied current is too low to induce action potentials (and to evoke any painful sensations to the participant), but it tends to change the resting membrane potential of the neurons underlying the electrode according to whether the anodal (excitation) or cathodal (inhibition) electrode is placed on the target area. It was found that increasing the excitability of the primary motor cortex with anodal tDCS boosts the learning of an implicit motor task, while cathodal stimulation of the primary motor cortex had no effects (Nitsche et al., 2003). Other studies have shown that anodal tDCS over the motor cortex can reduce neuromuscular fatigue and enhance endurance in both novices (Cogiamanian, Marceglia, Ardolino, Barbieri, & Priori, 2007; Oki et al., 2016; Williams, Hoffman, & Clark, 2013) and athletes (Sasada, Endoh, Ishii, & Komiyama, 2017; Vitor-Costa et al., 2015). Furthermore, other perceptual abilities linked to sport performance, for example visual motion tracking, can be enhanced by stimulation of visual, extrastriate areas (Antal et al., 2004).

Further non-invasive brain stimulation techniques have been recently introduced and may be exploited for boosting motor performance in sports. For example, transcranial alternate current stimulation (tACS) is a noninvasive method that allows neuronal excitability and spontaneous brain oscillations to be modulated via low-intensity (<1 mA) alternating (rhythmic) currents applied on the scalp surface (Moisa, Polania, Grueschow, & Ruff, 2016). Frequency of stimulation can be tuned to the natural frequency of the underlying oscillation (e.g., 20 Hz, beta motor rhythms), inducing online and after-effect improvements (up to 2 SD effect size) of motor performance (Ciechanski & Kirton, 2017; Moisa et al., 2016). A particularity of this technique is that it can be synchronized not only to the spontaneous frequencies of the brain, but also to the frequency of stimuli occurring in the external environment (e.g., visual or auditory patterns), thus allowing for a multimodal entrainment of the learning brain.

Conclusion

In the present chapter, we have provided a partial overview of the neuroscientific knowledge of sports performance. Despite this, the complexity of the factors that may determine how a plastic brain can reach excellence in sports is almost overwhelming. Some of the researches described here have been criticized for the artificiality of the stimuli and for the scarce ecological validity of the laboratory settings, which cannot explain the complexity and richness of natural stimuli in field environments (Mann, Dicks, Cañal-Bruland, & van der Kamp, 2013). In order to control for variables involved in motor, cognitive and perceptual tasks, neuroscience researchers need to reduce the complexity of the experimental set-up, often making it very dissimilar from what people encounter in real life. Furthermore, most techniques for studying brain activity require the subject to refrain from whole body movements (if not staying completely still as for functional magnetic resonance imaging, fMRI), thus making the study of sport-related functions particularly problematic. While we give credits to these reserves, we contest the simplistic criticisms that, since cognitive neuroscience study can hardly test athletes in natural environments, it cannot provide any helpful information to applicative disciplines. We rather claim for integrative efforts that allow elucidating which aspects of real-life situations are crucial for triggering naturalistic processing of sport-related actions and using this information in neuroscientific studies.

Glossary

Action potential: Electrical signals that represent the sum of the registered activity of thousands of cells by means of electrodes. The method of the evoked potential was applied by Marshall, Woolsey and Bard to reconstruct the neuronal map of the body surface representation in the monkey brain (Marshall, Woolsey, & Bard, 1941).

Affordance: "The *affordances* of the environment are what it *offers* the animal, what it *provides* or *furnishes*, either for good or ill. The verb to *afford* is found in the dictionary, but the noun affordance is not. I have made it up. I mean by it something that refers to both the environment and the animal in a way that no existing term does. It implies the complementarity of the animal and the environment. … An important fact about the affordances of the environment is that they are in a sense objective, real, and physical, unlike values and meanings, which are often supposed to be subjective, phenomenal, and mental. But, actually, an affordance is neither an objective property nor a subjective property; or it is both if you like. An affordance cuts across the dichotomy of subjective-objective and helps us to understand its inadequacy. It is equally a fact of the environment and a fact of behavior. It is both physical and psychical, yet neither. An affordance points both ways, to the environment and to the observer". Gibson, J.J. (1986).

After-effects: Effects of repeated presentation of a stimulus on motor and perceptual processes that outlast the duration of the stimulus itself; they may refer to unwanted persistence of compensatory movements when transferring to an environment that does not require such compensations or to alterations of perceptual processing in the direction opposite to the adapting stimulus.

Anticipatory Muscular Adjustments (APA): Activations of postural muscles that precede (50–150 ms) the activation of the prime mover of a body's segment. APAs are interpreted as feed-forward parallel commands aimed at minimizing the equilibrium disturbance provoked by a movement. The first that described these anticipated muscular contraction was Belenkiy and collaborators in 1967 (Belenkiy et al., 1967).

Biological motion: A point-light display with a static or dynamic visual that consists of small, circular light sources placed on the major joints that allow movement. Although these lights are individual, participants are able to perceive motion and to recognize different types of action, including the related emotions expressed.

Mirror neurons: A class of neurons, first discovered in the premotor cortex of monkeys, which are activated during both observation and execution of a given action.

Motor expertise: Ability in performing specific actions that has been acquired during extensive direct experience with performing the actions as compared with visual familiarity with the same stimuli. It may regard either general ability of people in performing everyday actions or domain-specific skills of musicians, dancer or athletes in performing actions that other people are less or not able to perform. Regarding the domain of sports, the definition of expertise is not uniform. It may vary from country to country and from sport to sport. Typically, in psychological and neuroscientific fields, expertise is defined on the basis of years of practice and weekly hours and type of practice, and these estimations are used to match the expertise level of players, who practice sports, and that of experienced observers, who watch sports actions (e.g., team supporters) or are trained in judging the actions (e.g., coaches, judges, journalists).

Representational momentum: A tendency to mislocalize the perceived position of a moving living or non-living entity further along its trajectory. This effect is held to demonstrate the tendency of our brain to form anticipatory representations of changes in the world by using internal models of the rules that govern these changes. These internal models are created after perceptual and motor experience.

Temporal occlusion paradigm: A psychological paradigm for the investigation of perceptual processing in which the presentation of a dynamic stimulus is interrupted at different delays from its onset, thus probing the capability to create anticipatory representation of the perceived stimulus.

Transcranial Magnetic Stimulation (TMS): A technique for the study of the brain which applies short lasting magnetic fields over the scalp locations corresponding to given brain areas. These magnetic fields induce changes of the electrical status of neurons below the stimulating coil, altering their functions. These alterations can be revealed by evoked muscular contractions (measured with electromyography), altered brain states (measured with other neuroimaging or electrophysiological methods) or modification of behavioral responses (measured as variation of accuracy or reaction times while performing given tasks).

References

Abernethy, B., & Zawi, K. (2007). Pickup of essential kinematics underpins expert perception of movement patterns. *Journal of Motor Behavior, 39*, 353–367.

Abreu, A. M., Macaluso, E., Azevedo, R. T., Cesari, P., Urgesi, C., & Aglioti, S. M. (2012). Action anticipation beyond the action observation network: A functional magnetic resonance imaging study in expert basketball players. *The European Journal of Neuroscience, 35*, 1646–1654.

Aglioti, S. M., Cesari, P., Romani, M., & Urgesi, C. (2008). Action anticipation and motor resonance in elite basketball players. *Nature Neuroscience, 11*, 1109–1116.

Antal, A., Nitsche, M. A., Kincses, T. Z., Kruse, W., Hoffmann, K.-P., & Paulus, W. (2004). Facilitation of visuo-motor learning by transcranial direct current stimulation of the motor and extrastriate visual areas in humans. *The European Journal of Neuroscience, 19*, 2888–2892.

Ashford, D., Davids, K., & Bennett, S. J. (2007). Developmental effects influencing observational modelling: A meta-analysis. *Journal of Sports Sciences, 25*, 547–558.

Avenanti, A., Annella, L., Candidi, M., Urgesi, C., & Aglioti, S. M. (2013). Compensatory plasticity in the action observation network: Virtual lesions of STS enhance anticipatory simulation of seen actions. *Cerebral Cortex, 23*, 570–580.

Avenanti, A., Candidi, M., & Urgesi, C. (2013). Vicarious motor activation during action perception: Beyond correlational evidence. *Frontiers in Human Neuroscience, 7*, 185.

Avenanti, A., & Urgesi, C. (2011). Understanding "what" others do: Mirror mechanisms play a crucial role in action perception. *Social Cognitive and Affective Neuroscience, 6*, 257–259.

Bertucco, M., & Cesari, P. (2008). Dimensional analysis and ground reaction forces for stair climbing: Effects of age and task difficulty. *Gait & Posture, 29*(2), 326–331.

Bertucco, M., & Cesari, P. (2010). Does movement planning follow Fitts' law? Scaling anticipatory postural adjustments with movement speed and accuracy. *Neuroscience, 171*(1), 205–213.

Borroni, P., Montagna, M., Cerri, G., & Baldissera, F. (2005). Cyclic time course of motor excitability modulation during the observation of a cyclic hand movement. *Brain Research, 1065*, 115–124.

Brault, S., Bideau, B., Craig, C. M., & Kulpa, R. (2010). Balancing deceit and disguise: How to successfully fool the defender in a 1 vs. 1 situation in rugby. *Human Movement Science, 29*, 412–425.

Brown, L. E., Wilson, E. T., & Gribble, P. L. (2009). Repetitive transcranial magnetic stimulation to the primary motor cortex interferes with motor learning by observing. *Journal of Cognitive Neuroscience, 21*, 1013–1022.

Camponogara, I., Komeilipoor, N., & Cesari, P. (2015). When distance matters: Perceptual bias and behavioral response for approaching sounds in peripersonal and extrapersonal space. *Neuroscience, 304*, 101–108.

Camponogara, I., Rodger, M., Craig, C., & Cesari, P. (2016). Expert players accurately detect an opponent's movement intentions through sound alone. *Journal of Experimental Psychology Human Perception & Performance, 43*(2), 342–359.

Camponogara, I., Turchet, L., Carner, M., Marchioni, D., & Cesari, P. (2016). To hear or not to hear: Sound availability modulates sensory-motor integration. *Frontiers in Neuroscience, 10*, 22.

Cañal-Bruland, R., & Schmidt, M. (2009). Response bias in judging deceptive movements. *Acta Psychologica, 130*, 235–240.

Cañal-Bruland, R., van der Kamp, J., & van Kesteren, J. (2010). An examination of motor and perceptual contributions to the recognition of deception from others' actions. *Human Movement Science, 29*, 94–102.

Cazzato, V., Mele, S., & Urgesi, C. (2016). Different contributions of visual and motor brain areas during liking judgments of same- and different-gender bodies. *Brain Research, 1646*, 98–108.

Censor, N., & Cohen, L. G. Ã. (2011). Using repetitive transcranial magnetic stimulation to study the underlying neural mechanisms of human motor learning and memory. *The Journal of Physiology, 589*, 21–28.

Cesari, P. (2005) An invariant guiding stair descent by young and old adults. *Experimental Aging Research, 31*(4), 441–455.

Cesari, P., & Newell, K. M. (1999). The scaling of human grip configurations. *Journal of Experimental Psychology. Human Perception and Performance, 25*(4), 927–935.

Cesari, P., & Newell, K. M. (2000a). Body scaling of grip configurations in children aged 6–12 years. *Developmental Psychobiology, 36*(4), 301–310.

Cesari, P., & Newell, K. M. (2000b). Body-scaled transitions in human grip configurations. *Journal of Experimental Psychology. Human Perception and Performance, 26*(5), 1657–1668.

Cesari, P., & Newell, K. M. (2002). Scaling the components of prehension. *Motor Control, 6*(4), 347–365.

Cesari, P., Camponogara, I., Papetti, S., Rocchesso, D., & Fontana, F. (2014). Might as well jump: Sound affects muscle activation in skateboarding. *PLoS ONE, 9*(3), e90156.

Cesari, P., Formenti, F., & Olivato, P. (2003). A common perceptual parameter for stair climbing for children, young and old adults. *Human Movement Science, 22*(1), 111–124.

Cesari, P., Pizzolato, F., & Fiorio, M. (2011). Grip-dependent cortico-spinal excitability during grasping imagination and execution. *Neuropsychologia, 49*, 2121–2130.

Chen, Y. H., & Cesari, P. (2015). Elite athletes refine their internal clocks. *Motor Control, 19*, 90–101.

Chen, Y. H., Pizzolato, F., & Cesari, P. (2013). Observing expertise-related actions leads to perfect time flow estimations. *PLoS One, 8*(2), e55294.

Chen, Y. H., Pizzolato, F., & Cesari, P. (2014). Time flies when we view a sport action. *Experimental Brain Research, 232*, 629–635.

Chen, Y. H., Verdinelli, I., & Cesari, P. (2016). Elite athletes refine their internal clocks: A Bayesian analysis. *Motor Control, 20*, 255–265.

Ciechanski, P., & Kirton, A. (2017). Transcranial direct-current stimulation can enhance motor learning in children. *Cerebral Cortex, 27*, 2758–2767.

Classen, J., Liepert, J., Wise, S. P., Hallett, M., & Cohen, L. G. Ã. (1998). Rapid plasticity of human cortical movement representation induced by practice. *Journal of Neurophysiology, 79*, 1117–1123.

Cogiamanian, F., Marceglia, S., Ardolino, G., Barbieri, S., & Priori, A. (2007). Improved isometric force endurance after transcranial direct current stimulation over the human motor cortical areas. *The European Journal of Neuroscience, 26*, 242–249.

Correia, V., Araújo, D., Vilar, L., & Davids, K. (2012). From recording discrete actions to studying continuous goal-directed behaviours in team sports. *Journal of Sports Sciences, 31*(5), 546–553.

Craig, C. M. (2013). Understanding perception and action in sport: How can virtual reality technology help? *Sports Technology, 6*, 161–169.

Cutting, J. E., & Kozlowski, L. T. (1977). Recognizing friends by their walk: Gait perception without familiarity cues. *Bulletins Psychonomic Society, 9*, 353–356.

Davis, N. J. (2013). Neurodoping: Brain stimulation as a performance-enhancing measure. *Sports Medicine, 43*, 649–653.

Decety, J., & Grezes, J. (1999). Neural mechanisms subserving the perception of human actions. *Trends in Cognitive Science, 3*, 172–178.

Dessing, J. C., & Craig, C. M. (2010). Bending it like Beckham: How to visually fool the goalkeeper. *PLoS One, 5*, e13161.

Dias, J. W., & Rosenblum, L. D. (2016). Visibility of speech articulation enhances auditory phonetic convergence. *Attention, Perception & Psychophysics, 78*(1), 317–333.

Dicks, M., Button, C., & Davids, K. (2010). Availability of advance visual information constrains association-football goalkeeping performance during penalty kicks. *Perception, 39*, 1111–1124.

Dicks, M., Davids, K., & Button, C. (2010). Individual differences in the visual control of intercepting a penalty kick in association football. *Human Movement Science, 29*, 401–411.

di Pellegrino, G., Fadiga, L., Fogassi, L., Gallese, V., & Rizzolatti, G. (1992). Understanding motor events, a neurophysiological study. *Experimental Brain Research, 91*, 176–180.

Facchini, S., Muellbacher, W., Battaglia, F., Boroojerdi, B., & Focal, H. M. (2002). Focal enhancement of motor cortex excitability during motor imagery : A transcranial magnetic stimulation study. *Acta Neurologica Scandinavica, 105*, 146–151.

Fadiga, L., Craighero, L., & Olivier, E. (2005). Human motor cortex excitability during the perception of others' action. *Current Opinion in Neurobiology, 15*, 213–218.

Finisguerra, A., Amoruso, L., Makris, S., & Urgesi, C. (2016). Dissociated representations of deceptive intentions and kinematic adaptations in the observer's motor system. *Cerebral Cortex, 269*, 1–15.

Finisguerra, A., Canzoneri, E., Serino, A., Pozzo, T., & Bassolino, M. (2015) Moving sounds within the peripersonal space modulate the motor system. *Neuropsychologia, 70*, 421–428.

Finke, R. A., & Freyd, J. J. (1985). Transformations of visual memory induced by implied motions of pattern elements. *Journal of Experimental Psychology: Learning, Memory, and Cognition, 11*, 780–794.

Finke, R. A., & Shyi, G. C. (1988). Mental extrapolation and representational momentum for complex implied motions. *Journal of Experimental Psychology. Learning, Memory, and Cognition, 14*, 112–120.

Flach, R., Knoblich, G., & Prinz, W. (2004). The two-thirds power law in motion perception. *Visual Cognition, 11*, 461–481.

Fogassi, L., Gallese, V., Buccino, G., Craighero, L., Fadiga, L., & Rizzolatti, G. (2001). Cortical mechanism fr the visual guidance of hand grasping movements in the monkey: A reversible inactivation study. *Brain : A Journal of Neurology, 124*, 571–586.

Fogassi, L., Gallese, V., di Pellegrino, G., Fadiga, L., Gentilucci, M., Luppino, G., … Rizzolatti, G. (1992). Space coding by premotor cortex. *Experimental Brain Research, 89*(3), 686–690.

Foti, F., Martone, D., Orrù, S., Montuori, S., Imperlini, E., Buono, P. … Mandolesi, L. (2017). Are young children able to learn exploratory strategies by observation? *Psychological Research*, 1–12.

Fourkas, A. D., Bonavolontà, V., Avenanti, A., & Aglioti, S. M. (2008). Kinesthetic imagery and tool-specific modulation of corticospinal representations in expert tennis players. *Cerebral Cortex, 18*, 2382–2390.

Freyd, J. J. (1983). Representing the dynamics of a static form. *Memory & Cognition, 11*, 342–346.

Gazzola, V., & Keysers, C. (2009). The observation and execution of actions share motor and somatosensory voxels in all tested subjects: Single-subject analyses of unsmoothed fMRI data. *Cerebral Cortex, 19*, 1239–1255.

Gibson, J. J. (1979). *The Ecological Approach to Visual Perception*. Boston: Houghton Mifflin.

Graziano, M. S. A. (1999). Where is my arm? The relative role of vision and proprioception in the neuronal representation of limb position. *Proceedings of the National Academy of Sciences of the United States of America, 96*, 10418–10421.

Gruetzmacher, N., Panzer, S., Blandin, Y., Shea, C. H., & Charles, H. (2011). Observation and physical practice: Coding of simple motor sequences. *Quarterly Journal of Experimental Psychology, 64*, 1111–1123.

Handford, C., Davids, K., Bennett, S., & Button, C. (1997). Skill acquisition in sport: some applications of an evolving practice ecology. *Journal of Sports Sciences, 15*, 621–640.

Haxby, J. V, Hoffman, E. A, & Gobbini, M. I. (2002). Human neural systems for face recognition and social communication. *Biological Psychiatry, 51*, 59–67.

Hayes, S. J., Elliott, D., & Bennett, S. J. (2010). General motor representations are developed during action-observation. *Experimental Brain Research, 204*, 199–206.

Holmes, P., & Calmels, C. (2008). A neuroscientific review of imagery and observation use in sport. *Journal of Motor Behavior, 40*, 433–445.

Hommel, B., Müsseler, J., Aschersleben, G., & Prinz, W. (2001). The theory of event coding (TEC): A framework for perception and action planning. *The Behavioral and Brain Sciences, 24*, 849–78–937.

Hubbard, T. L. (2005). Representational momentum and related displacements in spatial memory: A review of the findings. *Psychonomic Bulletin & Review, 12*, 822–851.

Ingvar, D. H. (1985). "Memory of the future": An essay on the temporal organization of conscious awareness. *Human Neurobiology, 4*, 127–136.

Ishihara, T., Sugasawa, S., Matsuda, Y., & Mizuno, M. (2017). Relationship of tennis play to executive function in children and adolescents. *European Journal of Sport Science, 17*, 1074–1083.

Jackson, R. C., Warren, S., & Abernethy, B. (2006). Anticipation skill and susceptibility to deceptive movement. *Acta Psychologica, 123*, 355–371.

James, W. ([1890] 1950). *The Principles of Psychology*. New York, NY: Dover.

Jeannerod, M. (2003). The mechanism of self-recognition in humans. *Behavioural Brain Research, 142*, 1–15.

Johansson, G. (1973). Visual perception of biological motion and a model for its analysis. *Perception and Psychophysics, 46*, 201–211.

Kaas, J. H., Nelson, R. J., Sur, M., Lin, C. S., & Merzenich, M. M. (1979). Multiple representations of the body within the primary somatosensory cortex of primates. *Science, 204*, 521–523.

Karni, A., Meyer, G., Rey-Hipolito, C., Jezzard, P., Adams, M. M., Turner, R.,, & Ungerleider, L. G. (1998). The acquisition of skilled motor performance: Fast and slow experience-driven changes in primary motor cortex. *Proceedings of National Academy of Science United States of America, 95*, 861–868.

Kilner, J. M., & Lemon, R. N. (2013). What we know currently about mirror minireview neurons. *Current Biology, 23*, 1057–1062.

Kleim, J. A., Chan, S., Pringle, E., Schallert, K., Procaccio, V., Jimenez, R., & Cramer, S. C. (2006). BDNF val66met polymorphism is associated with modified experience-dependent plasticity in human motor cortex. *Nature Neuroscience, 9*, 735–737.

Kohler, E., Keysers, C., Umilta`, M. A., Fogassi, L., Gallese, V., & Rizzolatti, G. (2002). Hearing sounds, understanding actions, action representation in mirror neurons. *Science, 297*, 846–848.

Komatsu, H. (2006). The neural mechanisms of perceptual filling-in. *Nature Reviews Neuroscience, 7*, 220–231.

Komeilipoor, N., Rodger, W. M., Cesari, P., & Craig, M. C. (2015). Movement and perceptual strategies to intercept virtual sound sources. *Frontiers in Neuroscience, 9*, 149.

Komeilipoor, N., Rodger, W. M., Craig, C., & Cesari, P. (2015). (Dis-)Harmony in movement: Effects of musical dissonance on movement timing and form. *Experimental Brain Research, 233*(5), 1585–1595.

Kozlowski, L. T., & Cutting, J. E. (1977). Recognizing the sex of a walker from point-lights display. *Perception and Psychophysics, 21*, 575–580.

Kraskov, A., Dancause, N., Quallo, M. M., Shepherd, S., & Lemon, R. N. (2009). Corticospinal neurons in macaque ventral premotor cortex with mirror properties: A potential mechanism for action suppression? *Neuron, 64*, 922–930.

Lee, D. (1974). Visual information during locomotion. In R. B. MacLeod & J. H. L. Pick (Eds.), *Perception: Essays in honor of James J. Gibson* (pp. 250–267). Ithaca, NY: Cornell University Press.

Lee, D., Young, M. F., Reddish, P. E., Lough, S., & Clyton, T. M. H. (1983). Visual timing in hitting an accelerating ball. *Quarterly Journal of Experimental Psychology A, Human Experimental Psychology, 35A*, 333–346.

Makris, S., & Urgesi, C. (2015). Neural underpinnings of superior action prediction abilities in soccer players. *Social Cognitive and Affective Neuroscience, 10*, 342–351.

Mann, D., Dicks, M., Cañal-Bruland, R., & van der Kamp, J. (2013). Neurophysiological studies may provide a misleading picture of how perceptual-motor interactions are coordinated. *i-Perception, 4*, 78–80.

Marshall, W. H., Woolsey, C. N., & Bard, P. (1941). Observations on cortical somatics sensory mechanisms of cat and monkey. *Journal of Neurophysiology, 4*, 1–24.

Mattar, A. A, & Gribble, P. L. (2005). Motor learning by observing. *Neuron, 46*, 153–160.

Milner, A. D., & Goodale, M. A. (2002). The visual brain in action. In A. Noe, & E. Thompson (Eds.), *Vision and mind: Selected readings in the philosophy of perception*. Cambridge, MA: MIT Press.

Moisa, X. M., Polania, X. R., Grueschow, M., & Ruff, X. C. C. (2016). Brain network mechanisms underlying motor enhancement by transcranial entrainment of gamma oscillations. *Journal of Neuroscience, 36*, 12053–12065.

Molenberghs, P., Cunnington, R., & Mattingley, J. B. (2012). Brain regions with mirror properties: A meta-analysis of 125 human fMRI studies. *Neuroscience and Biobehavioral Reviews, 36*, 341–349.

Moro, V., Urgesi, C., Pernigo, S., Lanteri, P., Pazzaglia, M., & Aglioti, S. M. (2008). The neural basis of body form and body action agnosia. *Neuron, 60*, 235–246.

Motes, M. A, Hubbard, T. L., Courtney, J. R., & Rypma, B. (2008). A principal components analysis of dynamic spatial memory biases. *Journal of Experimental Psychology: Learning, Memory, and Cognition, 34*, 1076–1083.

Muellbacher, W., Ziemann, U., Wissel, J., Dang, N., Kofler, M., Facchini, S., … Hallett, M. (2002). Early consolidation in human primary motor cortex. *Nature, 415*, 640–644.

Mukamel, R., Ekstrom, A. D., Kaplan, J., Iacoboni, M., & Fried, I. (2010). Single-neuron responses in humans during execution and observation of actions. *Current Biology, 20*(8), 750–756.

Murphy, S. M. (1994). Imagery interventions in sport. *Medicine and Science in Sports and Exercise, 26*, 486–494.

Naish, K. R., Houston-Price, C., Bremner, A., & Holmes, N. (2014). Effects of action observation on corticospinal excitability: Muscle specificity, direction, and timing of the mirror response. *Neuropsychologia, 64C*, 331–348.

Nielsen, J. B., & Cohen, L. G. Ã. (2008). The Olympic brain. Does corticospinal plasticity play a role in acquisition of skills required for high-performance sports? *The Journal of Physiology, 586*, 65–70.

Nitsche, M. A., Schauenburg, A., Lang, N., Liebetanz, D., Exner, C., Paulus, W., & Tergau, F. (2003). Facilitation of implicit motor learning by weak transcranial direct current stimulation of the primary motor cortex in the human. *Journal of Cognitive Neuroscience, 15*, 619–626.

Oki, K., Mahato, N. K., Nakazawa, M., Amano, S., France, C. R., Russ, D. W., & Clark, B. C. (2016). Preliminary evidence that excitatory transcranial direct current stimulation extends time to task failure of a sustained, submaximal muscular contraction in older adults. *The Journals of Gerontology Series A: Biological Sciences and Medical Sciences, 71*, 1109–1112.

Ong, N. T., & Hodges, N. J. (2010). Absence of after-effects for observers after watching a visuomotor adaptation. *Experimental Brain Research, 205*, 325–334.

Pascual-Leone, A., Grafman, J., & Hallett, M. (1994). Modulation of cortical motor output maps during development of implicit and explicit knowledge. *Science (New York, N.Y.), 263*, 1287–1289.

Pascual-Leone, A., Tarazona, F., Keenan, J., Tormos, J. M., Hamilton, R., & Catala, M. D. (1999). Transcranial magnetic stimulation and neuroplasticity. *Neuropsychologia, 37*, 207–217.

Pearce, A. J., Thickbroom, G. W., Byrnes, M. L., & Mastaglia, F. L. (2000). Functional reorganisation of the corticomotor projection to the hand in skilled racquet players. *Experimental Brain Research, 130*(2), 238–243.

Peelen, M. V., & Downing, P. E. (2007). The neural basis of visual body perception. *Nature Reviews. Neuroscience, 8*, 636–648.

Perez, M. A., Wise, S. P., Willingham, D. T., & Cohen, L. G. (2007). Neurophysiological mechanisms involved in transfer of procedural knowledge. *The Journal of Neuroscience : The Official Journal of the Society for Neuroscience, 27*, 1045–1053.

Perrett, D. I., Xiao, D., Barraclough, N. E., Keysers, C., & Oram, M. W. (2009). Seeing the future: Natural image sequences produce "anticipatory" neuronal activity and bias perceptual report. *Quarterly Journal of Experimental Psychology (2006), 62*, 2081–2104.

Pessoa, L., Thompson, E., & Noë, A. (1998). Finding out about filling-in: A guide to perceptual completion for visual science and the philosophy of perception. *The Behavioral and Brain Sciences, 21*, 723–748, 802.

Pizzolato, F., Fiorio, M., & Cesari, P. (2012). Motor system modulation for movement direction and rotation angle during motor imagery. *Neuroscience, 218*, 154–160.

Porro, C. A, Facchin, P., Fusi, S., Dri, G., & Fadiga, L. (2007). Enhancement of force after action observation: Behavioural and neurophysiological studies. *Neuropsychologia, 45*, 3114–3121.

Previc, F. H. (1998). The neuropsychology of 3-D space. *Psychological Bulletin, 124*, 123–164.

Prinz, W. (1997). Perception and action planning. *European Journal of Cognitive Psychology, 9*, 129–154.

Ramnani, N., & Miall, R. C. (2004). A system in the human brain for predicting the actions of others. *Nature Neuroscience, 7*, 85–90.

Ripoll, H., Kerlirzin, Y., Stein, J. F., & Reine, B. (1995). Analysis of information processing, decision making, and visual strategies in complex problem solving sport situations. *Human Movement Science, 14*, 325–349.

Rizzolatti, G., Fadiga, L., Fogassi, L., & Gallese, V. (1997). The space around us. *Science, 277*, 190–191.

Rizzolatti, G., & Luppino, G. (2001). The cortical motor system. *Neuron, 31*, 889–901.

Rowe, R., Horswill, M. S., Kronvall-Parkinson, M., Poulter, D. R., & McKenna, F. P. (2009). The effect of disguise on novice and expert tennis players' anticipation ability. *Journal of Applied Sport Psychology, 21*, 178–185.

Runeson, S., & Frykholm, G. (1983). Kinematic specification of dynamics as an informational basis for person-and-action perception: Expectation, gender recognition, and deceptive intention. *Journal of Experimental Psychology: General, 112*, 585–615.

Sakata, H., Taira, M., Murata, A., & Mine, S. (1995). Neural mechanisms of visual guidance of hand action in the parietal cortex of the monkey. *Cerebral Cortex, 5*, 429–438.

Sasada, S., Endoh, T., Ishii, T., & Komiyama, T. (2017). Polarity-dependent improvement of maximal-effort sprint cycling performance by direct current stimulation of the central nervous system. *Neuroscience Letters, 657*, 97–101.

Savelsbergh, G. J. P., Williams, A. M., Van der Kamp, J., & Ward, P. (2002). Visual search, anticipation and expertise in soccer goalkeepers. *Journal of Sports Sciences, 20*, 279–287.

Schütz-Bosbach, S., & Prinz, W. (2007). Prospective coding in event representation. *Cognitive Processing, 8,* 93–102.

Sebanz, N., & Shiffrar, M. (2009). Detecting deception in a bluffing body: The role of expertise. *Psychonomic Bulletin & Review, 16,* 170–175.

Serino, A., Annella, L., & Avenanti, A. (2009). Motor properties of peripersonal space in humans. *PLoS One, 4*(8), e6582.

Shea, C. H., Wright, D. L., Wulf, G., & Whitacre, C. (2000). Physical and observational practice afford unique learning opportunities. *Journal of Motor Behavior, 32,* 27–36.

Smeeton, N. J., & Huys, R. (2011). Anticipation of tennis-shot direction from whole-body movement: The role of movement amplitude and dynamics. *Human Movement Science, 30,* 957–965.

Springer, A., Parkinson, J., & Prinz, W. (2013). Action simulation: Time course and representational mechanisms. *Frontiers in Psychology, 4,* 1–20.

Stefan, K., Classen, J., Celnik, P., & Cohen, L. G. Ã. (2008). Concurrent action observation modulates practice-induced motor memory formation. *The European Journal of Neuroscience, 27,* 730–738.

Stepniewska, I., Preuss, T. M., & Kaas, J. H. (2006). Ipsilateral cortical connections of dorsal and ventral premotor areas in New World owl monkeys. *Journal of Comparative Neurology, 495,* 691–708.

Sumi, S. (1984). Upside-down presentation of the Johansson moving light-spot pattern. *Perception, 13,* 238–286.

Taschereau-Dumouchel, V., Hétu, S., Michon, P.-E., Vachon-Presseau, E., Massicotte, E., De Beaumont, L., Jackson, P. L. (2016). BDNF Val66Met polymorphism influences visuomotor associative learning and the sensitivity to action observation. *Scientific Reports, 6,* 34907.

Tidoni, E., Borgomaneri, S., di Pellegrino, G., & Avenanti, A. (2013). Action simulation plays a critical role in deceptive action recognition. *Journal of Neuroscience, 33,* 611–623.

Tomeo, E., Cesari, P., Aglioti, S. S. M., & Urgesi, C. (2013). Fooling the kickers but not the goalkeepers: Behavioral and neurophysiological correlates of fake action detection in soccer. *Cerebral Cortex (New York, NY: 1991), 23,* 2765–2778.

Turchet, L., Camponogara, I., & Cesari, P. (2014). Interactive footstep sounds modulate the perceptual-motor aftereffect of treadmill walking. *Experimental Brain Research, 233*(1), 205–214.

Turchet, L., Camponogara, I., Nardello, F., Zamparo, P., & Cesari, P. (2018). Interactive footsteps sounds modulate the sense of effort without affecting the kinematics and metabolic parameters during treadmill-walking. *Applied Acoustics, 129,* 379–385.

Turchet, L., Serafin, S., & Cesari, P. (2013). Walking pace affected by interactive sounds simulating stepping on different terrains. *ACM Transactions on Applied Perception, 10*(4), 23:1–23:14., DOI: 10.1145/2536764.2536770

Urgesi, C., Candidi, M., Ionta, S., & Aglioti, S. M. (2007). Representation of body identity and body actions in extrastriate body area and ventral premotor cortex. *Nature neuroscience, 10,* 30–31.

Urgesi, C., Maieron, M., Avenanti, A., Tidoni, E., Fabbro, F., & Aglioti, S. M. (2010). Simulating the future of actions in the human corticospinal system. *Cerebral cortex (New York, NY: 1991), 20,* 2511–2521.

Urgesi, C., Moro, V., Candidi, M., & Aglioti, S. M. (2006). Mapping implied body actions in the human motor system. *The Journal of Neuroscience, 26,* 7942–7949.

Urgesi, C., Savonitto, M. M, Fabbro, F., & Aglioti, S. M. (2012). Long- and short-term plastic modeling of action prediction abilities in volleyball. *Psychological Research, 76,* 542–560.

van der Kamp, J. (2006). A field simulation study of the effectiveness of penalty kick strategies in soccer: Late alterations of kick direction increase errors and reduce accuracy. *Journal of Sports Sciences, 24,* 467–477.

Verfaillie, K., & Daems, A. (2002). Representing and anticipating human actions in vision. *Visual Cognition, 9,* 217–232.

Vestberg, T., Gustafson, R., Maurex, L., Ingvar, M., & Petrovic, P. (2012). Executive functions predict the success of top-soccer players. *PLoS One, 7,* e34731.

Vestberg, T., Reinebo, G., Maurex, L., Ingvar, M., & Petrovic, P. (2017). Core executive functions are associated with success in young elite soccer players. (L. P. Ardigò, Ed.) *PLoS One, 12,* e0170845.

Vicario, C. M., Makris, S., & Urgesi, C. (2017). Do experts see it in slow motion? Altered timing of action simulation uncovers domain-specific perceptual processing in expert athletes. *Psychological Research, 81,* 1201–1212.

Vigneswaran, G., Philipp, R., Lemon, R. N., & Kraskov, A. (2013). M1 corticospinal mirror neurons and their role in movement suppression during action observation. *Current Biology : CB, 23,* 236–243.

Vitor-Costa, M., Okuno, N. M., Bortolotti, H., Bertollo, M., Boggio, P. S., Fregni, F, Altimari, L. R. (2015). Improving cycling performance: Transcranial direct current stimulation increases time to exhaustion in cycling. (A. Antal, Ed.) *PLoS One, 10,* e0144916.

Vrij, A. (2004). Why professionals fail to catch liars and how they can improve. *Legal and Criminological Psychology, 9,* 159–181.

Williams, A. M. (2000). Perceptual skill in soccer: Implications for talent identification and development. *Journal of Sports Sciences, 18*, 737–750.

Williams, P. S., Hoffman, R. L., & Clark, B. C. (2013). Preliminary evidence that anodal transcranial direct current stimulation enhances time to task failure of a sustained submaximal contraction. (F. Hug, Ed.) *PLoS One, 8*, e81418.

Wilson, M., & Knoblich, G. G. (2005). The case for motor involvement in perceiving conspecifics. *Psychological Bulletin, 131*, 460–473.

Woods, E.A., Hernandez, A. E., Wagner, V. E., & Beilock, S. L. (2014). Expert athletes activate somatosensory and motor planning regions of the brain when passively listening to familiar sports sounds. *Brain and Cognition, 87*, 122–133.

Yoshikawa, S., & Sato, W. (2008). Dynamic facial expressions of emotion induce representational momentum. *Cognitive, Affective & Behavioral Neuroscience, 8*, 25–31.

Young, W., Rodger, M., & Craig, C. M. (2013). Perceiving and reenacting spatiotemporal characteristics of walking sounds. *Journal of Experimental Psychology. Human Perception and Performance, 39*(2), 464–476.

Young, W. R., Shreve, L., Quinn, E. J., Craig, C., & Bronte-Stewart, H. (2016). Auditory cueing in Parkinson's patients with freezing of gait. What matters most: Action-relevance or cue-continuity? *Neuropsychologia, 87*, 54–62.

Zago, M., McIntyre, J., Senot, P., & Lacquaniti, F. (2008). Internal models and prediction of visual gravitational motion. *Vision Research, 48*, 1532–1538.

3

Fundamentals of Electroencephalography and Optical Imaging for Sport and Exercise Science

From the Laboratory to On-the-Playing-Field Acquired Evidence

Michela Balconi and Davide Crivelli

The present chapter will focus on the use of electroencephalography (*EEG*) and cerebral optical imaging (*functional Near-Infrared Spectroscopy, fNIRS*) techniques within the domain of sport and exercise sciences. After a brief introduction on brain functioning and how it is mirrored by electrophysiological and hemodynamic responses, we will present examples from literature concerning the application of EEG and fNIRS to study the correlates and consequences of sport activity and physical exercise, with a focus on both clinical and non-pathological domains. Finally, we will present a technical-methodological primer for the use of EEG and fNIRS, and discuss some troubleshooting practical advice to account for limitations and technical issues when using them as investigation tools for sport applied research.

Introduction to Electroencephalography and Optical Imaging: Brain Activity, Electrophysiology and Hemodynamic Responses

The human brain is a complex system allowing us to experience external and internal events, to automatically react or thoughtfully behave depending on situations and contextual information, and to attribute thoughts, emotions, and meaning to our own and others action. Besides those and other notable functions, our brains also show, together with our bodies, a highly critical and remarkable ability to learn and capitalize from experience to reach mastery and excellence in highly specialized skills. That is particularly important when focusing on peak performance and highly specialized activities, such as in sport practice.

Given the complexity of such system, it is not conceivable that meaningful events occurring in the world or within our bodies would generate a single related physiological event. They would rather generate a cascade of physiological events that would be mirrored by the modulation of different activities (e.g. electrical, metabolic, and hemodynamic). By accurately measuring such modulations and by linking them to behavior and psychological processes it is possible to open a window on how our brain functions during different tasks and to be informed even on how it supports (and is shaped by) our everyday activity.

Communication within the brain occurs by electrochemical connections. Neurons constituting neural structures exchange information and process them thanks to the combination of a complex pattern of excitatory and inhibitory signals. Simplifying, when we typically perceive something within our environment, sensory inputs are brought to primary cortical sensory areas to start their encoding and then transmitted to higher sensory and associative areas to be processed and integrated, so to understand what we are perceiving and properly respond (if needed). Similarly, our behavioral responses – from the simplest ones to the most complex and specialized sport gestures – depend on previous planning and programming processes integrating intention plans and information about the physical and relational context (e.g. the presence and number of other potential agents) and leading to a motor output based on a complex series of previous neural computations.

Neuronal communications take place at the level of synapses, where excitatory and inhibitory pre-synaptic neurons affect a post-synaptic neuron activity thanks to the mediation of neurotransmitters. The binding of neurotransmitters to specific receptors induces a graded modulation of the post-synaptic membrane potential, also known as postsynaptic potential. The summation of excitatory and inhibitory postsynaptic potential (respectively facilitating and inhibiting neuronal discharge) is thought to produce the form of electrophysiological activity that can be recorded non-invasively by electromagnetic methods, such as electroencephalography (EEG) and magnetoencephalography (MEG).

As above-mentioned, such series of electrochemical interactions – besides the modulation of electrophysiological activities at both the cell and the system levels – also induces a series of changes in metabolic and hemodynamic activities and the localized increase of blood supply. The link between functional activity, metabolic and energy demand, and blood flow was originally proposed by Roy and Sherrington as early as in 1890 (Roy & Sherrington, 1890). The relationship (and the dependence) between low-level neural activity and subsequent changes in the regional cerebral blood flow is now known as neurovascular coupling. The process linking neural activity and localized hemodynamic modulations goes through the following steps. When a neural population in a specific cortical area is activated by the processing of an external stimulus or an internal event, oxygen molecules are extracted from oxygenated hemoglobin to be consumed and to produce energy, and that leads to an initial increase of the concentration of de-oxygenated hemoglobin (deoxy-Hb) in blood and to a concurrent decrease of the amount of available oxygenated hemoglobin (oxy-Hb). Subsequently, capillaries and blood vessels dilate to allow a compensatory increase of regional blood supply. With the localized increase of blood flow increases, the concentration of oxygenated hemoglobin also becomes greater and exceeds the requests for local consumption of oxygen. In the end, this leads to a localized overconcentration of oxy-HB (and a concurrent decrease in concentration of deoxy-Hb) in correspondence to active cortical areas, which is the basis of the blood-oxygenation level dependent (BOLD) signal commonly used in functional magnetic resonance imaging (fMRI) and of the applications of optical imaging (functional Near-Infrared Spectroscopy, fNIRS) for the investigation of brain function.

Moving from a physiology to a methodological point of view, what about electrophysiological and optical imaging techniques as investigation tools for motor and cognitive brain function?

Electroencephalography

Electroencephalography allows for recording non-invasively from sensors placed on the scalp the summation of electrical phenomena generated inside the brain. While the activity of neurons is associated to two kinds of primary electrical events – action potentials and postsynaptic potentials – observed EEG is thought to mirror only the latter due do their specific spatial-temporal characteristics (action potentials indeed last approximately 1 ms, while the duration of postsynaptic potentials ranges between tens and hundreds of milliseconds). Further, three criteria are considered to be crucial for non-invasive recording of brain electromagnetic activity. Firstly, relative large population of neurons has to be active and exchange information so to generate a strong signal. Secondly, the activity of neurons constituting such population has to be synchronous. Thirdly, neurons within the active population have to be consistently arranged so that the effect of generated electromagnetic fields may accumulate. For further details, the interested reader may refer to the valuable book by Zani and Proverbio (2002) and to Crivelli and Balconi (2017).

Thus, when large populations of consistently arranged neurons activate together synchronously and – specifically for the EEG technique – are oriented perpendicularly with respect to the scalp, it is possible to record and analyze the informative outcome of intra-cerebral activity. Since the first reports of electroencephalographic recordings in humans by Hans Berger (1929) – the father of electroencephalography that discovered and labeled the first two observed EEG rhythms (α and β) – recording and quantification methods became finer and finer. Going down to specifics, the continuous or task-related modulation of such electrophysiological activity across time that takes the shape of a complex oscillatory signal can be analyzed in the frequency domain to obtain frequency-dependent measures and to investigate the presence and prevalence of known frequency bands such as delta (δ, 0.5–3.5 Hz), theta (θ, 4–7.5 Hz), alpha (α, 8–12.5 Hz), beta (β, 13–30 Hz), and gamma (γ, 30–50/80 Hz). Alternatively, transient responses time-locked to specific stimuli or events can be singled-out from the ongoing oscillatory activity (event-related potentials, ERPs, from EEG) and analyzed within the time domain to try and investigate specific stages of movement, cognitive, or affective processes.

To date, time-domain and frequency-domain measures can also be further analyzed by advanced processing methods allowing for the definition of the recurrent determinant patterns of activation for specific cognitive processes (microstate segmentation) and the estimation of cortical generators of scalp-recorded signals.

Optical Imaging

The application of Optical Imaging techniques to the study of brain function, instead of capitalizing on electromagnetic properties of active neurons, depends on their ability to track and measure changes in the amount of oxygenated and deoxygenated hemoglobin in relatively circumscribed portions of the cerebral cortex, and are then listed among the indirect hemodynamic imaging techniques such as fMRI, PET, and SPECT.

Optical Imaging techniques grounds on optical properties and different light absorption properties of chromophores within molecules constituting biological tissues. To date, the most diffused methodology is functional Near-Infrared Spectroscopy (fNIRS). Such technique takes advantage of the specific features of the interaction between near-infrared light (NIR) and constituents of skin, bone, muscles, fat, and blood. By using different NIR wavelengths, it is possible to discern and quantify the concentration of different elements of tissues such as hemoglobin in its two different states (oxygenated vs. deoxygenated), water, and lipids. NIR radiations within 650–950 nm wavelengths range are indeed primarily absorbed by hemoglobin while skin, bone, and other tissues are mostly transparent to them. The analysis of attenuation patterns for multiple NIR radiations and, in particular, differences in absorption spectra for oxygenated and deoxygenated hemoglobin (oxy-Hb, deoxy-Hb) now allows for estimating their relative local concentration, and then also the modulation of total hemoglobin concentration, in real-time.

As introduced above, due to the neurovascular coupling phenomenon, cortical activations are associated to localized hemodynamic changes and the consequent modification of optical properties of brain tissues may thus indirectly inform us on ongoing brain activity. In order to track NIR attenuation patterns and estimate the concentration of oxy-Hb and deoxy-Hb, fNIRS recording systems make use of three key components: a light source, a detector, and a multiplexer. Given the requisites for precision of stimulation needed by fNIRS applications, the light source – usually referred to as injector – needs to be able to emit a dynamic range of selected wavelengths with high and adjustable power levels and is usually constituted by a laser diode or a light emitting diode (LED). The light detector – usually simply referred to as detector – is probably the most critical element of the system and need to be highly sensitive to be able to detect even the slightest changes in absorbed/attenuated light depending on the relative presence of oxy- and deoxy-Hb. The multiplexer is finally needed to organize, split, and integrate light signals that are emitted by the injector and recollected from the detector after having travelled through surface and cortical tissues. Each injector-detector pair constitutes a single measurement channel. Recent fNIRS systems allow for measuring hemoglobin modulations from multiple points on the scalp subtending different cortical portions. By increasing the number of recording channels (i.e. source-detector pairs), it is possible to increase spatial sampling of hemodynamic changes associated to brain function and, thanks to advanced processing algorithms, even to create 2-D or 3-D reconstructions of the blood perfusion within the cortex.

Starting from the seminal works by Chance (1951) and Jöbsis (1977), who introduced the concept of differential spectroscopy and firstly reported differential spectral absorption of hemoglobin in vivo with NIR transillumination, technological advancements lead to the development of even more usable, informative, sensitive, and portable instruments for NIRS-based investigation. To date, three main kinds of fNIRS systems have been devised and can already be used in practice: continuous wave NIRS, time-resolved NIRS, and spatially-resolved NIRS. Continuous wave NIRS systems (the earliest developed method) allow for measuring only relative values of hemoglobin concentration but, at the same time, are also less expensive than other systems and can be miniaturized to the extent of a wireless instrument. Time-resolved NIRS systems are more sensitive and allow for measuring absolute values of hemoglobin concentration. Nonetheless, given technical complexity of such systems, they can't be miniaturized or made portable, are really expensive, and may be used only in laboratory settings. Finally, spatially-resolved NIRS systems allow for recording relative values of oxygenated and deoxygenated hemoglobin rather precisely, with a better control of noise at the expenses of a greater complexity of the instrument and of recording settings.

EEG and fNIRS: Compared Techniques

Given that EEG and fNIRS applications are based on different biosignals, they are also characterized by peculiar features in term of time and spatial resolution.

As for time-resolution, the EEG technique takes advantage of the extreme sensitivity and responsivity of ongoing brain electromagnetic activity, on the relatively (at least with respect to fNIRS) simplicity of circuitry and processing systems, and on computational advancements of PC processors to allow for recording data with a millisecond precision. Data sampling rates (SR) in monitoring clinical settings are usually set at 250 Hz (thus collecting 250 data points per second), but it is now more and more likely to find higher sampling rates (up to 1,000 Hz) – commonly used in experimental settings – even in clinics. For specific diagnostic applications, however, such as the recording of somatosensory potentials, even greater sampling rates can be found (up to 5,000 Hz, i.e. 5,000 collected data points per second).

While recently devised fNIRS systems allow for recording from multiple channels with relatively good sampling rate (up to 100 Hz), the nature of measures biosignal imposes a limitation on time-domain information that can be obtained. Cerebral hemodynamic responses linked to neural activations are indeed approximately delayed by one to two seconds with respect to the initial event and peak about four to six seconds later due to the time needed by underlying physiological processes. Because of that, the most commonly used systems record data at lower SR (e.g. 6.25 Hz, thus collecting approximately six data points per second). Nonetheless, advanced signal processing methods and advanced experimental design procedures might give the opportunity to effectively track relevant and informative signal changes in the order of hundreds of milliseconds (see Gratton & Fabiani, 2010; Quaresima & Ferrari, 2016).

Spatial resolution is instead the well-known Achilles' heel of electroencephalography. Due to scattering and diffusion of the electric signal in its path from cortical generators to the scalp surface and to the fact that scalp-recorded data are the outcome of electric activity potentially generated in various points of the brain (thus potentially mirroring the summation of the contribution of different systematically-active structures to the task), the localization power of EEG is commonly deemed as poor. It is possible to increase the resolution by increasing the number of electrodes used to capture the signal, thus increasing the spatial sampling density, but limitations due to the nature of the target biosignal cannot be nullified. At the expenses of a proper design of the recording setting and montage and additional precautions during the preparation of data collection, advanced techniques such as computing current source density (CSD) and estimating intracortical signal generators by source localization algorithms (e.g. the LORETA family of methods, BESA, MUSIC, and FOCUSS) give the researcher and clinician the opportunity to obtain better and more informative evidences even concerning spatial distribution and detection of EEG activity.

Contrary to the EEG, fNIRS applications takes advantage of the circumscribed distribution of hemodynamic modulations due to neurovascular coupling and of the specific sensitivity of optical measurement to even the slightest changes in both oxygenated and deoxygenated hemoglobin in the capillary components of cortical tissues. While the actual spatial resolution of an fNIRS recording partially depends on specific aspects of data recording and of the optode montage that is used (in particular the distance between light injectors and detectors, the scalp/cortical regions that are transilluminated, and technical settings of the recording system), it is generally reported in the centimeter range (i.e. approximately 1 cm). It is further worth noting that injected photons do not travel directly from the injectors to the detectors, but tend to follow a curve banana-shaped path. NIR light then shows a penetration depth within the tissues of about one half of the distance between optodes, and collected hemodynamic data then refer to a virtual channel placed within the tissues and in the middle of the gap separating the injector and the detector. Inter-optodes distance depends on the system but is usually approximately 3–4 cm. fNIRS is then thought to show a penetration power of about 2 cm, sufficient to reach cortical tissues layers.

Table 3.1 reports a synopsis of the comparison between EEG and fNIRS techniques.

Notwithstanding their differences, both those investigation tools proved to be very useful for understanding how our brains support us during sports and exercise activities and also when, where, and to what extent an athlete's brain is different from the brain of a common person. By helping us in getting a better look at sensory (visual, auditory, somatosensory, etc) motor, and cognitive processes contributing to the preparation, execution, and imagination of complex

Table 3.1 Comparison between EEG and fNIRS main characteristics

Feature	Technique	
	EEG	fNIRS
Recorded biosignal	Modulations of scalp-recorded electric potential	Fluctuations of oxygenated/deoxygenated hemoglobin following hemodynamic response
Signal sampling rate	250–5,000 Hz	≤100 Hz
Time resolution	Very good	Good
Spatial resolution	Poor	Good
Instrument size	Both small portable systems and bulky systems	Both small portable systems and bulky systems
Transportability	Feasible, more or less easy depending on the recording system	Feasible, more or less easy depending on the recording system
Telemetry	Feasible and available	Feasible and available
Cost	Variable, low/medium/high	Variable, medium/high

behaviors, they also helped to shed light on peculiar aspects of sport activity and its neurofunctional characteristics.

As underlined by Nakata and colleagues (2010), to perform skilled movements in real-life sport situations, an individual needs to be able to flexibly and efficiently adapt movements constituting the athletic gesture based on the perception of environmental information, discrimination of relevant stimuli, rapid decision-making processes, integration of afferent signals, and anticipatory action preparation. Set-shifting, behavioral inhibition, focusing, and attention mechanisms are all crucial to maintaining high-performance levels.

The next two sections will focus on sketching a brief review on main research evidences and clinical applications of EEG and fNIRS in sport and exercise science.

EEG in Sport and Exercise Science

In one of the first systematic review reports on EEG changes associated to exercise by Hatfield (1987), the author categorized EEG measurements as spontaneous recordings, averaged evoked potentials, and readiness potentials. Interestingly, such distinction can still be considered valid since EEG research continued to try and understand athletes' brains and correlations of sport-related functions by looking at task-specific modulations of frequency bands profile (with a particular interest for the alpha band), movement-related potentials, sensory evoked potentials, and cognitive event-related potentials.

EEG was firstly considered as an ideal psychophysiological measure in sport science due to its responsivity to changing psychological and contextual stimuli and to measurement sensitivity. Compared to early alternative techniques such as cardiovascular recordings via photoplethysmography and electrodermal activity measures, the millisecond resolution of ERPs and EEG measures opened novel and complementary opportunities for investigation. Further, with respect to alternative imaging techniques such as PET and fMRI, EEG recordings can be made under realistic conditions where sport gestures and performance can properly be produced and reproduced and recent wireless systems allow for investigating electrophysiological correlates of exercise activity even in the (playing) field.

Clinical and Rehabilitation Perspectives

The main application of electroencephalographic measures in clinical settings with specific reference to the domain of sport and exercise sciences has traditionally been the monitoring of sport-related concussions with diagnostic and "return-to-play" aims. Such phenomenon encompassed all ages and levels of competition, and also many different disciplines, from soccer and boxing to football and extreme sports. Because of that, concerns are more and more raised for potential effects of chronic repeated traumas and for both short- and long-term potential complications, often presenting at the beginning as subtle difficulties almost undetectable by standard paper-and-pencil assessment procedures. Further, because of inter-individual differences in brain structure and functioning and in subjective resilience, the clinical manifestations following an injury, their severity, and their clinical progression are highly variable thus making their assessment, monitoring, and management difficult. Athletes and individuals who suffered concussions may indeed display variable cognitive impairments, deficits in postural control, and other neurological symptoms (e.g. headache), which may in turn negatively affect academic and job achievements (Broglio & Puetz, 2008; Covassin, Swanik, & Sachs, 2003). In a scenario where shared assessment practices and really informative, meaningful, and efficient diagnostic and management instruments are still lacking, electrophysiological evaluations were considered a potentially valuable and clinically useful tool due to, among other specificities, its ease-of-use, its sensitivity to subtle changes in electrocortical activity, its portability, and the possibility to implement field-based recordings.

Among evidences concerning continuous EEG modulations and markers, the most commonly reported observations are a reduction in mean alpha frequency and an increase in the ratio between theta and alpha bands power (Arciniegas, 2011; Gosselin et al., 2009; Korn, Golan, Melamed, Pascual-Marqui, & Friedman, 2005). Nonetheless, we have to acknowledge that such evidences seem not to show specificity with respect to the cause of trauma. Focusing on sport-related concussions, it was shown that concussed athletes present early alterations of quantitative EEG indexes that tend to normalize after a few days (Barr, Prichep, Chabot, Powell, & McCrea, 2012; McCrea, Prichep, Powell, Chabot, & Barr, 2010). Similar alterations have been reported also by Cao and Slobounov (2011) in correspondence to occipital, temporal, and central areas, who applied advances processing procedures to EEG data and explored the potential of a novel measure of signal non-stationarity named Shannon-entropy of the peak frequency shifting (SEPFS).

The analysis of event-related responses pointed at the potential contribution of both cognitive- and movement-related potentials, while the investigation of sensory potentials resulted in still preliminary evidences. Event-related potentials overall are small time-locked electrophysiological responses, contrasting with the ampler continuous oscillatory EEG activity. While sensory evoked potentials are almost automatically elicited by exogenous stimuli and are mainly used to assess the integrity of sensory systems, motor and cognitive event-related potentials mirror different steps of information-processing and are locked to endogenous events (e.g. action preparation, error detection, attention orienting). P300, in particular, is a relatively large positive deflection occurring approximately 300 ms after the presentation of a stimulus (or later), and it is thought to mark the allocation of attention resources, the update of context and mental models, and/or stimulus categorization (Donchin & Coles, 1988). Such deflection has usually been studied via oddball experimental paradigms, where at least two stimuli are presented with different probabilities and responses to frequent and rare stimuli are then compared. Different authors reported that concussed athletes present smaller and/or later P300 deflections with respect to athletes without history of concussions or control subjects, thus suggesting a reduced ability to allocate attention resources and slowed information-processing. Though literature is not completely consistent, such observation have been obtained by using classical oddball paradigms (Baillargeon, Lassonde, Leclerc, & Ellemberg, 2012; Broglio, Pontifex, O'Connor, & Hillman, 2009; De Beaumont et al., 2009; Gaetz, Goodman, & Weinberg, 2000; Gosselin, Thériault, Leclerc, Montplaisir, & Lassonde, 2006; Thériault, De Beaumont, Gosselin, Filipinni, & Lassonde, 2009), Go/No-Go paradigms (Di Russo & Spinelli, 2010), and visual search paradigms (De Beaumont, Brisson, Lassonde, & Jolicoeur, 2007). Interestingly, it was proved that P300 morphological features (amplitude and/ or latency) are associated to self-reported symptoms, such as difficulty in concentrating and subjective cognitive deficits (Gaetz, Goodman, & Weinberg, 2000; Gosselin, Thériault, Leclerc, Montplaisir, & Lassonde, 2006).

By looking at the error-related negativity – an early event-related deflection mirroring action monitoring and error-detection mechanisms that are crucial to optimize everyday and sport behavior – Pontifex and colleagues (2009) observed a reduction of the deflection depending also on the number of sustained concussive incidents in a sample of athletes with history of concussions. Slobounov and colleagues (Slobounov, Sebastianelli, & Moss, 2005; Slobounov, Sebastianelli, & Simon, 2002) instead focused also on proper movement-related potentials – electrophysiological deflection that precede the execution of voluntary movements and are linked action preparation, programming, and initiation – and reported that concussed athletes presented reduced movement-related activity compared to the non-concussed group during a simple motor task. Notably, such markers of alterations of motor planning, initiation, and monitoring processes were present well after the concussive injury, when standard assessment procedures would have not raised concerns for return-to-play.

Research Lines

Experimental research based on EEG measurements in sport science mainly focused on the following topic: the identification of functional biomarkers associated to performance, and the investigation of EEG correlates of skilled sport behavior.

Correlates and Biomarkers for Skilled Sport Behavior and Performance

As early as 1961, Pineda and Adkisson first reported evidences for a systematic modulation of EEG activity following an exhaustive treadmill walk (Pineda & Adkisson, 1961). The authors asked participants walk at a constant speed of 3 mph and recorded pre-exercise and post-exercise alpha activity from four bipolar electrodes. Though the measurement of the alpha component was not so fine, they observed an increase in the prevalence of the frequency band and of its amplitude from two to three minutes after physical activity to 30–40 minutes later, in particular in correspondence to frontal areas. Those first evidences of exercise-induced electrophysiological changes made the authors hypothesize that exercise induced a lack of attentiveness and that participants entered a "median" state of consciousness. The observation of the rise of alpha activity following physical exercise was confirmed even by investigations in the following years but, because of substantial differences in signal processing methods and induction procedures, results showed limited generalization. Further, the induced inattention hypothesis was challenged by a subsequent evidences on the sensitivity of alpha frequencies to the internal vs. external focus of attention (depending also on recording sites) with beta frequencies as more sensitive to proper cognitive and affective information-processing (Ray & Cole, 1985). Later and methodologically finer studies on the effect of physical exercise on EEG (and in particularly alpha) activity reported inconsistent results, with evidences both on the increase (Gutmann et al., 2015; Robertson & Marino, 2015) and the decrease (Ludyga, Gronwald, & Hottenrott, 2016; Schneider, Brümmer, Abel, Askew, & Strüder, 2009) of alpha activity after exercise periods.

In more recent years, the analysis of EEG frequency components has been especially applied to investigate neural correlates of sport practice relying on focusing skills such as shooting (Kerick, Douglass, & Hatfield, 2004; Loze, Collins, & Holmes, 2001), archery (Landers et al., 1994; Salazar et al., 1990), golf (Del Percio et al., 2008), and dart-throwing (Radlo, Steinberg, Singer, Barba, & Melnikov, 2002), and in particular of preparation and pre-shot phases. By measuring modulations of signal power for the alpha and beta frequency bands over sensorimotor cortical areas, it was shown that expert athletes present less alpha activity during movement preparation and focusing periods usually in association to better subsequent performances (Babiloni et al., 2008, 2009; Del Percio et al., 2009), but and also an upper-alpha left asymmetry and a greater-alpha/lesser-beta pattern of activation with respect to novices (see Haufler, Spalding, Santa Maria, & Hatfield, 2000). Again, differences in EEG profiles and topographical distribution of such electrophysiological modulations have been reported depending on practiced sport (see, for example: Del Percio et al., 2011 for karate; Taliep & John, 2014 for golf; Del Percio et al., 2009 for pistol shooting), and data in favor of the neural efficiency hypothesis linked to reduced cortical activation and alpha blocking reactions in expert athletes have been reported by Del Percio and colleagues (2010, 2011).

Interestingly, some authors reported asymmetries in brain activation during preparatory periods (Janelle et al., 2000; Salazar et al., 1990). For example, to study elite marksmen ability to focus on the target and prepare for shooting, besides the investigation of overall alpha power, researchers also focused on asymmetries recorded over temporal areas (T3 and T4 electrode sites) (see, for example, Haufler, Spalding, Santa Maria, & Hatfield, 2000). Temporal areas asymmetry also proved to be influenced and to present following sport training. Landers and colleagues (1994) and Kerick and colleagues (2004) respectively showed that archery and pistol training induced a novel systematic relevant task-related (during aiming) increase of alpha activity in correspondence to the T3 electrode and not in correspondence to its right homologous. Those evidences are in line with the cerebral lateralization hypothesis, which suggests that the activation of the right hemisphere may more directly mirror somatic processes involved in sport and physical exercise, and such lateralized activity may act as a marker of the effect of aerobic and physical activity (Tucker, 1981).

Markers of sport activity and athletes' peculiarities were found even studying the theta band. In particular, better performances of expert golfers and rifle shooting professionals with respect to novices proved to be associated to higher frontal-midline theta power (Baumeister, Reinecke, Liesen, & Weiss, 2008; Doppelmayr, Finkenzeller, & Sauseng, 2008).

Movement-related potentials (MRP) are transient electrophysiological deflections locked to the onset of a voluntary movement that are analyzed to investigate different stages of intentionalization, preparation, programming, and execution of actions. The first reported movement-related component is known as Bereitschaftspotential or Readiness Potential, and it is also the first MRP that is generated by the sensorimotor system during planning and preparation of a movement (Deecke, Scheid, & Kornhuber, 1969). An early slowly rising component of the Readiness Potential (starting approximately 1,500–2,000 ms before the actual movement) is followed by a steeper component know as late Readiness Potential and linked to actual programming of actions and motor outputs. Subsequently, a pre-motion positivity (PMP) and the motor potential (MP) respectively mark the signal for movement initiation and the final motor output to the spinal cord. Among the cortical generators of such electrophysiological components we can list supplementary motor areas (SMA), pre-SMA, premotor and motor areas (MI), primary somatosensory areas (SI), and anterior cingulate cortex (ACC). For an extensive presentation of movement-related potentials, please refer to Shibasaki and Hallet (2006) and Santucci and Balconi (2009).

Notably, a reduction of latency or amplitude in such electrophysiological deflections is commonly thought to mirror increased neural efficiency (i.e. cortical structures are able to keep high-performance levels with minimal energy consumption). The first report hinting at sensorimotor heightened efficiency in trained athletes showed that a small group of kendo practitioners and gymnasts generated smaller and later-rising (with almost 1 seconds of difference in latencies) pre-movement components than control participants (Kita, Mori, & Nara, 2001). Subsequent studies confirmed those initial observations and highlighted how such increased efficiency depends even on training and can be specifically observed when acting with trained arms or body parts (e.g. right fingers for elite shooters) or enacting trained movements (Del Percio et al., 2008; Di Russo, Pitzalis, Aprile, & Spinelli, 2005).

Early accounts on the modulation of sensory evoked potential and cognitive event-related potentials induced by prolonged physical activity showed partially inconsistent results. Latency or amplitude of visual evoked potential (VEP) components seemed not to be relevantly changed after marathon race notwithstanding a behavioral performance decrease at a visual vigilance task (Gliner, Matsen-Twisdale, Horvath, & Maron, 1979). At the same time, strong acute exercise stress proved to induce relevant changes even in athletes in later components of flash-evoked and pattern-reversal VEP (Reeves, Justesen, Levinson, Riffle, & Wike, 1985). Namely, N100 and P300 deflections showed post-exercise reduced latencies consistent with a slight reduction in reaction times. Systematic training in ball games, instead, seems to modulate and empower visual cognitive processing likely due to the specific requirements of a given sports. A study on tennis and squash players highlighted a reduction in P100 latencies with respect to other sports athletes and control subjects (Delpont, Dolisi, Suisse, Bodino, & Gastaud, 1991). Similar modifications seem also to characterize other sports highly relying on visual detection and processing such as fencing (Taddei, Viggiano, & Mecacci, 1991), volleyball (Ozmerdivenli et al., 2005), and karate (Del Percio et al., 2007).

The analyses of early components of somatosensory evoked potentials – mirroring the functionality of somatosensory pathways and, in particular, the activity of 3b and SI areas – yielded contrasting results, with sport-specific evidences against (even if only a few) and in favor of a modulation of such responses due to sport practice (Bulut, Ozmerdivenli, & Bayer, 2003; Murakami, Sakuma, & Nakashima, 2008). Finally, only a few studies focused on very early components of auditory evoked potentials (and not on middle-latency higher sensory components) with contrasting results concerning the positive effect of sport practice on synaptic transmission times in the superior olivary complex (see Magnié et al., 1998). It is, however, worth noting that the scarcity of empirical studies and differences in sports that have been analyzed (negative results are indeed relative to cycling) may account for those contrasting results.

To investigate motivation, attention orienting, and expectancy building processes, it is possible to record and analyze the contingent negative variation (CNV), a cognitive endogenous event-related response that can be collected and quantified between an initial warning stimulus and a second cued imperative stimulus (Brunia, 1988). Hung and colleagues (2004) in particular compared professional table tennis players and non-athletes reporting that elite athletes showed larger CNVs and a peculiar distribution of the attention N100 ERP component. Such response pattern suggested that elite table tennis athletes were able to maintain notable speeded response while keeping an open distribution of their attention resources. Such increased control for the uncertainty of spatial location of stimuli may help them in achieving high performances in their peculiar sport.

Electrophysiological correlates of the involvement of higher cognitive functions in sport and exercise practice have also been studied by looking at the P300 ERP component in athletes. Such event-related deflection, as above-noted, is thought to mirror the updating of mental models and contextual information, categorization processes, and the amount of attention resources directed to a stimulus/task (Donchin & Coles, 1988). The latency of P300 component seem to be reduced in athletes (Rossi, Zani, Taddei, & Pesce, 1992), with some potential evidence on the dependence of such modulation based on expertise (Radlo, Janelle, Barba, & Frehlich, 2001; Rossi & Zani, 1991) and movement/arm-specificities of different sports (Iwadate, Mori, Ashizuka, Takayose, & Ozawa, 2005). Similarly, chronic training and sport-related aerobic fitness have been positively linked to greater P300 deflections (Chang, Tsai, Chen, & Hung, 2013; Getzmann, Falkenstein, & Gajewski, 2013; Taddei, Bultrini, Spinelli, & Di Russo, 2012), but also to greater N100 and P100 (Berchicci et al., 2015), and/or N200 (Taddei, Bultrini, Spinelli, & Di Russo, 2012; Winneke, Godde, Reuter, Vieluf, & Voelcker-Rehage, 2012) ERP amplitudes, even across the lifespan.

Again, an interesting modulation of frontal P300 as marker of response inhibition (in this case ERPs were collected during a Go/No-Go task) was observed in baseball players and fencers with respect to control subjects (Di Russo, Taddei, Apnile, & Spinelli, 2006; Nakamoto & Mori, 2008). Such enhanced behavior inhibition skill may be peculiarly present in baseball athletes and fencers due to the fact that, in such sports, it is particularly important to be able to stop movements as quickly as possible and change behavior plans.

A final basic research line in sport and exercise sciences has to do with the effect on cognitive event-related potential of acute physical exercise, even across the lifespan. Studies of the effect of single sessions overall highlighted after-effects of moderate exercise on the amplitude and latency of the P300 component, namely inducing an increase in amplitude and a decrease in latency of such deflection (see, for example, Hillman et al., 2009; Kamijo, Nishihira, Higashiura, & Kuroiwa, 2007; Pontifex, Parks, Henning, & Kamijo, 2015; Tsai et al., 2014).

EEG Correlates of Physical Exercise Under Extreme Conditions

Further classic applied research lines in sport sciences focused on specific extreme conditions, such as heat and modified gravity, and investigated relative EEG correlates of physical exercise.

Research on EEG correlates of sport activity and exercise in the heat is mainly guided by the intent to assess both changes in physiology processes, the development and experience of fatigue, and the safety and the potential of training in such extreme condition. Hyperthermia during exercise seems to affect primary brain functioning instead of impairing muscles efficiency or strength. Such effect presents as a gradual EEG slowing whereas electromyography recordings do not present relevant modulations depending on environmental heat (Nielsen & Nybo, 2003). Further, modulations of electroencephalographic activity are associated to athletes' perception of exertion.

Prolonged, high-intensity cycling in hot environments (30°C) proved to induce a post-exercise reduction of global beta activity, possibly mirroring inhibitory signals from the thalamus/hypothalamus to higher cortical areas involved in sensory and motor processing (De Pauw et al., 2013). Consistently, studies focusing on brain electrophysiological activity during exercising highlighted the following: an initial increase of prefrontal beta activity and a subsequent progressive power decline with the rise of body temperature likely due to the hypothalamus, which plays a critical role in the control of the autonomic and behavioral thermoregulatory responses by integrating efferent and afferent signals (Nielsen, Hyldig, Bidstrup, González-Alonso, & Christoffersen, 2001); an increase of the ratio between alpha and beta activity due to a relevant reduction of beta oscillations (Ftaiti, Kacem, Jaidane, Tabka, & Dogui, 2010); and also reduced alpha power during extremely prolonged light-intensity exercise – namely during an ultramarathon (Doppelmayr, Sauseng, Doppelmayr, & Mausz, 2012).

The effect of gravity changes on brain electroencephalographic activity has instead been studied with the ultimate aim to develop proper physical and cognitive countermeasures to be used during space missions and to assure safe human survival in space. Published reports of studies actually performed during space missions are still very few, also because of the cost of such studies and limitations imposed by the extreme situation. Because of that, the majority of data on the modulation of EEG activity under modified gravity conditions have actually been performed in alternative settings such as parabolic flight and prolonged bed rest. During parabolic flights it is indeed possible to repeatedly recreate transient microgravity conditions (approximately 20 seconds at 0g) preceded and followed by brief hypergravity conditions (1.8g). Prolonged bed rest, with either downward or upward tilted head, has been alternatively used to investigate human adaptation occurring with microgravity during space flights (Adams, Caiozzo, & Baldwin, 2003).

The first reports of electroencephalographic recording during space missions (US and Russian) date back to the 60s, with both evidences on an increase in alpha, beta, and theta power during space flight and negative evidences for the presence of abnormalities in continuous EEG (see Maulsby, 1966). Methodological issues and potential confounding factors due to the recording environment, however, limited the precision of those first experiments. Recent studies highlighted an increase in alpha power during eyes-closed recording over posterior and sensorimotor areas during a space flight mission (Cheron et al., 2006). In addition, alpha peak frequency was shifted from 9.9 Hz to 10.4 Hz and participants showed remarkable suppression of alpha activity when changing from an eyes-closed to an eyes-open condition. A common account for those modifications suggests that they are associated to changes in representation of space, since the lack of gravity eliminates the vertical axis and thus changes the integration of visual and vestibular inputs.

Studies of brain activity during parabolic flights, instead, reported partially contrasting results likely due to high inter-individual variability of responses to microgravity (Pletser & Quadens, 2003). Still, untrained participants showed higher EEG asymmetry than astronauts during parabolic flights (De Metz, Quadens, & De Graeve, 1994), and the induced microgravity condition has been associated to reduced beta oscillatory activity (Schneider et al., 2008; Wiedemann, Kohn, Roesner, & Hanke, 2011). Those latter evidences have been either interpreted as mirroring stress and emotional reactions to the condition and lower arousal levels (Schneider et al., 2008; Wiedemann, Kohn, Roesner, & Hanke, 2011), or as mirroring cortical inhibition induced by baroreceptor stimulations due to body fluid shifts in microgravity (Lipnicki, 2009). The effect of hypergravity, estimated by analyzing the 1.8g periods of parabolic flights, seems instead marked by a decrease in alpha power (in particular upper alpha) or theta power (respectively, Schneider et al., 2008; Wiedemann, Kohn, Roesner, & Hanke, 2011), either mirroring a protective decrease of brain functioning to address falling oxygen saturation or heightened arousal. Extreme hyper-gravity conditions recreated thanks to centrifugal cabins in the end led to loss of consciousness associated to slowed cortical rhythms (see, for example, Wilson, Reis, & Tripp, 2005).

Finally, studies on prolonged bed rest highlighted, for example, an increase in alpha, beta, and theta power together with a gradual reduction of EEG peak frequency and greater theta and delta power during downward tilted bed rest suggesting an increment in cortical inhibition (see, for example, Vaitl, Gruppe, Stark, & Pössel, 1996). Such results and their informativity with respect to proper microgravity conditions, however, should still be taken with caution since biases associated to changes in cerebral hemodynamic and shifts of the brain within the skull due to different body position might relevantly connote and affect recorded data.

fNIRS in Sport and Exercise Science

Traditionally, the use of optical imaging techniques for sport sciences and sport medicine took advantage of its peculiar capacity to non-invasively inform us about the status of soft tissues via transillumination with no relevant unwanted effects and without discomfort for the examinee. In particular, within those fields, imaging techniques based on near-infrared light have been used to investigate both the structure of muscle tissues (and potential abnormalities following injuries) and the functionality of athletes' muscles (with research, monitoring, or clinical assessment aims). Such applications have been used as potential alternatives to electromyography examinations of muscle tissues, which in turn need to invasively place needle electrodes within the examined tissue.

To date, the analysis of skeletal muscle oxygenation and oxidative energy metabolism by near-infrared spectroscopy still is one of primary applications for the technique (Hamaoka, McCully, Niwayama, & Chance, 2011; Neary, 2004), but fNIRS-based investigation of brain functioning in relation to sport activity and exercise is becoming more and more diffused. The exploration of brain activity allows for describing and understanding how processes supporting sport performance and related to athletic gestures are shaped and begin, and those pieces of information are extremely useful to complement those obtained by analyzing their output in terms of muscle and movement efficiency.

Further, fNIRS has, compared to other diffused metabolic and hemodynamic imaging tools (such as fMRI and PET), many strong points. With recent fNIRS systems, in particular continuous-wave systems, it is possible to record modulations of oxygenated and deoxygenated hemoglobin associated to cortical activity from multiple channels even outside the laboratory, thus obtaining a rather precise spatial-temporal mapping of activation patterns even in the field. Besides the peculiar feature of portability, fNIRS systems, with respect to alternative above-mentioned imaging techniques, are also less costly, less invasive, and give the opportunity to track and measure cortical functioning even *during* proper sport and complex physical exercise tasks. Though interesting preliminary usability reports have been published (see Tashiro et al., 2008), fMRI and PET examinations in sport research are still mainly used to assess pre-/post-exercise differences in brain activity, motor imagery related to athletic gestures, and neural correlates of complex movements and re-created simplified versions of actions produced during sport activities, due to technical and methodological limitations.

Clinical and Rehabilitation Perspectives

Though the application of brain imaging fNIRS in sport medicine and with clinical aims for the diagnosis and rehabilitation of sport-related injuries can be still deemed to be really at its dawn, functional optical imaging systems recently began to be studied as alternative potential tools for the assessment of the functionality of cortical structures involved in action planning and execution, and for monitoring and supporting rehabilitative interventions.

To date, despite its intrinsic limitation to measuring only cortical activity, brain fNIRS is considered a promising technique for the study and assessment of mild traumatic injuries since such clinical picture is thought to be primarily characterized by subtle functional deficits rather than structural alterations. Nonetheless, only a few relevant preliminary reports focused on sport-related concussions have been published. Kontos and colleagues (2014), for example, analyzed cortical activations as measured by fNIRS during different computerized cognitive tasks in a sample of participants who sustained sport-related concussions and a sample of age-matched controls. In the injured participants group, optical imaging data highlighted a reduction of cortical activation during tasks tapping on verbal and visual-spatial memory, executive functions, and working memory. Such evidences for the clinical utility of portable fNIRS systems was suggested even by Helmich and colleagues (2016). The authors focused on postural instability rather than on cognitive deficits since it is another primary characteristic of people who suffered from long-term symptoms after mild traumatic brain injury. Young adults who sustained sport-related concussions and presented persistent post-concussion symptoms, who had an history of concussions but no persistent symptomatology, and control participants were asked to perform a balance control task on stable *vs.* unstable surfaces and with eyes open *vs.* closed. Blood oxygenation data highlighted that concussed participants with persistent symptoms had to rely more than the other two groups on right prefrontal structures to maintain the balance, in particular during the most effortful condition. Such alteration likely mirrored increased demand of attention resources to properly face the task notwithstanding the increased neuromuscular cost.

fNIRS examination of cortical motor structures following stroke (and even other cortical injuries with different etiology), instead, highlighted an upregulation of the activity of ipsilateral motor areas when moving the affected hemisoma, together with decreased concentration of oxygenated hemoglobin and/or increased blood concentration of deoxygenated hemoglobin in contralateral affected areas (Bhambhani, Maikala, Farag, & Rowland, 2006; Kato, Izumiyama, Koizumi, Takahashi, & Itoyama, 2002; Murata, Sakatani, Katayama, & Fukaya, 2002). Such unbalanced activation pattern – which has been theorized in the form of the inter-hemispheric rivalry model – seems to be susceptible to rehabilitation. Indeed, it was shown that rehabilitative interventions for upper (e.g. hand grip) and lower limb motor skills (e.g. walking, running) are able to induce measurable modifications of compensatory (though sometimes maladaptive) asymmetries – i.e. a rise of the concentration of oxy-Hb in contralateral affected cortical areas and a decrease in the concentration of deoxy-Hb in ipsilateral pre-/motor regions (see, for example, Takeda et al., 2007).

Still taking into account the domain of motor rehabilitation, Holper and colleagues (2010) published a proof-of-concept study presenting an integrated fNIRS and Virtual Reality (VR) protocol based on observation, imitation, and execution of simple action in a virtual environment. Preliminary results showed that the integrated system and the tasks allowed for a proper activation of perception-action coupling mechanisms and for recording their functional correlates. Further, they highlighted that fNIRS recording does not impede interaction with the VR environment, a crucial point for the development of integrated VR/fNIRS-based applications for neurorehabilitation, neurofeedback, or brain-computer interfaces.

Recent Research Lines

fNIRS (and its applications to study brain functioning) is a rather recent technique with respect to electrophysiological and other brain imaging tools. The development of multichannel recording systems pushed related research activity further with respect to many research topics, such as markers of cognitive functioning and correlates of affective and social interaction processes, up to the most recent hyperscanning investigations – i.e. advanced empirical protocols focused on the coordinated analyses of two inter-agents and their physiological activities. Again, such recent developments, together with remarkable improvements in systems miniaturization, helped in making the technique even more suitable for many applications in real-life natural situations (e.g. during real-world spatial exploration while walking) and strengthened the notion of its noteworthy applicability (Quaresima & Ferrari, 2016).

Initial reports and research lines based on brain optical imaging in the specific field of sport and exercise sciences are still limited, though also constantly growing in number. At the same time, the fNIRS technique already proved to be useful and informative for studying basic motor functions and processes. For example, increased oxygenated hemoglobin concentration was observed in correspondence to motor cortices during execution of transitive and intransitive complex gestures, while premotor and posterior parietal areas were similarly activated in case of both execution and observation of gestures, supporting the hypothesis of a partial common coding and substrate for observation and execution of actions (Balconi & Cortesi, 2016; Balconi, Cortesi, & Crivelli, 2017; Balconi, Crivelli, & Cortesi, 2017; Balconi, Vanutelli, Bartolo, & Cortesi, 2015; Crivelli, Sabogal Rueda, & Balconi, 2018). In the present section, we will review some of the main relevant findings available in literature and relative to the functional correlates of the execution of skilled sport behavior and the effect of sport and physical exercise on cortical hemodynamic responses.

Preparation and execution of movements are associated to the activation of a sensorimotor network. Such cortical activations may be quantified by fNIRS measurements as a decrease in the localized concentration of deoxygenated hemoglobin and a concurrent increase of 2/3-fold magnitude in oxygenated hemoglobin concentration (Perrey, 2008), thus resulting in the well-known circumscribed increase of cerebral blood flow. Basic research findings also showed how specific characteristics of executed actions – such as the frequency of repetition, the intensity of the movement, and its complexity – may modulate concurrent cortical activations as measured by fNIRS with greater activity over motor, premotor, and prefrontal areas during more complex and effortful movements (see, for example, Holper, Biallas, & Wolf, 2009). Prefrontal structures, in particular, seems to be preferentially recruited during real everyday tasks with respect to simulated ones (Okamoto et al., 2004) and that once again stresses the importance of realistic setting to understand actual functional substrates of our behavior, in particular for sport research.

Consistently, given the flexibility and usability of fNIRS compared to other imaging methods, optical imaging has been used to highlight the cortical network supporting our ability to walk and run by recording brain activity while participants actually walked or run on treadmills. Miyai and colleagues (2001) reported notable cortical oxygenation changes in bilateral sensorimotor and pre-supplementary motor cortex during a real walking task and Suzuki and colleagues (2004) – by contrasting walking and running at different speeds (3 km/h *vs.* 5 km/h *vs.* 9 km/h) – reported that moving speed may affect sensorimotor cortical activation. Namely, while walking was associated to bilateral activation of sensorimotor cortices (as shown also by Miyai and colleagues), running was associated to greater activation of prefrontal and premotor structures, likely mirroring increased allocation of attention and monitoring resources to properly execute the complex set of body movements. Again, a similar increase of prefrontal and premotor activity was observed as a function of increasing walking speed in a sample of elderly people, particularly in individuals with greater gait difficulties (Harada, Miyai, Suzuki, & Kubota, 2009), and also during cycling at a submaximal work intensity (Ide, Horn, & Secher, 1999). Such evidence seems to corroborate the above-cited attention demand explanation for prefrontal involvement.

fNIRS studies on the effect of physical activity on brain functioning – with a peculiar focus on fatigue and resistance exercises – have usually been performed by assessing responses to mild, sub-maximal, and exhaustive exercises. Overall, empirical evidences suggest that the concentration of oxygenated hemoglobin increases in cortical structures following the increased metabolic demand due to the activity and that extended supramaximal exercise is then associated to a relevant reduction of oxygenation in correspondence to ipsilateral and contralateral pre-/motor cortices (Nielsen, Boesen, & Secher, 2001; Rooks, Thom, McCully, & Dishman, 2010; Rupp & Perrey, 2007; Subudhi, Miramon, Granger, & Roach, 2009). Besides the modification of oxy/deoxy-Hb in sensorimotor areas, it has been reported that intense exhaustive physical exercise lead to a notable decrease in oxygenation even in correspondence to prefrontal cortical regions (Rupp & Perrey, 2007; Subudhi, Miramon, Granger, & Roach, 2009), thus supporting the hypothesis that the phenomenon of fatigue is more complex than previously thought and is related not only to muscle structures, but also to the activity of central hubs involved in programming and initiation of peripheral movements. Interestingly, the rise of cerebral activity observed during exercise often contrasts with the gradual reduction of muscle tissues oxygenation with workload, and reduction of oxygenation during intense prolonged physical activity often precede the occurrence of fatigue and failure of motor performance, perhaps mirroring a protective central mechanism.

The comparison of fNIRS measures between trained athletes and novices during exercise at various workloads is another explored research topic. Concentration of oxy/deoxy-Hb and total hemoglobin indeed proved to vary sensibly depending on participants fitness, with lower cortical oxygenation indices and lower total blood volume in trained individuals with respect to untrained ones at low and moderate exercise intensities; higher concentration of oxy-Hb, deoxy-Hb and blood volume in trained *vs.* untrained individuals at maximal exhaustive intensities; a remarkable drop of oxygenated hemoglobin and blood volume at supra-maximal very hard intensities only in untrained individuals; and a clear increase of deoxygenated hemoglobin (suggesting an unbalance between oxygen demand and oxygen supply) in trained people at supra-maximal intensities (Rooks et al., 2010). Among the hypotheses developed to account for the observed lowered oxygenation values in trained people during sub-maximal effort, it was interestingly suggested that specific training might lead to the down-regulation of signals concerning fatigue from muscle afferents and from arterial baroreceptors (or maybe an alternative desensitization of central structures to such signaling), which in turn might explain the lack of increase in cortical structures activation (i.e. lower central blood flow and oxygenation) despite the physical effort.

Finally, as for hemodynamic changes in pre-/motor areas associated to progressive learning and consolidation of motor skills, research suggests that cortical activation as measured by fNIRS and relative to the execution of complex actions tends to decrease while expertise and performances increase with practice (Hatakenaka, Miyai, Mihara, Sakoda, & Kubota, 2007; Ikegami & Taga, 2008), in agreement with the release of executive control over behavior and processes of neuroplastic adaptation of cortical maps.

Electroencephalography (EEG) and Optical Imaging (fNIRS): A Comparative Primer

In this section, we will try and present a brief and practice-focused primer for the use of EEG and fNIRS recording systems. In particular, we will focus on four main issues – participants' preparation, data recording, signal processing, and principal measures and indices. Many points and advices pertain to both techniques and they will then be considered together. Where needed, we will instead discuss them at the light of methodological requirements and technical specificities peculiarly characterizing electroencephalography and functional near-infrared spectroscopy.

Here, we aim at giving a simple basic introduction, we then suggest the interested reader to further explore the topics by referring, for example, to the following books and papers: Ferrari and Quaresima (2012); Handy (2009); Keil and colleagues (2014); Perrey (2008); Senior, Russel, and Gazzaniga (2006) Thompson and colleagues (2008); and Wolf, Ferrari, and Quaresima (2007).

Preparing the Participant

In agreement with the Declaration of Helsinki and its subsequent revisions, any investigation with human participants has to abide by shared principles of respect and quality. In both experimental and clinical settings, it is particularly important to inform the participants (or the examinee) on procedures (e.g. light skin abrasion), instruments (e.g. sensors and recording systems), and/or products (e.g. conductive gels, pastes) that will be used and on the freedom to individually decide whether to participate or not (in particular for experimental studies). Participants' respect, safety, and interests must also always be safeguarded and put before collective potential benefits, especially when research involve impaired patients or people unable to understand and take actions (e.g. following severe sport injuries). In addition, any empirical study or clinical examination must also respect any higher standard norm or further specification requested by national methodological and ethical guidelines.

Said that, aside from proper participant information and collection of written consent, it is important to try and keep both physical and relational settings as clean and comfortable as possible so to avoid inducing (or increasing) stress in participants or influencing their behavior and their performances. That is particularly important when using electrophysiological, psychophysiological, or imaging techniques since recordings may be biased by confounding factors and altered physiological states. In those cases, giving time to participants to accustom to the placement of sensors and the examination setting is a useful expedient to lower unwanted biological noise and other intervenient factors.

Taking into consideration EEG and recent fNIRS applications, both techniques rely on sensors that are placed on participants' scalp. Shared rules for sensors placement are, to date, almost the same for both techniques, and ground on international coordinate systems. Procedures for preparing sensors sites, instead, are slightly different and will then be discussed separately.

Sensors Placement

International coordinates systems for sensors placement are shared guidelines that localize and label various scalp positions with reference to specific anatomical landmarks – i.e. nasion, inion, and left/right preauricular points (see Figure 3.1). Labels used to define scalp positions are constituted by letters and numbers: letters broadly refer to scalp regions (e.g. F = frontal, T = temporal, P = parietal, C = central, O = occipital, with mixed labeling in correspondence to borderlands such as FC = frontal-central, PO = parietal-occipital, and so on) and numbers define the scalp side (even numbers correspond to the right hemisphere and odd numbers to the left one, with the exception of midline sites placed sagittally over the interhemispheric fissure, which are identified by a lowercase z) and the distance from the scalp midline (the greater the number, the greater distance from the midline).

The most diffused systems are the 10–20 International System (IS), the 10–10 IS (also known as the 10% system), and the 10–5 IS (also known as the 5% system). Numbers reported in the name of each system represent percentage values that define the distance between sensor positions. The reference measures from which such percentages are calculated are the distances between nasion and inion and from the two pre-auricular points. The lower is the inter-electrode gap, the greater is the number of defined sensor positions (and then the scalp spatial sampling): the 10–20 IS (Jasper, 1958) includes 21 standard positions, the 10–10 IS (Chatrian, Lettich, & Nelson, 1985, 1988) includes up to 81 standard positions, and the 10–5 IS (Oostenveld & Praamstra, 2001) includes up to 345 standard position. Figure 3.2 presents a comparison between the two most used coordinates systems in sport and exercise sciences. While EEG recordings may equally refer to either one of the three systems depending on the aim, the amount of needed information, and the context of the examination, fNIRS recordings based on cap-mounted optodes usually refer to the 10–10 IS. In such system, indeed, the distance between sensor positions is approximately 3 cm: an optimal injector-detector distance for recent optical imaging instruments to guarantee a stable and informative measure of cortical blood oxygenation/deoxygenation. Alternatively, older fNIRS systems (primarily devised to investigate prefrontal cortices activation) used fixed-design injectors/detectors dispositions where optodes were premounted on flexible silicone patches according

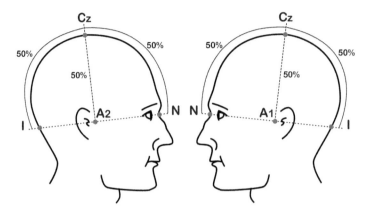

Figure 3.1 Anatomical landmarks for the definition of international coordinates systems for sensors placement. N: nasion; I: inion; A1: left preauricular points; A2: right preauricular points.

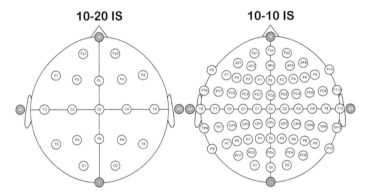

Figure 3.2 Simplified representation and comparison between the two most used coordinates systems for EEG and fNIRS sensors placement in sport and exercise sciences. Left: 10–20 International System; right: 10–10 International System. Please, note the slightly different nomenclature of sensors sites.

to predefined signal acquisition patterns. It is worth underlining once again that actual fNIRS recording channels are virtual points within biological tissues (cortical level) and in the middle of the gap between injectors and detectors due to the banana-shape principle.

Noteworthy, different methods and algorithms have been developed to track the correspondence between international standardized sensors positions and anatomical (e.g. cortical structures) or functional (e.g. Brodmann areas) regions of interests (see Giacometti, Perdue, & Diamond, 2014; Jurcak, Tsuzuki, & Dan, 2007; Koessler et al., 2009; Towle et al., 1993).

Preparing Sensors Sites: EEG

Placing EEG sensors (usually made of Ag/AgCl or gold) needs appropriate preparation of the scalp skin. Electric signal transmission is allowed and facilitated by the use of conductive gels or pastes (depending on used electrodes) but the skin has to be mildly abraded so to lower electrical impedance and allow for a high quality recording. Impedance values for each electrode should be kept below 5 kΩ. Such operation is usually done after having moved participants' hair away, by using soft cotton buds and light abrasive preparation gels. Special attention should also be paid when adding the conductive gel, since an excess might lead to bridging – i.e. creation of an unwanted electrical contact between two or more electrodes consequent to gel oozing.

Besides electrodes over participants' scalp, EEG recording (as all electrophysiological techniques like EMG and ECG) also needs reference and ground electrodes to be placed and prepared. The ground electrode is used for safety reasons and to lower potential recording noise (e.g. power line noise). The reference electrode(s) are instead used to actually compute the differential EEG signal. EEG waveforms derive from the subtraction of electrical activity recoded in correspondence to "inactive" sites from the modulations of electrical potential recorded at the scalp (and then plausibly linked to the summation of brain electrical activity). Such procedure cleans the recorded signal from common confounding factors like, for example, slow generalized voltage shifts due to sweating, changes in skin potential, and progressive drying of conductive gel. Common reference placements are earlobes (single or linked), the tip of the nose, or scalp portions over mastoid bones, but others exist.

Finally, EEG recordings are associated to concurrent measurement of electrical activity related to eye movements. The electrooculogram (EOG) is collected to keep track of saccades and blinks, which both produce highly interfering electrical signals that have to be identified and eliminated from EEG measurements. EOG is recorded from sensors placed above and below the eye (vertical EOG, forehead and cheek) and next to the outer canthi of the eyes (horizontal EOG).

Preparing Sensors Sites: fNIRS

Given the nature of recorded signal and of the recording method, fNIRS examinations do not require skin preparation to obtain informative and clean data. It is however really important that both injectors and detectors are correctly placed and touch the skin of the scalp so to avoid surface scattering, diffusion, and loss of emitted near-infrared light. To do that, hair must be accurately moved away and optodes must be kept perpendicular to the scalp. When needed, transparent gels are sometimes used to help keeping the hair away from optodes. In addition, following optodes positioning, it is important to cover them with dark clothes so to reduce potential biases due to environmental light and to absorb superficially travelling photons. Recently, some fNIRS systems manufacturers has begun to distribute special additional opaque caps that can be placed over the optodes to cover them and that can be fit to individual head shape to optimize recordings.

Data Recording

The definition of recording montages (i.e. the disposition of sensors over the scalp) is usually guided by the actual aim of the recording, clinical/research interests, and limitations imposed by the recording systems (e.g. maximum number of available channels). As a general rule of thumb, the higher the number of channels, the better, more robust, and more informative the recording. Furthermore, it is also important – in particular for EEG, and especially when electromagnetic source localization analyses are planned – that the sensors are evenly and equally distributed on the scalp. As for fNIRS data, recording it is in addition necessary to respect the injectors-detectors distance that is communicated by the system manufacturer and that depends on system settings. Usually, such distance is approximately 3 cm. As a consequence – when devising an fNIRS recording montage – it is not only important to define which cortical regions to transilluminate, but also to design optodes disposition patterns in agreement with that critical distance.

Since the advent of personal computers to collect and store data, all recorded analogue biosignal has to be digitalized. Digitalization implies that recording systems actually capture and send for storage only a certain amount of data by sampling them from the continuous original biosignal. Sampling rate (SR) is the parameter that defines how many data will be saved for each second: the higher is the SR, the more accurate and realistic is the reconstructed digital signal. The common rule that is used to decide the SR is the Nyquist theorem, which – by simplifying – states that the SR must be at least twice the highest frequency component of the signal that will be analyzed to avoid aliasing and distortion in the digital signal. For example, if you are interested in recording EEG oscillations up to 100 Hz frequency, the SR has to be at least 200 Hz. To date, apart from peculiar applications where higher sampling may be needed (e.g. sensory evoked potentials), EEG is usually sampled at 250, 500, or 1,000 Hz to allow for high quality signal. fNIRS data, due to the nature and time features of the recoded hemodynamic response, are usually collected using low sampling rates. Even if every commercial system has its own preferred settings, and with the most recent optical imaging systems it is possible to set the SR up to 100 Hz in order to try and track even the slightest signal change (Perrey, 2008), data are usually sampled at approximately 6 Hz. In normal situations, hemodynamic responses due to neurovascular coupling indeed rise and fall in approximately 8–10 seconds, which is approximately 0.1–0.125 Hz, well below the commonly-used SR.

In addition to the SR, input filters are other important parameters to be set at the beginning of the recording. Input filters are used to begin reducing the unwanted effect of environmental noise on digitalized signals. While in commercial fNIRS equipments they are usually pre-set by the manufacturer depending on characteristics of the circuitry, of used wavelengths, and of the components generating and re-capturing NIR light, they can be freely set by the technician/clinician/researcher in most EEG systems. Modifying input signal can strongly affect the recorded and digitalized signal, and then such operation should be made with caution.

As above noted, in EEG application before starting to record the electrical biosignal it is important to lower impedance values for each sensor (and, in particular, the ground electrode). Similarly, in fNIRS application, it is important to complete a sensors calibration procedure before every recording. Such automatized procedure allows for adapting light emission and signal collection based on recording-specific factors related to the context, the participant, and optodes positioning. Going down to specifics, it aims at setting channel-specific gains to equally amplify collected signals.

A further critical issue in EEG and fNIRS examinations is the use of markers (or triggers). Markers are time-locked labels used to define the occurrence, beginning and/or end of an event – such as the presentation of a stimulus, the beginning of a task or of a form of stimulation, the execution of a movement, or the increase of a biological parameter (e.g. a pre-defined heart-rate threshold). Markers are used in signal processing to segment the flow of recorded data and organize subsequent analyses.

Signal Processing

EEG Signal Processing

Recorded EEG signals are usually first re-filtered offline (i.e. subsequent to the recording) by using more stringent bandpass filters. A bandpass filter allow for attenuating frequency components of the recorded signal that stands above or below defined cut-offs frequencies, and definable as noise. After offline signal filtering, the application of artifacts correction algorithms is becoming more and more popular. Such automated or semi-automated procedure is primarily used to detect ocular artifacts such as blinks and saccades and then compute correction factors to subtract their unwanted influence on proper EEG data.

Data are then usually segmented with respect to relevant markers, and baseline reference intervals have to be defined. Subsequently, residual artifacts are visually identified and thus rejected so to avoid measurement and analysis biases. Artifact-free segments may then be averaged to increase signal-to-noise ratio and obtain more robust and reliable results. Depending on the kind of analyses and measures one is interested in, data are further processed in the time or the frequency domain. Time-domain processing has to do with time-locked or event-locked responses such as sensory evoked, event-related, and movement related potentials. Frequency domain processing has to do with task-related or resting-state oscillatory EEG activity and frequency components constituting the recorded biosignal.

When focusing on time-domain measures, relevant electrophysiological deflections have to be detected in averaged waveforms related to the presentation of a peculiar stimulus or the occurrence of a repeatable event (such as a movement) and then quantified in terms of their amplitude (measured in microvolts) and latency (measured in milliseconds and relative to the time from the segment onset to peak of the deflection), or even the area under the curve. When focusing on frequency-domain measures, oscillatory components of the EEG signal are usually computed by applying the Fast Fourier Transform (FFT) to the recorded data, which is used to convert data in the frequency-domain and calculate the relative power spectra. Power spectra allow for identifying the EEG frequency profile and analyze modulations of oscillatory activity (e.g. increase or decrease of a specific EEG band). Further advanced processing possibilities include joint time-frequency analysis (based, for example, on the wavelet transform), functional and effective connectivity analyses, and signal source localization to estimate intra-cortical generators of the activity recorded at the scalp. For a first further presentation of advanced analyses possibilities, please refer to Sanei and Chambers (2007).

fNIRS Signal Processing

Offline processing of fNIRS signal recorded by the majority of commercial systems follows, more or less, the same procedures and steps described for EEG data. Firstly, recorded data are bandpass filtered, even if the cut-off frequencies are different. Following the application of filters to reduce noise components, recording artifacts – usually presenting in the form of spikes – are searched and rejected from the fNIRS signal to avoid biasing the measurements. Subsequently, resting and task-related periods (in experimental blocks-designs) or periods related to resting and stimuli presentation (in event-related experimental designs) are defined based on markers position.

At this point, the optical signal is processed and converted, according to a modified version of the Beer-Lambert law, to calculate resting, task-related, and/or stimulus-related concentration of oxygenated hemoglobin (oxy-Hb), deoxygenated hemoglobin (deoxy-Hb), and total hemoglobin (tHB). Please refer to Perrey (2008) and Wolf and colleagues (2007) for further specifications.

Based on such concentration values, the most recent signal processing software packages allow for computing and graphically presenting modulations of oxy-Hb, deoxy-Hb, or tHb over reconstructed 3D brain models. It is possible to obtain both static and dynamic (i.e. video) results representations. As for EEG and other imaging techniques, advanced brain connectivity analysis opportunities have also been developed and are constantly improved, even if they are still primarily used with experimental aims.

Measures and Indices

EEG and fNIRS recording allows for computing a wide range of functional measures and indices, and each of them offer interesting pieces of information on brain functioning. Here, we will briefly present a selection of measures that have been used (or may be used) to investigate sport and exercise activity, while leaving further explorations to the interested reader.

Movement Related Indices

Within the domain of electrophysiological time-locked responses, action-related processes are primarily linked to movement-related potentials and action-monitoring potentials. Movement-related potentials are electrophysiological deflections that rise before or approximately in correspondence to movement execution and are linked to intentionalization, preparation, programming, and initiation of voluntary actions (see Figure 3.3). The first slowly increasing component is the Readiness Potential (initially known as Bereitschaftspotential (Deecke, Scheid, & Kornhuber, 1969). It is thought to mirror action intentionalization and preparation, rises approximately 1.5 seconds before a movement is executed, and is constituted by two subcomponents: the early-RP is slower and associated to preSMA, SMA, and premotor activity, the late-RP is the subsequent steeper segment of the deflection occurring in the last 500 ms before movement onset and associated to the activity of contralateral premotor and motor areas. By using signal subtraction techniques, it is also possible to compute a derived measure known as Lateralized Readiness Potential and used to investigate lateralized responses. The RP is then followed by the pre-motion positivity (PMP), a slight positive-going deflection occurring approximately 50–100 ms before muscles activation. It is lateralized with respect to the movement, occurs over pre-/motor regions, and is thought to mark the signal for movement initiation. Finally, the motor potential (MP) is thought to represent the final motor output to the spinal cord. It is a small further steep negative deflection occurring almost in correspondence of muscles activation and over contralateral motor areas. We suggest the works by Shibasaki and Hallett (2006) and by Jahanshahi and Hallett (2003) for further information.

Post-movement action-monitoring mechanisms are instead thought to be marked by the occurrence of the error-related negativity (ERN). The ERN is a negative deflection occurring between 70 and 120 ms after giving a behavioral response or initiating an action, and it occurs when the performed action or response was wrong. The scalp distribution of this error signal is mainly localized over frontal midline areas and source localization studies suggested that its generators are within the anterior cingulate cortex. Since it has been associated to mechanisms supporting behavior appropriateness checking that are initiated in parallel with the programming of the response, this event-related potential might offer interesting pieces of information on sport/exercise-induced modulations of such behavior monitoring mechanism.

As already reviewed in *Section 2.2*, slow electrocortical responses and proper cognitive event-related potentials – like the Contingent Negative Variation and the P300 deflection – have also been used to investigate the contribution of cognitive processes in sport and exercise activity with various results.

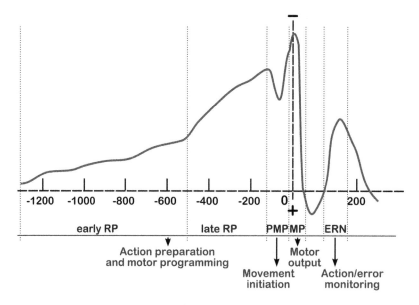

Figure 3.3 Schematic representation of movement-related potentials and components associated to action monitoring. RP: Readiness Potential; PMP: Pre-Motion Positivity; MP: Motor Potential; ERN: error-related negativity.

Task-Related Indices

Task-related measures can be obtained from both EEG and fNIRS recordings and are usually computed as a function of the difference between electrophysiological or hemodynamic brain activity recorded during a task or activity – such as different physical exercises, specific phases of the athletic gesture preparation or execution, and so on – and during a resting baseline period.

As for EEG, alpha band activity – and in particular its upper subcomponent know as *upper-alpha* or *alpha2* (10–13 Hz) – recorded over sensorimotor regions has been linked to action-related processes (Babiloni et al., 1999; Klimesch, Russegger, Doppelmayr, & Pachinger, 1998; Kuhlman, 1978; Manganotti et al., 1998; Pfurtscheller, Neuper, & Krausz, 2000). In particular, a task-related decrease of upper-alpha power is associated to action execution, perception, and imagination and showed somatotopic correspondence to executed movements and involved cortical areas. Such activity – which is recorded over sensorimotor regions instead of being posteriorly distributed like the classical visual alpha rhythm – is also alternatively known as Mu rhythm. Recently, it was shown that specific frequency-domain EEG activity may mark the experience of acting even when it is illusory (Balconi, Crivelli, & Bove, 2018) and the understanding of motor acts even when they are sub-optimally performed (Crivelli et al. 2018), with interesting implications for motor training and rehabilitation.

As for fNIRS, when focusing on brain activity, the analysis is commonly based on task-related changes in oxygenated hemoglobin (oxy-Hb), deoxygenated hemoglobin (deoxy-Hb), and/or total hemoglobin (tHB), and relevant pieces of information are obtained by comparing their spatial location, distribution, and modulation with respect to different experimental conditions. The accurate analysis of oxy-Hb, deoxy-Hb, and tHB modifications allows for investigating spatial-temporal dynamics of cortical hemodynamic responses and thus obtaining information on active sensorimotor or higher structures and networks during peculiar physical activities, sport disciplines, or specific exercise conditions (such as, for example, environment temperature, prolonged effort, exhaustive workloads). In addition to hemoglobin concentration values, it is also possible to calculate and analyze differential indices know as *d-values*. When computing such measures, task *vs.* baseline differences are weighted on individual variability of resting hemodynamic responses. The *d-values* are then deemed as stable indices partly accounting for inter-individual differences (see also Matsuda & Hiraki, 2006; Schroeter, Zysset, Kruggel, & von Cramon, 2003; Shimada & Hiraki, 2006).

Limitations and Troubleshooting for Sport Applied Research

Previous practical introduction to electrophysiological and optical imaging examinations briefly presented principal steps in recording and analyzing EEG and fNIRS data and relative methodological precautions. Such procedures and recommendations are important in laboratory settings, but even more critical and valid when devising an examination in the field, where unpredictable events will likely affect data recording together with peculiar factors of the investigation of sport and exercise activity (e.g. body movements and sweating).

Biological and environmental noise and limitations due to the context, to the physical activity under investigation, or to the practiced sport discipline (think to the different challenges posed by studying, for example, correlates of performance during endurance running or cycling) may raise both practical and technical-methodological issues that have to be properly faced. The next synopsis of troubleshooting suggestions (see Table 3.2) is a preliminary tentative tool thought to help the sport researcher approaching EEG and fNIRS recordings to solve basic potential problems in particular under the most problematic situation – i.e. field recording of dynamic physical activity.

Michela Balconi and Davide Crivelli

Table 3.2 Synopsis of common recording problems and potential solutions

Common problems	Possible solutions
a) EEG recording	
The signal is low or too noisy	If the problem affects all recording channels, double check the wiring and impedance values for reference and ground electrodes. If recording issues concern only one or a few channels, double check their connections and impedance values.
Different recording channels show remarkably different values	Double check the wiring and impedance values. If the problem still occurs, check channels calibration values and, if needed, perform a recalibration procedure for the recording system.
The signal presents systematic high-frequency noise	Prepare again the ground electrode site, double check ground impedance.
The signal presents broad and ample artifacts consistently affecting all recording channels	Artifacts are likely due to head/body movements, they can be lowered and controlled by braiding electrodes cables, using electrode caps, and properly preparing electrode sites.
Recording channels present diffused slow signal drifts	Global drifts are likely due to increased sweating, they can be lowered and controlled by properly preparing electrode sites and/or by using special active electrodes.
Two or more electrodes present highly coherent and ample recording artifacts	Artifacts are likely due to bridging, they can be controlled by checking whether gel or electrode paste actually created an electric bridge between two electrodes due to oozing, eliminating the conductive medium in excess, and preparing again the involved electrode sites.
b) fNIRS recording	
The signal is low and unresponsive	If the problem affects all recording channels, double check signal amplification settings, cable connections, and optodes covering, then run the calibration procedure again. If recording issues concern only one or a few channels, double check the placement of optodes constituting such channels, prepare again the sites by moving away participants' hair (even using a transparent gel), and run again the calibration procedure.
Different recording channels show remarkably different values	Double check the placement and covering of optodes constituting such channels, and run again the calibration procedure to adjust gain values.
The signal presents broad and ample artifacts consistently affecting all recording channels	Not so likely, but artifacts may be due to head/body movements and can be lowered and controlled by carefully securing optodes cables and using special fitting covering caps.
Recording channels present slow signal drifts	Global drifts are likely due to non-ideal optode-skin contact. They can be minimized by properly placing injectors and detectors and by keeping them perpendicular with respect to the scalp.

References

Adams, G. R., Caiozzo, V. J., & Baldwin, K. M. (2003). Skeletal muscle unweighting: Spaceflight and ground-based models. *Journal of Applied Physiology*, *95*(6), 2185–2201. doi:10.1152/japplphysiol.00346.2003.

Arciniegas, D. B. (2011). Clinical electrophysiologic assessments and mild traumatic brain injury: State-of-the-science and implications for clinical practice. *International Journal of Psychophysiology*, *82*(1), 41–52. doi:10.1016/j.ijpsycho.2011.03.004.

Babiloni, C., Carducci, F., Cincotti, F., Rossini, P. M., Neuper, C., Pfurtscheller, G., & Babiloni, F. (1999). Human movement-related potentials vs desynchronization of EEG alpha rhythm: A high-resolution EEG study. *NeuroImage*, *10*(6), 658–665. doi:10.1006/nimg.1999.0504.

Babiloni, C., Del Percio, C., Iacoboni, M., Infarinato, F., Lizio, R., Marzano, N., ... Eusebi, F. (2008). Golf putt outcomes are predicted by sensorimotor cerebral EEG rhythms. *The Journal of Physiology*, *586*(1), 131–139. doi:10.1113/jphysiol.2007.141630.

Babiloni, C., Del Percio, C., Rossini, P. M., Marzano, N., Iacoboni, M., Infarinato, F., ... Eusebi, F. (2009). Judgment of actions in experts: A high-resolution EEG study in elite athletes. *NeuroImage*, *45*(2), 512–521. doi:10.1016/j.neuroimage.2008.11.035.

Baillargeon, A., Lassonde, M., Leclerc, S., & Ellemberg, D. (2012). Neuropsychological and neurophysiological assessment of sport concussion in children, adolescents and adults. *Brain Injury*, *26*(3), 211–220. doi:10.3109/02699052.2012.654590.

Balconi, M., & Cortesi, L. (2016). Brain activity (fNIRS) in control state differs from the execution and observation of object-related and object-unrelated actions. *Journal of Motor Behavior*, *48*(4), 289–296. doi:10.1080/00222895.2015.1092936.

Balconi, M., Cortesi, L., & Crivelli, D. (2017). Motor planning and performance in transitive and intransitive gesture execution and imagination: Does EEG (RP) activity predict hemodynamic (fNIRS) response? *Neuroscience Letters*, *648*, 59–65. doi:10.1016/j.neulet.2017.03.049.

Balconi, M., Crivelli, D., & Bove, M. (2018). 'Eppur si move': The association between electrophysiological and psychophysical signatures of perceived movement illusions. *Journal of Motor Behavior*, *50*(1), 37–50. doi:10.1080/00222895.2016.1271305.

Balconi, M., Crivelli, D., & Cortesi, L. (2017). Transitive versus intransitive complex gesture representation: a comparison between execution, observation and imagination by fNIRS. *Applied Psychophysiology and Biofeedback*, *42*(3), 179–191. doi:10.1007/s10484-017-9365-1.

Balconi, M., Vanutelli, M. E., Bartolo, A., & Cortesi, L. (2015). Transitive and intransitive gesture execution and observation compared to resting state: The hemodynamic measures (fNIRS). *Cognitive Processing*, *16*(S1), 125–129. doi:10.1007/s10339-015-0729-2.

Barr, W. B., Prichep, L. S., Chabot, R., Powell, M. R., & McCrea, M. (2012). Measuring brain electrical activity to track recovery from sport-related concussion. *Brain Injury*, *26*(1), 58–66. doi:10.3109/026990 52.2011.608216.

Baumeister, J., Reinecke, K., Liesen, H., & Weiss, M. (2008). Cortical activity of skilled performance in a complex sports related motor task. *European Journal of Applied Physiology*, *104*(4), 625–631. doi:10.1007/s00421-008-0811-x.

Berchicci, M., Pontifex, M. B., Drollette, E. S., Pesce, C., Hillman, C. H., & Di Russo, F. (2015). From cognitive motor preparation to visual processing: The benefits of childhood fitness to brain health. *Neuroscience*, *298*, 211–219. doi:10.1016/j.neuroscience.2015.04.028.

Berger, H. (1929). Über das Elektrenkephalogramm des Menschen. *Archiv Für Psychiatrie Und Nervenkrankheiten*, *87*, 527–570. doi:10.1007/BF01797193.

Bhambhani, Y., Maikala, R., Farag, M., & Rowland, G. (2006). Reliability of near-infrared spectroscopy measures of cerebral oxygenation and blood volume during handgrip exercise in nondisabled and traumatic brain-injured subjects. *Journal of Rehabilitation Research and Development*, *43*(7), 845–856.

Broglio, S. P., Pontifex, M. B., O'Connor, P., & Hillman, C. H. (2009). The persistent effects of concussion on neuroelectric indices of attention. *Journal of Neurotrauma*, *26*(9), 1463–1470. doi:10.1089/neu.2008.0766.

Broglio, S. P., & Puetz, T. W. (2008). The effect of sport concussion on neurocognitive function, self-report symptoms and postural control. *Sports Medicine*, *38*(1), 53–67. doi:10.2165/00007256-200838010-00005.

Brunia, C. H. M. (1988). Movement and stimulus preceding negativity. *Biological Psychology*, *26*(1–3), 165–178. doi:10.1016/0301-0511(88)90018-X.

Bulut, S., Ozmerdivenli, R., & Bayer, H. (2003). Effects of exercise on somatosensory-evoked potentials. *The International Journal of Neuroscience*, *113*(3), 315–322. doi:10.1080/00207450390162119.

Cao, C., & Slobounov, S. (2011). Application of a novel measure of EEG non-stationarity as "Shannon-entropy of the peak frequency shifting" for detecting residual abnormalities in concussed individuals. *Clinical Neurophysiology*, *122*(7), 1314–1321. doi:10.1016/j.clinph.2010.12.042.

Chance, B. (1951). Rapid and sensitive spectrophotometry. III. A double beam apparatus. *Review of Scientific Instruments*, *22*(8), 634–638. doi:10.1063/1.1746021.

Chang, Y. K., Tsai, Y. J., Chen, T. T., & Hung, T. M. (2013). The impacts of coordinative exercise on executive function in kindergarten children: An ERP study. *Experimental Brain Research*, *225*(2), 187–196. doi:10.1007/s00221-012-3360-9.

Chatrian, G.-E., Lettich, E., & Nelson, P. L. (1985). Ten percent electrode system for topographic studies of spontaneous and evoked EEG activity. *The American Journal of EEG Technology*, *25*, 83–92.

Chatrian, G.-E., Lettich, E., & Nelson, P. L. (1988). Modified nomenclature for the "10%" Electrode System. *Journal of Clinical Neurophysiology*, *5*(2), 183–186.

Cheron, G., Leroy, A., De Saedeleer, C., Bengoetxea, A., Lipshits, M., Cebolla, A., … McIntyre, J. (2006). Effect of gravity on human spontaneous 10-Hz electroencephalographic oscillations during the arrest reaction. *Brain Research*, *1121*(1), 104–116. doi:10.1016/j.brainres.2006.08.098.

Covassin, T., Swanik, C. B., & Sachs, M. L. (2003). Epidemiological considerations of concussions among intercollegiate athletes. *Applied Neuropsychology*, *10*(1), 12–22. doi:10.1207/S15324826AN1001_3.

Crivelli, D., & Balconi, M. (2017). Event-Related Electromagnetic Responses. In *Reference Module in Neuroscience and Biobehavioral Psychology*. doi:10.1016/B978-0-12–809324-5.03053-4.

Crivelli, D., Pedullà, L., Bisio, A., Sabogal Rueda, M. D., Brichetto, G., Bove, M., & Balconi, M. (2018). When "extraneous" becomes "mine". Neurophysiological evidence of sensorimotor integration during observation of suboptimal movement patterns performed by people with Multiple Sclerosis. *Neuroscience*, Advance Online Publication. doi:10.1016/j.neuroscience.2018.07.003.

Crivelli, D., Sabogal Rueda, M. D., & Balconi, M. (2018). Linguistic and motor representations of everyday complex actions: an fNIRS investigation. *Brain Structure and Function*, *223*(6), 2989–2997. doi:10.1007/s00429-018-1646-9

De Beaumont, L., Brisson, B., Lassonde, M., & Jolicoeur, P. (2007). Long-term electrophysiological changes in athletes with a history of multiple concussions. *Brain Injury*, *21*(6), 631–644. doi:10.1080/02699050701426931.

De Beaumont, L., Thoret, H., Mongeon, D., Messier, J., Leclerc, S., Tremblay, S., … Lassonde, M. (2009). Brain function decline in healthy retired athletes who sustained their last sports concussion in early adulthood. *Brain*, *132*(3), 695–708. doi:10.1093/brain/awn347.

De Metz, K., Quadens, O., & De Graeve, M. (1994). Quantified EEG in different G situations. *Acta Astronautica*, *32*(2), 151–157.

De Pauw, K., Roelands, B., Marusic, U., Tellez, H. F., Knaepen, K., & Meeusen, R. (2013). Brain mapping after prolonged cycling and during recovery in the heat. *Journal of Applied Physiology*, *115*(9), 1324–1331. doi:10.1152/japplphysiol.00633.2013.

Deecke, L., Scheid, P., & Kornhuber, H. H. (1969). Distribution of readiness potential, pre-motion positivity, and motor potential of the human cerebral cortex preceding voluntary finger movements. *Experimental Brain Research*, *7*(2), 158–168. doi:10.1007/BF00235441.

Del Percio, C., Babiloni, C., Bertollo, M., Marzano, N., Iacoboni, M., Infarinato, F., … Eusebi, F. (2009). Visuo-attentional and sensorimotor alpha rhythms are related to visuo-motor performance in athletes. *Human Brain Mapping*, *30*(11), 3527–3540. doi:10.1002/hbm.20776.

Del Percio, C., Babiloni, C., Marzano, N., Iacoboni, M., Infarinato, F., Vecchio, F., … Eusebi, F. (2009). "Neural efficiency" of athletes' brain for upright standing: A high-resolution EEG study. *Brain Research Bulletin*, *79*(3–4), 193–200. doi:10.1016/j.brainresbull.2009.02.001.

Del Percio, C., Brancucci, A., Vecchio, F., Marzano, N., Pirritano, M., Meccariello, E., … Eusebi, F. (2007). Visual event-related potentials in elite and amateur athletes. *Brain Research Bulletin*, *74*(1–3), 104–112. doi:10.1016/j.brainresbull.2007.05.011.

Del Percio, C., Infarinato, F., Iacoboni, M., Marzano, N., Soricelli, A., Aschieri, P., … Babiloni, C. (2010). Movement-related desynchronization of alpha rhythms is lower in athletes than non-athletes: A high-resolution EEG study. *Clinical Neurophysiology*, *121*(4), 482–491. doi:10.1016/j.clinph.2009.12.004.

Del Percio, C., Infarinato, F., Marzano, N., Iacoboni, M., Aschieri, P., Lizio, R., … Babiloni, C. (2011). Reactivity of alpha rhythms to eyes opening is lower in athletes than non-athletes: A high-resolution EEG study. *International Journal of Psychophysiology*, *82*(3), 240–247. doi:10.1016/j.ijpsycho.2011.09.005.

Del Percio, C., Rossini, P. M., Marzano, N., Iacoboni, M., Infarinato, F., Aschieri, P., … Eusebi, F. (2008). Is there a "neural efficiency" in athletes? A high-resolution EEG study. *NeuroImage*, *42*(4), 1544–1553. doi:10.1016/j.neuroimage.2008.05.061.

Delpont, E., Dolisi, C., Suisse, G., Bodino, G., & Gastaud, M. (1991). Visual evoked potentials: Differences related to physical activity. *International Journal of Sports Medicine*, *12*(03), 293–298. doi:10.1055/s-2007-1024684.

Di Russo, F., Pitzalis, S., Aprile, T., & Spinelli, D. (2005). Effect of practice on brain activity: An investigation in top-level rifle shooters. *Medicine and Science in Sports and Exercise*, *37*(9), 1586–1593. doi:10.1249/01.mss.0000177458.71676.0d.

Di Russo, F., & Spinelli, D. (2010). Sport is not always healthy: Executive brain dysfunction in professional boxers. *Psychophysiology*, *47*(3), 425–434. doi:10.1111/j.1469–8986.2009.00950.x.

Di Russo, F., Taddei, F., Apnile, T., & Spinelli, D. (2006). Neural correlates of fast stimulus discrimination and response selection in top-level fencers. *Neuroscience Letters*, *408*(2), 113–118. doi:10.1016/j.neulet.2006.08.085.

Donchin, E., & Coles, M. G. H. (1988). Is the P300 component a manifestation of context updating? *Behavioral and Brain Sciences, 11*, 351–374.

Doppelmayr, M., Finkenzeller, T., & Sauseng, P. (2008). Frontal midline theta in the pre-shot phase of rifle shooting: Differences between experts and novices. *Neuropsychologia, 46*(5), 1463–1467. doi:10.1016/j.neuropsychologia.2007.12.026.

Doppelmayr, M., Sauseng, P., Doppelmayr, H., & Mausz, I. (2012). Changes in EEG during Ultralong Running. *Journal of Human Performance in Extreme Environments, 10*(1), 4. doi:10.7771/2327–2937.1047.

Ferrari, M., & Quaresima, V. (2012). A brief review on the history of human functional near-infrared spectroscopy (fNIRS) development and fields of application. *NeuroImage, 63*(2), 921–935. doi:10.1016/j.neuroimage.2012.03.049.

Ftaiti, F., Kacem, A., Jaidane, N., Tabka, Z., & Dogui, M. (2010). Changes in EEG activity before and after exhaustive exercise in sedentary women in neutral and hot environments. *Applied Ergonomics, 41*(6), 806–811. doi:10.1016/j.apergo.2010.01.008.

Gaetz, M., Goodman, D., & Weinberg, H. (2000). Electrophysiological evidence for the cumulative effects of concussion. *Brain Injury, 14*(12), 1077–1088. doi:10.1080/02699050050203577.

Getzmann, S., Falkenstein, M., & Gajewski, P. D. (2013). Long-term cardiovascular fitness is associated with auditory attentional control in old adults: Neuro-behavioral evidence. *PLoS ONE, 8*(9), e74539. doi:10.1371/journal.pone.0074539.

Giacometti, P., Perdue, K. L., & Diamond, S. G. (2014). Algorithm to find high density EEG scalp coordinates and analysis of their correspondence to structural and functional regions of the brain. *Journal of Neuroscience Methods, 229*, 84–96. doi:10.1016/j.jneumeth.2014.04.020.

Gliner, J. A., Matsen-Twisdale, J. A., Horvath, S. M., & Maron, M. B. (1979). Visual evoked potentials and signal detection following a marathon race. *Medicine and Science in Sports, 11*(2), 155–159.

Gosselin, N., Lassonde, M., Petit, D., Leclerc, S., Mongrain, V., Collie, A., & Montplaisir, J. (2009). Sleep following sport-related concussions. *Sleep Medicine, 10*(1), 35–46. doi:10.1016/j.sleep.2007.11.023.

Gosselin, N., Thériault, M., Leclerc, S., Montplaisir, J., & Lassonde, M. (2006). Neurophysiological anomalies in symptomatic and asymptomatic concussed athletes. *Neurosurgery, 58*(6), 1151–1160. doi:10.1227/01.NEU.0000215953.44097.FA.

Gratton, G., & Fabiani, M. (2010). Fast optical imaging of human brain function. *Frontiers in Human Neuroscience, 52*. doi:10.3389/fnhum.2010.00052.

Gutmann, B., Mierau, A., Hülsdünker, T., Hildebrand, C., Przyklenk, A., Hollmann, W., & Strüder, H. K. (2015). Effects of physical exercise on individual resting state EEG alpha peak frequency. *Neural Plasticity*, 1–6. doi:10.1155/2015/717312.

Hamaoka, T., McCully, K. K., Niwayama, M., & Chance, B. (2011). The use of muscle near-infrared spectroscopy in sport, health and medical sciences: Recent developments. *Philosophical Transactions of the Royal Society A: Mathematical, Physical and Engineering Sciences, 369*(1955), 4591–4604. doi:10.1098/rsta.2011.0298.

Handy, T. C. (Ed.). (2009). *Brain Signal Analysis. Advances in Neuroelectric and Neuromagnetic Methods.* Cambridge, MA: The MIT Press.

Harada, T., Miyai, I., Suzuki, M., & Kubota, K. (2009). Gait capacity affects cortical activation patterns related to speed control in the elderly. *Experimental Brain Research, 193*(3), 445–454. doi:10.1007/s00221-008-1643-y.

Hatakenaka, M., Miyai, I., Mihara, M., Sakoda, S., & Kubota, K. (2007). Frontal regions involved in learning of motor skill—A functional NIRS study. *NeuroImage, 34*(1), 109–116. doi:10.1016/j.neuroimage.2006.08.014.

Hatfield, B. D., & Landers, D. M. (1987). Psychophysiology in exercise and sport research: An overview. *Exercise and Sport Sciences Reviews, 15*, 351–387.

Haufler, A. J., Spalding, T. W., Santa Maria, D. L., & Hatfield, B. D. (2000). Neuro-cognitive activity during a self-paced visuospatial task: Comparative EEG profiles in marksmen and novice shooters. *Biological Psychology, 53*(2–3), 131–160. doi:10.1016/S0301-0511(00)00047-8.

Helmich, I., Berger, A., & Lausberg, H. (2016). Neural control of posture in individuals with persisting postconcussion symptoms. *Medicine & Science in Sports & Exercise, 48*(12), 2362–2369. doi:10.1249/MSS.0000000000001028.

Hillman, C. H., Pontifex, M. B., Raine, L. B., Castelli, D. M., Hall, E. E., & Kramer, A. F. (2009). The effect of acute treadmill walking on cognitive control and academic achievement in preadolescent children. *Neuroscience, 159*(3), 1044–1054. doi:10.1016/j.neuroscience.2009.01.057.

Holper, L., Biallas, M., & Wolf, M. (2009). Task complexity relates to activation of cortical motor areas during uni-and bimanual performance: A functional NIRS study. *NeuroImage, 46*(4), 1105–1113. doi:10.1016/j.neuroimage.2009.03.027.

Holper, L., Muehlemann, T., Scholkmann, F., Eng, K., Kiper, D., & Wolf, M. (2010). Testing the potential of a virtual reality neurorehabilitation system during performance of observation, imagery and imitation of motor actions recorded by wireless functional near-infrared spectroscopy (fNIRS). *Journal of NeuroEngineering and Rehabilitation*, 7(1), 57. doi:10.1186/1743-0003-7-57.

Hung, T. M., Spalding, T. W., Santa Maria, D. L., & Hatfield, B. D. (2004). Assessment of reactive motor performance with event-related brain potentials: Attention processes in elite table tennis players. *Journal of Sport & Exercise Psychology*, 26(2), 317–337.

Ide, K., Horn, A., & Secher, N. H. (1999). Cerebral metabolic response to submaximal exercise. *Journal of Applied Physiology*, 87(5), 1604–1608.

Ikegami, T., & Taga, G. (2008). Decrease in cortical activation during learning of a multi-joint discrete motor task. *Experimental Brain Research*, 191(2), 221–236. doi:10.1007/s00221-008-1518-2.

Iwadate, M., Mori, A., Ashizuka, T., Takayose, M., & Ozawa, T. (2005). Long-term physical exercise and somatosensory event-related potentials. *Experimental Brain Research*, 160(4), 528–532. doi:10.1007/s00221-004-2125-5.

Jahanshahi, M., & Hallett, M. (2003). *The Bereitschaftspotential: Movement-related cortical potentials*. New York, NY: Kluwer Academic/Plenum Publishers.

Janelle, C. M., Hillman, C. H., Apparies, R. J., Murray, N. P., Meili, L., Fallon, E. A., & Hatfield, B. D. (2000). Expertise differences in cortical activation and gaze behavior during rifle shooting. *Journal of Sport and Exercise Psychology*, 22(2), 167–182.

Jasper, H. H. (1958). The ten–twenty electrode system of the International Federation. *Electroencephalography and Clinical Neurophysiology*, 10, 367–380.

Jöbsis, F. F. (1977). Noninvasive, infrared monitoring of cerebral and myocardial oxygen sufficiency and circulatory parameters. *Science*, 198(4323), 1264–1267.

Jurcak, V., Tsuzuki, D., & Dan, I. (2007). 10/20, 10/10, and 10/5 systems revisited: Their validity as relative head-surface-based positioning systems. *NeuroImage*, 34(4), 1600–1611. doi:10.1016/j.neuroimage.2006.09.024.

Kamijo, K., Nishihira, Y., Higashiura, T., & Kuroiwa, K. (2007). The interactive effect of exercise intensity and task difficulty on human cognitive processing. *International Journal of Psychophysiology*, 65(2), 114–121. doi:10.1016/j.ijpsycho.2007.04.001.

Kato, H., Izumiyama, M., Koizumi, H., Takahashi, A., & Itoyama, Y. (2002). Near-infrared spectroscopic topography as a tool to monitor motor reorganization after hemiparetic stroke: A comparison with functional MRI. *Stroke*, 33(8), 2032–2036.

Keil, A., Debener, S., Gratton, G., Junghöfer, M., Kappenman, E. S., Luck, S. J., … Yee, C. M. (2014). Committee report: Publication guidelines and recommendations for studies using electroencephalography and magnetoencephalography. *Psychophysiology*, 51(1), 1–21. doi:10.1111/psyp.12147.

Kerick, S. E., Douglass, L. W., & Hatfield, B. D. (2004). Cerebral cortical adaptations associated with visuomotor practice. *Medicine & Science in Sports & Exercise*, 36(1), 118–129. doi:10.1249/01. MSS.0000106176.31784.D4.

Kita, Y., Mori, A., & Nara, M. (2001). Two types of movement-related cortical potentials preceding wrist extension in humans. *Neuroreport*, 12(10), 2221–2225.

Klimesch, W., Russegger, H., Doppelmayr, M., & Pachinger, T. (1998). A method for the calculation of induced band power: Implications for the significance of brain oscillations. *Electroencephalography and Clinical Neurophysiology*, 108(2), 123–130.

Koessler, L., Maillard, L., Benhadid, A., Vignal, J. P., Felblinger, J., Vespignani, H., & Braun, M. (2009). Automated cortical projection of EEG sensors: Anatomical correlation via the international 10–10 system. *NeuroImage*, 46(1), 64–72. doi:10.1016/j.neuroimage.2009.02.006.

Kontos, A. P., Huppert, T. J., Beluk, N. H., Elbin, R. J., Henry, L. C., French, J., … Collins, M. W. (2014). Brain activation during neurocognitive testing using functional near-infrared spectroscopy in patients following concussion compared to healthy controls. *Brain Imaging and Behavior*, 8(4), 621–634. doi:10.1007/s11682-014-9289-9.

Korn, A., Golan, H., Melamed, I., Pascual-Marqui, R., & Friedman, A. (2005). Focal cortical dysfunction and blood-brain barrier disruption in patients with Postconcussion syndrome. *Journal of Clinical Neurophysiology*, 22(1), 1–9. doi:10.1097/01.WNP.0000150973.24324.A7.

Kuhlman, W. N. (1978). Functional topography of the human mu rhythm. *Electroencephalography and Clinical Neurophysiology*, 44(1), 83–93. doi:10.1016/0013–4694(78)90107-4.

Landers, D. M., Han, M.-W., Salazar, W., Petruzzello, S. J., Kubitz, K. A. K., & Gannon, T. L. (1994). Effects of learning on electroencephalographic and electrocardiographic patterns in novice archers. *International Journal of Sport Psychology*, 25(3), 313–330.

Lipnicki, D. M. (2009). Baroreceptor activity potentially facilitates cortical inhibition in zero gravity. *NeuroImage, 46*(1), 10–11. doi:10.1016/j.neuroimage.2009.01.039.

Loze, G. M., Collins, D., & Holmes, P. S. (2001). Pre-shot EEG alpha-power reactivity during expert air-pistol shooting: A comparison of best and worst shots. *Journal of Sports Sciences, 19*(9), 727–733. doi:10.1080/02640410152475856.

Ludyga, S., Gronwald, T., & Hottenrott, K. (2016). Effects of high vs. low cadence training on cyclists' brain cortical activity during exercise. *Journal of Science and Medicine in Sport, 19*(4), 342–347. doi:10.1016/j.jsams.2015.04.003.

Magnié, M. N., Bermon, S., Martin, F., Madany-Lounis, M., Gastaud, M., & Dolisi, C. (1998). Visual and brainstem auditory evoked potentials and maximal aerobic exercise: Does the influence of exercise persist after body temperature recovery? *International Journal of Sports Medicine, 19*(4), 255–259.

Manganotti, P., Gerloff, C., Toro, C., Katsuta, H., Sadato, N., Zhuang, P., ... Hallett, M. (1998). Task-related coherence and task-related spectral power changes during sequential finger movements. *Electroencephalography and Clinical Neurophysiology, 109*(1), 50–62.

Matsuda, G., & Hiraki, K. (2006). Sustained decrease in oxygenated hemoglobin during video games in the dorsal prefrontal cortex: A NIRS study of children. *NeuroImage, 29*(3), 706–711. doi:10.1016/j.neuroimage.2005.08.019.

Maulsby, R. L. (1966). Electroencephalogram during orbital flight. *Aerospace Medicine, 37*(10), 1022–1026.

McCrea, M., Prichep, L., Powell, M. R., Chabot, R., & Barr, W. B. (2010). Acute effects and recovery after sport-related concussion. *Journal of Head Trauma Rehabilitation, 25*(4), 283–292. doi:10.1097/HTR.0b013e3181e67923.

Miyai, I., Tanabe, H. C., Sase, I., Eda, H., Oda, I., Konishi, I., ... Kubota, K. (2001). Cortical mapping of gait in humans: A near-infrared spectroscopic topography study. *NeuroImage, 14*(5), 1186–1192. doi:10.1006/nimg.2001.0905.

Murakami, T., Sakuma, K., & Nakashima, K. (2008). Somatosensory evoked potentials and high-frequency oscillations in athletes. *Clinical Neurophysiology, 119*(12), 2862–2869. doi:10.1016/j.clinph.2008.09.002.

Murata, Y., Sakatani, K., Katayama, Y., & Fukaya, C. (2002). Increase in focal concentration of deoxyhaemoglobin during neuronal activity in cerebral ischaemic patients. *Journal of Neurology, Neurosurgery, and Psychiatry, 73*(2), 182–184.

Nakamoto, H., & Mori, S. (2008). Effects of stimulus-response compatibility in mediating expert performance in baseball players. *Brain Research, 1189*(1), 179–188. doi:10.1016/j.brainres.2007.10.096.

Nakata, H., Yoshie, M., Miura, A., & Kudo, K. (2010). Characteristics of the athletes' brain: Evidence from neurophysiology and neuroimaging. *Brain Research Reviews, 62*(2), 197–211. doi:10.1016/j.brainresrev.2009.11.006.

Neary, J. P. (2004). Application of Near Infrared Spectroscopy to exercise sports science. *Canadian Journal of Applied Physiology, 29*(4), 488–503.

Nielsen, B., Boesen, M., & Secher, N. H. (2001). Near-infrared spectroscopy determined brain and muscle oxygenation during exercise with normal and resistive breathing. *Acta Physiologica Scandinavica, 171*(1), 63–70. doi:10.1046/j.1365-201X.2001.00782.x.

Nielsen, B., Hyldig, T., Bidstrup, F., González-Alonso, J., & Christoffersen, G. R. J. (2001). Brain activity and fatigue during prolonged exercise in the heat. *Pflügers Archiv, 442*(1), 41–48. doi:10.1007/s004240100515.

Nielsen, B., & Nybo, L. (2003). Cerebral changes during exercise in the heat. *Sports Medicine, 33*(1), 1–11. doi:10.2165/00007256-200333010-00001.

Okamoto, M., Dan, H., Shimizu, K., Takeo, K., Amita, T., Oda, I., ... Dan, I. (2004). Multimodal assessment of cortical activation during apple peeling by NIRS and fMRI. *NeuroImage, 21*(4), 1275–1288. doi:10.1016/j.neuroimage.2003.12.003.

Oostenveld, R., & Praamstra, P. (2001). The five percent electrode system for high-resolution EEG and ERP measurements. *Clinical Neurophysiology, 112*(4), 713–719.

Ozmerdivenli, R., Bulut, S., Bayar, H., Karacabey, K., Ciloglu, F., Peker, I., & Tan, U. (2005). Effects of exercise on visual evoked potentials. *The International Journal of Neuroscience, 115*(7), 1043–1050. doi:10.1080/00207450590898481.

Perrey, S. (2008). Non-invasive NIR spectroscopy of human brain function during exercise. *Methods, 45*(4), 289–299. doi:10.1016/j.ymeth.2008.04.005.

Pfurtscheller, G., Neuper, C., & Krausz, G. (2000). Functional dissociation of lower and upper frequency mu rhythms in relation to voluntary limb movement. *Clinical Neurophysiology, 111*(10), 1873–1879.

Pineda, A., & Adkisson, M. A. (1961). Electroencephalographic studies in physical fatigue. *Texas Reports on Biology and Medicine, 19*, 332–342.

Pletser, V., & Quadens, O. (2003). Degraded EEG response of the human brain in function of gravity levels by the method of chaotic attractor. *Acta Astronautica*, *52*(7), 581–589.

Pontifex, M. B., O'Connor, P. M., Broglio, S. P., & Hillman, C. H. (2009). The association between mild traumatic brain injury history and cognitive control. *Neuropsychologia*, *47*(14), 3210–3216. doi:10.1016/j.neuropsychologia.2009.07.021.

Pontifex, M. B., Parks, A. C., Henning, D. A., & Kamijo, K. (2015). Single bouts of exercise selectively sustain attentional processes. *Psychophysiology*, *52*(5), 618–625. doi:10.1111/psyp.12395.

Quaresima, V., & Ferrari, M. (2016). Functional Near-Infrared Spectroscopy (fNIRS) for assessing cerebral cortex function during human behavior in natural/social situations: A concise review. *Organizational Research Methods*. Advance online publication. doi:10.1177/1094428116658959.

Radlo, S. J., Janelle, C. M., Barba, D. A., & Frehlich, S. G. (2001). Perceptual decision making for baseball pitch recognition: Using P300 latency and amplitude to index attentional processing. *Research Quarterly for Exercise and Sport*, *72*(1), 22–31. doi:10.1080/02701367.2001.10608928.

Radlo, S. J., Steinberg, G. M., Singer, R. N., Barba, D. A., & Melnikov, A. (2002). The influence of an attentional focus strategy on alpha brain wave activity, heart rate and dart-throwing performance. *International Journal of Sport Psychology*, *33*(2), 205–217.

Ray, W. J., & Cole, H. W. (1985). EEG alpha activity reflects attentional demands, and beta activity reflects emotional and cognitive processes. *Science*, *228*(4700), 750–752.

Reeves, D. L., Justesen, D. R., Levinson, D. M., Riffle, D. W., & Wike, E. L. (1985). Endogenous hyperthermia in normal human subjects: I. Experimental study of evoked potentials and reaction time. *Physiological Psychology*, *13*(4), 258–267. doi:10.3758/BF03326531.

Robertson, C. V, & Marino, F. E. (2015). Prefrontal and motor cortex EEG responses and their relationship to ventilatory thresholds during exhaustive incremental exercise. *European Journal of Applied Physiology*, *115*(April), 1939–1948. doi:10.1007/s00421-015-3177-x.

Rooks, C. R., Thom, N. J., McCully, K. K., & Dishman, R. K. (2010). Effects of incremental exercise on cerebral oxygenation measured by near-infrared spectroscopy: A systematic review. *Progress in Neurobiology*, *92*(2), 134–150. doi:10.1016/j.pneurobio.2010.06.002.

Rossi, B., & Zani, A. (1991). Timing of movement-related decision processes in clay-pigeon shooters as assessed by event-related brain potentials and reaction times. *International Journal of Sport Psychology*, *22*, 128–139.

Rossi, B., Zani, A., Taddei, F., & Pesce, C. (1992). Chronometric aspects of information processing in high level fencers as compared to non-athletes: An ERPs and RT study. *Journal of Human Movemennt Studies*, *23*, 17–28.

Roy, C. S., & Sherrington, C. S. (1890). On the regulation of the blood-supply of the brain. *The Journal of Physiology*, *11*(1–2), 85–158.

Rupp, T., & Perrey, S. (2007). Prefrontal cortex oxygenation and neuromuscular responses to exhaustive exercise. *European Journal of Applied Physiology*, *102*(2), 153–163. doi:10.1007/s00421-007-0568-7.

Salazar, W., Landers, D. M., Petruzzello, S. J., Han, M.-W., Crews, D. J., & Kubitz, K. A. (1990). Hemispheric asymmetry, cardiac response, and performance in elite archers. *Research Quarterly for Exercise and Sport*, *61*(4), 351–359. doi:10.1080/02701367.1990.10607499.

Sanei, S., & Chambers, J. A. (2007). *EEG Signal Processing*. Chichester: John Wiley & Sons, Ltd.

Santucci, E., & Balconi, M. (2009). The multicomponential nature of movement-related cortical potentials: Functional generators and psychological factors. *Neuropsychological Trends*, *5*, 59–84.

Schneider, S., Brümmer, V., Abel, T., Askew, C. D., & Strüder, H. K. (2009). Changes in brain cortical activity measured by EEG are related to individual exercise preferences. *Physiology and Behavior*, *98*(4), 447–452. doi:10.1016/j.physbeh.2009.07.010.

Schneider, S., Brümmer, V., Carnahan, H., Dubrowski, A., Askew, C. D., & Strüder, H. K. (2008). What happens to the brain in weightlessness? A first approach by EEG tomography. *NeuroImage*, *42*(4), 1316–1323. doi:10.1016/j.neuroimage.2008.06.010.

Schroeter, M. L., Zysset, S., Kruggel, F., & von Cramon, D. Y. (2003). Age dependency of the hemodynamic response as measured by functional near-infrared spectroscopy. *NeuroImage*, *19*(3), 555–564. doi:10.1016/S1053-8119(03)00155-1.

Senior, C., Russell, T., & Gazzaniga, M. S. (Eds.). (2006). *Methods in Mind*. Cambridge, MA: The MIT Press.

Shibasaki, H., & Hallett, M. (2006). What is the Bereitschaftspotential? *Clinical Neurophysiology*, *117*(11), 2341–2356. doi:10.1016/j.clinph.2006.04.025.

Shimada, S., & Hiraki, K. (2006). Infant's brain responses to live and televised action. *NeuroImage*, *32*(2), 930–939. doi:10.1016/j.neuroimage.2006.03.044.

Slobounov, S., Sebastianelli, W., & Moss, R. (2005). Alteration of posture-related cortical potentials in mild traumatic brain injury. *Neuroscience Letters*, *383*(3), 251–255. doi:10.1016/j.neulet.2005.04.039.

Slobounov, S., Sebastianelli, W., & Simon, R. (2002). Neurophysiological and behavioral concomitants of mild brain injury in collegiate athletes. *Clinical Neurophysiology*, *113*(2), 185–193. doi:10.1016/S1388–2457(01)00737-4.

Subudhi, A. W., Miramon, B. R., Granger, M. E., & Roach, R. C. (2009). Frontal and motor cortex oxygenation during maximal exercise in normoxia and hypoxia. *Journal of Applied Physiology*, *106*(4), 1153–1158. doi:10.1152/japplphysiol.91475.2008.

Suzuki, M., Miyai, I., Ono, T., Oda, I., Konishi, I., Kochiyama, T., & Kubota, K. (2004). Prefrontal and premotor cortices are involved in adapting walking and running speed on the treadmill: An optical imaging study. *NeuroImage*, *23*(3), 1020–1026. doi:10.1016/j.neuroimage.2004.07.002.

Taddei, F., Bultrini, A., Spinelli, D., & Di Russo, F. (2012). Neural correlates of attentional and executive processing in middle-age fencers. *Medicine and Science in Sports and Exercise*, *44*(6), 1057–1066. doi:10.1249/MSS.0b013e31824529c2.

Taddei, F., Viggiano, M. P., & Mecacci, L. (1991). Pattern reversal visual evoked potentials in fencers. *International Journal of Psychophysiology*, *11*(3), 257–260.

Takeda, K., Gomi, Y., Imai, I., Shimoda, N., Hiwatari, M., & Kato, H. (2007). Shift of motor activation areas during recovery from hemiparesis after cerebral infarction: A longitudinal study with near-infrared spectroscopy. *Neuroscience Research*, *59*(2), 136–144. doi:10.1016/j.neures.2007.06.1466.

Taliep, M. S., & John, L. (2014). Sport expertise: The role of precise timing of verbal-analytical engagement and the ability to detect visual cues. *Perception*, *43*(4), 316–332. doi:10.1068/p7530.

Tashiro, M., Itoh, M., Fujimoto, T., Masud, M. M., Watanuki, S., & Yanai, K. (2008). Application of positron emission tomography to neuroimaging in sports sciences. *Methods*, *45*(4), 300–306. doi:10.1016/j.ymeth.2008.05.001.

Thériault, M., De Beaumont, L., Gosselin, N., Filipinni, M., & Lassonde, M. (2009). Electrophysiological abnormalities in well functioning multiple concussed athletes. *Brain Injury*, *23*(11), 899–906. doi:10.1080/02699050903283189.

Thompson, T., Steffert, T., Ros, T., Leach, J., & Gruzelier, J. (2008). EEG applications for sport and performance. *Methods*, *45*(4), 279–288. doi:10.1016/j.ymeth.2008.07.006.

Towle, V. L., Bolaños, J., Suarez, D., Tan, K., Grzeszczuk, R., Levin, D. N., … Spire, J.-P. (1993). The spatial location of EEG electrodes: Locating the best-fitting sphere relative to cortical anatomy. *Electroencephalography and Clinical Neurophysiology*, *86*(1), 1–6.

Tsai, C. L., Chen, F. C., Pan, C. Y., Wang, C. H., Huang, T. H., & Chen, T. C. (2014). Impact of acute aerobic exercise and cardiorespiratory fitness on visuospatial attention performance and serum BDNF levels. *Psychoneuroendocrinology*, *41*(1), 121–131. doi:10.1016/j.psyneuen.2013.12.014.

Tucker, D. M. (1981). Lateral brain function, emotion, and conceptualization. *Psychological Bulletin*, *89*(1), 19–46.

Vaitl, D., Gruppe, H., Stark, R., & Pössel, P. (1996). Simulated micro-gravity and cortical inhibition: A study of the hemodynamic-brain interaction. *Biological Psychology*, *42*(1–2), 87–103.

Wiedemann, M., Kohn, F. P. M., Roesner, H., & Hanke, W. R. L. (2011). *Self-organization and pattern-formation in neuronal systems under conditions of variable gravity*. Berlin, Heidelberg: Springer Berlin Heidelberg. doi:10.1007/978-3-642-14472-1.

Wilson, G. F., Reis, G. A., & Tripp, L. D. (2005). EEG correlates of G-induced loss of consciousness. *Aviation, Space, and Environmental Medicine*, *76*(1), 19–27.

Winneke, A. H., Godde, B., Reuter, E.-M., Vieluf, S., & Voelcker-Rehage, C. (2012). The association between physical activity and attentional control in younger and older middle-aged adults. *GeroPsych*, *25*(4), 207–221. doi:10.1024/1662–9647/a000072.

Wolf, M., Ferrari, M., & Quaresima, V. (2007). Progress of near-infrared spectroscopy and topography for brain and muscle clinical applications. *Journal of Biomedical Optics*, *12*(6), 062104. doi:10.1117/1.2804899.

Zani, A., & Proverbio, A. M. (Eds.). (2002). *The cognitive electrophysiology of mind and brain*. New York: Academic Press.

4

Sport-Related EEG Activity

What Have We Learned from a Quarter-Century's Worth of Research?

Karla A. Kubitz

This chapter reviews the published literature examining sport-related EEG activity over the past quarter-century. Using several search engines to probe multiple databases with the key terms "EEG" and "sport", 13 reviews and 92 research studies were identified. Reviews and research studies were limited to those published in academic journals, in English, and between 1983 and 2016. The majority of the published reviews (Cheron et al., 2016; Cooke, 2013; Etnier & Gapin, 2014; Hatfield, Haufler, Hung, & Spalding, 2004; Hatfield & Kerick, 2007; Hatfield & Landers, 1983; Janelle & Hatfield, 2008; Lawton, Saarela, & Hatfield, 1998; Mancevska, Gligoroska, Todorovska, Dejanova, & Petrovska, 2016; Yarrow, Brown, & Krakauer, 2009) focused on the sport-related EEG research studies available at the time. Three of the published reviews (Gentili, Oh, Bradberry, Hatfield, & Contreras-Vidal, 2010; Mann & Janelle, 2012; Thompson, Steffert, Ros, Leach, & Gruzelier, 2008) focused technological considerations for sport-related EEG researchers. Significant conclusions for the most recent (i.e., those published within the past decade) of the published EEG research-focused reviews are described below.

Yarrow et al. (2009) reviewed the pre-2009 literature and drew two conclusions. First, they concluded that the literature supports the notion that experts demonstrate more efficient cortical processing. Second, they concluded that the literature supports a predictive relationship between sport-related EEG activity and performance.

Gentili et al. (2010) reviewed the pre-2010 literature and drew four conclusions. They concluded that the literature supported the existence of important relationships between sport-related EEG activity and performance. Second, they concluded that the literature supported the existence of differences in sport-related EEG activity between experts and novices. Third, they concluded that the literature supported the existence of learning effects. Fourth, they concluded that the literature supported the existence of specific locations and frequency bands of importance.

Cooke (2013) reviewed the pre-2013 literature and drew two main conclusions. First, the literature indicated differences in external information processing. Second, the literature indicated differences in verbal-analytic information processing.

Etnier and Gapin (2014) reviewed the pre-2014 literature and drew three conclusions. First that the sport-related EEG literature supported the existence of expert/novice differences in EEG activity. Second, that the literature supported the importance of left hemisphere activity. Third, Etnier and Gapin (2014) concluded that the sport-related EEG literature supported the importance of slow potential activity, specifically the contingent negative variation (CNV) waveform.

Mancevska et al. (2016) reviewed the pre-2016 literature and drew several important conclusions. First, they concluded that the literature supported a shift from left brain to right brain activity during sport performance. Second, they concluded that the literature supported the importance of reduced EEG coherence as a concomitant of optimal performance. Third, they concluded that the literature supported the importance of studying event-related potentials related to sport performance.

There were several similar conclusions in these reviews. Four of the reviews (Etnier & Gapin, 2014; Janelle & Hatfield, 2008; Lawton et al., 1998; Mancevska et al., 2016) concluded that the literature supported the existence of hemispheric differences in EEG activity during the pre-performance period. Three of the reviews (Hatfield et al., 2004; Janelle & Hatfield, 2008; Lawton et al., 1998) concluded that the literature supported the existence of decreased EEG activation during the pre-performance period. Two of the reviews (Etnier & Gapin, 2014; Gentili et al., 2010) concluded that the literature supported the existence of differences sport-related EEG activity between experts and novices. Two of the reviews (Etnier & Gapin, 2014; Mancevska et al., 2016) concluded that the literature supported the relevance of event-related potentials for understanding sport-related EEG activity.

Based on the aforementioned reviews of the sport-related EEG research studies (see Table A1 for methodological details on the sport-related EEG studies) over the past quarter-century, this chapter focuses on eight questions, including:

1   How does EEG activity change across the pre-performance period?
2   How is EEG activity different during good and poor performances?
3   How is EEG activity different in experts and novices?
4   How is EEG activity different in competitive athletes and non-athletes?
5   How is EEG activity different in disabled and non-disabled athletes?
6   How does practice/learning change EEG activity?
7   Is EEG activity during a sport task different from EEG activity during other tasks (e.g., balancing on a stabilometer)?
8   Is sport-related EEG activity changed by socio-environmental manipulations (e.g., adding competition)?

How Does EEG Activity Change across the Pre-Performance Period?

Several early (pre-2001) studies recorded theta and/or alpha activity (i.e., using power, ERD/ERS, and/or asymmetry metrics) during the pre-performance period. For example, Hatfield, Landers, and Ray (1984, Study 1) used a within-subject design to examine shooting-related EEG activity. Participants were 17 elite-level shooters who performed an air rifle shooting task. Hatfield et al. recorded spontaneous EEG activity, specifically alpha activity before shooting. They found that alpha power at T3 increased and alpha power at T4 remained constant across time during the pre-performance period. In like manner, Hatfield, Landers, and Ray (1987) used a within-subject design to examine shooting-related EEG activity. Participants were 15 expert marksmen who performed self-paced 40 shots to a target. Hatfield et al. recorded spontaneous EEG activity, specifically theta, alpha, and beta activity, before shooting. In addition, they recorded heart rate. They found no significant differences in heart rate or alpha activity across time during the pre-performance period. However, there was a trend for heart rate and for alpha activity (at T3) to increase across this period. Continuing, the focus on shooting, Janelle et al. (2000) used a between-subject design to examine shooting-related EEG activity. Participants were 12 expert shooters and 13 non-expert shooters who performed 40 shots in a standing position using the Noptel Shooter Training system. Janelle et al. recorded spontaneous EEG activity, specifically alpha activity. They also recorded visual point of gaze (as an index of Quiet Eye duration). The results revealed that experts had higher performance scores and longer quiet eye periods than novices. Both experts and novices exhibited increased left hemisphere alpha power and decreased right hemisphere alpha power during shooting. Focusing on a different sport, Salazar et al. (1990) used a multi-factorial design to examine archery-related EEG activity. Participants were 13 male and 15 female archers who performed four tasks, including shooting with normal bow; shooting with light bow; bow drawing without aiming; and aiming without bow drawing. Salazar et al. recorded spontaneous EEG activity, specifically 5–31 Hz activity. The results indicated that power at 10 and 12 Hz (i.e., T3 alpha activity) increased across the pre-performance period. However, power at T4 remained constant across the same period. Continuing this line of inquiry, Crews and Landers (1993) used a within-subject design to examine golf-related EEG activity. Participants were 34 highly skilled golfers who performed a putting task. Crews and Landers recorded both spontaneous and event-related EEG activity, including theta, alpha, beta1, beta2, and 40 Hz activity. They found that left hemisphere alpha power increased and right hemisphere alpha power decreased across time during the pre-performance period.

Numerous recent studies also recorded theta and/or alpha activity (i.e., using power, ERD/ERS, and/or asymmetry metrics) during the pre-performance period. The majority focused on alpha activity. For example, Loze, Collins, and Holmes (2001) used a within-subject design to examine shooting-related EEG activity. Participants were six expert air-pistol shooters who performed a shooting task. Loze et al. recorded spontaneous EEG activity, specifically alpha activity. The results revealed that there was a lower level of alpha power at T4 than at T3 (i.e., asymmetry was negative) during the pre-performance period. In like manner, Kerick, McDowell, and Hung (2001) used a within-subject design to examine shooting-related EEG activity. Participants were eight skilled marksmen who performed shooting, postural control, and movement control tasks. Kerick et al. recorded event-related EEG activity, specifically alpha ERD. They reported that high alpha power (at T3) increased across the pre-performance period and that there were no changes during this period at T4, C3, or C4. Similarly, Holmes, Collins, and Calmels (2006) used a within-subject design to compare EEG activity across the pre-performance period. Participants were six expert shooters who performed 40 shots (using the SCATT Shooter Training system) and three observation tasks. Holmes et al. recorded event-related EEG activity, specifically alpha ERD. The results showed that alpha desynchronization (in the right hemisphere) increased (i.e., alpha power decreased) across the pre-performance period in the shooting condition. Focusing on archery, Twigg, Sigurnjak, Southall, and Shenfield (2014) used a within-subject design to examine shooting-related EEG activity. Participants were two experienced archers who shot 12 arrows each. Twigg et al. recorded spontaneous EEG activity, specifically 1–30 Hz activity. They reported that alpha activity increased across the pre-performance period. Although most of these studies focused on alpha activity, there was one study that focused on theta activity. Specifically, Doppelmayr, Finkenzeller, and Sauseng (2008) used a between-subject design to examine shooting-related EEG activity. Participants were eight expert shooters and 10 novice shooters who performed 10 blocks of five shots each. Doppelmayr et al. recorded spontaneous EEG activity, specifically frontal midline theta activity. Furthermore, they performed source localization using the LORETA algorithm. The results indicated that frontal midline theta (at Fz) increased across the pre-performance period.

A small group of studies recorded other EEG measures, including higher frequency EEG activity, EEG coherence, event-related potentials, or self-organizing neural networks during the pre-performance period. As mentioned previously, Janelle et al. (2000) used a between-subject design to examine shooting-related EEG activity. In addition to the findings described earlier in this section, they also reported that experts had higher performance scores and longer quiet eye periods than novices. Moreover, both experts and novices exhibited increased left hemisphere beta power and decreased right hemisphere beta power during shooting. As mentioned previously, Twigg et al. (2014) used a within-subject design to examine shooting-related EEG activity. In addition to the findings described earlier in this section, they also reported that beta activity decreased across the pre-performance period. Focusing on coherence, Wu, Lo, Lin, Shih, and Hung (2007) used a within-subject design to examine sport-related EEG activity. Participants were 12 highly skilled basketball players who shot 50 baskets. Wu et al. recorded spontaneous

EEG activity, specifically low alpha, high alpha, and low beta coherence. The results indicated that high alpha and low beta coherence decreased across the pre-performance period. Focusing on event-related potentials, Konttinen and Lyytinen (1992) used a mixed-model design to examine sport-related EEG activity. Participants were three skilled marksmen and three novice shooters who performed a simulated rifle shooting task. Konttinen and Lyytinen recorded event-related EEG activity, specifically slow potential waveforms. Additionally, they recorded heart rate and respiration. The results indicated that, for all shooters, heart rate decreased and slow potential negativity (at C3 and C4) increased across the pre-performance period. Focusing on self-organizing neural networks, Stikic et al. (2014, Study 1) used a within-subject design to examine shooting-related EEG activity. Participants were 51 adult volunteers (i.e., without any marksmanship training) who performed a simulated shooting task using the Virtual Battle Space2 Tactical Warfare Simulator. Stikic et al. recorded spontaneous EEG activity, specifically self-organizing neural networks. In particular, they used the B-Alert model to classify cognitive states according to engagement and workload. The results showed that a neural network successfully indexed engagement and workload during a simulated shooting task. The nodes that were activated most often included nodes 8, 6, and 11. Node 8 represented low EEG-engagement, node 6 represented high EEG-engagement, and node 11 represented both EEG-engagement and EEG workload.

In summary, there were 15 studies that examined changes in sport-related EEG activity across the pre-performance period. Most (n=10) of these examined changes in alpha activity across the pre-performance period. There seems to be a consensus that alpha activity (particularly in the left hemisphere) increases across the pre-performance period. All but one of the studies examining alpha activity reported increased left hemisphere alpha activity across the pre-performance period. The exception, Holmes et al. (2006) reported increased right hemisphere alpha ERD (i.e., decreased alpha activity) across the pre-performance period. Only six studies examined measures other than alpha activity, including theta (n=1), beta (n=2), EEG coherence (n=1), slow potentials (n=1), and self-organizing neural networks (n=1). Consequently, it was impossible to draw conclusions regarding changes in any of the other EEG measures (i.e., other than alpha activity) across the pre-performance period.

How Is EEG Activity Different During Good and Poor Performances?

Quite a few studies recorded theta activity (i.e., using power, ERD/ERS, and/or asymmetry metrics) during good and poor performances. Among them, Salazar et al. (1990) used a multi-factorial design to compare EEG activity during good and poor performances. Participants were 13 male and 15 female archers who performed four tasks, including shooting with normal bow; shooting with light bow; bow drawing without aiming; and aiming without bow drawing. Salazar et al. recorded spontaneous EEG activity, specifically 5–31 Hz activity. The results showed that 7 Hz theta power (i.e., at T3) was lower during good performance than during poor performance. Along the same lines, Kao, Huang, and Hung (2013) used a within-subject design to compare EEG activity during good and poor performances. Participants were 18 skilled golfers who performed 100 putts. Putts were divided into 15 best and 15 worst outcomes. Kao et al. (2013) recorded spontaneous EEG activity, specifically frontal midline theta activity. The results indicated that there was a lower level of frontal midline theta activity (at Fz, Cz, and Pz) in the best relative to the worst shots. Similarly, Chuang, Huang, and Hung (2013) used a within-subject design to compare EEG activity during good and poor performance. Participants were 15 skilled basketball players who performed basketball free throw shots. Chuang et al. recorded spontaneous EEG activity, specifically low theta and high theta band activity. They reported that theta1 power (at Fz) and theta2 power (at Fz and F4) remained stable during the pre-performance period for successful shots. In contrast, theta power was unstable for unsuccessful shots. Likewise, Dyke et al. (2014) used a within-subject design to compare EEG activity during good and poor performances.

Participants were 13 novice golfers who performed 30 putts. Putts were divided into five most and five least accurate. Dyke et al. recorded spontaneous EEG activity, specifically theta, low alpha, high alpha, low beta, high beta, and gamma activity. They reported higher levels of theta activity (in the left temporal area) before the more accurate putts. Taking a different, model-building approach, di Fronso et al. (2016) used a within-subject design to compare EEG activity during good and poor performances. The study tested the predictions of the 'multi-action plan' (MAP) model. The MAP model predicted specific within-subject differences in EEG activity (and perceived control) between four types of shots, including Type I/Efficient shots, Type II/Effortful shots, Type III/Impaired shots, and Type IV/Inefficient shots. A single elite air pistol shooter performed 40 self-paced shots. Di Fronso et al. recorded event-related EEG activity, specifically theta, low alpha, and high alpha event-related synchrony. Types I and II had the best shooting scores. In addition, consistent with the MAP model, Type I/Efficient shots were characterized by increased theta synchrony (i.e., more theta activity) and Type II/Effortful shots were characterized by decreased theta synchrony (i.e., less theta activity). Also testing the MAP model, Bertollo et al. (2016) used a within-subject design to compare EEG activity during good and poor performances. Participants were 10 elite shooters who performed 120 shots. Bertollo et al. recorded event-related EEG activity, specifically theta, low alpha, and high alpha event-related synchrony. The results, once again, supported the MAP model. That is, Type I/Efficient shots were characterized by increased theta synchrony (i.e., more theta activity). Type II/Effortful and Type III/Impaired shots were characterized by decreased theta synchrony (i.e., less theta activity).

Several early (pre-2001) studies recorded alpha activity (i.e., using power, ERD/ERS, and/or asymmetry metrics) during good and poor performances. Among them, Bird (1987) used a within-subject design to compare EEG activity during good and poor performances. A single elite marksman performed a shooting task. Bird recorded spontaneous EEG activity, specifically EEG peak frequency. The results indicated that the average frequency was lower (about 12–14 Hz) in good than in poor shots (about 14–16 Hz). As mentioned previously, Salazar et al. (1990) used a multi-factorial design to compare EEG activity during good and poor performances. In addition to the findings described earlier in this section, they also reported that 12 Hz alpha power (i.e., at T3) was lower during good performance than during poor performance. Continuing the focus on shooting, Hillman, Apparies, Janelle, and Hatfield (2000) used a within-subject design to compare EEG activity during good and poor performance. Participants were seven expert shooters who performed a simulated rifle shooting task. Hillman et al. recorded spontaneous EEG activity, specifically alpha and beta activity. They found that good performances (i.e., executed shots) were accompanied by lower alpha power than poor performances (i.e., rejected shots).

Numerous recent studies recorded alpha activity (i.e., using power, ERD/ERS, and/or asymmetry metrics) during good and poor performances. Among these, Loze et al. (2001) used a within-subject design to compare EEG activity during good and poor performances. Participants were six expert air-pistol shooters who performed a shooting task. Loze et al. recorded spontaneous EEG activity, specifically alpha activity and found differences in EEG activity between good and bad shots. Alpha power (at Oz) was higher before good shots and lower before bad shots. Similarly, Bablioni et al. (2008) used a within-subject design to compare EEG activity during good and poor performances. Participants were 12 expert golfers who performed 10 blocks of 10 putts each (while standing on a balance platform) using a putting green simulator. Bablioni et al. recorded spontaneous EEG activity, specifically alpha and beta activity. Furthermore, they performed source localization using the Laplacian transformation algorithm and measured body sway. The results showed that the amplitude of high frequency alpha power (at Cz) was lower in the successful than in the unsuccessful putts. In addition, alpha power and performance were positively related. That is, putts were closer to the hole when there were larger decreases in alpha power and farther away from the hole when there were smaller decreases in alpha power. Likewise, Cooke et al. (2014) used a mixed-model design to compare sport-related EEG activity between good and poor performances. Participants were 10 expert golfers and 10 novice golfers who performed 60 putts. Cooke et al. recorded spontaneous EEG activity, specifically theta, low alpha, high alpha, and beta activity. In addition, they recorded number of putts holed, self-reported pressure, movement kinematics, heart rate, and EMG activity. The results indicated that experts had less low alpha power and less high alpha power (at frontal and central sites) for holed putts than for missed putts. Focusing on ERD/ERS, Del Percio, Bablioni, Bertollo et al. (2009) used a mixed-model design to compare EEG activity across good and poor performances. Participants were 18 expert shooters and 10 non-athletes who performed 120 shots. Del Percio, Bablioni, Bertollo et al. recorded event-related EEG activity, specifically low alpha and high alpha ERD. They performed source localization using the Laplacian transformation algorithm. The results revealed that high-frequency alpha ERD was less (i.e., alpha power was higher) for high score shots than for low score shots. As mentioned previously, Bertollo et al. (2016) used a within-subject design to compare EEG activity during good and poor performances. In addition to the findings described earlier in this section, they also reported that Type I/Efficient shots were characterized by increased low alpha synchrony (i.e., more alpha activity). Moreover, Type II/Effortful and Type III/Impaired shots were characterized by decreased low alpha synchrony (i.e., less alpha activity).

A few studies recorded beta and/or gamma activity during good and poor performances. Each of these studies have been mentioned previously. Among these, Salazar et al. (1990) used a multi-factorial design to compare EEG activity during good and poor performances. In addition to the findings described earlier in this section, they also reported that beta power (i.e., 28 Hz power at T3) was lower during good performance than during poor performance. Similarly, Hillman et al. (2000) used a within-subject design to compare EEG activity during good and poor performance. In addition to the findings described earlier in this section, they also reported that good performances (i.e., executed shots) were accompanied by lower beta power than poor performances (i.e., rejected shots). Likewise, Dyke et al. (2014) used a within-subject design to compare EEG activity during good and poor performances. In addition to the findings described earlier in this section, they also reported higher levels of low beta activity (in the left temporal area) before the more accurate putts.

Several recent studies recorded EEG coherence during good and poor performances. Among them, Wu et al. (2007) used a within-subject design to compare EEG activity during good and poor performances. Participants were 12 highly skilled basketball players who shot 50 baskets. Wu et al. recorded spontaneous EEG activity, specifically low alpha, high alpha, and low beta coherence. They found coherence was lower across all frequency bands for good shots than for poor shots. Furthermore, Gallicchio, Cooke, and Ring (2015) used a mixed-model design to compare sport-related EEG activity between experts and novices. Participants were 10 expert golfers and 10 novice golfers who performed 60 putts. Gallicchio et al. recorded spontaneous EEG activity, specifically left and right hemisphere alpha coherence. They found less left hemisphere high alpha coherence for successful than for unsuccessful putts. There were no differences in right hemisphere high alpha coherence between successful and unsuccessful putts. Likewise, Bablioni et al. (2011) used a within-subject design to compare EEG activity during good and poor performances. Participants were 12 expert golfers who performed 100 self-paced putts using a golf green simulator. Bablioni et al. recorded spontaneous EEG activity, specifically low alpha and high alpha coherence. Furthermore, they performed source localization using the Laplacian transformation algorithm. They reported that intra-hemispheric coherence (in parietal and frontal sites) was higher during successful putts than during unsuccessful putts. As mentioned previously, Dyke et al. (2014) used a within-subject design to compare EEG activity during good and poor performances. In addition to the findings described earlier in this section, they also reported no significant differences in EEG coherence between the more and the less accurate putts.

Several studies recorded event-related potentials during good and poor performances. Among those, Konttinen and Lyytinen (1992) used a mixed-model design to compare EEG activity across good and poor performances. Participants were three skilled marksmen and three novice shooters who performed a simulated rifle shooting task. Konttinen and Lyytinen recorded event-related EEG activity, specifically slow potential waveforms. In addition, they recorded heart rate and respiration. They reported that the experts' best shots were accompanied by less negativity (at Fz) than their worst shots. Similarly, Konttinen, Lyytinen, and Konttinen (1995) used a within-subject design to compare EEG activity during good and poor performances. Participants were six elite marksmen and six pre-elite marksmen who performed a simulated rifle shooting task. Konttinen et al. recorded event-related EEG activity, specifically slow potential waveforms. They found that there was less slow potential negativity/more frontal slow potential positivity during good versus poor performances. Extending these findings, Konttinen and Lyytinen (1993a) used a within-subject design to compare EEG activity during good and poor performances. Participants were 12 expert shooters who performed a simulated rifle shooting task. Konttinen and Lyytinen recorded event-related EEG activity, specifically slow potential waveforms. They also recorded heart rate and respiration. They found individual differences in slow potential waveforms during shooting. There was a unique slow potential profile (i.e., a certain amount of negativity and/or positivity) for each shooter, a profile that differed across their good and poor performances.

In summary, there were 23 studies that examined differences in sport-related EEG activity between good and poor performances. Most (n=13) of these examined changes in theta and/or alpha activity between good and poor performances. A few studies examined changes in beta activity (n=3), EEG coherence (n=4), or slow potentials (n=3). Across these studies, two points of agreement emerged. First, there seems to be a consensus that beta activity is lower in good performances than in poor performances. All three of the studies reviewed reported that beta activity was lower in good performances than in poor performances. Second, there seems to be a consensus that slow potential shifts are less negative in good performances than in poor performances. All but one of the studies reviewed reported that slow potential shifts were less negative in good performances than in poor performances. The exception (Konttinen & Lyytinen, 1993a) reported individual differences in slow potentials between good and poor performances. Finally, the findings were mixed regarding differences in theta activity, alpha activity, and EEG coherence between good and poor performances.

How Is EEG Activity Different in Experts and Novices?

A small group of studies recorded theta activity (i.e., using power, ERD/ERS, and/or asymmetry metrics) in expert and novice performers. Among those, Haufler, Spalding, Maria, and Hatfield (2000) used a mixed-model design to compare sport-related EEG activity between experts and novices. Participants were 15 elite shooters and 21 novice shooters who performed simulated a simulated rifle shooting task. Haufler et al. recorded spontaneous EEG activity, specifically theta, low alpha, high alpha, beta, and gamma activity. They reported that experts performed better on the shooting task than novices. Moreover, experts had more left (and right) hemisphere theta activity during shooting than novices. Continuing the focus on shooters, Doppelmayr et al. (2008) used a between-subject design to compare shooting-related EEG activity in experts and novices. Participants were eight expert shooters and 10 novice shooters who performed 10 blocks of five shots each. Doppelmayr et al. recorded spontaneous EEG activity, specifically frontal midline theta activity. They also performed source localization using the LORETA algorithm. They reported that frontal midline theta activity (at Fz) was higher for experts than for novices (during last 3s before the shot). Focusing on golfers, Baumeister, Reinecke, Liesen, and Weiss (2008) used a between-subject design to compare sport-related EEG activity in experts and novices. Participants were nine experienced golfers and nine novice golfers who performed five blocks of 10 putts each on an indoor carpet putting green. Baumeister et al. recorded spontaneous EEG activity, specifically theta, alpha1, alpha2, beta1, and beta2 activity and EEG asymmetry. In addition, they measured anxiety (using the State-Trait Anxiety Inventory) and stress (using a visual analog scale). The results revealed that experts performed better than novices. Performance differences were accompanied by EEG differences. Experts had higher theta (at Fz and Pz) than novices. Continuing the focus on golfers, Cooke et al. (2014) used a mixed-model design to compare sport-related EEG activity between experts and novices. Participants were 10 expert golfers and 10 novice golfers who performed 60 putts. Cooke et al. recorded spontaneous EEG activity, specifically theta, low alpha, high alpha, and beta activity. In addition, they recorded number of putts holed, self-reported pressure, movement kinematics, heart rate, and EMG activity. The results indicated that experts had less theta power during the pre-putt period than novices.

Another small group of studies recorded alpha activity (i.e., using power, ERD/ERS, and/or asymmetry metrics) in expert and novice performers. Each of these studies has been mentioned previously. Among them, Haufler et al. (2000) used a mixed-model design to compare sport-related EEG activity between experts and novices. In addition to the findings mentioned earlier in this section, they also reported that experts performed better on the shooting task than novices. Moreover, experts had more left hemisphere low alpha activity and more left hemisphere high alpha activity during shooting than novices. Similarly, Baumeister et al. (2008) used a between-subject design to compare sport-related EEG activity in experts and novices. In addition to the findings described earlier in this section, experts had higher alpha1 (at Pz), and alpha2 (at Pz) than novices. Likewise, Cooke et al. (2014) used a mixed-model design to compare sport-related EEG activity between experts and novices. In addition to the findings described earlier in this chapter, they also reported that experts had more high alpha power during the pre-putt period than novices. Continuing this line of inquiry, Janelle et al. (2000) used a between-subject design to compare sport-related EEG activity in experts and novices. Participants were 12 expert shooters and 13 non-expert shooters who performed 40 shots in a standing position using the Noptel Shooter Training system. Janelle et al. recorded spontaneous EEG activity, specifically alpha activity. Additionally, they recorded visual point of gaze (as an index of Quiet Eye duration). They found that experts had longer quiet eye periods and better performance than novices. However, there were no between-group differences in alpha activity. Likewise, Taliep and John (2014) used a between-subject design to compare sport-related EEG activity in experts and novices. Participants were eight skilled and 10 less skilled cricket batsmen. The cricket batsmen watched 24 bowling deliveries and decided whether they were in-swinger or out-swinger deliveries. Taliep et al. recorded event-related EEG activity, specifically alpha ERD. The results indicated that expert batsmen showed more alpha synchronization (i.e., more alpha activity) than novices during the pre-performance period. These differences were statistically significant from −1500s to −250s before ball release.

A few studies recorded beta and/or gamma activity in expert and novice performers. Each of these studies has been mentioned previously. Among these, Haufler et al. (2000) used a mixed-model design to compare sport-related EEG activity between experts and novices. In addition to the findings mentioned earlier in this section, they also reported that experts performed better on the shooting task than novices. Moreover, experts had less left and right hemisphere (except for T3) beta activity and less left and right hemisphere gamma activity during shooting than novices. Similarly, Janelle et al. (2000) used a between-subject design to compare sport-related EEG activity in experts and novices. In addition to the findings described earlier in this section, they also reported that there were no between-group differences in beta activity. Likewise, Cooke et al. (2014) used a mixed-model design to compare sport-related EEG activity between experts and novices. In addition to the findings described earlier in this section, they also reported that experts had more beta power during the pre-putt period than novices.

In addition, a few studies recorded SMR activity in expert and novice performers. For example, Wolf et al. (2014) used a between-subject design to compare sport-related EEG activity in different levels of expertise. Participants were 14 expert table tennis players, 15 amateur table tennis players, and 15 young elite table tennis players who watched 40 videos of table tennis strokes. Participants were asked to imagine themselves responding to the strokes. Wolf et al. recorded event-related EEG activity, specifically sensorimotor ERD. They reported that SMR desynchronization was greater (i.e., there was less SMR activity) in elite athletes (over the motor cortex) than in amateur athletes. In addition, Cheng et al. (2015) used a between-subject design to compare sport-related EEG activity in experts and novices. Participants were 14 expert dart throwers and 11 novice dart throwers who performed 60 self-paced dart throws. Cheng et al. recorded spontaneous EEG activity, specifically sensorimotor ERD. In addition, they recorded EMG activity from forearm flexor muscles. They found that experts had higher SMR activity and higher beta1 activity during the pre-performance period than novices.

Numerous studies recorded EEG coherence in expert and novice performers. Among those, Deeny, Hillman, Janelle, and Hatfield (2003) used a between-subject design to compare sport-related EEG activity in experts and novices. Participants were 10 expert shooters and nine less skilled shooters who completed a shooting task. Deeny et al. recorded spontaneous EEG activity, specifically low alpha, high alpha, and beta coherence. The results showed that experts had lower low alpha (between T3 and Fz), high alpha (between all left hemisphere sites and Fz), and low beta coherence (between T3 and Fz) than novices. Extending the results of the earlier study, Deeny, Haufler, Saffer, and Hatfield (2009) used a between-subject design to compare sport-related EEG activity in experts and novices. Participants were 15 expert shooters and 21 novice shooters who performed 40 self-paced shots using the Noptel Shooter Training System. Deeny et al. recorded spontaneous EEG activity, specifically theta, low alpha, high alpha, low beta, high beta, and gamma coherence. Additionally, they recorded variability in aiming point. They found difference in shooting scores between experts and novices. These differences were accompanied by lower EEG coherence (most evident in the right hemisphere) in experts than in novices. In addition, EEG coherence (in low alpha at F4-P4, F4-O2, F3-P3, and F3-O1) was positively correlated with movement variability during aiming. Additionally, Gallicchio et al. (2015) used a mixed-model design to compare sport-related EEG activity between experts and novices. Participants were 10 expert golfers and 10 novice golfers who performed 60 putts. Gallicchio et al. recorded spontaneous EEG activity, specifically left and right hemisphere alpha coherence. They reported that there was less left hemisphere high alpha coherence (between T7 and Fz) during the pre-performance period in experts than in novices. However, there were no differences in right hemisphere high alpha coherence between experts and novices. Continuing this line of inquiry, Harung (2011) used a between-subject design to compare sport-related EEG activity in different levels of expertise. Participants were 33 Olympic/world class and 33 competitive athletes who performed two paired reaction time tasks (i.e., tasks that included a warning stimulus followed by an imperative stimulus). Harung recorded spontaneous EEG activity, specifically 6–40 Hz EEG coherence. The results showed that 6–40 Hz EEG coherence were higher in world class than in average athletes. Taking a slightly different approach, Wolf, Brölz, Keune, and Wesa (2015) used a between-subject design to compare sport-related EEG activity in experts and novices. Participants were 14 expert table tennis players and 15 amateur table tennis players who watched 40 videos of table tennis strokes and imagined themselves responding to the strokes. Wolf et al. recorded spontaneous EEG activity, specifically theta coherence. The results indicated that experts had higher T4-Fz theta coherence than amateurs.

A few studies recorded event-related potentials in expert and novice performers. Among these, Radlo, Janelle, Barba, and Frehlich (2001) used a between-subject design to compare sport-related EEG activity in experts and novices. Participants were 10 advanced baseball players and 10 intermediate-level baseball players who completed a baseball pitch discrimination task. Radlo et al. recorded event-related EEG activity, specifically the P300 event-related potential. Additionally, they recorded reaction times. The results revealed that advanced players had shorter reaction times and more correct responses (when judging baseball pitches) than intermediate-level players. This was accompanied by differences in the P300 event-related potential waveform. Advanced players had longer P300 latencies and smaller P300 amplitudes than intermediate-level players. In addition, Hack, Memmert, and Rupp (2009) used a between-subject design to compare sport-related EEG activity in experts and novices. Participants were 10 experienced basketball referees and 10 novice basketball referees who judged pictures of basketball game situations varying on the presence/absence of a foul. Hack et al. recorded event-related EEG activity, specifically the N1 and P300 waveforms. They found that the event-related potentials were different for experienced and novice referees. Experienced referees had higher N1 and P3 amplitudes relative to novice referees. In addition, experienced referees had shorter P3 latencies (at Pz) than novice referees. However, there were no differences in foul judgment accuracy between the two groups.

A few early studies recorded slow potentials in expert and novice performers. Among them, Fattapposta et al. (1996) used a between-subject design to compare sport-related EEG activity in experts and novices. Participants were eight elite pentathletes and eight novice pentathletes who completed the Skilled Performance Task (i.e., an interactive bi-manual motor-perceptual task). Fattapposta et al. recorded event-related EEG activity, specifically movement-related cortical potentials. In particular, they focused on the Bereitschaftspotential and skilled performance positivity waveforms. They reported better performance in the expert than in the novices. This was accompanied by smaller Bereitschaftspotential and larger skilled performance positivity waveforms in experts than in novices. Similarly, Konttinen, Lyytinen, and Viitasalo (1998) used a between-subject design to compare sport-related EEG activity in experts and novices. Participants were six elite marksmen and six pre-elite marksmen who performed a simulated rifle shooting task. Konttinen et al. recorded event-related EEG activity, specifically slow potentials. The results of the study were that elite and pre-elite shooters used different rifle-holding strategies and had differences in slow potential activity. For elite shooters, frontal (Fz) slow potential positivity was associated with decreased rifle stability. For pre-elite shooters, frontal (Fz) slow potential positivity was associated with increased rifle stability. Continuing this line of inquiry, Konttinen, Lyytinen, and Era (1999) used a between-subject design to compare sport-related EEG activity in experts and novices. Participants were six elite marksmen and six pre-elite marksmen who performed a simulated rifle shooting task. Konttinen et al. recorded event-related EEG activity, specifically slow potentials. They also recorded body sway during shooting. The results of the study were that there was were different relationships in the elite and the pre-elite shooters between slow potentials and body sway. For elite shooters, decreased frontal slow potential positivity was associated with greater stability. For pre-elite shooters, decreased central (C4) slow potential Negativity was associated with greater stability. Similarly, Konttinen, Landers, and Lyytinen (2000) used a between-subject design to compare sport-related EEG activity in experts and novices. Participants were six elite marksmen and six pre-elite marksmen who performed a simulated rifle shooting task. Konttinen et al. recorded event-related EEG activity, specifically slow potentials. The results of the study were that pre-trigger slow potentials (at Fz) were more positive among elite shooters than among pre-elite shooters.

Several recent studies also recorded slow potentials in expert and novice performers. Among them, Mann, Coombes, Mousseau, and Janelle (2011) used a between-subjects design to compare sport-related EEG activity in experts and novices. Participants were 10 expert golfers and 10 near-expert golfers who performed two blocks of 45 putts each. Mann et al. recorded event-related EEG activity, specifically movement-related cortical potentials (i.e., the Bereitschaftspotential). In addition, Mann et al. recorded the Quiet Eye duration and EMG activity from right forearm extensor muscles. They reported that experts made more putts and had a longer quiet eye period than near-experts. This was accompanied by greater negativity in the Bereitschaftspotentials of the experts than of the novices. This difference was clear at C4 for the early and late components and at P4 for the early component only. Moreover, there were no expert/near-expert differences for any of the C3, P3, or Cz components. Likewise, Nakamoto and Mori (2012) used a between-subject design to compare sport-related EEG activity in experts and novices. Participants were seven expert baseball players and seven novice baseball players who performed an anticipation timing (Go/No-go) reaction time task in two conditions, timing unchanged and timing changed. Nakamoto et al. recorded event-related EEG activity, specifically movement-related cortical potentials. They focused on the contingent negative variation (CNV) waveform. They found that experts made fewer timing errors during the anticipation timing task. In addition, experts had shorter latencies for the CNV waveform and increased amplitudes for the N200 and P300 waveforms. As mentioned previously, Harung (2011) used a between-subject design to compare sport-related EEG activity in different levels of expertise. Participants were 33 Olympic/world class and 33 competitive athletes who performed two paired reaction time tasks (i.e., tasks that included a warning stimulus followed by an imperative stimulus). Harung recorded slow potential waveforms (i.e., the CNV waveform). The results showed that the amplitudes of the late CNV waveform (in frontal and central areas) were higher in world class than in average athletes. Along the same line, Hung, Spalding, Maria, and Hatfield (2004) used a between-subject design to compare sport-related EEG activity in experts and novices. Participants were 15 highly skilled table tennis players and 15 non-athletic college students who completed a cued reaction time task (i.e., Posner's cued attention task). Hung et al. recorded event-related EEG activity, specifically slow potentials. In particular, they focused on lateralized readiness potentials, which reflect cortical preparation for cued hand movement. The results indicated that skilled table tennis players had faster reaction times to both correctly and incorrectly cued stimuli than novices. They also had larger lateralized readiness potentials than novices.

Last, two studies recorded different EEG metrics in expert and novice performers. First, Del Percio, Brancucci et al. (2007) used a multi-factorial design to compare sport-related EEG in experts and novices. Participants were 17 elite karate athletes, 14 amateur karate athletes, and 15 non-athletes who observed 180 pictures different karate attacks and decided whether the attacks were right/left side attacks. Del Percio et al. recorded event-related EEG activity, specifically visual evoked potentials. The results revealed that the elite karate athletes had a smaller amplitude visual evoked potential waveform (at 300–450 ms) for the karate than for the fencing attacks. Second, Hung, Haufler, Lo, Mayer-Kress, and Hatfield (2008) used a between-subject design to compare sport-related EEG activity between experts and novices. Participants were 15 expert shooters and 21 novice shooters who performed 40 shots (with a 5s aiming period) in a standing position. Hung et al. recorded spontaneous EEG activity, specifically EEG dimensionality (i.e., D2). D2 is an "estimate of the number of active cell assemblies that produce the [EEG] signal through their independent oscillations" (Hung et al., 2008, p. 753). D2 was calculated using the Dataplore software. The results of the study were that experts showed higher performance accuracy and lower D2 than novices. In addition, shooting performance and D2 were negatively correlated (in experts). That is, better shooting performance was associated with a lower level of D2. Novices showed the opposite relationship, a positive correlation between shooting performance and D2. Third, Stikic et al. (2014, Study 2) used a within-subject design to examine golfing-related EEG activity. Participants were 11 experienced golfers and 11 novice golfers who performed 10 sessions of 10 putts each. They recorded spontaneous EEG activity, specifically self-organizing neural networks (using the B-Alert model generated in Study 1). The results of Study 2 showed EEG-engagement and EEG workload were higher than average during the pre-performance period and decreased afterwards. The results of Study 2 showed that node 11 (both EEG engagement and EEG workload) and node 6 (EEG-engagement) were activated most often during golfing. That is, golfing activated two of the same nodes (i.e., 6 and 11) that shooting did (in Study 1) but did not activate node 8 (low EEG-engagement).

In summary, there were 32 studies that examined differences in sport-related EEG activity between experts and novices. The majority of these examined differences in alpha activity (n=5), EEG coherence (n=5), or slow potentials (n=8) between experts and novices. A few studies examined differences in theta activity (n=4), beta activity (n=3), SMR activity (n=2), event-related potentials (n=2), evoked potentials (n=1), EEG dimensionality (n=1), and self-organizing neural networks (n=1). Across these studies, two points of agreement emerged. First, there seems to be a consensus that theta activity and alpha activity are higher in experts than in novices. Three out of the four studies reviewed reported that theta activity was higher in experts than in novices. The exception (Andrew Cooke et al., 2014) reported lower theta in experts than in novices. Four out of the five studies reviewed reported that alpha activity was higher in experts than in novices. The exception (Janelle et al., 2000) reported no significant differences in alpha activity between experts and novices. Second, there seems to be a consensus that EEG coherence is lower in experts than in novices. Three out of the five studies reviewed reported that EEG coherence was lower in experts than in novices. The exceptions (Harung, 2011; Wolf et al., 2015) reported that EEG coherence was higher in experts than in novices. Finally, the findings were mixed regarding differences in beta activity, SMR activity, and event-related potentials between experts and novices.

How Is EEG Activity Different in Competitive Athletes and Non-athletes?

A small group of studies recorded theta activity (i.e., using power, ERD/ERS, and/or asymmetry metrics) in competitive athletes and non-athletes. Among them, Ziółkowski et al. (2014) used a between-subject design to compare sport-related EEG activity in competitive athletes and non-athletes. Participants were 36 amateur boxers and 52 college student volunteers who completed three one-minute periods, including maintaining eyes open, maintaining eyes closed, and maintaining visual focus. Ziółkowski et al. recorded spontaneous EEG activity, specifically delta, theta, alpha, SMR, beta, and high beta activity. They found that there was less theta activity in competitive athletes than in non-athletes. Similarly, Wang et al. (2015) used a between-subject design to compare sport-related EEG activity in competitive athletes and non-athletes. Participants were 12 experienced badminton players and 13 non-athletes who performed visuospatial attention and working memory tasks. Wang et al. recorded spontaneous EEG activity, specifically theta, alpha, and beta activity. The results showed that athletes (i.e., badminton players) had faster reaction times and were more accurate than non-athletes. This performance difference was accompanied by increased theta activity in competitive athletes relative to non-athletes. Likewise, Ermutlu, Yücesir, Eskikurt, Temel, and İşoğlu-Alkaç (2015) used a between-subject design to examine EEG activity different athletes. Participants were 12 dancers, 12 fast ball sport athletes, and 12 non-athletes who completed a five-minute period of 'awake' relaxation. Ermutlu et al. recorded spontaneous EEG activity, specifically delta, theta, alpha, and beta activity. The results indicated that ball players had a higher level of slower frequency EEG (i.e., both theta and delta activity) than did dancers or non-athletes. In addition, Luchsinger, Sandbakk, Schubert, Ettema, and Baumeister (2016) used a mixed-model design to compare sport-related EEG activity between athletes and non-athletes. Participants were nine biathletes and eight non-athletes who performed 100 shots using the SCATT Shooter Training system. Luchsinger et al. recorded spontaneous EEG activity, specifically frontal theta activity. In addition, they measured perceived exertion (using a Borg scale) and self-reported concentration (using a visual analog scale). They reported that biathletes had more frontal theta activity during shooting than did non-athletes.

Another small group of studies recorded alpha activity (i.e., using power, ERD/ERS, and/or asymmetry metrics) in competitive athletes and non-athletes. Leading off this group of studies, Del Percio, Bablioni, Bertollo et al. (2009) used a mixed-model design to compare sport-related EEG activity between athletes and non-athletes. Participants were 18 expert shooters and 10 non-athletes who performed 120 shots. Del Percio, Bablioni, Bertollo et al. recorded event-related EEG activity, specifically low alpha and high alpha ERD. They performed source localization using the Laplacian transformation algorithm. The results revealed that low- and high-frequency alpha ERD was less in shooters than in non-athletes. Similarly, Del Percio, Bablioni, Marzano et al. (2009) used a between-subject design to compare sport-related EEG activity in competitive athletes and non-athletes. Participants were 10 elite karate athletes, 10 elite fencing athletes, and 12 non-athletes who performed an eyes-open balancing task (i.e., balancing on two feet and balancing on one foot) on a stabilometer. Del Percio, Bablioni, Marzano et al. recorded event-related EEG activity, specifically alpha ERD. They performed source localization using the Laplacian transformation algorithm and also recorded body sway during balancing. They reported that 8–10 Hz alpha ERD was lower (in left and right central as well as mid and right parietal areas) during balancing in competitive athletes than in non-athletes. In addition, 10–12 Hz alpha ERD (in right frontal, left and right central, and mid parietal areas) was lower during balancing in competitive athletes than in non-athletes. Extending this line of research, Del Percio et al. (2010) used a between-subject design to compare sport-related EEG activity in competitive athletes and non-athletes. Participants were 10 elite karate athletes and 12 non-athletes who performed wrist extensions of the right and left hands. Del Percio et al. recorded event-related EEG activity, specifically low alpha and high alpha ERD. They performed source localization using the LORETA algorithm. The results indicated that 8–10 Hz and 10–12 Hz alpha ERD was lower (in lateral and medial pre-motor areas) during right handed wrist movements in competitive athletes than in non-athletes. In addition, Bablioni et al. (2010) used a between-subject design to compare sport-related EEG activity in competitive athletes and non-athletes. Participants were 16 elite karate athletes, 15 amateur karate athletes, and 17 non-athletes who judged videos of karate movements. Bablioni et al. recorded spontaneous EEG activity, specifically low alpha and high alpha ERD and performed source localization using the LORETA algorithm. They reported that elite athletes were more accurate in judging karate videos than novice athletes. They also experienced less low and high frequency alpha ERD (in Broadmann's dorsal area) compared to novice athletes. Additionally, Del Percio, Infarinato et al. (2011) used a between-subject design to compare sport-related EEG activity in competitive athletes and non-athletes. Participants were 18 elite karate athletes and 28 non-athletes who completed periods of resting with eyes open and eyes closed. Del Percio, Infarinato et al. recorded event-related EEG activity, specifically low alpha and high alpha ERD. They performed source localization using the Laplacian transformation algorithm. The results showed that competitive athletes had less low and high frequency alpha ERD (at frontal, parietal, and occipital sites) when moving from eyes open to eyes closed than did the non-athletes. As mentioned previously, Ermutlu et al. (2015) used a between-subject design to examine EEG activity different athletes. In addition to the findings described earlier in this section, they also reported that dancers had a higher level of alpha activity than did ball players or non-athletes.

A few studies recorded beta and/or gamma activity in competitive athletes and non-athletes. Each of these studies have been mentioned previously. For example, Wang et al. (2015) used a between-subject design to compare sport-related EEG activity in competitive athletes and non-athletes. In addition to the findings described earlier in this section, they also reported that athletes (i.e., badminton players) had faster reaction times and were more accurate than non-athletes. This performance difference was accompanied by decreased beta activity in competitive athletes relative to non-athletes. Likewise, Ermutlu et al. (2015) used a between-subject design to examine EEG activity different athletes. In addition to the findings described earlier in this section, they also reported that dancers had a higher level of beta activity than did ball players or non-athletes.

A single study recorded SMR activity in in competitive athletes and non-athletes. As mentioned previously, Ziółkowski et al. (2014) used a between-subject design to compare sport-related EEG activity in competitive athletes and non-athletes. In addition to the findings described earlier in this section, they also reported that there was more SMR activity in competitive athletes than in non-athletes.

A few studies recorded EEG coherence in competitive athletes and non-athletes. For example, Del Percio, Iacoboni et al. (2011) used a between-subject design to compare sport-related EEG activity in experts and novices. Participants were 18 elite shooters and 10 non-athletes who performed 120 pistol shots. Del Percio et al. recorded spontaneous EEG activity, specifically theta, low alpha, high alpha, low beta, high beta, and gamma coherence. Moreover, they performed source localization using the Laplacian transformation algorithm. They reported that both intra-hemispheric and inter-hemispheric low alpha, high alpha, high beta, and gamma coherence were stable across the pre-performance period in elite shooters. Both intra-hemispheric and inter-hemispheric coherences were unstable across the pre-performance period in non-athletes. Similarly, Velikova et al. (2012) used a mixed model design to compare sport-related EEG activity between competitive athletes and non-athletes during eyes-open and eyes-closed conditions. Participants were 13 expert fencers and 13 non-athletes who completed several conditions, including maintaining eyes open, maintaining eyes closed, making in-phase movements, and making anti-phase movements. Velikova et al. recorded spontaneous EEG activity, specifically delta, theta, alpha2, alpha2, beta1, beta2, beta3, and gamma coherence. They performed source localization using the LORETA algorithm. The results showed that fencers had higher alpha2 coherence (between the posterior cingulate cortex and the right angular gyrus) and higher delta coherence (between the left middle frontal gyrus and the left temporal gyrus) than non-athletes.

More than a few, studies recorded event-related potentials in competitive athletes and non-athletes. Among them, Rossi, Zani, Taddei, and Pesce (1992) used a mixed-model design to compare sport-related EEG activity between athletes and non-athletes. Participants were 11 expert fencers and 10 non-athletes who performed an auditory discrimination (Go/No-Go) reaction time task. Rossi et al. recorded event-related EEG activity, specifically including the N2 and P300 waveforms. The results indicated that the fencers evidenced faster reaction times and shorter latencies for the N2 and P300 waveforms than the non-athletes. Following along these lines, Di Russo, Taddei, Apnile, and Spinelli (2006) used a between-subject design to compare sport-related EEG activity in competitive athletes and non-athletes. Participants were 12 expert fencers and 12 non-athletes who completed 400 trials of a discriminative (Go/No-go) reaction time task. Di Russo et al. recorded event-related EEG activity, specifically including the P1, N1, P2, N2, and P300 waveforms. They performed source localization using the Brain Electrical Source Analysis algorithm. They found that the competitive athletes had faster reaction times (for the discrimination task) than the non-athletes. In addition, there were significant event-related potential differences between competitive athletes and non-athletes. The amplitude for the N1 waveform was larger in competitive athletes than in non-athletes. Similarly, the amplitude for the No-go (the inhibition) N2 and P3 amplitudes were larger in competitive athletes than in non-athletes. Likewise, Taddei, Bultrini, Spinelli, Di Russo, and Francesco (2012) used a between-subject design to compare sport-related EEG activity in competitive athletes and non-athletes. Participants were 10 older fencers, 10 younger fencers, 10 older non-athletes, and 10 younger non-athletes who performed a simple reaction time task and a discrimination (Go/No-Go) reaction time task. Taddei et al. recorded event-related EEG activity, specifically including the P1, N1, P2, N2, and P300 waveforms. They performed source localization using the Brain Electrical Source Analysis algorithm. The results revealed that competitive athletes had faster reaction times and more false alarms than non-athletes. These differences were accompanied by between-subject differences in event-related potentials. Specifically, the competitive athletes had shorter latencies and larger amplitudes for the P1 and the N2 waveforms than the non-athletes. In addition, the competitive athletes had larger amplitude P3 waveforms (in the inhibition/No-Go condition) than non-athletes.

Several studies recorded slow potentials in competitive athletes and non-athletes. Among them, Kita, Mori, and Nara (2001) used a between-subject design to compare sport-related EEG activity in competitive athletes and non-athletes. Participants were four kendo players, two gymnasts, and nine non-athletes who performed brief, self-paced wrist extensions of the right hand. Kita et al. recorded event-related EEG activity, specifically movement-related cortical potentials. They focused on the Bereitschaftspotential, the negative slope, and the motor potential. In addition, they recorded EMG activity (from the right wrist extensor muscles). They reported that the integrated amplitude of the EMG was larger in the competitive athletes than in the non-athletes. In addition, the Bereitschaftspotentials were smaller, in the competitive athletes than in the non-athletes. More recently, Del Percio et al. (2008) used a between-subject design to compare sport-related EEG activity in competitive athletes and non-athletes. Participants were 11 elite fencing athletes, 11 elite karate athletes, and 11 non-athletes who observed 200 pictures (of either fencing or karate attacks) and decided whether the attacks looked like right or left side attacks. Del Percio et al. recorded event-related EEG activity, specifically movement-related cortical potentials. They focused on the readiness and the motor potential waveforms and performed source localization using the Laplacian transformation algorithm. The results indicated significant between-subject differences in movement-related cortical amplitudes during the karate/fencing attack judging task. The amplitudes of the readiness potential and the motor potential (at C3 and Cz) were smaller in competitive athletes than in non-athletes. In addition, Nakamoto and Mori (2008) used a between-subject design to compare sport-related EEG activity in competitive athletes and non-athletes. Participants were nine college baseball players and nine non-athletes who performed an anticipation timing (Go/No-go) reaction time task with varying levels of stimulus response compatibility (i.e., compatible with baseball batting and not compatible with baseball batting). Nakamoto et al. recorded event-related EEG activity, specifically movement-related cortical potentials. They focused on the CNV. They reported that competitive athletes had faster reaction times than non-athletes (in Go trials) and shorter lateralized readiness potential onsets. Likewise, Hatta, Nishihira, Higashiura, Kim, and Kaneda (2009) used a between-subject design to compare sport-related EEG activity in competitive athletes and non-athletes. Participants were eight elite kendo players and eight non-athletes who performed 70 trials each of a left and right hand grip task (i.e., squeezing a dynamometer). Hatta et al. recorded event-related EEG activity, specifically movement-related cortical potentials. They focused on the Bereitschaftspotential, the negative slope, and the motor potential. Additionally, they recorded EMG activity from forearm extensor muscles. The results showed that the onset of the Bereitschaftspotential (for the non-dominant handgrip) was shorter in the competitive athletes than in the non-athletes. In addition, the peak amplitude of the motor potential was larger in the kendo players than in the non-athletes.

Last, more than a few studies recorded evoked potentials in competitive athletes and non-athletes. Among them, Thomas and Mitchell (1996) used a between-subject design to compare sport-related EEG activity in competitive athletes and non-athletes. Participants were 10 endurance runners, seven elite gymnasts, and seven non-athletes who completed a period of somatosensory stimulation (using a Nihon Kohden Electromyograph with stimulating electrodes attached to the wrist). Thomas et al. recorded event-related EEG activity, specifically somatosensory evoked potentials (i.e., the P9, P11, P13/14, N20, P25, and N30 waveforms). They also measured reaction times. They found no significant between-subject differences in any of the components of the somatosensory waveform or in the reaction times. Continuing this line of inquiry, Thomas, Harden, and Rogers (2005) used a between-subject design to compare sport-related EEG activity in competitive athletes and non-athletes. Participants were 25 elite cricketers and 10 non-athletes who completed a period of visual stimulation (i.e., watching an alternating checkerboard pattern). Thomas et al. recorded event-related EEG activity, specifically visual evoked potentials (i.e., the N70, P100, and N145 waveforms). In addition, they measured choice reaction times. They found no differences in choice reaction time task performance between competitive athletes and non-athletes. However, the latencies for the visual evoked potential waveform (i.e., the N70) were shorter for the competitive athletes than for the non-athletes. Delpont, Dolisi, Suisse, Bodino, and Gastaud (1991) used a between-subject design to examine EEG activity in competitive athletes and non-athletes. Participants were 24 skilled tennis players, 24 skilled rowers, and 24 non-athletes who completed a period of visual stimulation (i.e., watching an alternating checkerboard pattern). Delpont et al. recorded event-related EEG activity, specifically visual evoked potentials. They reported that the tennis players had shorter visual evoked potential latencies (i.e., for the two P100s) than did the rowers or the control subjects. Similarly, Taddei, Viggiano, and Mecacci (1991) used a between-subject design to compare sport-related EEG activity in competitive athletes and non-athletes. Participants were eight expert fencers and eight non-athletes who completed a period of visual stimulation (i.e., watching an alternating checkerboard pattern) in two conditions – a large visual field and small visual field. Taddei et al. recorded event-related EEG activity, specifically visual evoked potentials (i.e., the P60-N75, N75-P100, and P100-N145 waveforms). The results showed that the latencies for the N75 waveform were shorter in the right hemisphere in the competitive than in the non-athletes. In addition, the amplitudes for the N75-P100 waveforms were larger in the left hemisphere in the competitive athletes than in the non-athletes. The latencies for the P100 waveform were shorter in the competitive athletes (in both hemispheres) than in the non-athletes. In addition, Martin, Delpont, Suisse, and Dolisi (1993) used a between-subject design to compare sport-related EEG activity in competitive athletes and non-athletes. Participants were 24 tennis players, 24 rowers, and 24 non-athletes who completed a period of monaural stimulation (i.e., listening to 'clicks' presented to right and left ears). Martin et al. recorded event-related EEG activity, specifically brainstem auditory evoked potentials. They reported that the latencies for five (out of 13) of the brainstem auditory evoked potentials examined were shorter in the competitive athletes (i.e., the tennis players) than in the non-athletes. In addition, the amplitudes for one (out of nine) brainstem auditory evoked potentials were larger in the competitive athletes (i.e., the tennis players) than in the non-athletes.

In summary, there were 27 studies that examined differences in sport-related EEG activity between competitive athletes and non-athletes. The majority of these examined differences in theta activity (n=4), alpha activity (n=6), slow potentials (n=4), or evoked potentials (n=5) between competitive athletes and non-athletes. A few studies examined differences in beta activity (n=2), SMR activity (n=1), EEG coherence (n=2), and event-related potentials (n=3). Across these studies, three points of agreement emerged. First, there seems to be a consensus that theta and alpha activity are higher in competitive athletes than in non-athletes. Three out of the four studies reviewed reported that theta activity was higher in competitive athletes than in non-athletes. The exception reported (Ziółkowski et al., 2014) that theta activity was lower in competitive athletes than in non-athletes. Moreover, all of the studies reviewed reported that alpha activity was higher in competitive athletes than in non-athletes. Second, there seems to be a consensus that event-related potential latencies are shorter and/or their amplitudes are larger in competitive athletes than in non-athletes. All of the studies reviewed reported that event-related potential latencies were shorter and/or their amplitudes were larger in competitive athletes than in non-athletes. Third, there seems to be a consensus that evoked potential latencies are shorter in competitive athletes than in non-athletes. All five of the studies reviewed reported that evoked potential latencies were shorter in competitive athletes than in non-athletes.

How Is EEG Activity Different in Disabled and Non-disabled Athletes?

A few studies recorded EEG activity in disabled and non-disabled athletes. For example, Kim and Woo (2013) used a between-subject design to examine EEG activity disabled and non-disabled shooters. Participants were 12 disabled air pistol shooters and 22 non-disabled elite shooters who performed 20 self-paced shots using the SCATT Shooter Training system. Kim and Woo recorded spontaneous EEG activity, specifically alpha activity and alpha asymmetry (R-L). They reported that there were no differences in shooting performance between disabled and non-disabled shooters. Nonetheless, there were EEG-related differences between the two groups of shooters. Disabled shooters had more left hemisphere activation (i.e., less left hemisphere alpha activity) than non-disabled shooters. Shooting scores were correlated (r's @.6) with alpha asymmetry scores. In addition, Kim, Lee, Kim, and Woo (2013) used a between-subject design to examine EEG activity disabled and non-disabled shooters. Participants were 12 disabled air pistol shooters and 22 non-disabled elite shooters who performed 20 self-paced shots using the SCATT Shooter Training system. Kim et al. recorded spontaneous EEG activity, specifically theta, low alpha, high alpha, beta, and gamma coherence. They found no differences in shooting performance between disabled and non-disabled shooters. Still, there were EEG-related differences between the two groups of shooters. Disabled shooters had higher theta (at Fz/T4), low alpha (at Fz/C4, Fz/T4, and Fz/T3), beta, and gamma (at frontal and central sites) coherence during the pre-performance period than non-disabled shooters.

In summary, there were two studies that examined differences in sport-related EEG activity between disabled and non-disabled athletes. Both studies reported differences in sport-related EEG activity between disabled and non-disabled athletes. Specifically, Kim and Woo (2013) found less left hemisphere alpha activity in disabled than in non-disabled athletes and Kim et al. (2013) found higher coherence (i.e., theta, alpha, beta, and gamma coherence) in disabled than in non-disabled athletes. Given the paucity of research, it's impossible to answer the question about disabled and non-disabled athletes at this point in time.

How Does Practice/Learning Change EEG Activity?

Several studies examined the effects of practice/learning on EEG activity. Among those, Landers et al. (1994) used a within-subject design to examine EEG activity pre- and post-training. Participants were 11 novice archers who performed an archery shooting task (shooting arrows at a target) before and after a 15-w archery training class. Landers et al. recorded spontaneous EEG activity, specifically 4–30 Hz activity. They focused on EEG asymmetry and also measured heart rate. The results revealed that performance improved and heart rate deceleration increased from pre- to post-test. In addition, alpha power at T3 increased after archery training and alpha power at T4 did not. Furthermore, there were no significant hemispheric differences (no asymmetry) at the pretest. However, there were significant hemispheric differences (negative asymmetry) at the post-test. Similarly, Kerick, Douglass, and Hatfield (2004) used a multi-factorial design to compare EEG activity pre- and post-training and across two different tasks. Participants were 11 novice pistol shooters who performed a shooting and a postural simulation task at two different time periods (i.e., before and after a 12–14 week training period). Kerick et al. recorded spontaneous EEG activity, specifically high alpha activity. They reported that performance increased across time during the training period. This was accompanied by an increase in event-related high alpha power during shooting (at T3 but not T4) across time during the training period. Likewise, Domingues et al. (2008) used a within-subject design to examine EEG activity performance across learning trials. Participants were 23 novice pistol shooters who performed four blocks of 10 shots each. Domingues et al. recorded spontaneous EEG activity, specifically alpha activity. They found that accuracy increased across learning trials. This performance effect was accompanied by decreased alpha power (at F3 and F4 and F7 and F8) across learning trials.

In summary, there were only three studies that examined the effects of learning on sport-related EEG activity. All three reported changes in alpha activity from pre- to post-tests. Landers et al. (1994) reported increased left hemisphere alpha activity from before to after 15 weeks of archery training. Kerick et al. (2004) reported increased left hemisphere alpha activity from before to after 12–14 weeks of shooting training. Domingues et al. (2008), however, reported increased left and right hemisphere (i.e., at F3, F4, F7, and F8) activity across a series of practice sessions (i.e., 4 blocks of 10 shots each). Given the paucity of research, it's impossible to definitively answer the question about learning and EEG activity at this point in time. However, the research to date suggests that learning results in increased sport-related alpha activity (specifically left hemisphere alpha activity).

Is EEG Activity during a Sport Task Different from EEG Activity during Other Tasks (e.g., Balancing on a Stabilometer)?

Several early (pre-2000) studies compared the effects of different tasks on EEG activity. For example, Hatfield et al. (1984, Study 2) used a within-subject design to compare sport-related EEG activity during different tasks. Participants were 15 collegiate shooters who performed an air rifle shooting and two non-shooting tasks (i.e., a verbal-analytic task and a visuospatial task). Hatfield et al. recorded spontaneous EEG activity, specifically alpha activity and alpha asymmetry. The results revealed that EEG activity during shooting was not significantly different from EEG during the visuospatial task. Using a similar approach, Salazar et al. (1990) used a multi-factorial design to compare sport-related EEG activity during different tasks. Participants were 13 male and 15 female archers who performed four tasks, including shooting with normal bow, shooting with light bow, bow drawing without aiming, and aiming without bow drawing. Salazar et al. recorded spontaneous EEG activity, specifically 5–31 Hz activity. They reported that there were significant differences in EEG activity across conditions. For the relaxation condition, there were significant within-subject differences for 6–12 Hz EEG activity. For the full-draw (2 kg bow) condition, there were significant within-subject differences for 10–16 Hz EEG activity. For the next full-draw (18 kg bow) condition, there were significant within-subject differences for 10–14 Hz EEG activity. Finally, for the shooting condition, there were significant within-subject differences for 12–14 Hz EEG activity. Using a different approach, Konttinen and Lyytinen (1993b) used a within-subject design to compare sport-related EEG activity in four different tasks. Participants were eight novice shooters who performed four different shooting tasks varying on motor and visual components. Konttinen et al. recorded event-related EEG activity, specifically slow potentials. They recorded heart rate, respiration, and rifle stability. They found differences in slow potentials across the different tasks. Participants evidenced less slow potential negativity (i.e., more slow potential positivity) during the more motor/less visual targeting-related task and more slow potential negativity during the less motor/more visual targeting-related task. In addition, Haufler et al. (2000) used a mixed-model design to compare sport-related EEG activity across several tasks. Participants were 15 elite shooters and 21 novice shooters who performed simulated rifle shooting and visuospatial and verbal tasks. Haufler et al. recorded spontaneous EEG activity, specifically theta, low alpha, high alpha, beta, and gamma activity. They reported that EEG asymmetry during shooting was lower than in the dot localization task (for experts only). In addition, EEG asymmetry during shooting was like that in the word finding task. This was not true for novices. EEG asymmetry was similar across tasks for novices. Along this line, Kerick et al. (2001) used a within-subject design to compare sport-related EEG activity during different tasks. Participants were eight skilled marksmen who performed shooting, posture control, and movement control tasks. Kerick et al. recorded event-related EEG activity, specifically event-related alpha activity. The results indicated that event-related alpha power was higher before shooting than the posture or movement control tasks.

In summary, five studies compared sport-related EEG activity with EEG activity during other tasks. A couple of these (Hatfield et al., 1984; Haufler et al., 2000) compared EEG activity during shooting with EEG activity during verbal-analytic and visuospatial tasks. Both reported that EEG activity during shooting was most like EEG activity during visuospatial tasks. Moreover, Salazar et al. (1990) found difference in EEG activity between shooting an arrow, aiming an arrow at a target, and holding a drawn bow (without aiming at a target). Likewise, Kerick et al. (2001) found more alpha activity before shooting than before movement control or posture control tasks. Finally, using a different metric, Konttinen and Lyytinen (1993b) found less slow potential negativity during a more motor/less visual targeting type task and more slow potential negativity during a less motor/more visual targeting type task.

Karla A. Kubitz

Is Sport-Related EEG Activity Changed by Socio-Environmental Manipulations (e.g., Adding Competition)?

A few studies examined the effects of pre-task stimulation on EEG activity. Focusing on pre-task audio-visual stimulation, Del Percio, Marzano et al. (2007) used a multi-factorial design to compare sport-related EEG activity between athletes and non-athletes and across two levels of pre-task audio-visual stimulation. Participants were 14 elite fencing athletes and 14 non-athletes who observed 80 pictures (of either fencing or karate attacks). The picture judging task was performed in two conditions, with and without pre-task (10 Hz) audio-visual stimulation. Del Percio et al. recorded event-related EEG activity, specifically alpha ERD. They also measured reaction times. They reported that pre-task audio-visual stimulation (at a 10 Hz frequency) improved reaction times and increased alpha power. Focusing on pre-task exercise, Luchsinger et al. (2016) used a mixed-model design to compare sport-related EEG activity across resting and post-exercise performances. Participants were nine biathletes and eight non-athletes who performed 100 shots using the SCATT Shooter Training system. The shooting task was performed in two conditions, resting and post-exercise (i.e., five-minute in-line skating). Luchsinger et al. recorded spontaneous EEG activity, specifically frontal theta activity. In addition, they measured perceived exertion (using a Borg scale) and self-reported concentration (using a visual analog scale). They reported no significant effects of exercise on frontal theta activity in either biathletes or non-athletes.

In addition, a few studies examined the effects of attentional manipulations on EEG activity. For example, Radlo, Steinberg, Singer, Barba, and Melnikov (2002) used a between-subject design to compare the effects of different attention-focusing strategies on sport-related EEG activity. Participants were 20 novice dart throwers who performed 10 blocks of four dart throws in one of two conditions. Dart throws were performed either using an internal attention-focusing strategy or using an external attention-focusing strategy. Radlo et al. recorded spontaneous EEG activity, specifically alpha power. They also recorded heart rate and EMG activity. The results showed that dart throwers using the external attention-focusing strategy performed better (i.e., had less absolute error) than those using the internal attention-focusing strategy. They also had lower heart rates and a lower level of alpha activity than those in the internal attention condition. Along the same lines, Zhu, Poolton, Wilson, Maxwell, and Masters (2011) conducted two studies examining the effects of self-monitoring-related manipulations on sport-related EEG activity. Study 1 used a between-subject design to compare sport-related EEG activity high self-monitoring and low self-monitoring athletes. Participants were 16 novice golfers (varying on tendency to self-monitor) who performed a putting task. Zhu et al. recorded spontaneous EEG activity, specifically alpha1 and alpha2 coherence. In addition, they measured the athletes' tendencies to self-monitor (using the Movement Specific Reinvestment Scale). They reported that participants who tended to self-monitor had more T3-Fz alpha coherence than those who did not tend to self-monitor. Extending the results of Study 1, Zhu et al. (2011)'s second study used a between-subject design to compare sport-related EEG activity during implicit and explicit practice. Implicit practice has been shown to be associated with "reduced verbal-analytical involvement in movement control" (Zhu et al., 2011, p. 67) in comparison with explicit practice. Participants were 18 novice golfers randomly assigned to implicit and explicit practice conditions who performed a putting task. Zhu et al. recorded spontaneous EEG activity, specifically alpha1 and alpha2 coherence. The results indicated that participants who experienced explicit practice on golf putting task had a higher level of alpha (T3-Fz) coherence than those who experienced implicit practice. In addition, Reinecke et al. (2011) indirectly manipulated attentional focus. That is, they used a within-subject design to compare sport-related EEG activity during different tasks. Participants were 11 collegiate golfers who performed self-paced putts in two conditions, inside and outside. Reinecke et al. recorded spontaneous EEG activity, specifically theta, alpha1, alpha2, and beta1 activity. They also measured state anxiety (using the State-Trait Anxiety Inventory). The results showed no significant differences in state anxiety between the two conditions. Nonetheless, participants had higher F4 theta activity during putting than during rest and higher F4 theta activity when putting in the field than when putting in the lab.

A single study examined the effects of winning on EEG activity. Hunt, Rietschel, Hatfield, and Iso-Ahola (2013) used a between-subject design to examine EEG activity winning athletes and losing athletes. Participants were 17 collegiate/ROTC volunteers who completed 40 shots using the NOPTEL Shooter Training system in a head-to-head competition with another participant. Participants were assigned to either the 'winning' group (n=10) or 'losing' group (n=7) depending on whether they won or lost the competition. Hunt et al. recorded spontaneous EEG activity, specifically delta, theta, alpha, low alpha, high alpha, beta, and gamma activity. They also measured confidence levels. They found that winners had the same level of performance, and a higher level of confidence, as losers. This was accompanied by less high alpha power and less theta power (in both hemispheres) in winners than in losers. The differences in alpha and theta power were clear during all pre-shot epochs.

Several studies examined the effects of applying pressure (i.e., making tasks competitive) on EEG activity. For example, Cooke et al. (2014) used a mixed-model design to compare sport-related EEG activity across high and low pressure conditions. Participants were 10 expert golfers and 10 novice golfers who performed 60 putts. The putting task was performed under two conditions, low-pressure (non-competitive) and high-pressure (competitive). Cooke et al. recorded spontaneous EEG activity, specifically theta, low alpha, high alpha, and beta activity. They also recorded number of putts holed, self-reported pressure, movement kinematics, heart rate, and EMG activity. They reported few effects of the high/low pressure manipulation. Although there were differences in self-reported pressure and heart rate, there were no within-subject differences in number of putts holed. There were also no differences in movement kinematics, in EMG activity, or in spontaneous EEG activity between the high and low pressure conditions. Similarly, Gallicchio et al. (2015) used a mixed-model design to compare sport-related EEG activity across high and low pressure conditions. Participants were 10 expert golfers and 10 novice golfers who performed 60 putts. The putting task was performed in two conditions, low-pressure (non-competitive) and high-pressure (competitive). Gallicchio et al. recorded spontaneous EEG activity, specifically left and right hemisphere alpha coherence. They also recorded number of putts holed. They found no effects of the high/low pressure manipulation. There were no within-subject differences in number of putts holed or in left or right hemisphere alpha coherence. In addition, Hatfield et al. (2013) used a within-subject design to compare sport-related EEG activity during high and low pressure conditions. Participants were 19 ROTC student volunteers who performed 40 shots using the Noptel Shooter Training system in competitive (included time constraints and rewards/penalties) and non-competitive conditions. Hatfield et al. recorded event-related EEG activity, specifically alpha ERD/ERD. They also recorded movement kinematics, state anxiety, and cortisol levels. The results revealed that self-reported anxiety, salivary cortisol, and alpha coherence (between Fz and all other recording sites) were higher when shooting competitively than when shooting alone. In addition, shooting competitively was also associated with lower 10–13 Hz alpha activity.

Several studies examined the effects of manipulating task type, task difficulty, or type of feedback on EEG activity. Focusing on the effects of task difficulty, Collins, Powell, and Davies (1990) used a within-subject design to compare sport-related EEG activity during different tasks. Participants were eight male karate experts who performed easy and difficult board breaking tasks. Collins et al. recorded spontaneous EEG activity, specifically alpha activity. The results showed no significant between-task differences in EEG activity. Comparing different sport athletes, Rossi and Zani (1991) used a within-subject design to compare sport-related EEG activity during different tasks. Participants were four skilled skeet-shooters and four skilled trap-shooters who performed an auditory discrimination task with two levels of difficulty, easy and difficult. Rossi et al. recorded event-related EEG activity, specifically including the N2 and P300 waveforms.

They reported that the skeet-shooters had earlier latencies for the N2 and P300 waveforms than the trap-shooters. In addition, Vrbik, Bene, and Vrbik (2015) used a within-subject design to examine sport-related EEG activity in athletes doing different types of archery. Participants were four experienced, recurve bow archers and four experienced, compound bow archers who shot 12 arrows. Vrbik et al. recorded spontaneous EEG activity, specifically attention' and 'meditation' scores (i.e., as derived from Mindwave Mobile Software algorithms). They reported EEG-related differences between compound bow shooters and recurve bow shooters. Compound bow shooters had higher EEG attention and lower EEG meditation scores pre, during, and post shooting compared to recurve bow shooters. Similarly, Rossi et al. (1992) used a mixed-model design to compare sport-related EEG activity across easy and difficult tasks. Participants were 11 expert fencers and 10 non-athletes who performed an auditory discrimination (Go/No-Go) reaction time task with two levels, easy and difficult. Rossi et al. recorded event-related EEG activity, specifically including the N2 and P300 waveforms. They also measured reaction times. They reported that both reaction times and N2 and P300 latencies were longer for the difficult task. Along the same lines, Kerick, Hatfield, and Allender (2007) used a within-subject design to compare sport-related EEG activity during different tasks. Participants were 14 experienced shooters who performed a simulated shooting task, involving decision (enemy/no-enemy) and no-decision conditions. Requiring the enemy/no-enemy decision before shooting increases task difficulty. Kerick et al. recorded spontaneous EEG activity, specifically theta and upper alpha activity. They reported that theta peak amplitude was higher (at P3 and Pz) and alpha peak amplitude was lower (at C3) in choice relative to no-choice tasks. Focusing on the effect of 'false' feedback, Kerick, Iso-Ahola, and Hatfield (2000) used a within-subject design to examine EEG activity during different types of feedback. Participants were 17 novice rifle shooters who performed 40 shots in a seated position (with the rifle supported by a shooting stand). The shooting task was performed in four different conditions, including no-feedback (about performance), false/low performance feedback, false/moderate performance feedback, and false/high performance feedback. Kerick et al. recorded spontaneous EEG activity, specifically alpha asymmetry. In addition, they measured subjective performance (using the Subjective Performance Questionnaire) and affect (using the Positive and Negative Affect Scale). The results indicated that performance was worse and affect was more negative in the false/low performance feedback condition than in the no-feedback and false/moderate performance feedback conditions. This was not accompanied by significant differences across feedback conditions in alpha (F3/F4) asymmetry.

Several studies examined the effects of performing with an audience on EEG activity. For example, Shelley-Tremblay, Shugrue, and Kline (2006) used a within-subject design to compare sport-related EEG activity during high and low pressure conditions. Participants were 20 novice golfers who performed 20 putts. The putting task was performed in a low pressure (no audience) condition and in a high pressure (audience watching) condition. Shelley-Tremblay et al. recorded spontaneous EEG activity, specifically alpha, beta1, and beta2 activity. They also measured mood states (using the Profile of Mood States questionnaire). They found that putting accuracy decreased in the audience condition relative to the no-audience condition. This performance decrement was accompanied by an increase in beta activity in the audience condition. Interestingly, beta activity was positively related (r's @.6) to error/distance from hole. The higher the level of beta activity (i.e., at C3, C4, and T4), the farther the distance from the hole. Similarly, Rietschel et al. (2011) used a within-subject design to compare EEG activity in high and low pressure (i.e., presence/absence of social evaluation). Participants were 13 college student volunteers who completed 60 trials of a visuo-motor pointing task in two conditions. The task was performed alone and with social evaluation (i.e., two confederates standing just behind the participant). Rietschel et al. recorded spontaneous EEG activity, specifically low alpha, high alpha, and gamma coherence. In addition, they recorded heart rate and skin conductance. The results indicated that arousal was higher and performance was better in the social evaluation condition. Specifically, heart rate was higher, skin conductance levels were higher, self-reported stress was higher, and the variability of the aiming trajectory was lower in the social evaluation condition. This was accompanied by increased beta coherence (in the frontal, left central, parietal, and occipital areas) and increased gamma coherence (in the temporal areas) in the social evaluation condition. It was also accompanied by decreased beta coherence (in the right temporal areas) in social evaluation condition.

In summary, 19 studies examined the effects of four broad types of socio-environmental manipulations on sport-related EEG activity. First, there were two studies that examined the effects of pre-task stimulation on sport-related EEG activity. Only pre-task audio-visual stimulation (Del Percio, Marzano et al., 2007) had an impact on reaction time and alpha activity in athletes judging fencing attacks. Second, there were five studies that examined the effects of either task type or task difficulty on sport-related EEG activity. Among these, Collins et al. (1990) found no differences in alpha activity for harder compared to easier tasks. In contrast, Rossi et al. (1992) found increased event-related potential latencies (i.e., N2 and P300 latencies) for harder compared to easier tasks. Likewise, Kerick et al. found more theta activity and less alpha activity in difficult compared to easy tasks. Moreover, Rossi and Zani (1991) found earlier event-related potential latencies (i.e., N2 and P300 latencies) for skeet-shooters compared to trap-shooters; and Vrbik et al. (2015) found EEG differences between compound bow shooters and recurve bow shooters. Third, there were four studies that examined the effects of attentional manipulations on sport-related EEG activity. One study found that focusing externally decreased alpha activity and improved performance. Another study found that putting outdoors increased theta activity compared to putting indoors. Two other studies found that participants that tended to do more self-monitoring and participants that used explicit practice strategies had higher levels of EEG coherence. Fourth, there were several studies (n=8) that examined the effects of either competition or of some other way of 'pressuring' athletes. Of these, four studies manipulated pressure/competition and found effects on performance and EEG activity. Among these, Hunt et al. (2013) found that winning a competition was associated with less theta and alpha activity than losing the competition. Similarly, Hatfield et al. (2013) found that shooting competitively resulted in increased state anxiety, increased salivary cortisol, decreased alpha activity, and increased alpha coherence in comparison with shooting non-competitively. Additionally, Shelley-Tremblay et al. (2006) found that performing in front of an audience negatively impacted performance (and mood states) and also increased beta activity. Further, Rietschel et al. (2011) also examined the effects of performing in front of an audience. They found that performing in front of an audience improved performance (and self-reported stress) and increased beta and gamma coherence (i.e., in most, but not all of the areas measured). However, there were also three studies that reported nonsignificant effects of pressure/competition manipulations. That is, Cooke et al. (2014) and Gallicchio et al. (2015) manipulated pressure/competition as golfers attempted to sink putts. Neither of these studies reported significant effects of the pressure/competition manipulations. Likewise, Kerick et al. (2000) found that false feedback (i.e., informing participants that they performed worse than they did) impaired shooting performance (and negatively impacted affect), but did not impact EEG asymmetry. Across these studies, the consensus seems to be that manipulations that increase the athlete's stress levels and/or change the athlete's attentional focusing strategy impact sport-related EEG activity.

Conclusion

This chapter reviewed the literature examining sport-related EEG activity over the past quarter-century and focused on eight questions, including questions related to changes in EEG activity across the pre-performance period, differences in EEG activity between good and poor performances, differences in EEG activity between experts and novices, differences in EEG activity between competitive athletes and non-athletes, differences in EEG activity between disabled and non-disabled athletes, effects of practice on sport-related EEG activity, effects of different tasks on sport-related EEG activity, and effects of socio-environmental manipulations on sport-related EEG activity. Ninety-two research studies were reviewed and five main conclusions were drawn.

1   There seems to be a consensus that alpha activity (particularly in the left hemisphere) increases across the pre-performance period. With regard to increasing left hemisphere alpha activity, Janelle and Hatfield (2008) noted that the "hypothesis was that superior performance would be characterized by attenuation of activity in the left temporal region in light of the automaticity of expert performance and the need to reduce possible interference from analysis and overthinking" (p. S50).

2   There seems to be a consensus that beta activity is lower, and that slow potential shifts are less negative, in good performances than in poor performances. With regard to lower beta activity in good versus poor performances, it is worth noting that beta activity has been interpreted as indicative of cognitive effort and/or as increased anxiety (Crews & Landers, 1993). Moreover, Shelley-Tremblay et al. (2006) noted that the "positive correlations [between beta activity and distance from the hole] in all cases indicate that greater beta activity was correlated with ... less accuracy" (p. 364).

3   There seems to be a consensus that theta activity and alpha activity are higher, and that EEG coherence is lower, in experts than in novices. With regard to higher theta and alpha activity in experts versus novices, Kerick et al. (2007) noted that

> theta and alpha provide unique but complementary information that together yield an enhanced ability to monitor cognitive load. More specifically, the theta peak appears related to working memory for stimulus encoding and decision making, whereas the progressive increase in alpha appears related to focused motor preparation.
>
> *(p. B163)*

With regard to lower EEG coherence in experts versus novices, Cooke (2013) noted that

> the increased accuracy of experts compared to novices in both shooting and golf... could be reflected by ... a reduction in EEG alpha power coherence between the left temporal and frontal midline regions of the brain during preparation for action in both shooting and golf.
>
> *(p. 132)*

4   There seems to be a consensus that theta and alpha activity are higher, that event-related potential latencies are shorter and/or their amplitudes are larger, and that evoked potential latencies are shorter in competitive athletes than in non-athletes. With regard to shorter event-related potential latencies and larger amplitudes, it is worth noting that event-related potentials have been interpreted as a "reflection of neural synchronization" (Del Percio, Brancucci et al., 2007, p. 110). Moreover, Del Percio, Brancucci et al. (2007) noted that "peculiar mechanisms of occipital neural synchronization can be observed in elite athletes during visuo-spatial demands, possibly to underlie sustained visuo-spatial attention and self-control" (p. 104).

5   There seems to be a consensus that manipulations that increase the salience of competition/ winning, increase the athlete's stress levels and/or change the athlete's attentional focusing strategy impact sport-related EEG activity. Among the studies reporting significant effects (Hatfield et al., 2013; Hunt et al., 2013; Shelley-Tremblay et al., 2006), the direction of the effects seemed to be towards increased activation (i.e., less theta activity, less alpha activity, and more beta activity).

In conclusion, a recurent theme in the studies reviewed was the notion of 'efficiency/economy'. Early on, Hatfield et al. (1987) mentioned "information processing efficiency" (p. 542) as part of the rationale for their study. Following their lead, Hatfield and Kerick (2007) said that the "relevance of this work to the sport practitioner lies in the overwhelming support in the scientific literature for the notion that high-level performance is marked by economy of brain activity that underlies mental processes" (p. 106). Similarly, Baumeister et al. (2008) noted that the "fndings suggest that with increasing skill level, golfers have developed task solving strategies ... and an economy in neural activity" (p. 630). Likewise, Janelle and Hatfield (2008) reported that the "corpus of research that has been conducted to date ... clearly supports the notion of efficiency or economy of cortical processes" (p. S 49). Additionally, Mann et al. (2011) said that the "significant relationship between right-central (i.e., C4) cortical activation and QE duration ... speaks to the cognitive advantage of the expert and supports the notion of relative sensorimotor efficiency of expert athletes" (p. 231). In line with the previous literature, the main conclusions of this chapter (i.e., increased alpha across the pre-performance period in elite athletes, lower beta and less negative slow potential shifts in good performances, higher alpha and theta activity in experts/competitive athletes, and lower EEG coherence in experts) are consistent with the hypothesized relationship between efficient/economical sport-related EEG activity and optimal performance in sport.

Appendix A

Table A1. Methodological details for sport-related EEG studies

Study	Focus	Participants	Design	Task	EEG Variables	Other Variables
Bablioni et al. (2008)	good and poor performance	12 expert golfers	within-subject	performed 10 blocks of 10 putts each (while standing on a balance platform) using a putting green simulator	alpha and beta band activity	body sway
Bablioni et al. (2010)	athletes and non-athletes	16 elite karate athletes, 15 amateur karate athletes, and 17 non-athletes	between-subject	judged videos of karate movements varying with regard to technical and athletic level displayed	low alpha and high alpha band activity (+/-2 Hz individual peak frequency)	
Bablioni et al. (2011)	good and poor performance	12 expert golfers	within-subject	performed 100 self-paced putts using a golf green simulator	low alpha and high alpha band coherence	
Baumeister et al. (2008)	experts and novices	nine experienced golfers and nine novice golfers	between-subject	performed five blocks of 10 putts each using an indoor carpet type putting green	theta, alpha1, alpha2, beta1, and beta2 band activity and EEG asymmetry	anxiety (using the STAI) and stress (using a visual analogue scale)
Bertollo et al. (2016)	good and poor performance	10 elite shooters	within-subject	performed 120 shots	theta, low alpha, and high alpha band ERD/ERS	
Bird (1987)	good and poor performance	one elite marksman	within-subject	performed a shooting task	peak frequency	
Cheng et al. (2015)	experts and novices	14 expert dart throwers and 11 novice dart throwers	between-subject	performed 60 self-paced dart throws	SMR band ERD/ERS	EMG from forearm flexor muscles
Chuang et al. (2013)	good and poor performance	15 skilled basketball players	within-subject	performed basketball free throw shots	low theta and high theta band activity	
Collins et al. (1990)	different tasks	eight male karate experts	within-subject	performed easy and difficult board breaking tasks	alpha band activity	

Study	Factor	Sample	Model	Task	EEG measure	Other measures
Collins, Powell, and Davies (1991)	different tasks	22 physically active volunteers	within-subject	performed repetitions of three motor tasks, including jumping onto a box, doing leg extensions on a leg extension machine, and kicking a soccer ball between two cones	alpha band activity	movement kinematics, ECG, and EMG
Cooke et al. (2014)	experts and novices as a between-subjects factor and high and low pressure as a within-subjects factor	10 expert golfers and 10 novice golfers	mixed-model	performed 60 putts under two conditions, low-pressure (non-competitive) and high-pressure (competitive)	theta, low alpha, high alpha, and beta band activity	
Crews and Landers (1993)	experts and novices before and during putting	34 highly skilled golfers	within-subject	performed a putting task	theta, alpha, beta1, beta2, and 40 Hz band activity and slow potentials	
Deeny et al. (2009)	experts and novices	15 expert shooters and 21 novice shooters	between-subject	performed 40 self-paced shots using the Noptel Shooter Training System	theta, low alpha, high alpha, low beta, high beta, and gamma band coherence	aiming point
Deeny et al. (2003)	experts and novices	10 expert shooters and nine less skilled shooters	between-subject	Shooting	low alpha, high alpha, and beta band coherence	
Del Percio et al. (2008)	athletes and non-athletes	11 elite fencing athletes, 11 elite karate athletes, and 11 non-athletes	between-subject	observed 200 pictures (of either fencing or karate attacks) and made decisions about whether the attacks were right/left side attacks	single trial epochs	
Del Percio et al. (2010)	athletes and non-athletes	10 elite karate athletes and 12 non-athletes	between-subject	performed wrist extensions of the right and left hands	low alpha and high alpha band activity (+/-2 Hz individual peak frequency)	EMG from operant hand

(Continued)

Study	Focus	Participants	Design	Task	EEG Variables	Other Variables
Del Percio, Bablioni, Bertollo et al. (2009)	athletes and non-athletes as a between-subject factor and good and poor performance as a within-subject factor	18 expert shooters and 10 non-athletes	mixed-model	performed 120 shots	low alpha and high alpha band ERD/ERS	
Del Percio, Bablioni, Marzano et al. (2009)	athletes and non-athletes	10 elite karate athletes, 10 elite fencing athletes and 12 non-athletes	between-subject	performed an eyes-open balancing task (i.e., balancing on two feet and balancing on one foot) using a stabilometer	alpha band ERD/ERS	sway index
Del Percio, Brancucci et al. (2007)	experts and novices as one between-subject factor and athletes and non-athletes as another between-subject factor experts and novices	17 elite karate athletes, 14 amateur karate athletes, and 15 non-athletes	multi-factorial	observed 180 pictures of different types of karate attacks and made decisions about whether the attacks were right/left side attacks	visual evoked potentials	
Del Percio, Iacoboni et al. (2011)	experts and novices	18 elite shooters and 10 non-athletes	between-subject	performed 120 pistol shots	theta, low alpha, high alpha, low beta, high beta, and gamma band coherence	
Del Percio, Infarinato et al. (2011)	athletes and nonathletes	18 elite karate athletes and 28 non-athletes	between-subject	completed periods of resting with eyes open and resting with eyes closed	low alpha and high alpha band activity (+/-2 Hz individual peak frequency)	
Del Percio, Marzano et al. (2007)	athletes and non-athletes as a between-subjects factor and with/without pre-task audio-visual stimulation as a within-subjects factor	14 elite fencing athletes and 14 non-athletes	multi-factorial	observed 80 pictures (of either fencing or karate attacks) in two conditions, with and without pre-task (10 Hz) audio-visual stimulation	alpha band ERD/ERS	reaction time

Study	Comparison	Sample	Design	Task	Measure	
Delpont et al. (1991)	athletes and non-athletes	24 skilled tennis players, 24 skilled rowers and 24 non-athletes	between-subject	completed a period of visual stimulation (i.e., watching an alternating checkerboard pattern)	visual evoked potentials	perceived control
di Fronso et al. (2016)	good and poor performance	one elite air pistol shooter	within-subject	performed 40 self-paced shots	theta, low alpha, and high alpha band ERD/ERS	
Di Russo, Pitzalis, Aprile, and Spinelli (2005)	experts and novices	12 professional clay-target shooters and 12 novice shooters	between-subject	performed three blocks of 50 self-paced finger flexion (i.e., keypad press) movements	movement-related cortical potentials, specifically the Bereitschaftspotential, the negative slope, and the motor potential	
Di Russo et al. (2006)	athletes and non-athletes	12 expert fencers and 12 non-athletes	between-subject	completed 400 trials of a discriminative (Go/No-go) reaction time task	including the P1, N1, P2, N2, and P300 waveforms	
Domingues et al. (2008)	performance across learning trials	23 novice pistol shooters	within-subject	performed four blocks of 10 shots each	alpha band activity	
Doppelmayr et al. (2008)	experts and novices	eight expert shooters and 10 novice shooters	between-subject	performed 10 blocks of five shots each	frontal theta band activity	
Dyke et al. (2014)	good and poor performance	13 novice golfers	within-subject	performed 30 putts. Putts were divided into five most and five least accurate	theta, low alpha, high alpha, low beta, high beta, and gamma band coherence	
Ermutlu et al. (2015)	different types of athletes	12 dancers, 12 fast ball sport athletes and 12 non-athletes	between-subject	completed a five-minute period of 'awake' relaxation	delta, theta, alpha, and beta band activity	
Fattapposta et al. (1996)	experts and novices	eight elite pentathletes and eight novice pentathletes	between-subject	completed the Skilled Performance Task (i.e., an interactive bi-manual motor-perceptual task)	movement-related cortical potentials, specifically the Bereitschaftspotential and the skilled performance positivity potential	EMG from forearm flexor muscles

(Continued)

Study	Focus	Participants	Design	Task	EEG Variables	Other Variables
Gallicchio et al. (2015)	experts and novices as a between-subjects factor and high and low pressure as a within-subjects factor	10 expert golfers and 10 novice golfers	mixed-model	performed 60 putts under two conditions, low-pressure (non-competitive) and high-pressure (competitive)	alpha band coherence	
Hack et al. (2009)	experts and novices	10 experienced basketball referees and 10 novice basketball referees	between-subject	judged pictures of basketball game situations varying with regard to the presence/absence of a foul	including the N1 and P300 waveforms	
Harung (2011)	different levels of expertise	33 Olympic/world class and 33 competitive athletes	between-subject	performed two paired reaction time tasks (i.e., tasks that included a warning stimulus followed by an imperative stimulus)	6–40 Hz EEG coherence, alpha/gamma ratio, and slow potentials (i.e., the CNV)	GSR and self-reported peak experiences
Hatfield et al. (2013)	high and low pressure conditions	19 ROTC student volunteers	within-subject	performed 40 shots using the Noptel Shooter Training System in two conditions, competitive (included time constraints and rewards/penalties) and non-competitive	alpha band ERD/ERS	movement kinematics, state anxiety, and cortisol levels
Hatfield et al. (1984, Study 1)	before and during shooting	17 elite-level shooters	within-subject	performed an air rifle shooting task	alpha band activity and EEG alpha asymmetry	
Hatfield et al. (1984, Study 2)	different tasks	15 collegiate shooters	within-subject	performed an air rifle shooting and two non-shooting tasks, a verbal-analytic task and a visuospatial task	alpha band activity and EEG alpha asymmetry	
Hatfield et al. (1987)	before and during shooting	15 expert marksmen	within-subject	performed self-paced 40 shots to a target	theta, alpha, and beta band activity	ECG

Study	Group comparison	Sample	Design	Task	Measures
Hatta et al. (2009)	athletes and non-athletes	eight elite kendo players and eight non-athletes	between-subject	performed 70 trials each of a left and right hand grip task (i.e., squeezing a dynamometer)	EMG from forearm extensor muscles
Haufler et al. (2000)	experts and novices as a between-subjects factor and different tasks as a within-subjects factor	15 elite shooters and 21 novice shooters	mixed-model	performed simulated rifle shooting, as well as visuo-spatial and verbal tasks	movement-related cortical potentials, specifically the Bereitschaftspotential, the negative slope, and the motor potential; theta, low alpha, high alpha, beta, and gamma band activity
Hillman et al. (2000)	good and poor performance	seven expert shooters	within-subject	performed simulated rifle shooting	alpha and beta band activity
Holmes et al. (2006)	good and poor performance	six expert shooters	within-subject	performed a 40 shots (using the SCATT Shooter Training system) and three observation tasks	alpha band ERD/ERS
Hung et al. (2008)	experts and novices	15 expert shooters and 21 novice shooters	between-subject	performed 40 shots in a standing position with a 5s aiming period	EEG dimensionality (i.e., D2)
Hung et al. (2004)	experts and novices	15 highly skilled table tennis players; 15 non-athletic college students	between-subject	completed a cued reaction time task (i.e., Posner's cued attention task)	Slow potentials, including lateralized readiness potentials
Hunt et al. (2013)	winning athletes and losing athletes	17 collegiate/ROTC volunteers	between-subject	performed 40 shots using the NOPTEL Shooter Training system in a head-to-head competition with another participant. Participants were assigned to either the 'winning' group (n=10) or 'losing' group (n=7) depending on whether they won or lost the competition	delta, theta, alpha, low alpha, high alpha, beta, and gamma band activity; self-reported confidence

(Continued)

Study	Focus	Participants	Design	Task	EEG Variables	Other Variables
Janelle et al. (2000)	experts and novices	12 expert shooters and 13 nonexpert shooters	between-subject	performed 40 shots in a standing position using the Noptel Shooter Training system	alpha and beta band activity	visual point of gaze (as an index of Quiet Eye duration)
Kao et al. (2013)	good and poor performance	18 skilled golfers	within-subject	performed 100 putts. Putts were divided into 15 best and 15 worst outcomes	frontal theta band activity	
Kerick et al. (2004)	pre- and post-training as a within-subjects factor and two different tasks as another within-subjects factor	11 novice pistol shooters	multi-factorial	performed a shooting and a postural simulation task at two different time periods (i.e., before and after a 12–14 week training period)	high alpha band activity	
Kerick et al. (2007)	different tasks	14 experienced shooters	within-subject	performed a simulated shooting task, involving decision (enemy/no-enemy) and no-decision conditions	theta and upper alpha band activity	perceived workload
Kerick et al. (2000)	different types of feedback	17 novice rifle shooters	within-subject	performed 40 shots in a seated position (with the rifle supported by a shooting stand) in four different conditions, including no-feedback (about performance), low feedback, moderate feedback, and high feedback	EEG alpha asymmetry	subjective performance (using the Subjective Performance Questionnaire) and affect (using the PANAS)
Kerick et al. (2001)	different tasks	eight skilled marksmen	within-subject	performed shooting, postural control, and movement control tasks	alpha band ERD/ERS	

Study	Comparison/factor	Sample	Design	Task	Measure	Other measure
Kim and Woo (2013)	disabled and non-disabled shooters	12 disabled air pistol shooters; 22 non-disabled elite shooters	between-subject	performed 20 self-paced shots using the SCATT Shooter Training system	alpha band activity and EEG alpha asymmetry (R-L)	
Kim et al. (2013)	disabled and non-disabled shooters	12 disabled air pistol shooters and 22 non-disabled elite shooters	between-subject	performed 20 self-paced shots using the SCATT Shooter Training system	theta, low alpha, high alpha, beta, and gamma band coherence	
Kita et al. (2001)	athletes and non-athletes	four kendo players, two gymnasts, and nine non-athletes	between-subject	performed brief, self-paced wrist extensions of the right hand	movement-related cortical potentials, specifically the Bereitschaftspotential, the negative slope, and the motor potential	EMG (from the right wrist extensor muscles)
Konttinen and Lyytinen (1992)	experts and novices as a between-subject factor and good and poor performance as a within-subjects factor	three skilled marksmen and three novice shooters	mixed-model	performed simulated rifle shooting	slow potentials	heart rate and respiration
Konttinen and Lyytinen (1993a)	good and poor performance	12 expert shooters	within-subject	performed simulated rifle shooting	slow potentials	heart rate and respiration
Konttinen and Lyytinen (1993b)	four tasks, varying with regard to motor and visual targeting requirements	eight novice shooters	within-subject	performed four different shooting tasks varying with regard to motor and visual components	slow potentials	rifle stability and heart rate and respiration
Konttinen et al. (2000)	experts and novices	six elite marksmen; six pre-elite marksmen	between-subject	performed simulated rifle shooting	slow potentials	
Konttinen et al. (1999)	experts and novices	six elite marksmen and six pre-elite marksmen	between-subject	performed simulated rifle shooting	slow potentials	body sway
Konttinen et al. (1995)	good and poor performance	six elite marksmen and six pre-elite marksmen	within-subject	performed simulated rifle shooting	slow potentials	

(Continued)

Study	Focus	Participants	Design	Task	EEG Variables	Other Variables
Konttinen et al. (1998)	experts and novices	six elite marksmen and six pre-elite marksmen	between-subject	performed simulated rifle shooting	slow potentials	
Landers et al. (1994)	pre- and post-training as a within-subjects factor	11 novice archers	within-subject	performed an archery shooting task at two different time periods (i.e., before and after a 15-w archery training class)	4–30 Hz activity	
Loze et al. (2001)	good and poor performance	six expert air-pistol shooters	within-subject	performed a shooting task	alpha band activity	
Luchsinger et al. (2016)	athletes and non-athletes as a between-subjects factor and resting and post-exercise performance as a within-subject factor	nine biathletes and eight non-athletes	mixed-model	performed 100 shots using the SCATT Shooter Training System in two conditions, resting and post-exercise (i.e., five-minute inline skating)	frontal theta band activity	perceived exertion (using a Borg scale) and self-reported concentration (using a visual analogue scale)
Mann et al. (2011)	experts and novices as a between-subject factor and good and poor performance as a within-subjects factor	10 expert golfers and 10 near-expert golfers	mixed-model	performed two blocks of 45 putts each	movement-related cortical potentials, specifically the Bereitschaftspotential	Quiet Eye duration and EMG from right forearm extensor muscles
Martin et al. (1993)	athletes and non-athletes	24 tennis players, 24 rowers, and 24 non-athletes	between-subject	completed a period of monaural stimulation (i.e., listening to 'clicks' presented to right and left ears)	brainstem auditory evoked potentials	
Nakamoto and Mori (2008)	athletes and non-athletes	nine college baseball players and nine college non-baseball players	between-subject	performed an anticipation timing (Go/Nogo) reaction time task with varying levels of stimulus response compatibility (i.e., compatible with baseball batting and not compatible with baseball batting)	movement-related cortical potentials, specifically the CNV	

Study	Comparison	Sample	Design	Task	EEG/ERP measure	Other measure
Nakamoto and Mori (2012)	experts and novices	seven expert baseball players and seven novice baseball players	between-subject	performed an anticipation timing (Go/Nogo) reaction time task in two conditions, timing unchanged and timing unexpectedly changed	movement-related cortical potentials, specifically the CNV	reaction time
Radlo et al. (2001)	experts and novices	10 advanced baseball players and 10 intermediate-level baseball players	between-subject	completed a baseball pitch discrimination task	P300	
Radlo et al. (2002)	internal and external attentional focus strategy	20 novice dart throwers	between-subject	performed 10 blocks of four dart throws in one of two conditions. Dart throws were performed either using an internal attention focusing strategy or using an external attention focusing strategy	alpha power	heart rate and EMG activity
Reinecke et al. (2011)	different tasks	11 collegiate golfers	within-subject	performed self-paced putts in two conditions, inside and outside	theta, alpha1, alpha2, and beta1 band activity	state anxiety (using the STAI)
Rietschel et al. (2011)	good and poor performance	13 college student volunteers	within-subject	completed 60 trials of a visuomotor pointing task in two conditions, performing alone and performing with social evaluation (i.e., two confederates standing just behind the participant)	low alpha, high alpha, and gamma band coherence	heart rate and skin conductance
Rossi and Zani (1991)	different tasks	four skilled skeet-shooters and four skilled trap-shooters	within-subject	performed an auditory discrimination task with two levels of difficulty, easy and difficult	including the N2 and P300 waveforms	reaction time

(Continued)

Study	Focus	Participants	Design	Task	EEG Variables	Other Variables
Rossi et al. (1992)	athletes and nonathlates as a between-subjects factor and easy and difficult tasks as a within-subjects factor	11 expert fencers and 10 non-athletes	mixed-model	performed an auditory discrimination (Go/NoGo) reaction time task with two levels, easy and difficult	including the N2 and P300 waveforms	reaction time
Salazar et al. (1990)	different tasks as one within-subjects factor and good and poor performance as another within-subjects factor	13 male and 15 female archers	multi-factorial	performed four tasks, including shooting with normal bow; shooting with light bow; bow drawing without aiming; and aiming without bow drawing	5–31 Hz activity	
Shelley-Tremblay et al. (2006)	high and low pressure conditions	20 novice golfers	within-subject	performed 20 putts with and without an audience	alpha, beta1, and beta2 band activity	mood states (using the Profile of Mood States)
Stikic et al. (2014, Study 1)	before and during shooting	51 adult volunteers (i.e., volunteers without any marksmanship training)	within-subject	performed a simulated shooting task using the Virtual Battle Space2 Tactical Warfare Simulator	self-organizing neural networks;	
Stikic et al. (2014, Study 2)	before and during shooting	11 experienced golfers and 11 novice golfers	within-subject	performed 10 sessions of 10 putts each	self-organizing neural networks;	
Taddei et al. (2012)	athletes and non-athletes	10 older fencers, 10 younger fencers, 10 older non-athletes, and 10 younger non-athletes	between-subject	performed a simple reaction time task and a discrimination (Go/NoGo) reaction time task	including the P1, N1, P2, N2, and P300 waveforms	
Taddei et al. (1991)	athletes and non-athletes	eight expert fencers and eight non-athletes	between-subject	completed a period of visual stimulation (i.e., watching an alternating checkerboard pattern) in two conditions, large visual field and small visual field	visual evoked potentials, including the P60-N75, N75-P100, and P100-N145 waveforms	

Author (year)	Comparison	Sample	Design	Task	Neural measure	Additional measure
Taliep and John (2014)	experts and novices	eight skilled and 10 less skilled cricket batsmen	between-subject	watched 24 bowling deliveries and decided whether they were in-swinger or out-swinger deliveries	alpha band event-related desynchronization	reaction times
Thomas and Mitchell (1996)	athletes and non-athletes	10 endurance runners, seven elite gymnasts, and seven non-athletes	between-subject	completed a period of somatosensory stimulation (using a Nihon Kohden Electromyograph with stimulating electrodes attached to the wrist)	somatosensory evoked potentials, including the P9, P11, P13/14, N20, P25, and N30 waveforms	reaction time
Thomas et al. (2005)	athletes and non-athletes	25 elite cricketers and 10 non-athletes	between-subject	completed a period of visual stimulation (i.e., watching an alternating checkerboard pattern)	visual evoked potentials including the N70, P100, and N145 waveforms	choice reaction time
Twigg et al. (2014)	before and during shooting	two experienced archers	within-subject	shot 12 arrows	1–30 Hz activity	
Velikova et al. (2012)	eyes open versus eyes closed conditions	13 expert fencers	within-subject	completed several different conditions, including maintaining eyes open, maintaining eyes closed, making in-phase movements, and making anti-phase movements	delta, theta, alpha2, alpha2, beta1, beta2, beta3, and gamma band coherence	
Vrbik et al. (2015)	good and poor performance	four experienced, recurve bow archers and four experienced, compound bow archers	within-subject	shot 12 arrows	'attention' and 'meditation' scores (i.e., as derived from Mindwave Mobile Software algorithms)	HRV
Wang et al. (2015)	experts and novices	12 experienced badminton players and 13 non-athletes	between-subject	performed visuo-spatial attention and working memory tasks	theta, alpha, and beta band activity	self-reported physical activity
Wolf et al. (2014)	different levels of expertise	14 expert table tennis players, 15 amateur table tennis players, and 15 young elite table tennis players	between-subject	watched 40 videos of table tennis strokes and were asked to imagined themselves responding to the strokes	SMR band ERD/ERS	

(Continued)

Study	Focus	Participants	Design	Task	EEG Variables	Other Variables
Wolf et al. (2015)	experts and novices	14 expert table tennis players and 15 amateur table tennis players	between-subject	watched 40 videos of table tennis strokes and imagined themselves responding to the strokes	EEG alpha asymmetry and theta band coherence	
Wu et al. (2007)	good and poor performance	12 highly skilled basketball players	within-subject	shot 50 baskets	low alpha, high alpha, and low beta band coherence	
Zhu et al. (2011, Study 1)	high reinvestment/ self-monitoring and low reinvestment/self-monitoring athletes	16 novice golfers	between-subject	performed a putting task	alpha1 and alpha2 band coherence	self-reported movement self-monitoring
Zhu et al. (2011, Study 2)	implicit and explicit practice	18 novice golfers randomly assigned to implicit and explicit practice conditions	between-subject	performed a putting task	alpha1 and alpha2 band coherence	
Ziółkowski et al. (2014)	athletes and non-athletes	36 amateur boxers and 52 college student volunteers	between-subject	completed three one-minute periods, including maintaining eyes open, maintaining eyes closed, and maintaining visual focus	delta, theta, alpha, SMR, beta, and high beta band activity	

References

Bablioni, C., Claudio, D. P., Iacoboni, M., Infarinato, F., Lizio, R., Marzano, N., … Eusebi, F. (2008). Golf putt outcomes are predicted by sensorimotor cerebral EEG rhythms. *The Journal of Physiology*, 586(1), 131–139. doi:10.1113/jphysiol.2007.141630

Bablioni, C., Infarinato, F., Marzano, N., Iacoboni, M., Dassù, F., Soricelli, A., … Del Percio, C. (2011). Intra-hemispheric functional coupling of alpha rhythms is related to golfer's performance: A coherence EEG study. *International Journal of Psychophysiology*, 82(3), 260–268. doi:10.1016/j.ijpsycho.2011.09.008

Bablioni, C., Marzano, N., Infarinato, F., Iacoboni, M., Rizza, G., Aschieri, P., … Del Percio, C. (2010). Neural efficiency of experts' brain during judgment of actions: A high-resolution EEG study in elite and amateur karate athletes. *Behavioural Brain Research*, 207(2), 466–475. doi:10.1016/j.bbr.2009.10.034

Baumeister, J., Reinecke, K., Liesen, H., & Weiss, M. (2008). Cortical activity of skilled performance in a complex sports related motor task. *European Journal of Applied Physiology*, 104, 625–631. doi:10.1007/s00421-008-0811-x

Bertollo, M., di Fronso, S., Filho, E., Conforto, S., Schmid, M., Bortoli, L., … Robazza, C. (2016). Proficient brain for optimal performance: The MAP model perspective. *PeerJ*, 4, e2082. doi:10.7717/peerj.2082

Bird, E. (1987). Psychophysiological processes during rifle shooting. *International Journal of Sport Psychology*, 18, 9–18.

Cheng, M. Y., Hung, C. L., Huang, C.-J., Chang, Y. K., Lo, L. C., Shen, C., & Hung, T.-M. (2015). Expert-novice differences in SMR activity during dart throwing. *Biological Psychology*, 110, 212–218. doi:10.1016/j.biopsycho.2015.08.003

Cheron, G., Petit, G., Cheron, J., Leroy, A., Cebolla, A., Cevallos, C., … Dan, B. (2016). Brain oscillations in sport: Toward EEG biomarkers of performance. *Frontiers in Psychology*, 7(FEB). doi:10.3389/fpsyg.2016.00246

Chuang, L., Huang, C. J., & Hung, T. M. (2013). The differences in frontal midline theta power between successful and unsuccessful basketball free throws of elite basketball players. *International Journal of Psychophysiology*, 90, 321–328. doi:10.1016/j.ijpsycho.2013.10.002

Collins, D., Powell, G., & Davies, I. (1990). An electroencephalographic study of hemispheric processing patterns during karate performance. *Journal of Sport and Exercise Psychology*, 12, 223–234. doi:10.1123/jsep.12.3.223

Collins, D., Powell, G., & Davies, I. (1991). Cerebral activity prior to motion task performance: An electro-encephalographic study. Journal of Sports Sciences, 9(3), 313–324.

Cooke, A. (2013). Readying the head and steadying the heart: A review of cortical and cardiac studies of preparation for action in sport. *International Review of Sport and Exercise Psychology*, 6(1), 122–138. doi:10.1080/1750984X.2012.724438

Cooke, A., Kavussanu, M., Gallicchio, G., Willoughby, A., Mcintyre, D., & Ring, C. (2014). Preparation for action: Psychophysiological activity preceding a motor skill as a function of expertise, performance outcome, and psychological pressure. *Psychophysiology*, 51(4). doi:10.1111/psyp.12182

Crews, D. J., & Landers, D. M. (1993). Electroencephalographic measures of attentional patterns prior to the golf putt. *Medicine and Science in Sports and Exercise*, 25(1), 116–126. doi:10.1249/00005768-199301000-00016

Deeny, S. P., Haufler, A. J., Saffer, M., & Hatfield, B. D. (2009). Electroencephalographic coherence during visuo-motor performance: A comparison of cortico-cortical communication in experts and novices. *Journal of Motor Behavior*, 41(2), 106–116. doi:10.3200/JMBR.41.2.106-116

Deeny, S. P., Hillman, C. H., Janelle, C. M., & Hatfield, B. D. (2003). Cortico-cortical communication and superior performance in skilled marksmen: An EEG coherence analysis. *Journal of Sport & Exercise Psychology*, 25(2), 188–204. doi:10.1123/jsep.25.2.188

Del Percio, C., Bablioni, C., Bertollo, M., Marzano, N., Iacoboni, M., Infarinato, F., … Cibelli, G. (2009). Visuo-attentional and sensorimotor alpha rhythms are related to visuo-motor performance in athletes. *Human Brain Mapping*, 30(11), 3527–3540. doi:10.1002/hbm.20776

Del Percio, C., Bablioni, C., Marzano, N., Iacoboni, M., Infarinato, F., Vecchio, F., … Eusebi, F. (2009). Neural efficiency of athletes' brain for upright standing: A high-resolution EEG study. *Brain Research Bulletin*, 79, 193–200. doi:10.1016/j.brainresbull.2009.02.001

Del Percio, C., Brancucci, A., Vecchio, F., Marzano, N., Pirritano, M., Meccariello, E., … Eusebi, F. (2007). Visual event-related potentials in elite and amateur athletes. *Brain Research Bulletin*, 74(1–3), 104–112. doi:10.1016/j.brainresbull.2007.05.011

Del Percio, C., Iacoboni, M., Lizio, R., Marzano, N., Infarinato, F., Vecchio, F., … Lizio, R. (2011). Functional coupling of parietal alpha rhythms is enhanced in athletes before visuomotor performance: A coherence electroencephalographic study. *Neuroscience*, 175, 198–211. doi:10.1016/j.Neuroscience.2010.11.031

Del Percio, C., Infarinato, F., Iacoboni, M., Marzano, N., Soricelli, A., Aschieri, P., … Iacoboni, M. (2010). Movement-related desynchronization of alpha rhythms is lower in athletes than non-athletes: A high-resolution EEG study. *Clinical Neurophysiology*, 121, 482–491. doi:10.1016/j.clinph.2009.12.004

Del Percio, C., Infarinato, F., Marzano, N., Iacoboni, M., Aschieri, P., Lizio, R., … Bablioni, C. (2011). Reactivity of alpha rhythms to eyes opening is lower in athletes than non-athletes: A high-resolution EEG study. *International Journal of Psychophysiology*, 82(3), 240–247. doi:10.1016/j.ijpsycho.2011.09.005

Del Percio, C., Marzano, N., Tilgher, S., Fiore, A., Di Ciolo, E., Aschieri, P., … Eusebi, F. (2007). Pre-stimulus alpha rhythms are correlated with post-stimulus sensorimotor performance in athletes and non-athletes: A high-resolution EEG study. *Clinical Neurophysiology*, 118(8), 1711–1720. doi:10.1016/j.clinph.2007.04.029

Del Percio, C., Rossini, P. M., Marzano, N., Iacoboni, M., Infarinato, F., Aschieri, P., … Eusebi, F. (2008). Is there a "neural efficiency" in athletes? A high-resolution EEG study. *NeuroImage*, 42(4), 1544–1553. doi:10.1016/j.neuroimage.2008.05.061

Delpont, E., Dolisi, C., Suisse, G., Bodino, G., & Gastaud, M. (1991). Visual evoked potentials: Differences related to physical activity. *International Journal of Sports Medicine*, 12(3), 293–298. doi:10.1055/s-2007-1024684

di Fronso, S., Robazza, C., Filho, E., Bortoli, L., Comani, S., & Bertollo, M. (2016). Neural markers of performance states in an Olympic athlete: An EEG case study in air-pistol shooting. *Journal of Sports Science and Medicine*, 15, 214–222.

Di Russo, F., Pitzalis, S., Aprile, T., Spinelli, D., Di Russo, F., Pitzalis, S., … Spinelli, D. (2005). Effect of practice on brain activity: an investigation in top-level rifle shooters. Medicine and Science in Sports and Exercise, 37(9), 1586–1593.

Di Russo, F., Taddei, F., Apnile, T., & Spinelli, D. (2006). Neural correlates of fast stimulus discrimination and response selection in top-level fencers. *Neuroscience Letters*, 408(2), 113–118. doi:10.1016/j.neulet.2006.08.085

Domingues, C. A., Machado, S., Cavaleiro, E, G., Furtado, V., Cagy, M., Ribeiro, P., & Piedade, R. (2008). Alpha absolute power: Motor learning of practical pistol shooting. *Arquivos de Neuro-Psiquiatria*, 66, 336–340. doi:10.1590/S0004-282X2008000300010

Doppelmayr, M., Finkenzeller, T., & Sauseng, P. (2008). Frontal midline theta in the pre-shot phase of rifle shooting: Differences between experts and novices. *Neuropsychologia*, 46, 1463–1467. doi:10.1016/j.neuropsychologia.2007.12.026

Dyke, F., Godwin, M. M., Goel, P., Rehm, J., Rietschel, J. C., Hunt, C. A., & Miller, M. W. (2014). Cerebral cortical activity associated with non-experts' most accurate motor performance. *Human Movement Science*, 37, 21–31. doi:10.1016/j.humov.2014.06.008

Ermutlu, N., Yücesir, I., Eskikurt, G., Temel, T., & İşoğlu-Alkaç, Ü. (2015). Brain electrical activities of dancers and fast ball sports athletes are different. *Cognitive Neurodynamics*, 9, 257–263. doi:10.1007/s11571-014-9320-2

Etnier, J. L., & Gapin, J. I. (2014). Electroencephalograph (EEG). In R. Eklund (Ed.), *Encyclopedia of Sport and Exercise Psychology* Vol 1 (1st ed., pp. 241–243). Thousand Oaks, CA: SAGE Publications. doi:10.4135/9781483332222.n96

Fattapposta, F., Amabile, G., Cordischi, M. V., Di Venanzio, D., Foti, A., Pierelli, F., … Morrocutti, C. (1996). Long-term practice effects on a new skilled motor learning: An electrophysiological study. *Electroencephalography and Clinical Neurophysiology*, 99(6), 495–507. doi:10.1016/S0013-4694(96)96560-8

Gallicchio, G., Cooke, A., & Ring, C. (2015). Lower left temporal-frontal connectivity characterizes expert and accurate performance: High-alpha T7-Fz connectivity as a marker of conscious processing during movement. *Sport, Exercise, and Performance Psychology*, 5(1), 14–24. doi:10.1037/spy0000055

Gentili, R. J., Oh, H., Bradberry, T. J., Hatfield, B. D., & Contreras-Vidal, J. (2010). Signal processing for non-invasive brain biomarkers of sensorimotor performance and brain monitoring. *Signal Processing. InTech*. Open Access Publisher.

Hack, J., Memmert, D., & Rupp, A. (2009). Attentional mechanisms in sports using brain-electrical event related potentials. *Research Quarterly for Exercise and Sport*, 80(4), 727–738.

Harung, H. S. (2011). Higher psycho-physiological refinement in world-class Norwegian athletes: Towards a brain measure of performance capacity in sport. *Scandinavian Journal of Medicine and Science in Sports*, 21(1), 32–41.

Hatfield, B. D., Costanzo, M. E., Goodman, R. N., Lo, L. C., Oh, H., Rietschel, J. C., … Haufler, A. J. (2013). The influence of social evaluation on cerebral cortical activity and motor performance: A study of a real life competition. *International Journal of Psychophysiology*, 90, 240–249. doi:10.1016/j.ijpsycho.2013.08.002

Hatfield, B. D., Haufler, A. J., Hung, T. M., & Spalding, T. W. (2004). Electroencephalographic studies of skilled psychomotor performance. *Journal of Clinical Neurophysiology*, 21(3), 144–156. doi:10.1097/00004691-200405000-00003

Hatfield, B. D., & Kerick, S. E. (2007). The psychology of superior sport performance. In G. Tenenbaum & R. Eklund (Eds.), *Handbook of Sport Psychology* (3rd ed., pp. 84–109). Hoboken, NJ: John Wiley & Sons, Inc.

Hatfield, B. D., & Landers, D. M. (1983). Psychophysiology: A new direction for sport psychology. *Journal of Sport Psychology*, 5(3), 243–259. doi:10.1123/jsp.5.3.243

Hatfield, B. D., Landers, D. M., & Ray, W. J. (1984). Cognitive-processes during self-paced motor-performance - an electroencephalographic profile of skilled marksmen. *Journal of Sport Psychology*, 6, 42–59. doi:10.1123/jsp.6.1.42

Hatfield, B. D., Landers, D. M., & Ray, W. J. (1987). Cardiovascular-CNS interactions during a self-paced, intentional attentive state: Elite marksmanship performance. *Psychophysiology*, 24(5), 542–549. doi:10.1111/j.1469-8986.1987.tb00335.x

Hatta, A., Nishihira, Y., Higashiura, T., Kim, S. R., & Kaneda, T. (2009). Long-term motor practice induces practice-dependent modulation of movement-related cortical potentials (MRCP) preceding a self-paced non-dominant handgrip movement in kendo players. *Neuroscience Letters*, 459(3), 105–108. doi:10.1016/j.neulet.2009.05.005

Haufler, A. J., Spalding, T. W., Santa Maria, D. L., & Hatfield, B. D. (2000). Neuro-cognitive activity during a self-paced visuospatial task: Comparative EEG profiles in marksmen and novice shooters. *Biological Psychology*, 53, 131–160. doi:10.1016/S0301-0511(00)00047-8

Hillman, C. H., Apparies, R. J., Janelle, C. M., & Hatfield, B. D. (2000). An electrocortical comparison of executed and rejected shots in skilled marksmen. *Biological Psychology*, 52, 71–83. doi:10.1016/S0301-0511(99)00021-6

Holmes, P. S., Collins, D., & Calmels, C. (2006). Electroencephalographic functional equivalence during observation of action. *Journal of Sports Sciences*, 24(6), 605–616. doi:10.1080/02640410500244507

Hung, T. M., Haufler, A. J., Lo, L. C., Mayer-Kress, G., & Hatfield, B. D. (2008). Visuo-motor expertise and dimensional complexity of cerebral cortical activity. *Medicine and Science in Sports and Exercise*, 40(4), 752–759. doi:10.1249/MSS.0b013e318162c49d

Hung, T. M., Spalding, T. W., Santa Maria, D. L., & Hatfield, B. D. (2004). Assessment of reactive motor performance with event-related brain potentials: Attention processes in elite table tennis players. *Journal of Sport and Exercise Psychology*, 26, 317–337. doi:10.1123/jsep.26.2.317

Hunt, C. A., Rietschel, J. C., Hatfield, B. D., & Iso-Ahola, S. E. (2013). A psychophysiological profile of winners and losers in sport competition. *Sport, Exercise, and Performance Psychology*, 2(3), 220–231. doi:10.1037/a0031957

Janelle, C. M., & Hatfield, B. D. (2008). Visual attention and brain processes that underlie expert performance: Implications for sport and military psychology. *Military Psychology*, 20(Suppl. 1), S39–S69. doi:10.1080/08995600701804798

Janelle, C. M., Hillman, C. H., Apparies, R. J., Murray, N. P., Meili, L., Fallon, E. A., & Hatfield, B. D. (2000). Expertise differences in cortical activation and gaze behavior during rifle shooting. *Journal of Sport and Exercise Psychology*, 22, 167–182. doi:10.1123/jsep.22.2.167

Kao, S. C., Huang, C. J., & Hung, T. M. (2013). Frontal midline theta is a specific indicator of optimal attentional engagement during skilled putting performance. *Journal of Sport & Exercise Psychology*, 35(5), 470–478. doi:10.1123/jsep.35.5.470

Kerick, S. E., Douglass, L. W., & Hatfield, B. D. (2004). Cerebral cortical adaptations associated with visuomotor practice. *Medicine and Science in Sports and Exercise*, 36(1), 118–129. doi:10.1249/01.MSS.0000106176.31784.D4

Kerick, S. E., Hatfield, B. D., & Allender, L. (2007). Event-related cortical dynamics of soldiers during shooting as a function of varied task demand. *Aviation, Space, and Environmental Medicine*, 78(5 Supplement), B153–B164.

Kerick, S. E., Iso-Ahola, S. E., & Hatfield, B. D. (2000). Psychological momentum in target shooting: Cortical, cognitive-affective, and behavioral responses. *Journal of Sport & Exercise Psychology*, 22(1), 1–20. doi:10.1123/jsep.22.1.1

Kerick, S. E., McDowell, K., & Hung, T. M. (2001). The role of the left temporal region under the cognitive motor demands of shooting in skilled marksmen. *Biological Psychology*, 58, 263–277. doi:10.1016/S0301-0511(01)00116-8

Kim, W., Lee, G., Kim, J., & Woo, M. (2013). A comparison of cortico-cortical communication during air-pistol shooting in elite disabled and non-disabled shooters. *Personality and Individual Differences*, 54, 946–950. doi:10.1016/j.paid.2013.01.010

Kim, W., & Woo, M. (2013). An electrocortical comparison of elite shooters with and without disability during visuo-motor performance. *Perceptual & Motor Skills*, 117(2), 498–510. doi:10.2466/25.15.PMS.117x25z1

Kita, Y., Mori, A., & Nara, M. (2001). Two types of movement-related cortical potentials preceding wrist extension in humans. *Neuroreport*, 12(10), 2221–2225. doi:10.1097/00001756-200107200-00035

Konttinen, N., Landers, D. M., & Lyytinen, H. (2000). Aiming routines and their electrocortical concomitants among competitive rifle shooters. *Scandinavian Journal of Medicine and Science in Sports*, 10, 169–177. doi:10.1034/j.1600-0838.2000.010003169.x

Konttinen, N., & Lyytinen, H. (1992). Physiology of preparation: Brain slow waves, heart rate, and respiration preceding triggering in rifle shooting. *International Journal of Sport Psychology*, 23, 110–127.

Konttinen, N., & Lyytinen, H. (1993a). Brain slow waves preceding time-locked visuo-motor performance. *Journal of Sports Sciences*, 11(3), 257–266.

Konttinen, N., & Lyytinen, H. (1993b). Individual variability in brain slow wave profiles in skilled sharpshooters during the aiming period in rifle shooting. *Journal of Sport and Exercise Psychology*, 15, 275–289.

Konttinen, N., Lyytinen, H., & Era, P. (1999). Brain slow potentials and postural sway behavior during sharpshooting performance. *Journal of Motor Behavior*, 31(1), 11–20. doi:10.1080/00222899909601888

Konttinen, N., Lyytinen, H., & Konttinen, R. (1995). Brain slow potentials reflecting successful shooting performance. *Research Quarterly for Exercise and Sport*, 66(1), 64–72. doi:10.1080/02701367.1995.10607656

Konttinen, N., Lyytinen, H., & Viitasalo, J. (1998). Rifle-balancing in precision shooting: Behavioral aspects and psychophysiological implication. *Scandinavian Journal of Medicine and Science in Sports*, 8, 78–83.

Landers, D. M., Han, M., Salazar, W., Petruzzello, S. J., Kubitz, K. A., & Gannon, T. L. (1994). Effects of learning on electroencephalographic and electrocardiographic patterns in novice archers. *International Journal of Sport Psychology*, 25(3), 313–330.

Lawton, G. W., Saarela, P., & Hatfield, B. D. (1998). Electroencephalography and mental states associated with elite performance. *Journal of Sport and Exercise Psychology*, 20, 35–53. doi:10.1123/jsep.20.1.35

Loze, G. M., Collins, D., & Holmes, P. S. (2001). Pre-shot EEG alpha-power reactivity during expert air-pistol shooting: A comparison of best and worst shots. *Journal of Sports Sciences*, 19(9), 727–733. doi:10.1080/02640410152475856

Luchsinger, H., Sandbakk, Ø., Schubert, M., Ettema, G., & Baumeister, J. (2016). A comparison of frontal theta activity during shooting among biathletes and cross-country skiers before and after vigorous exercise. *Plos One*, 11(3), e0150461. doi:10.1371/journal.pone.0150461

Mancevska, S., Gligoroska, J. P., Todorovska, L., Dejanova, B., & Petrovska, S. (2016). Psychophysiology and the sport science. *Research in Physical Education, Sport and Health ISSN*, 5(2), 101–105. Retrieved from www.pesh.mk

Mann, D. T. Y., Coombes, S. A., Mousseau, M. B., & Janelle, C. M. (2011). Quiet eye and the Bereitschaftspotential: Visuo-motor mechanisms of expert motor performance. *Cognitive Processing*, 12(3), 223–234. doi:10.1007/s10339-011-0398-8

Mann, D. T. Y., & Janelle, C. M. (2012). Psychophysiology: Equipment in research and practice. In W. Edmonds & G. Tennbaum (Eds.), *Case Studies in Applied Psychophysiology* (1st ed., pp. 257–274). Malden, MA: John Wiley & Sons, Inc. doi:10.1002/9781119959984.ch16

Martin, F., Delpont, E., Suisse, G., & Dolisi, C. (1993). Brainstem auditory evoked potentials: Differences related to physical activity. *International Journal of Sports Medicine*, 14(8), 427–432.

Nakamoto, H., & Mori, S. (2008). Effects of stimulus-response compatibility in mediating expert performance in baseball players. *Brain Research*, 1189(1), 179–188. doi:10.1016/j.brainres.2007.10.096

Nakamoto, H., & Mori, S. (2012). Experts in fast-ball sports reduce anticipation timing cost by developing inhibitory control. *Brain and Cognition*, 80(1), 23–32. doi:10.1016/j.bandc.2012.04.004

Radlo, S. J., Janelle, C. M., Barba, D. A., & Frehlich, S. G. (2001). Perceptual decision making for baseball pitch recognition: Using P300 latency and amplitude to index attentional processing. *Research Quarterly for Exercise and Sport*, 72(1), 22–31. doi:10.1080/02701367.2001.10608928

Radlo, S. J., Steinberg, G. M., Singer, R. N., Barba, D. A., & Melnikov, A. (2002). The influence of an attentional focus strategy on alpha brain wave activity, heart rate, and dart-throwing performance. *International Journal of Sport Psychology*, 33, 205–217.

Reinecke, K., Cordes, M., Lerch, C., Koutsandréou, F., Schubert, M., Weiss, M., & Baumeister, J. (2011). From lab to field conditions: A pilot study on EEG methodology in applied sports sciences. *Applied Psychophysiology & Biofeedback*, 36, 265–271. doi:10.1007/s10484-011-9166-x

Rietschel, J. C., Goodman, R. N., King, B. R., Lo, L. C., Contreras-Vidal, J. L., & Hatfield, B. D. (2011). Cerebral cortical dynamics and the quality of motor behavior during social evaluative challenge. *Psychophysiology*, 48(4), 479–487. doi:10.1111/j.1469-8986.2010.01120.x

Rossi, B., & Zani, A. (1991). Timing of movement-related decision processes in clay-pigeon shooters as assessed by event-related brain potentials and reaction times. *International Journal of Sport Psychology*, 22, 128–139.

Rossi, B., Zani, A., Taddei, F., & Pesce, C. (1992). Chronometric aspects of information processing in high level fencers as compared to nonathletes: An ERPS and RT study. *Journal of Human Movement Studies*, 23(1), 17–28.

Salazar, W., Landers, D. M., Petruzzello, S. J., Han, M., Crews, D. J., & Kubitz, K. A. (1990). Hemispheric asymmetry, cardiac response, and performance in elite archers. *Research Quarterly for Exercise and Sport*, 61(4), 351–359. doi:10.1080/02701367.1990.10607499

Shelley-Tremblay, J., Shugrue, J., & Kline, J. (2006). Changes in EEG laterality index effects of social inhibition on putting in novice golfers. *Journal of Sport Behavior*, 29(4), 353–373.

Stikic, M., Berka, C., Levendowski, D. J., Rubio, F. R., Tan, V., Korszen, S., … Wurzer, D. (2014). Modeling temporal sequences of cognitive state changes based on a combination of EEG-engagement, EEG-workload, and heart rate metrics. *Frontiers in Neuroscience*, 8, 1. doi:10.3389/fnins.2014.00342

Taddei, F., Bultrini, A., Spinelli, D., Di Russo, F., & Francesco, D. R. (2012). Neural correlates of attentional and executive processing in middle-age fencers. *Medicine and Science in Sports and Exercise*, 44(6), 1057–1066. doi:10.1249/MSS.0b013e31824529c2

Taddei, F., Viggiano, M. P., & Mecacci, L. (1991). Pattern reversal visual evoked potentials in fencers. *International Journal of Psychophysiology*, 11, 257–260. doi:10.1097/WNP.0b013e3182276574

Taliep, M. S., & John, L. (2014). Sport expertise : The role of precise timing of verbal – analytical engagement and the ability to detect visual cues. *Perception*, 43, 316–332. doi:10.1068/p7530

Thomas, N. G., & Mitchell, D. (1996). Somatosensory-evoked potentials in athletes. *Medicine and Science in Sports and Exercise*, 28(4), 473–481. doi:10.1097/00005768-199604000-00012

Thomas, N. G., Harden, L. M., & Rogers, G. G. (2005). Visual evoked potentials, reaction times and eye dominance in cricketers. *Journal of Sports Medicine & Physical Fitness*, 45, 428–433.

Thompson, T., Steffert, T., Ros, T., Leach, J., & Gruzelier, J. H. (2008). EEG applications for sport and performance. *Methods*, 45, 279–288. doi:10.1016/j.ymeth.2008.07.006

Twigg, P., Sigurnjak, S., Southall, D., & Shenfield, A. (2014). Exploration of the effect of electroencephalograph levels in experienced archers. *Measurement and Control*, 47(6), 185–190. doi:10.1177/0020294014539281

Velikova, S., Gonzales-Rosa, J., Castellani, C., Rossi, M., Tettamanti, A., Gatti, R., … Leocani, L. (2012). EEG connectivity in high-performance fencers. *International Journal of Psychophysiology*, 85(3), 297. doi:10.1016/j.ijpsycho.2012.06.023

Vrbik, A., Bene, R., & Vrbik, I. (2015). Heart rate values and levels of attention and relaxation in expert archers during shooting. *Hrvatski Športskomedicinski Vjesnik*, 30, 21–29.

Wang, C. H., Tsai, C. L., Tu, K. C., Muggleton, N. G., Juan, C. H., & Liang, W. K. (2015). Modulation of brain oscillations during fundamental visuo-spatial processing: A comparison between female collegiate badminton players and sedentary controls. *Psychology of Sport & Exercise*, 16, 121–129. doi:10.1016/j.psychsport.2014.10.003

Wolf, S., Brölz, E., Keune, P., & Wesa, B. (2015). Motor skill failure or flow-experience? Functional brain asymmetry and brain connectivity in elite and amateur table tennis players. *Biological Psychology*, 105, 95–105. doi:10.1016/j.biopsycho.2015.01.007

Wolf, S., Brolz, E., Scholz, D., Ramos-Murguialday, A., Keune, P. M., Hautzinger, M., … Strehl, U. (2014). Winning the game: Brain processes in expert, young elite and amateur table tennis players. *Frontiers in Behavioral Neuroscience*, 8(October), 1–12. doi:10.3389/fnbeh.2014.00370

Wu, C. C., Lo, L. C., Lin, J. J., Shih, H. H., & Hung, T. M. (2007). The relationship between basketball free throw performance and EEG coherence. *International Journal of Sport and Exercise Psychology*, 5(4), 448–450. doi:10.1080/1612197X.2007.9671846

Yarrow, K., Brown, P., & Krakauer, J. W. (2009). Inside the brain of an elite athlete: The neural processes that support high achievement in sports. *Nature reviews. Neuroscience*, 10(8), 585–596. doi:10.1038/nrn2700

Zhu, F. F., Poolton, J. M., Wilson, M. R., Maxwell, J. P., & Masters, R. (2011). Neural co-activation as a yardstick of implicit motor learning and the propensity for conscious control of movement. *Biological Psychology*, 87, 66–73. doi:10.1016/j.biopsycho.2011.02.004

Ziółkowski, A., Gorkovenko, A., Pasek, M., Włodarczyk, P., Zarańska, B., Dornowski, M., & Graczyk, M. (2014). EEG correlates of attention concentration in successful amateur boxers. *Neurophysiology*, 46(5), 422–427. doi:10.1007/s11062-015-9468-3

Neuroimaging
Techniques and Applications in Sports

Chantel Mayo and Jodie R. Gawryluk

Standing just outside the edge of sideline in your opponents' end, you grasp the basketball tightly between your two palms. You quickly scan the field to get a sense of where your teammates are positioned, where their defenders are, and where the net is in relation to everyone else, sending visual information from your retina to your lateral geniculate nucleus to your primary visual cortex in your occipital lobe. The ref's whistle sounds and it's time to start the play. You slam your hand sharply against the ball, notifying your team it's time to go—the neurons in your motor cortex communicate with the motor neurons in your spinal cord via the corticospinal tract; these motor neurons have direct connections to your muscles. You see your teammate cut toward the net; identifying information like your white home jersey is sent to the inferior cortex in the temporal lobe via the ventral stream, while your teammate's position is tracked and sent to the superior cortex in the parietal lobe via the dorsal stream. At the same time, your attention shifts to your other teammate who has escaped their defender just outside the three-point line. You think: Option (1) you can send the ball to teammate #1. They are right under the net and they would probably get it in, as they have been successful under the net all night; however, their defender is only a step behind. Option (2) alternatively, you can send the ball to teammate #2—they are further away from the net, but their shot is wide open. Mediated by your prefrontal cortex, you only have seconds to weigh your options. As the seconds count down, your medial frontal cortex evaluates your options in context. Option 2 emerges as your preferred option—no defense, wide-open shot. Your prefrontal cortex sends the instructions to your motor regions including your primary motor cortex. Again, your neurons send motor information to your motor neurons in your spinal cord via your corticospinal tract. Your muscles contract and you send the ball to teammate #2, hoping for three points.

The complexity of the human brain is astounding. The brain can be divided into various hierarchical regions from the hindbrain, which controls essential physiological functions (e.g., breathing), to the forebrain, which contributes to higher order functions (e.g., abstract thinking). The brain is composed of both grey and white matter; grey matter consists mostly of cell bodies and dendrites, while white matter consists mostly of myelinated axons. Together, the grey and white matter comprises a series of interconnected brain networks, which contribute to healthy brain function.

How do we understand which regions and networks of the brain are involved in the complex set of behaviors required in sports? Specifically, are the brains of some athletes bigger than others? Are there differences at a microstructural level? Are different regions recruited during a task given an athlete's training in sport? One of the key methodologies that have been employed to date to address questions like these is magnetic resonance imaging.

Magnetic Resonance Imaging

MRI has become an essential technique in diagnostic radiology as well as the scientific study of the brain. This is largely because MRI techniques can non-invasively reveal anatomic detail (as well as indicate the regions involved in a specific task) with high spatial resolution (sub mm). The underlying principles of MRI are based in nuclear magnetic resonance (NMR; Brown & Semelka, 2010). NMR relies on an inherent property of atomic nuclei called spin. In nuclei with an odd number of protons/neutrons (e.g., the overall spin results in a magnetic moment and angular momentum. In the presence of an external magnetic field (B_0), nuclei with spin will begin to precess about and align parallel or anti-parallel to the direction of an applied magnetic field. In a typical sample composed of many nuclei, slightly more nuclei align parallel to the direction of the magnetic field, which results in the development of bulk magnetization. The strength of the external magnetic field dictates the frequency at which the nuclei precess. This is known as the Larmour Frequency (ω), where, $\omega = \gamma Bo$, and γ represents the magnetogyric ratio for a particular nucleus (each type of nuclei has a characteristic value for γ).

In MRI, hydrogen nuclei (which consist of one unpaired proton) are most commonly focused on because they are abundant in body tissues composed of water and fat (Jezzard & Clare, 2001). In a homogeneous magnetic field, all hydrogen nuclei in the brain would have the same precession frequency. In order to create an image of the brain, the different regions must be distinguishable. This is accomplished by the application of three linear magnetic field gradients that are superimposed in orthogonal directions; the slice selecting gradient, the frequency encoding gradient, and the phase encoding gradient. The slice selecting gradient is used to introduce different magnetic field strengths in different locations, thereby leading the hydrogen nuclei in different areas to have different precession frequencies that can be targeted. In order to determine the origin of a signal within a slice, frequency and phase encoding gradients are used. For frequency encoding, a gradient is applied that causes the precession frequency of nuclei to change along the axis in which the gradient is applied, thereby causing the nuclei in different areas to emit signals of different frequencies. For phase encoding, a gradient is applied for a fixed period of time that creates changes in phase along a slice.

In order to measure a signal from the bulk magnetization of the precessing nuclei, an oscillating electromagnetic field known as a radio frequency (RF) pulse is applied (Brown and Semelka, 2010). Specifically, the application of an RF pulse (where the frequency matches the precession of the spins) can lead the bulk magnetization vector to rotate from the longitudinal plane into the transverse plane. The strength and/or duration of the pulse can be used to determine the rotation. A pulse that causes a rotation of 90° is common, and is called an excitation pulse. Some pulse sequences also involve the subsequent application of a 180° pulse that causes the spins to regain phase coherence and recovers a measurable signal (referred to as a spin echo; Jezzard & Clare, 2001). Following the application of an RF excitation pulse, a receiving coil can measure the voltage created by the oscillating magnetic field of the sample as it returns to the previous state.

There are two types of relaxation that occur during the acquisition of MRI signal: longitudinal relaxation and transverse relaxation (Brown & Semelka, 2010; Jezzard & Clare, 2001). Longitudinal relaxation is also known as spin-lattice relaxation because energy is transferred to the surrounding molecular environment; the time constant of this process is known as T1. T1 varies depending on how efficiently energy is exchanged between hydrogen nuclei and their environment. Transverse relaxation is also known as spin-spin relaxation because energy is transferred to nearby nuclei. The time constant for this process is called T2. T2 results from relaxation due a loss of phase coherence between neighboring nuclei. A related measure, T2⋆ refers to measured phase decay that results from the additional presence of local inhomogeneities in the magnetic field.

Given that different tissue types have distinct relaxation rates, it is possible to derive images with different contrasts. For example, if the MRI signal is acquired when tissue differences in

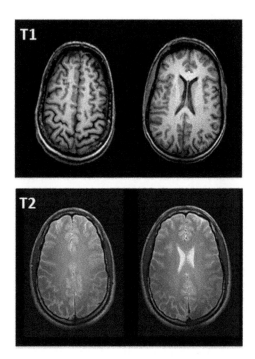

Figure 5.1 Images displaying T1 (top) and T2 (bottom) weighted MRI scans.

the longitudinal plane are maximized, the resulting image is considered T1 weighted. In this case, cerebral spinal fluid (CSF) appears dark (because it has a long T1 value), WM appears bright (because it has a short T1 value), and grey matter appears gray (because it has an intermediate T1 value). Conversely, if the MRI signal is measured when tissue differences in the transverse plane are maximized, the resulting image is considered T2 weighted. In this case, CSF appears bright (because it has a long T2 value) and white and grey matter appears dark (because they have short T2 values; Brown and Semelka, 2010). The resulting images can be used to examine the differences in the brain such as the total brain volume, the volume of specific brain structures, or cortical thickness (Figure 5.1).

Diffusion Tensor Imaging

A promising advanced MRI based tool that has been developed to examine white matter characteristics in particular is diffusion weighted MRI (Alexander, Lee, Lazar, & Field, 2007; Mori & Zhang, 2009). Diffusion weighted MRI is based on water diffusion within the brain (Soares, Marques, Alves, & Sousa, 2013). Diffusion of water occurs both within and between brain cells; these patterns of water diffusion vary in different types of tissue and are influenced by the presence of biological barriers (Gold, 2012; Mori & Zhang 2009; Soares et al., 2013). Water unconstrained by biological barriers diffuse equally, in all directions; this is known as random or isotropic diffusion. In contrast, biological barriers restrict water movement in a perpendicular direction; this is known as anisotropic diffusion (Gold, 2012).

A diffusion tensor is a mathematical model of this water diffusion in 3-dimensional space derived from diffusion measurements obtained through six or more diffusion gradient directions (Jones & Leemans, 2011; Jellison et al., 2004). It can be represented numerically in a diagonally symmetric three by three covariance matrix (Alexander et al., 2007; Jellison et al., 2004).

Diagonalization of this matrix generates three eigenvectors (ε_1, ε_2, ε_3,) and three corresponding eigenvalues (λ_1, λ_2, λ_3). Eigenvectors represent the direction of the maximum water diffusion, and eigenvalues represent the magnitude of the water diffusion for each vector (Jellison et al., 2004; Soares et al., 2013; Stebbins & Murphy, 2009).

It is typical to visualize the diffusion tensor as an ellipsoid shape (Jellison et al., 2004). In this case, the eigenvectors define the direction of the principle axes, while the eigenvalues define the radius of the ellipsoid (Alexander et al., 2007). With isotropic diffusion, the eigenvalues are approximately equal and the tensor approaches a spherical shape. With anisotropic diffusion, however, the eigenvalues are unequal, and the tensor becomes elliptical (i.e., deviates from the spherical shape; Alexander et al., 2007, Jellison et al., 2004).

Eigenvalues are influenced by changes in tissue microstructure (e.g., due to aging, brain trauma or disease). Thus, in modeling the diffusion weighted MRI data through this diffusion tensor imaging (DTI), researchers can detect *in* vivo microstructural changes in the brain that are not detected by conventional MRI (Alexander et al., 2007; deGois Vasconcelos, Dozzi Brucki, Parolin Jackowiski, Francisco, & Bueno, 2009; Gold, 2012; Jones & Leemans, 2011; Soares et al., 2013).

There are a number of common DTI measures used to assess microstructural changes in the brain. Four of the most commonly reported DTI indices include fractional anisotropy (FA), 2) mean diffusivity (MD), 3) axial diffusivity (AxD), and 4) radial diffusivity (RD):

FA. Measured on a scale from zero (isotropic diffusion) to one (anisotropic diffusion), FA is a measure of the degree of directionality of the water diffusion (Amlien & Fjell, 2014; deGois Vasconcelos et al., 2009; Mori & Zhang, 2009; Soares et al., 2013; Stebbins & Murphy, 2009).

MD. Unlike FA, MD does not provide any information regarding the direction associated with of the diffusion (Stebbins & Murphy, 2009). Instead, MD is a measure of the water diffusion rate (Soares et al., 2013).

AxD. AxD is a measure of the rate of water diffusion along the longitudinal axis. It is derived from the primary (i.e., largest) eigenvalue (Soares et al., 2013; Stebbins & Murphy, 2009).

RD. RD is a measure of the rate of water diffusion rate along the perpendicular axes. It is derived from the secondary and tertiary eigenvalues (Gold, 2012; Soares et al., 2013; Stebbins & Murphy, 2009).

Water diffusion is generally isotropic in CSF and nearly so in grey matter, but it is anisotropic in white matter (Alexander et al., 2007; Jones & Leemans, 2011). Because water diffusion is completely isotropic in CSF, it has very low FA. Although biological barriers such as cell membranes impede some of the water diffusion in grey matter, water diffusion is still largely isotropic, and thus, grey matter also has low FA (e.g., FA = 0.3; Keller et al., 2013). In contrast to CSF and grey matter, white matter is highly organized into parallel fiber bundles. While water is free to diffuse along the direction of the axonal fibers, water diffusion perpendicular to the fibers is greatly restricted by tightly packed axons and the myelin surrounding the axons. Therefore, white matter water diffusion is highly anisotropic and has high FA (deGois Vasconcelos et al., 2009; Stebbins & Murphy, 2009; Zhang, Xu, Zang, & Kantarci, 2014). Generally, water diffusion is highest in white matter with large number of parallel fibers (e.g., the corpus callosum; FA =0.8; Keller et al., 2013).

AxD and RD are more specific DTI indices of white matter integrity than MD or FA. AxD is thought to be influenced by axonal degeneration (Alexander et al., 2007). Decreased AxD has been reported in both mouse models and humans with damage to the axons, which may reflect increased barriers to diffusion in the axial axis (Gold, 2012; Stebbins & Murphy, 2009). RD is thought to be influenced by the myelin in white matter (Alexander et al., 2007). Increased RD has been reported to occur with loss of myelin in a number of animal studies, which may reflect increase diffusion in the perpendicular axis (Gold, 2012; Stebbins & Murphy, 2009).

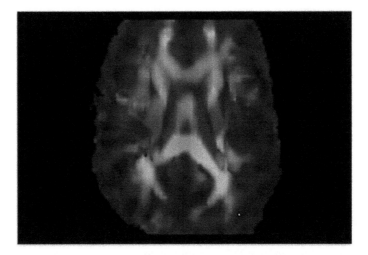

Figure 5.2   A diffusion weighted image with regions of high FA appearing bright. Dominant fiber direction is color coded with red indicating fibers running left to right (X plane); green indicating fibers running front to back (Y plane); blue indicating fibers running head to toe (Z plane).

Together, these DTI metrics may be used to examine differences between groups (e.g., types of athletes, level of athlete experience) or changes within the same athlete over time (Figure 5.2).

Functional Magnetic Resonance Imaging

Functional magnetic resonance imaging (fMRI) is used to visualize the neuroanatomical regions responsible for processing information. Since the conception of fMRI in the early 1990's (Ogawa et al., 1992), significant advances in research have broadened our understanding of how the brain functions under both healthy and diseased conditions (e.g., Dolan, 2008; Haller & Bartsch, 2009; Rosen, Buckner, & Dale, 1998).

Typically, fMRI relies on blood oxygen level dependent (BOLD) contrast. The source of BOLD contrast is derived from the difference between deoxygenated blood, which is paramagnetic (attracted to an external magnetic field) and oxygenated blood, which is diamagnetic (repelled from an applied magnetic field; Kim & Ugurbil, 2003).

Deoxygenated blood causes local magnetic field inhomogeneities, which lead to shorter T2$\star$ (faster transverse relaxation). For this reason, fMRI traditionally uses a T2$\star$ weighted pulse sequence in which oxygenated blood leads to increased signal intensity and deoxygenated blood leads to decreased signal intensity. Conventionally, it is thought that when a brain region becomes engaged there is an associated increase in metabolic demands that must be supported. Consequently, regional increases in cerebral blood flow and volume occur to deliver oxygenated blood to active neurons. As required, deoxygenated blood is produced, although a surplus of oxygenated blood remains, resulting in a small measurable increase in signal intensity (Matthews, 2001). FMRI can be collected while an individual performs a task in the scanner, or during resting state, which can reveal functional networks (e.g., the default mode network) that may differ between groups (e.g., athletes and non–athlete controls; athletes with concussion and healthy athletes) (Figure 5.3).

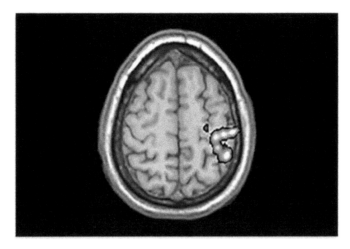

Figure 5.3   Image showing motor regions activate during a simple finger tapping test. fMRI activation pattern overlaid on T1 weighted structural MRI scan.

Table 5.1 Strengths and limitations of magnetic resonance imaging (MRI)

Strengths of MRI	Limitations of MRI
+ Non-invasive	– Temporal resolution limited (~ 50 ms)
+ Repeatable	– Susceptible to respiratory and cardiovascular artifacts)
+ High Spatial Resolution	– Susceptible to head motion artifacts
+ Ability to examine brain microstructure	– Localization of BOLD response to vasculature
+ Ability to examine brain function	– Lack of standardized methodology

Taken together, both structural and functional MRI possess strengths and limitations one should bear in mind when evaluating the literature that has employed this technique (Table 5.1).

Applications of Neuroimaging Techniques in Sport

To date, investigations into the neural correlates of athletic behavior have focused on (1) structural imaging using T1 and T2 weighted MRI, (2) structural imaging of white matter using DTI, and (3) the use of fMRI to visualize the brain at play. The findings are reviewed below according to the methodology employed.

MRI

Anatomical MRI studies to date have investigated differences between elite athletes and controls, as well as differences in brain structure resulting from involvement in different types of sports.

Recent research has revealed training-induced structural alterations in professional athletes. In particular, studies have shown larger grey matter volumes in athletes relative to non-exercising controls. For example, Schlaffke and colleagues (2014) found more grey matter volume in the supplementary motor area and dorsal pre-motor cortex in endurance athletes and martial artists relative to non-exercising controls. Additionally, Di and colleagues (2012), found that professional badminton players had more grey matter in the medial cerebellar region compared to healthy controls with no experience in badminton. Similarly, Hanggi and colleagues (2015) observed differences in grey matter volume in professional handball players compared with controls. Specifically, greater volume was observed in the right primary and secondary motor, bilateral supplementary motor area, cingulate motor area, and left intra parietal sulcus. Interestingly, the age at which the athlete began training was negatively related to grey matter volume in the bilateral primary and secondary motor area; a relationship which suggests that such structural changes are influenced by level of training and experience rather than a genetic predisposition.

As mentioned, a number of investigators have also examined whether the type of sport expertise influences brain structure. Wenzel and colleagues (2014), found higher cerebellar grey matter volume in "power" athletes (sprinters, jumpers, and throwers) to "endurance" (distance runners) athletes. Schlaffke and colleagues (2014) found that endurance athletes (aerobic sport) had higher grey matter volume in the hippocampus and parahippocampal gyrus of the medial temporal lobe relative to martial arts athletes (anaerobic sport).

In contrast with the majority of studies to date, which examined structural changes at the group-level, Taubert and colleagues (2015) compared professional track and field athletes to matched controls in a single-subject design. The findings revealed that total brain volumes were comparable between athletes and controls, although there were regional grey matter differences in the striatum and the thalamus, which remained two years later.

DTI

In addition to volumetric changes as assessed by MRI, there is evidence of microstructural brain changes in athletes as assessed by DTI. Specifically, Huang, Song, and Wang (2013) found decreased FA in the bilateral superior longitudinal fasciculus, inferior longitudinal fasciculus, and inferior occipito-frontal fascicle in world-class gymnasts compared to non-athlete controls; the authors hypothesize that such differences contribute to gymnasts' superior ability to localize the direction and speed of their movements. Hanggi and colleagues (2015) also observed microstructural differences in professional handball players relative to controls. Specifically, FA and A×D were increased in the right corticospinal tract. Interestingly, the years of handball training was negatively related with R×D in the right corticospinal tract, suggesting that specific training may induce neuroplastic, microstructural alterations.

Currently, there is a paucity of research on healthy athletes and even less on aging athletes. One recent study by Burzynska and colleagues (2016) examined white matter FA and hyperintensity burden and hippocampal volume in a single subject elderly athlete. Results indicated that the elderly athlete had a high amount of white matter hyperintensities and a lower hippocampal volume relative to a reference sample of 58 healthy low-active women, but had increased FA in the corpus callosum. The authors hypothesize that her relatively high FA may be related to the beneficial effects of exercise in old age; however it is important to recognize the limitations to generalizability given the single subject sample size.

fMRI

In addition to changes in brain structure in both grey and white matter, there is evidence of functional changes related to athletic activity. Many of the studies to date have focused on differences in brain activity related to level of athletic expertise.

In comparing expert and novice tennis players, Balser and colleagues (2014) found that experts performed better on spatial (direction of ball) and motor (response to action) anticipation tasks, with the experts having higher activation in the action-observation network (AON) regions such as a superior parietal lobe, the intraparietal sulcus, the inferior frontal gyrus, and the cerebellum. Accurate prediction of future movement allows athletes to anticipate and respond to the play appropriately and the fronto-parietal action-observation network (AON) is hypothesized to be involved in such early predictions.

Abreu and colleagues (2012) used fMRI to examine whether level of expertise influenced action prediction and found that although AON was activated in both expert and novice basketball players, correct prediction was related to higher posterior insular cortex activity in expert athletes and higher orbitofrontal activity in novice athletes. These findings suggest that novices may rely more heavily on higher-order strategies compared to expert athletes, who rely on body awareness.

However, there is evidence that accurate prediction is influenced by the familiarity with the sport within high-level athletes. Specifically, Balser et al. (2014) gathered fMRI data while groups of tennis and volleyball experts predicted the direction of both tennis and volleyball serves. The athletes had stronger activations of AON regions when they predicted serves in their respective sport, suggesting that years of sport-specific training improved sport-specific action prediction.

There is also evidence that an athlete's level of experience in sport influence neural activation. For example, Kim and colleagues (2014) examined differences in brain activity in elite, expert, and novice archers during simulated release of the bowstring. In elite and expert athletes, the greatest activity was observed in the dorsal pathways including the occipital lobe, the temporo-parietal lobe, and the dorsolateral pre-motor cortex, while novices had more widespread activity in the ventral pathways including the superior and inferior frontal area, ventral prefrontal cortex, pre-motor cortex, primary motor cortex, superior parietal lobule, and primary somatosensory cortex. The authors propose that the localized brain activity in the elite and expert athletes as compared to novice athletes reflect greater efficiency in the neural activities underlying shooting. Relatedly, Chang and colleagues (2011) found that non-archers recruited more brain regions including the cerebellum during a mental imagery archery task as compared to elite archers; again, the authors propose that such difference may underlie the consistency with which the elite archer performs. The mental imagery and mental rehearsal that precedes motor action in highly trained athletes are thought to differentiate them from novice athletes. Wei and Luo (2010) examined the pattern of activation in professional divers relative to controls during imagery related to diving as well as imagery related to simple motor skills. Here, the professional divers showed higher activation in the parahippocampal region during diving imagery, but not during the simple motor skills imagery, suggesting that the professional divers use imagery more efficiency than novices, but only for skills related to diving.

There is also evidence that long-term motor training may influence neural activation. Using fMRI, Naito and Hirose (2014) found that the size and intensity of neural activity in the medial-wall foot motor regions differed across two professional football (soccer) players, one amateur football (soccer) players, and two top swimmers, despite identical foot movements. Although all players made the same-sized foot movements, one player's motor activity in particular was lower than the others, suggesting that conserving motor-cortical neural resources may contribute to more efficient control of foot movement.

Future Directions in Sport Imaging

As is common in neuroimaging literature, the sample sizes in the studies described above are small—ranging from a single case study, to approximately 15 athletes in each group (e.g., athlete or control). Moving forward, to better characterize how athletes' brains differ in structure and function, future work would benefit from larger group sizes, to ensure sufficient power to detect small-scale changes in the brain.

Currently, the majority of studies use a single imaging technique. Combined imaging of athletes' brains through multiple modalities (e.g., MRI, DTI and fMRI) will provide researchers with simultaneous information about both structure and function of the brain, and will aid in better establishing the relationship between structure and function. A particular challenge in this work lies in the inability to perform exercises while undergoing MRI scanning. Here, complementary, alternative imaging techniques that can be brought to the sideline (e.g., functional near infrared spectroscopy; fNIRS) are ideal, but beyond the scope of the current chapter.

Another future direction in this line of research should aim to better characterize the changes in the brain that occur with exercise in different groups. For example, the difference between athletic individuals and similarly aged sedentary controls, or athletes with different levels of expertise in a given sport (amateur vs. professional athletes). If there are relative changes in brain structure or function as a result of exercise, these types of studies may hold promise for rehabilitation or prevention in select patient groups (e.g., traumatic brain injury). In particular, better identifying the *type* of exercise (aerobic vs. non-aerobic) that may be most beneficial from a rehabilitation or prevention perspective.

References

Abreu, A. M., Macaluso, E., Azevedo, R. T., Cesari, P., Urgesi, C., & Aglioti, S. M. (2012). Action anticipation beyond the action observation network: A functional magnetic resonance imaging study in expert football players. *European Journal of Neuroscience, 35,* 1646–1654.

Alexander, A. L., Lee, J. E., Lazar, M., & Field, A. S. (2007). Diffusion tensor imaging of the brain. *Neurotherapeutics, 7,* 316–329.

Amlien, I. K., & Fjell, A. M. (2014). Diffusion tensor imaging of white matter degeneration in Alzheimer's disease and mild cognitive impairment. *Neuroscience, 276,* 206–215.

Balser, N., Lorey, B., Pilgramm, S., Naumann, T., Kindermann, S., Stark, R., ... Munzert, J. (2014). The influence of expertise on brain activation of the action observation network during anticipation of tennis and volleyball serves. *Frontiers in Human Neuroscience, 8,* 1–13.

Brown, M. A., & Semelka, R. C., (2010). *MRI: basic principles and applications* (4th ed.), Hoboken, NJ: Wiley- Blackwell.

Burzynska, A. Z., Wong, C. N., Chaddock-Heyman, L., Olson, E. A., Gothe, N. P., Knecht, A., ... Kramer, A. F. (2016). White matter integrity, hippocampal volume, and cognitive performance of a world-famous nonagenarian track-and-field athlete. *Neurocase, 22,* 135–144.

Chang, Y., Lee, J. J., Seo, J. H., Song, H. J., Kim, Y. T., Lee, H. J., ... Kim, J. G. (2011). Neural correlates of motor imagery for elite archers. *NMR in Biomedicine, 24,* 366–372.

de Gois Vasconcelos, L., Dozzi Brucki, S. M., Parolin Jackowiski, A., Francisco, O., & Bueno, A. (2009). Diffusion tensor imaging for Alzheimer's disease: A review on concepts and potential clinical applicability. *Dementia & Neuropsychologia, 3,* 268–274.

Di, X., Zhu, S., Jin, H., Wang, P., Ye, Z., Zhou, K., ... Rao, H. (2012). Altered resting brain function and structure in professional badminton players. *Brain Connect, 2,* 225–233.

Dolan, R. J. (2008). Neuroimaging of cognition: Past, Present, and Future. *Neuron, 60,* 496–502.

Gold, B. T. (2012). White matter integrity and vulnerability to Alzheimer's disease: Preliminary findings and future directions. *Biochemica et Biophysica Acta, 1822,* 416–422.

Haller, S., & Bartsch, A. J. (2009). Pitfalls in FMRI. *European Radiology, 19,* 2689–2709.

Hanggi, J., Langer, N., Lutz, K., Birrer, K., Merillat, S., & Jancke, L. (2015). Structural brain correlates associated with professional handball playing. *PLoS One, 10,* 1–27.

Huang, R., Lu, M., Song, Z., & Wang, J. (2015). Long-term intensive training induced brain structural change in world class gymnasts. *Brain Structure and Function, 220,* 625–644.

Jellison, B. J., Field, A. S., Medow, J., Lazer, M., Salamat, M. S., & Alexander, A. L. (2004). Diffusion tensor imaging of cerebral white matter: A pictorial review of physics, fibre tract anatomy, and tumor imaging patterns. *American Journal of Neuroradiology, 25,* 356–369.

Jezzard, P., & Clare, S. (2001). Principles of nuclear magnetic resonance and MRI. In P. Jezzard, P. M. Matthews, & S. Smith (Eds.), *Functional MRI: An introduction to methods* (pp. 67–92). Oxford, UK: Oxford University Press.

Jones, D. K., & Leemans, A. (2011). Diffusion tensor imaging. *Methods in Molecular Biology, 711,* 127–144.

Keller, J., Rulseh, A. M., Komarek, A., Latnerova, I., Rusina, R., Brozova, H., & Vymazal, J. (2013). New non-linear color look-up table for visualization of brain fractional anisotropy based on normative measurements – principals and first clinical use. *PLoS One, 8,* 1–7.

Kim, S. G., & Ugurbil, K. (2003). High-resolution functional magnetic resonance imaging of the animal brain. *Methods, 30,* 28–41.

Kim, W., Chang, Y., Kim, J., Seo, J., Ryu, K., Lee, E., … Janelle, C. M. (2014). A fMRI study of differences in brain activity among elite, expert, and novice archers at the moment of optimal aiming. *Cognitive and Behavioural Neurology, 27,* 173–182.

Mori, S., & Zhang, J. (2009). Diffusion tensor imaging. In L. R. Squire (Ed.), *Encyclopedia of neuroscience* (pp. 531–538). London, UK: Elsevier Ltd.

Naito, E., & Hirose, S. (2014). Efficient foot motor control by Neymar's brain. *Frontiers in Human Neuroscience, 8,* 1–7.

Ogawa, S., Tank, D. W., Menon, R., Ellermann, J. M., Jim, S. G., Merkle, H., Ugurbil, K. (1992). Intrinsic signal changes accompanying sensory stimulation: functional brain mapping with magnetic resonance imaging. *PNAS, 89,* 5951–5955.

Rosen, B. R., Buckner, R. L., & Dale, A. M. (1998). Event-related functional MRI: past, present, and future. *PNAS, 95,* 773–780.

Schlaffke, L., Lissek, S., Lenz, M., Brune, M., Juckel, G., Hinrichs, … Schmidt-Wilcke, T. (2014). Sports and brain morphology – a voxel-based morphometry study with endurance athletes and martial artists. *Neuroscience, 259,* 35–42.

Stebbins, G. T., & Murphy, C. M. (2009). Diffusion tensor imaging in Alzheimer's disease and mild cognitive impairment. *Behavioural Neurology, 21,* 39–49.

Soares, J. M., Marques, P., Alves, V., & Sousa, N. (2013). A hitchhiker's guide to diffusion tensor imaging. *Frontiers in Neuroscience, 7,* 1–14.

Taubert, M., Wenzel, U., Draganski, B., Kiebel, S., Ragert, P., Krug, J., & Villringer, A. (2015). Investigating neuroanatomical features in top athletes at the single subject level. *PLoS One, 10,* 1–15.

Wei, G., & Luo, J. (2010). Sport expert's motor imagery: Functional imaging of professional motor skills and simple motor skills. *Brain Research, 1341,* 52–62.

Wenzel, U., Taubert, M., Ragert, P., Krug, J., & Villringer, A. (2014). Functional and structural correlates of motor speed in the cerebellar anterior lobe. *PLoS One, 9,* 1–8.

Zhang, B., Xu, Y., Zang, B., & Kantarci, K. (2014). The role of diffusion tensor imaging in detecting microstructural changes in prodromal Alzheimer's disease. *CNS Neuroscience & Therapeutics, 20,* 3–9.

fMRI in Sport and Performance Research

A Synthesis of Research Findings

Daniel T. Bishop and Michael J. Wright

Introduction

Functional magnetic resonance imaging, or fMRI, is a noninvasive neuroimaging technique for detecting changes in blood flow and oxygenation that occur as a function of changes in brain activity. Specifically, when a brain area is more active, it requires more oxygen. To meet this demand, there is an increase in blood flow to the active area and an associated increase in oxygen turnover, culminating in changes in the magnetic properties of our blood. An MRI scanner houses a very powerful electromagnet, with a typical magnetic field strength of 3 Tesla—about 50,000 times greater than the Earth's field. Protons within atomic nuclei are typically randomly oriented within our bodies, but temporarily align themselves with the scanner's magnetic field once within it. In fMRI studies, the orientation of these protons is perturbed by series of radio waves (RF pulses), before they then return to their resting state within the static field; the consequent release of energy results in a measureable signal—known as the blood oxygen level-dependent (BOLD) signal. The BOLD signal strength varies according to the protons' surroundings—i.e., the ratio of oxyhemoglobin to deoxyhemoglobin—which enables us to differentiate between grey matter, white matter and cerebrospinal fluid in the resulting images.

Although fMRI only provides us with a correlate of neural activity, its inception still represented a considerable step in our ability to investigate and understand neural function; for example, it is unquestionably more objective than self-report questionnaires. It also possesses excellent spatial resolution (approximately 3 mm at 3 Tesla) although its temporal resolution is limited; the blood response to increases in neuronal activity is in the order of a few seconds. However, because of its high spatial resolution, the technique has been successfully used to achieve a number of important aims, such as mapping the human retinotopic cortex (Engel et al., 1994), and demonstrating that attention modulates fundamental perceptual processing (O'Craven, Rosen, Kwong, Savoy, & Treisman, 2000; O'Craven, Rosen, Kwong, Treisman, & Savoy, 1997), although some have argued that fMRI has done little to advance our knowledge of cognitive processes, for example (Diener, 2010; Page, 2006); concerns that are highly pertinent to most sport and performance-based fMRI studies to date.

Thirteen years after the first fMRI publication (Kwong et al., 1992), Calvo-Merino and colleagues published their seminal investigation of action observation in expert ballet and capoeira dancers (Calvo-Merino, Glaser, Grèzes, Passingham, & Haggard, 2005). Since then, there has been a surge in sport and performance-related fMRI studies, with diverse objectives, methodological approaches, and outcomes. The end result has been a profusion of task-related activations in equally diverse brain regions. However, recent reviews and meta-analyses of the neuroscience literature pertaining to expertise in sport has lent some coherence to this burgeoning body of work (e.g., Moran, Guillot, MacIntyre, & Collet, 2012; Smith, 2016; Yang, 2015; Yarrow, Brown, & Krakauer, 2009). The result is that we now know a good deal more about brain activity related to sport performance than we did a decade ago. However, the present time is an appropriate juncture at which to re-examine what we (think we) know—not least in light of recent revelations pertaining to the validity of many fMRI studies that have been conducted in the past two decades (Eklund, Nichols, & Knutsson, 2016)

In this chapter, we will provide a critical overview of the body of literature that has been devoted to the use of fMRI in attempts to elucidate the neural processes that underpin performance in sport and related areas, in a variety of contexts including anticipation and prediction tasks, motor preparation, motor imagery, action observation, manipulation of affective state, and investigation of brain injury. We also discuss some of the limitations of fMRI, potential alternatives or complementary techniques, methodological considerations, and future research directions. In doing so, we have drawn on our own observations, those of the original authors, and recent reviews.

Investigations of Motor Expertise

Until fairly recently, it was believed that the brain was only capable of reorganization during its development—i.e., from fertilization to late adolescence. However, it has since been established that even the adult central nervous system is capable of adaptive changes and substantial cortical reorganization; and numerous studies have since shown that the neural representation of the adult cerebral cortex can change considerably as a result of practice (Bezzola, Mérillat, & Jäncke, 2012; Herholz & Zatorre, 2012; Nakata, Yoshie, Miura, & Kudo, 2010). Practice may bring about an increase or a decrease in brain activation associated with performance of a task, or it may result in a combination of activation increases and decreases across many brain areas, i.e., a functional reorganization of brain activity such as the expansion of brain activity or increases in the strength of activation (Kelly & Garavan, 2005). Increases in activity have been observed for task-specific areas such as motor cortex (Baeck et al., 2012), posterior parietal cortex (Kim et al., 2011; Stout, Passingham, Frith, Apel, & Chaminade, 2011), and lateral temporal cortex associated with the storage of those representations (Calvo-Merino et al., 2005). Conversely, a decrease in activity occurs in areas involved cognitive control and attentional processes, including prefrontal cortex (Petrini et al., 2011) and anterior cingulate cortex (Seo et al., 2012), arguably an increase in what has recently been referred to as 'neural efficiency'—a term that has most frequently been mooted in EEG studies (e.g., Babiloni et al., 2010; Del Percio et al., 2009; Kim et al., 2014; Ludyga, Gronwald, & Hottenrott, 2015; Zhu et al., 2011).

In order to examine cortical functional reorganization, fMRI researchers have typically recruited a group of participants with extensive experience of a given motor task (e.g., athletes, musicians, professional dancers) and a novice control group, to compare their brain activity during performance of a motor task related to the experts' skill. The bulk of this research has shown that motor expertise mediates brain activity during motor execution (Bernardi et al., 2013) and preparation (Milton, Solodkin, Hluštík, & Small, 2007), action observation (Kim et al., 2011; Olsson & Lundström, 2013), motor imagery (Chang et al., 2011; Wei & Luo, 2010), and anticipation tasks (Abreu et al., 2012; Balser, Lorey, Pilgramm, Naumann, et al., 2014; Bishop, Wright, Jackson, & Abernethy, 2013); it even does so for the comprehension of action language (Beilock, Lyons, Mattarella-Micke, Nusbaum, & Small, 2008; Lyons et al., 2010).

The findings are varied, in terms of the extent and locations of the activations observed. fMRI studies have shown that, compared with novices, motor experts showed increased activity in motor and premotor areas (e.g., Baeck et al., 2012; Wright, Bishop, Jackson, & Abernethy, 2013), areas related to attentional processes (Petrini et al., 2011; Seo et al., 2012), areas involved in episodic memory retrieval (Kim et al., 2011), and subcortical motor control regions such as the basal ganglia

(Bishop et al., 2013; Landau & D'Esposito, 2006). Conversely, it is also not uncommon to see relatively lower levels of neural activity in experts, when compared to novices—again, across multiple brain regions. For example, recent fMRI studies have shown that experts exhibit reduced brain activity in ventral and dorsal premotor cortex, supplementary motor area, superior parietal lobule, anterior cingulate cortex, basal ganglia, and cerebellum during motor tasks (Chang et al., 2011; Haslinger et al., 2005; Milton et al., 2007; Wright, Bishop, Jackson, & Abernethy, 2010)—further evidence for neural efficiency (Babiloni et al., 2010; Del Percio et al., 2008; Ludyga et al., 2015; Zhu et al., 2011).

Anticipation, Prediction, and Motor Preparation

In the first fMRI study of anticipation skill, Wright and Jackson (2007) asked nine novice tennis players watched video clips of tennis serves, from the returner's perspective; they also viewed sequences in which the player moved around the baseline area (as occurs between points), and static images. Their task was to predict the direction of the serve (left vs. right), by pressing one of two buttons on an MR-compatible button box; they pressed a middle button for the non-serve and static stimuli. Motion-sensitive regions of late visual cortices, namely MT/MST, and superior temporal sulcus in the posterior part of the temporal lobe, were active during observation of serve and non-serve stimuli, relative to the static controls. Serve sequences produced additional activation in bilateral inferior parietal lobule, right superior parietal lobule and in dorsal and ventral parts of inferior frontal gyrus; components of the 'mirror neuron system' (MNS; Rizzolatti & Craighero, 2004) that were not activated by non-serve sequences. From this, the authors concluded that neural processing of motion per se could be differentiated from the activity of the MNS. Wright and colleagues subsequently observed greater activation of MNS components in expert badminton players, relative to intermediate and novice players (Wright et al., 2010; Wright, Bishop, Jackson, & Abernethy, 2011). More recently, the same group of authors examined deceptive manoeuvres in soccer (Bishop et al., 2013; Wright et al., 2013). In addition to the expected stronger activations in MNS components, the authors also observed activation in experts, of a sub-region of anterior cingulate cortex—one that appears to have a role in conflict monitoring, i.e., detecting when there is a disparity between perception and action (Lütcke & Frahm, 2008; Lütcke, Gevensleben, Albrecht, & Frahm, 2009). This is an interesting finding, not least because of its appearance in these two deception-focused studies, which may ultimately tell us something about the ways in which experts deal with opponents' deliberately deceptive maneuvers.

Petrini et al. (2011) asked 11 drummers and 11 age- and gender-matched novices to make judgments as to whether point-light drumming movements with accompanying sound exhibited visual-auditory synchronization or asynchrony, for a series of edited clips in which the degree of synchrony was manipulated. In a second experiment, sound and video were always synchronized, but the natural covariation between sound intensity and velocity of the drumming strike was either maintained or eliminated. For both experiments, the authors observed a reduction in activation of motor and action representation regions of the drummers' brains when the sound matched the observed movements, and was comparable to that of novices when the two were mismatched. The authors suggested that brain functions in action-sound representation areas may be modulated by multimodal action expertise. This finding, and the manipulations used by Petrini et al., can readily be applied to a variety of sport performance contexts in which auditory information is a key determinant of the athlete's ability to execute the skill. Indeed, such audiovisual interaction has been demonstrated in table tennis (Bischoff et al., 2014).

In a study of basketball anticipatory skill, Abreu et al. (2012) used fMRI to determine whether expert basketballers' ability to predict the fate of free throws is underpinned by neural regions over-and-above the action observation network (AON). Indeed, the AON was comparably activated in novices and experts. Notably, athletes exhibited relatively greater activity in the extrastriate body area during the prediction task, which may have been due to their superior reading of the observed kinematics. There was also evidence for error monitoring (cf. Bishop et al., 2013; Wright et al., 2013), in right anterior insular cortex when they made errors. Correct action prediction was associated with greater posterior insular cortex activity in experts and stronger orbitofrontal activity in novices; the authors speculated that body awareness was important for the experts' performance monitoring, whereas the novices relied more on higher-order decision-making strategies. However, studies of embodied cognition suggest that the congruence of one's posture is crucial for the pickup of relevant information (Niedenthat, 2007), and so this assertion could be explored in light of this prevalent viewpoint.

Balser et al. (2014) explored whether motor expertise led to a differential activation pattern according to expertise level and the type of anticipation required. Expert and novice tennis players observed video clips in which forehand strokes were depicted; their task was to either indicate the predicted direction of ball flight (spatial anticipation) or to decide on an appropriate response to the observed action (motor anticipation). Not only did the experts perform better than novices on both tasks, but they also exhibited stronger neural activation in AON regions—namely, superior parietal lobe, intraparietal sulcus, inferior frontal gyrus, and the cerebellum. Novices displayed greater activation in the ventral premotor cortex, supplementary motor area, and superior parietal lobe during motor anticipation than during spatial anticipation. But in experts, there were no such difference, which the authors postulated was a reflection of the experts' use of more fine-tuned motor representations, which they have acquired and refined over years of training. Consistent with the findings discussed above, Balser et al.'s findings suggest that the neural processing of different anticipation tasks depends on the player's level of expertise.

fMRI has also been used to examine motor preparation prior to performance—albeit in the scanner. For example, in their investigation of golfers' motor preparation during pre-shot routines, Milton et al. (2007) found that, compared with novices, experienced golfers exhibited greater activation in the dorsal premotor cortex, occipital cortex, and superior parietal lobule. Conversely, the extent of activation in novices was more extensive, including regions as diverse as anterior medial prefrontal cortex, a region that is active during the assimilation of two separate cognitive operations in order to attain a behavioral goal (Ramnani & Owen, 2004); middle cingulate cortex, a region that subserves emotion processing (Vogt, Berger, & Derbyshire, 2003), basal ganglia (motor control and reward processing; Schultz, 2016); and anterior temporal lobe, which has been implicated in person-related processing, of a variety of stimuli and in a variety of contexts (Wong & Gallate, 2012). Milton et al. suggested that, through extensive practice, the experts had developed more efficient organization of neural resources, whereas the novices recruited considerably more of their resources in order to process irrelevant information (e.g., inhibition). However, given the diversity of activations described above, the explanation may not be so straightforward. There is no question that recruitment of greater resources, be they task-related or otherwise, is by definition 'less efficient'. However, because the novices' activations are in a number of regions that bear little relation to those required in order to perform experimental task, there may be other processes at work. For example, the concurrent enhanced activation in cingulate cortex and anterior temporal lobe may reflect novices' greater self-evaluative affective judgments during performance of the task. In their examination of expert and novice archers' preparation for motor execution, Kim et al. (2008) found comparable activation in anterior cingulate cortex—although the coordinates for this activation are similar to those found previously in studies of deception in soccer (Bishop et al., 2013; Wright et al., 2013); hence, it may reflect error processing, rather than self-evaluation.

Daniel T. Bishop and Michael J. Wright

Action Observation, Motor Imagery and Visuospatial Ability

Using positron emission tomography, Brown and colleagues (2006) showed that performance of complex dance steps exhibited strong overlap with observation, but investigators have since used fMRI to examine and compare the neural processes that underpin observational and physical experience when learning or perceiving complex motor skills (Calvo-Merino, Grèzes, Glaser, Passingham, & Haggard, 2006; Cross, Kraemer, Hamilton, Kelley, & Grafton, 2009). For example, in their pioneering study, Calvo-Merino et al. (2005) reported that expert ballet and capoeira dancers showed stronger bilateral activation in premotor cortex and intraparietal sulcus, and greater activation in right superior parietal lobule and left posterior superior temporal sulcus, when they watched videos of their own dance form, as compared with conditions in which they viewed the dance style for which they had not been trained (e.g., ballet dancers observing capoeira actions); the authors concluded that the observer's personal motor repertoire is crucial for understanding observed actions—a notion that has been corroborated since (Calvo-Merino et al., 2006; Cross, Hamilton, & Grafton, 2006).

Since Calvo-Merino et al.'s seminal study, a considerable body of work has been devoted to the investigation of the observation and execution of dance movements (Brown et al., 2006; Cross et al., 2006; Orgs, Dombrowski, Heil, & Jansen-Osmann, 2008). Observation of many dance forms (as well as other skilled whole-body actions such as gymnastics) elicits comparable activation in the brain to that elicited during actual physical execution (Calvo-Merino et al., 2006; Cross, Mackie, Wolford, & Hamilton, 2010; Cross, Stadler, Parkinson, Schütz-Bosbach, & Prinz, 2013).

Cross et al. (2006) investigated contemporary dancers' learning of a complex 30-minute contemporary dance piece, over a period of eight weeks. The dancers' brain activity was recorded for six consecutive weeks as they watched and imagined themselves performing short segments from the dance piece being learnt; they also viewed kinematically similar dance movements that had neither seen nor rehearsed (cf. Calvo-Merino et al., 2005). Throughout the rehearsal period the dancers understandably improved considerably in terms of their physical performance. But as they did so, activity within two core regions of the AON—the left inferior parietal lobule and the left ventral premotor cortex—exhibited activity that correlated strongly with the dancers' level of proficiency—evidence that, the more expert one becomes, then the more 'embodied' that action becomes.

Cross and colleagues (2009) asked novice dancers to learn novel dance sequences in a video game context. All participants physically practiced six sequences and passively observed a further six different sequences, over a five-day training period. Participants' brain activity was recorded immediately prior to, and after, training as they viewed the music videos for all practiced and observed dance sequences; they also watched videos for which they received no training. The authors found that observational experience yielded a performance advantage relative to those sequences for which participants received no training. Of even greater interest was the fact that responses within left IPL and right premotor cortex (two key components of the AON) were more comparable when observing danced and watched sequences compared to untrained sequences. This was one of the first neuroimaging studies to show that mere action observation can engender similar neural representations to those derived from physical practice (Cross et al., 2009), consistent with the functional equivalence hypothesis (Beilock & Lyons, 2009; Decety, 1996) and Bandura's (1986) early hypothesis.

To summarize the corpus of work stemming from Calvo-Merino et al.'s (2005) original study, Cross, Acquah, and Ramsey (2014) conducted a critical review of neuroscientific investigations of dance. Table 6.1 summarizes the findings from fMRI studies in Cross et al.'s review.

Table 6.1 Summary of fMRI studies in Cross et al's review and critical analysis

Study	Dance style	Sample	Primary research question	Finding
Calvo-Merino et al. 2005	Classical ballet; capoeira	10 ballet & nine capoeira experts; 10 non-dancers. All male	Is the brain's system for action observation precisely tuned to the individual's acquired motor repertoire?	Premotor, parietal, and posterior temporal cortices showed greater responses when participants observed actions within their motor repertoire (e.g., ballet dancers watching ballet moves).
Calvo-Merino et al. 2006	Classical ballet	24 M/F professional ballet dancers	Is activation of regions within the action AON representative specifically of motor knowledge or of a more general knowledge of an action (e.g., visual knowledge)?	Activation in premotor, parietal and cerebellar cortices specific to motor representation.
Calvo-Merino et al. 2008	Classical ballet	Six male non-dancers	How does variation in aesthetic responses to dance movements correlate with neural activation?	Medial visual cortices & right premotor cortex exhibited higher activation for liked movements. Stronger activation for whole body movements.
Cross et al. 2006	Contemporary Dance	10 M/F expert contemporary dancers	How do brain regions engaged in action observation and perception change as complex movements transition from unlearned to well-embodied?	Left PMv and IPL activity increased with increasing performance ability. AON activation more nuanced with expertise.
Cross, Kraemer, et al. 2009	Video game dance (step sequences in StepMania, an open source version of the popular video game Dance Dance Revolution™)	16 M/F non-dancers	How are physical and observational learning of complex, whole-body action sequences represented at brain and behavioral levels?	Learning (pre-posttest; as measured by video game scores) for physical practice (PP) > passive action observation (AO) > no practice. After training, a subset of AON regions (left IPL and right premotor cortex) did not discriminate when watching dance sequences learned via PP or AO.
Cross, Hamilton, et al. 2009	Video game dance (step sequences in StepMania, an open source version of the popular video game Dance Dance Revolution™)	16 M/F non-dancers (Additional analysis of Cross et al., 2009)	Is the AON tuned to learn from/ respond to only human actions, or might these brain regions also respond to symbolic, non-human cues for motor learning?	Individual AON components responded to PP and AO. Bilateral superior temporal sulcus preferentially responded to stimuli comprising a human form. Right PMv responded most to videos that participants had physically practiced (regardless of presence of human form).

(continued)

Study	Dance style	Sample	Primary research question	Finding
Cross et al. 2010	Static contortion postures	18 M/F non-dancers	How do body-sensitive brain regions respond to body postures within an observer's repertoire compared to those beyond their abilities (contorted postures)?	EBA & fusiform body area more responsive to contorted postures. Reduced activity within the AON & fusiform gyrus for repeated postures, independent of viewpoint.
Cross et al. 2011	Classical ballet/ contemporary dance	22 M/F Non-dancers	How is observers' aesthetic evaluation of dance related to their perceived physical ability to reproduce the movements they watch?	Participants reported preference for movements they would find difficult to execute. Interaction between liking and physical ability represented within occipitotemporal and parietal regions.
Cross et al. 2012	Club dancing/robotic breakdancing	45 M/F non-dancers (split across two independent experiments)	How do form (human vs. robot) and motion (rigid vs. fluid) cues interact and impact action perception within the AON?	Core AON regions responded more strongly to robotic, rigid movements, independent of form (robot or human).
Grosbras et al. 2012 fMRI & rTMS	Contemporary dance	16 M/F non-dancers	Which brain areas play a causal role in emotion processing during dance observation?	Emotional responses correlated negatively with activity in right posterior parietal cortex. rTMS over this area enhanced emotional responses to dance segments eliciting positive emotions.
Jola et al. 2013	Unedited 6.5 minute "padam" section of a Bharatanatyam performance (classical Indian dance) with music	12 M/F naïve observers unfamiliar with Indian dance and with no musical training	Is enhanced activity in audio, visual and audiovisual (AV) brain areas (e.g. superior temporal gyrus; STG) synchronized over time across subjects when they are presented with multisensory stimuli?	Brain activity significantly correlated across subjects in auditory (e.g., Heschl's gyrus), visual (e.g., lingual gyrus) and multisensory processing (e.g., STG) areas. No synchronization found in higher-order areas (e.g., areas implicated in cognition, action, and emotion tasks), suggesting that by presenting an unfamiliar dance, correspondence between subjects' is constrained to a sensory level.
Miura et al. 2010	Humanoid robot dance, human dance, moving objects (mosaics)	49 M/F participants (dance experience not reported)	What are the neural effects of motion smoothness and intersubjective variability in attitudes about art during dance observation?	Higher activity in brain areas sensitive to motion and body cues for smooth actions. AON activity was modulated by intersubjective variability in personal attitudes toward art.

In a study not included in Cross et al.'s (2014) review, Pilgramm et al. (2010) examined the influences of motor expertise and visual viewpoint (e.g., internal vs. external viewpoint) on the activity of the ventral and dorsal premotor cortex during motor observation, in groups of expert and novice dancers. They found a functional dissociation between the ventral and dorsal premotor cortex. Motor experts revealed increased activity in the ventral premotor cortex, which is involved in processing visuospatial object properties for grasping (Majdandzic, Bekkering, van Schie, & Toni, 2009), whereas visual viewpoint influenced activity in both ventral and dorsal premotor cortex; the latter is involved in using arbitrary rules to guide advance motor planning (Majdandzic et al., 2009). This suggests that (a) the experts were possibly more skilled in the 'mental rotation' required to observe another's movement, irrespective of viewpoint, and (b) viewpoint manipulations may be a fruitful means by which observational learning is consolidated.

In an fMRI study of expert divers' imagery ability, Wei and Luo (2010) found stronger activation in left parahippocampal gyrus and right fusiform gyrus during diving imagery as compared to gymnastic imagery; both of these structures are implicated in the retrieval of long-term spatial memories (Nadel & Peterson, 2013) and viewpoint-dependent object recognition and mental rotation (Wilson & Farah, 2006), respectively. In a subsequent investigation of generalized cognitive abilities in athletes, Sekiguchi et al. (2011) compared the levels of 20 top-level rugby players' brain activity during a mental rotation task to that of 20 matched novices. The aim of the task was to rapidly judge whether two concurrently presented shapes were identical. Although there were no group differences in task performance, the authors observed greater activation in right superior parietal lobe, lateral occipital cortex, and right medial prefrontal cortex in the experts. Sekiguchi et al. (2011) concluded that top-level rugby players used a different strategy to that of the novices; specifically, the postulated that the rugby players were able to take a 'bird's eye view' of the to-be-judged shapes—although the activation in right medial prefrontal cortex, part of the 'default-mode network' (Raichle & Snyder, 2007), implied that this strategy may have come at an additional cost, in terms of cognitive load. This is at odds with a more recent investigation of racing car drivers, who exhibited reduced activation in task-related areas, and increased functional connectivity between those regions, as they completed a visuospatial task (Bernardi et al., 2014). The notion of generalized visuospatial abilities as a potential determinant of sporting success is not a novel one, but fMRI studies such as these will help us to better understand the differences between experts and novices. It is straightforward to see how professional divers may require exceptional mental rotation ability, but the link between rugby and such ability is not so apparent, despite Sekiguchi et al.'s hypotheses.

The ability to imagine actions within one's sporting repertoire may also be reflected in one's interpretations of action language (Beilock et al., 2008). Tomasino, Maieron, Guatto, Fabbro, and Rumiati (2013) acquired fMRI data from ten expert volleyball players and ten novices, all of whom were presented with a series of sentences that described viable volleyball-specific motor acts and ones that are impossible; all were framed both in positive ("Do …!") or negative ("Don't …") commands. The participants' task was to silently read the commands and determine whether the actions were technically feasible or not. All participants' response times were shorter for the positive contexts than the negative ones. Positive and negative action-related commands modulated activity in left frontoparietal regions, as well as in the hand region of the primary motor and premotor cortices; specifically, in the athletes, the activity of left M1 hand area and of the left premotor cortex significantly decreased when participants processed impossible action sentences which were presented as positive commands ("Do…[an impossible action]"). This evidence suggests that coaches may be able to influence their athletes' ability to engage suitably in motor imagery, by judicious use of language.

fMRI Studies of Motor Expertise: A Meta-Analysis (Yang, 2015)

In an attempt to lend some coherence to fMRI investigation of motor expertise, Yang (2015) identified 39 studies in music and sport domains, in which the brain activity of motor experts and that of novices were compared during tasks related to motor experience, motor imagery, motor observation, motor planning, motor anticipation, and the comprehension of action language. Additionally, only those studies that reported whole-brain analyses, giving activation coordinates in Talairach (Talairach & Tournoux, 1988) or Montreal Neurological Institute (MNI) space, were analyzed. This resulted in 26 studies, which she entered into a meta-analysis; Table 6.2 details the studies (for a more detailed table, please refer to the original article). Yang applied four contrasts to the data—namely, all activations for which experts exhibited greater activation in motor tasks than in non-motor baseline tasks; the same as previous, but for novices; an expert-novice contrast for motor tasks, for activations that were stronger in the experts; and the same contrast, but for which novice activations were stronger. The author also conducted a fifth set of contrasts, in which different task types were compared. Specifically, she contrasted expert and novice activations for motor execution tasks, ones for motor (action) observation tasks, and those for which a prediction was required. Motor imagery task types were excluded, due to the low number of studies that met the inclusion criteria.

Yang (2015) used Ginger ALE 2.3.1 software (www.brainmap.org/ale; Eickhoff et al., 2009) to perform the meta-analysis, in standard Talairach space. Some of the findings were reported in MNI (Montreal Neurological Institute) coordinates (NB: there are two commonly used 'neural atlases' for mapping activations onto a template brain; see http://imaging.mrc-cbu.cam.ac.uk/imaging/MniTalairach for a brief but enlightening discussion of the differences between the two), but were transformed into Talairach space using the icbm2tal transformation (Lancaster et al., 2007). The ALE program considers each activation focus included in the meta-analysis as the center of a probability distribution, rather than a discrete locus within the brain. Hence, it assumes that the activation is most likely located at the reported coordinate, but that it might also be nearby; this is somewhat akin to the use of confidence intervals, as opposed to point estimates, in statistics.

Yang conducted random-effects analyses, which enable her to draw conclusions beyond the studies included in the meta-analysis, and compared the resultant ALE map with a null distribution, to distinguish random convergence and true convergence (i.e., instances where foci from different studies might have overlapped by chance vs. those that were likely to be genuine overlaps). The author then identified voxels in which activation maps converged more robustly than would have been expected under the null distribution. The resulting clusters, significant at the threshold of p <0.05 (False Discovery Rate [FDR] correction) with a default minimum cluster size of 200 mm^3, are summarized in Table 6.3.

In summary, Yang's (2015) findings showed that, in the case of action observation, motor experts exhibited stronger activation in the left precentral gyrus (BA 6). This is a region that comprises both premotor cortex and supplementary area, both of which are components of the AON (Rizzolatti, Cattaneo, Fabbri-Destro, & Rozzi, 2014; Rizzolatti & Maddalena Fabbri, 2007). Hence, the data seem to reliably show that there is an effect of expertise on activation of this network; specifically, as people become more proficient, then there is more extensive activation of these regions (cf. Cross et al., 2006) For all tasks combined, motor experts indicated stronger effects in both ventral and dorsal premotor areas than did novices. The premotor cortex plays an important role in the sensory guidance of motor behavior (Chouinard & Paus, 2006); dorsal premotor cortex is involved in execution of limb movements (Hoshi & Tanji, 2007), and ventral premotor cortex is important for matching an observed motor act with a concurrently or subsequently executed action (Hoshi & Tanji, 2007; Newman-Norlund, van Schie, van Zuijlen, & Bekkering, 2007). Hence, it is perhaps unsurprising, given the relative motor experience of the experts, that such differences are observed.

Motor experts also displayed stronger activation in posterior parietal cortex (PPC) during both motor execution and action prediction. This region is important for the production of planned movements that involve the hand and arm, such as reaching, grasping, and tool use (Vingerhoets,

Table 6.2 Studies included in Yang's (2015) meta-analysis

Authors	Year	Motor expertise	Task	No. of experts	No. of novices	Foci-expert	Foci-novice	Foci-contrast
Abreu et al.	2012	Playing basketball	Motor prediction	16	16	yes	yes	
Balser et al.	2014	Playing tennis	Motor prediction	16	16	yes	yes	yes
Baumann et al.	2007	Piano playing	Motor execution	7	7			yes
Berkowitz and Ansari	2010	Piano playing	Motor execution	13	15			yes
Bernardi et al.	2013	Driving racing-car	Motor execution	11	11			yes
Bishop et al.	2013	Playing soccer	Motor prediction	14	11			yes
Chang et al.	2011	Archery	Motor imagery	18	18	yes	yes	yes
Harris and de Jong	2014	Playing keyboard	Motor imagery	12	12			yes
Hasegawa et al.	2004	Piano playing	Motor observation	9	7	yes	yes	
Haslinger et al.	2004	Piano playing	Motor execution	12	12			yes
Haslinger et al	2005	Piano playing	Motor observation	12	12			yes
Kim et al.	2011	Archery	Motor observation	20	21	yes	yes	yes
Kim et al.	2008	Archery	Motor planning	8	8	yes	yes	
Landau and D'esposito	2006	Piano playing	Motor execution	9	8	yes	yes	yes
Lee and Noppeney	2011	Piano playing	Music listening	18	19			yes
Meister et al.	2005	Piano playing	Motor execution	12	12	yes	yes	yes
Olsson and Lundstrom	2013	Playing hockey	Motor observation	3	3	yes	yes	
Pau et al.	2013	Playing	Piano	14	15			yes
Petrini et al.	2011	Drumming	Motor prediction	11	11			yes
Pilgramm et al.	2010	Dancing	Motor observation	18	18			yes
Seo et al.	2012	Archery	Visuospatial memory	20	23	yes	yes	yes
Stout et al.	2011	Making tools	Motor observation	5	11	yes	yes	
Tomasino et al.	2013	Playing volleyball	Motor language processing	10	10			yes
Wei and Luo	2010	Diving	Motor imagery	12	12	yes	yes	
Wright et al.	2013	Playing soccer	Motor observation	17	17	yes	yes	yes
Wright et al.	2011	Playing badminton	Motor prediction	8	8			

Table 6.3 Results of Yang's (2015) meta-analysis

Volume	x	y	z	Hemisphere	Region	BA
Experts (13 studies, 256 foci)						
4552	−36	−46	38	Left	Inferior parietal lobule	40
	−24	−54	50	Left	Precuneus	7
	−30	−56	42	Left	Inferior parietal lobule	7
	−24	−58	50	Left	Precuneus	7
	−28	−54	50	Left	Precuneus	7
	−32	−48	52	Left	Superior parietal lobule	7
3216	40	−40	54	Right	Inferior parietal lobule	40
	34	−50	44	Right	Inferior parietal lobule	40
2312	−22	−12	54	Left	Middle frontal gyrus	6
	−36	−16	62	Left	Precentral gyrus	4
2192	26	−12	54	Right	Middle frontal gyrus	6
	24	−6	58	Right	Middle frontal gyrus	6
1072	−52	6	26	Left	Inferior frontal gyrus	9
1000	54	8	32	Right	Inferior frontal gyrus	9
552	0	12	48	Left	Superior frontal gyrus	6
	6	8	42	Right	Cingulate gyrus	32
488	22	−66	50	Right	Precuneus	7
480	−38	−6	36	Left	Precentral gyrus	6
472	4	−10	64	Right	Medial frontal gyrus	6
248	−32	16	4	Left	Claustrum	
248	12	−24	14	Right	Thalamus	
200	30	18	6	Right	Claustrum	
Novices (13 studies, 256 foci)						
5784	−24	−8	54	Left	Middle Frontal Gyrus	6
	−6	−2	58	Left	Medial Frontal Gyrus	6
	2	−6	64	Right	Medial Frontal Gyrus	6
	−2	4	46	Left	Medial Frontal Gyrus	32
	−2	12	46	Left	Medial Frontal Gyrus	6
4288	−30	−54	50	Left	Superior Parietal Lobule	7
	−34	−42	42	Left	Inferior Parietal Lobule	40
	−26	−56	54	Left	Precuneus	7
3368	32	−44	44	Right	Inferior Parietal Lobule	40
	30	−52	44	Right	Superior Parietal Lobule	7
2656	24	−14	54	Right	Middle Frontal Gyrus	6
872	10	−72	44	Right	Precuneus	7
848	40	0	32	Right	Precentral Gyrus	6
	50	4	30	Right	Inferior Frontal Gyrus	9
736	−12	−68	50	Left	Precuneus	7
336	−50	4	22	Left	Inferior Frontal Gyrus	9
240	30	−52	−24	Right	Cerebellum	
232	−50	−40	34	Left	Supramarginal Gyrus	40
Experts > novices (15 studies, 251 foci)						
3344	−50	0	38	Left	Precentral Gyrus	6
	−48	0	32	Left	Precentral Gyrus	6
	−56	6	32	Left	Precentral Gyrus	6
	−42	8	44	Left	Middle Frontal Gyrus	8
656	0	4	58	Left	Superior Frontal Gyrus	6
552	24	−16	52	Right	Precentral Gyrus	6
544	−30	−54	54	Left	Superior Parietal Lobule	7
536	32	−48	50	Right	Superior Parietal Lobule	7
448	48	10	30	Right	Inferior Frontal Gyrus	9
408	−44	−34	44	Left	Inferior Parietal Lobule	40
328	−34	−46	38	Left	Inferior Parietal Lobule	40
320	26	−10	64	Right	Precentral Gyrus	6

296	12	−68	42	Right	Precuneus	7
280	10	−74	38	Right	Precuneus	7
264	−52	6	−8	Left	Superior Temporal Gyrus	38
	−50	10	−6	Left	Superior Temporal Gyrus	22
264	−8	−12	56	Left	Medial Frontal Gyrus	6
232	−58	−30	14	Left	Superior Temporal Gyrus	42
Novices > experts (6 studies, 78 foci)						
336	−4	−80	−12	Left	Cerebellum	
312	52	−4	38	Right	Precentral Gyrus	6
224	6	−84	−4	Right	Lingual Gyrus	18
208	24	−2	14	Right	Lentiform Nucleus	
	22	2	16	Right	Lentiform Nucleus	
Motor execution						
Experts > novices (4 studies, 32 foci)						
328	−42	−32	46	Left	Inferior Parietal Lobule	40
Novices > experts (2 studies, 47 foci)						
352	−4	−80	−12	Left	Cerebellum	
248	24	−2	14	Right	Putamen	
Action observation						
Experts > novices (4 studies, 140 foci)						
320	−42	−2	28	Left	Precentral Gyrus	6
256	−56	8	30	Left	Inferior Frontal Gyrus	9
Novices > motor experts (N/A)						
Action prediction						
Experts > novices (3 studies, 50 foci)						
480	6	−74	−28	Right	Cerebellum	
228	−34	−48	38	Left	Inferior Parietal Lobule	40
Novices > motor experts (3 studies, 21 foci)						
204	0	−56	56	Left	Precuneus	7

Note: all coordinates are reported in Talairach space.

2014). The PPC receives input from auditory, visual, and somatosensory cortices, to localize the body and external objects in space during motor planning (Binkofski et al., 1999; Decety et al., 1994; Grèzes & Decety, 2002; Konen, Mruczek, Montoya, & Kastner, 2013), and projects outputs to dorsolateral prefrontal cortex and premotor cortex (Johnson, Farraina, Bianchi, & Caminiti, 1996). Therefore, extensive motor training may facilitate efficient motor planning during task performance, thereby increasing PPC activity (Calvo-Merino et al., 2005; Kim et al., 2011; Stout et al., 2011). Conversely, physical practice may increase automatization of task performance, thereby simplifying motor planning, with a concomitant decrease activity in PPC activity (e.g., Petrini et al., 2011). In Yang's (2015) meta-analysis, experts yielded stronger PPC activation than did novices, when performing learned actions (Bernardi et al., 2013; Pau, Jahn, Sakreida, Domin, & Lotze, 2013), observing other people performing actions (Haslinger et al., 2005), and when making predictions about a ball's movement as a function of anticipatory experience (Balser, Lorey, Pilgramm, Naumann, et al., 2014). This is consistent with the view that motor experts, as a result of extensive training, may be better at integrating somatosensory, auditory, and visual information in location monitoring and motor adjustment (Baeck et al., 2012).

Motor experts' more complex motor planning processes may fulfil various tasks related to their motor experience—what we might call positive skill transfer (Issurin, 2013). However, the relative decreases in several brain regions, including right precentral gyrus (BA 6), right lingual gyrus (BA 18), not only reflect specific findings from the studies included in Yang's (2015) review (Haslinger et al., 2005; Milton et al., 2007), but also lends support to the notion that motor experts have developed more efficient neural processes. This said, the motor expert group showed no decreases in PFC and ACC, which are involved in cognitive processes that govern motor performance, and so this efficiency may be restricted to motor regions. A viable explanation for this observation is that the experimental tasks are far removed from those that the experts have practiced for many years; ergo, the scanner task demands are qualitatively different.

Yang (2015) concluded that "motor expertise increases brain effects in areas related to action planning and action comprehension and decrease brain effects in right brain areas and areas related to motor control" (p. 392). She goes on to assert that intensive motor training strengthens the involvement of task-related areas, due to the development of a more elaborate task-related motor representation related to the tasks. She also noted that her meta-analysis solely comprised studies in which whole-brain analyses were performed—which she acknowledged as a weakness. Studies in which 'regions of interest' are specified prior to data collection are experimentally more rigorous and far less common than whole-brain approaches in sport and performance-related fMRI research, which may be a reflection of both the state of our knowledge base and the resulting confidence in our hypotheses—but this is something that will be rectified in time, as they both grow.

We will make some additional observations pertaining to Yang's summary; observations which we believe are noteworthy—hence their inclusion. The first of these is that Yang also made no observation pertaining to the fact that, in the three studies classified as 'motor prediction' (we have used the term 'action prediction'), there were human actors involved, with the explicit aim to predict the actor's future behavior, or the outcome of that behavior, from the actor's kinematics (Bishop et al., 2013; Wright et al., 2011). Hence, action observation was a key part of these studies also. This confusion is compounded by the fact that the study by Wright et al. (2013) is categorized as 'motor observation', when the participants were required to predict the actors' actions too.

Another noteworthy observation is the extent of activation manifested in some regions displayed in Table 6.3—notably the high volumes reported for both experts and novices, in regions such as inferior parietal lobule and middle frontal gyrus. This very likely reflects the diversity of coordinates derived from the constituent studies in the analysis, which is understandable, given not only the inadequacies of cluster-based analysis (Eklund et al., 2016), but also the potential variation in the approaches used to manipulate brain activations, the preprocessing of the fMRI data, and also its subsequent analysis (including threshold types and extents).

Finally, the laterality of the observed activations is also of interest. Although the data are incomplete with regard to participants' handedness, and the hand(s) used to respond where a response was required (e.g., in anticipation tasks), Yang's reporting of activations in experts suggests a strong rightward bias for motor activity, insofar as left precentral gyrus (i.e., motor cortex) was consistently activated. We might reasonably expect such activation, when 87–90% of the general population are right-handed (Raymond, Pontier, Dufour, & Møller, 1996); the chances are accordingly high that participants responded with right-hand digits, if given the opportunity to do so. This said, when compared with novices, experts displayed stronger activation in motor cortex bilaterally—although the cluster size was considerably greater for left M1 (more than a threefold difference). But the fact that novices displayed greater activation in left cerebellum and the right lentiform nucleus—which are collectively involved in the control of small, precise muscle movements on the left-hand side of the body – may be a finding that merits further investigation, as this difference seemed to be largely present for motor execution tasks only, suggesting poorer efficiency in their execution of the experimental tasks.

Emotional and Mental State Manipulations

In addition to the considerable body of work devoted to motor expertise and related processes, a small body of work has focused on the effect of emotional and mental state manipulations in the scanner. Given the inherently affective nature of competitive sport participation (Lazarus, 2000), we deemed it appropriate to provide a brief overview of some of these studies here.

The notion of optimal zones of functioning has received a good deal of research interest in sport (Hanin, 1995, 2000, 2003; Robazza, Pellizzari, Bertollo, & Hanin, 2008; Robazza, Pellizzari, & Hanin, 2004). Ferrell, Beach, Szeverenyi, Krch, and Fernhall (2006) used fMRI to examine the patterning of neural activation as competitive archers recalled, under hypnotic influence, performances for which they would describe themselves as having been 'in the zone'; they also did so for performance that they described as 'normal'. The authors found increased activation, for 'in-zone' performance relative to normal performance, for regions involved in fine motor control (cerebellum), spatial attention and perception (inferior parietal lobule), and reward processing (putamen and insula). Moreover, there was greater activation in occipital cortex, which suggests that the in-zone performances were easier to recall more vividly (visual cortex is active during visual imagery; Sparing et al., 2002); and in motor and premotor regions—again in the left hemisphere. Supplementary motor area was also activated bilaterally. Although this study represents an interesting step towards understanding a commonly reported phenomenon, any future research in this area should be more experimental in nature. Specifically, athlete participants' mental state should be manipulated via more established means of, for example, emotional state manipulation (e.g., using the International Affective Picture System [IAPS]; Lang, Bradley, & Cuthbert, 2008), immediately prior to their engagement in a sport-relevant task within the scanner. In combination with the participants' performance scores, we may begin to learn something about changes in neural activation that signify being 'in the zone'.

Combinations of affective auditory and visual stimuli are a reliable means by which participants' emotional states may be manipulated (Baumgartner, Esslen, & Jäncke, 2006; Loizou, Karageorghis, & Bishop, 2014). Accordingly, some researchers have used videos of personal athletic performance to manipulate the viewer's emotional state inside an MRI scanner. For example, Davis IV et al. (2008) recruited a group of elite swimmers, who were asked to view a video recording of a personal performance failure, both before and after what the authors called a 'cognitive intervention'; this intervention required the participants to (a) express their feelings generated from watching the failed race; (b) express self-referent cognitions related to the actual motor performance, both attitudinal and behavioral (e.g., "I am slow", "I need to work on my stroke length"); and (c) consider and imagine their performance changes for the next race. In a blocked fMRI design, participants saw their personal failure video two times at each scanner visit (i.e., pre- and post-intervention), along with two viewings of a neutral video (contrast condition). They also provided regular self-ratings of their negative affect, using an on-screen visual analog scale (0–7) as a guide.

There were main effects of both the session (pre- vs. post-intervention) and the video type (failure vs. neutral) on participants affect ratings. Specifically, they rated their affect when viewing the 'failure videos' as more negative than when viewing the neutral videos—and also provided more negative ratings during the first viewing of the failure video (i.e., pre-intervention). The authors concluded that this implied that the brief (20 mins) intervention was successful. There was also greater activation in right premotor cortex and left sensorimotor cortex during the second viewing of the failure video, whereas there was greater evidence of visual recall and negative emotion processing during the first viewing—namely, in parahippocampal gyrus and rostral anterior cingulate cortex. There was also evidence for increased thought processes (dorsolateral prefrontal cortex). Moreover, there was a negative correlation between negative affect and activity in motor and premotor regions, which the authors interpreted in light of evidence for motor retardation in depression (Sabbe, Hulstijn, van Hoof, Tuynman-Qua, & Zitman, 1999).

There was an important oversight in Davis IV et al.'s (2008) experimental design; one to which the authors did not refer. Whilst it is not possible to counterbalance pre- and post-intervention conditions, for obvious reasons, the fact that participants watched the same failure video four times in total over the course of the experiment may explain the increases in motor activity—i.e. a shift away from emotion-related processes, to ones of motor reenactment, perhaps as a function of observational learning practice. It may also explain the apparent reduction in emotion processing, for the same reason. Hence, although this study has yielded potentially informative data, a single-subject, multiple-baseline design might be more appropriate for future investigations. Nonetheless, in a follow-up study, Davis IV et al. (2012) compared successful and unsuccessful Olympic athletes. Eleven of the latter group (n = 14) did not qualify for a Games, whereas the majority of the former (n = 12) had won an Olympic or World Championship medal; they viewed success and failure videos, respectively. The authors collected salivary samples, to assess the ratio of testosterone and cortisol, in addition to affective and fMRI measures. There were robust effects on this ratio, in terms of pre-to-post changes: the ratio increased (i.e., improved) for the successful athletes, whereas it decreased for the unsuccessful ones. Moreover, this was mirrored in increases in premotor and sensorimotor cortices for the former—lending greater credibility to Davis IV et al.'s (2008) earlier findings.

Affective responses to sporting footage are not restricted to viewing oneself. For example, copious anecdotal evidence suggests that being a supporter is one way of vicariously experiencing the highs and the lows of professional soccer. Hye Ju et al. (2009) recruited nine South Korean undergraduates, who viewed 30-second video clips depicting their national team winning (n = 5) and losing (n = 5) during the 2002 World Cup, hosted in their country, as they lay in an MRI scanner. Although the activations that they reported were somewhat eclectic, if we assume that the conditions under which data were collected for each of the two conditions were comparable, then a clear pattern emerged. There was considerably lower widespread activation in the 'losing' condition, which the authors interpreted as some form of suppression of negative emotional responses. Given the makeup of the sample, this may represent a cultural difference that differentiates Korean participants, for example, from their North American counterparts. If such suppression was demonstrated to either positively or negatively affect subsequent task performance within the scanner, then this might be a finding of great relevance for athletic pursuits.

In an fMRI investigation of intensely pleasurable responses to soccer goals being scored, McLean et al. (2009) also recruited nine participants—this time, all supporters of the same Scottish soccer team. They viewed thirty 4-second clips that showed each of the following: their team scoring a goal, the same team missing a goal opportunity, and the team in open play. In the subsequent analysis, the authors contrasted (a) goals versus open play, (b) missed chances versus open play, (c) goals versus missed chances, and (d) goals and missed chances versus open play. Superior temporal gyrus, inferior frontal gyrus, and amygdala were commonly activated by all four of the contrasts. Additionally, anterior cingulate was activated by contrasts (a) and (c), and putamen, a reward processing region, was activated for all contrasts except contrast (c). In other words, all contrasts in which an anticipatory element was compared with a non-anticipatory one (i.e., open play). The authors concluded that such video sequences could be used to identify reward processing regions of the brain. This finding may also be successfully applied to sport performance. If anticipatory states can be engendered in the dressing room, then this might be manifested in adaptive behavioral changes on the pitch, such as increased coverage of the pitch by midfield players; such inherent 'exploratory/foraging' behaviors are an innate consequence of greater activity in regions such as the putamen (Panksepp, 1998).

In an extension of a previous behavioral study (Bishop, Karageorghis, & Kinrade, 2009), Bishop and colleagues (Bishop, Wright, & Karageorghis, 2014) asked 12 young athletes to listen to 90-second excerpts of a popular music track, each of which was played at one of three different tempi (99 bpm, 129 bpm [original tempo], and 161 bpm) and one of two different sound intensities (55 dBA [moderate] or 75 dBA [loud]), prior to completing a choice reaction time (CRT) task in which they had to respond with a button press to a target stimulus appearing in one of three on-screen locations. They hypothesized that, in accordance with Bishop et al.'s (2009) findings, there would be a neural mechanism underpinning previously observed improvements in post-music listening choice reaction times (Bishop et al., 2009). Hypotheses were made with regard to CRT task performance, due to the large sample size that would be required to derive significant effects for RT data.

There was a 'residual' effect of listening to music per se, as the participants performed the CRT task. Specifically, the authors observed greater activation in the cerebellum, which suggests that listening to music may serve a useful preparatory function for motor performance (e.g., Karageorghis & Drew, 1996). But, perhaps more interestingly, there was an effect of the music manipulations on brain activations. Notably, when the participants had heard music played at the fast tempo, as compared to when they heard the same music played at the slow tempo, there was greater activation in inferior temporal cortex, an integral component of the ventral visual stream, used for object recognition (Corbetta & Shulman, 2002; Milner & Goodale, 1995). However, given the nature of the experimental task—i.e., to identify the location of one solitary target, which was identical on all trials—it does not appear to be the case that object recognition is required; hence, it could be the case that the recognition involved pertained to the location. Nonetheless, there was additional evidence for enhanced visual processing as a result of listening to fast, as opposed to slow, music, in primary visual cortex. There was also an effect of music intensity (i.e., volume) on brain activity during subsequent CRT performance. Notably, there was continued evidence of greater visual processing (middle temporal cortex), spatial perception and visuomotor integration (inferior parietal lobule), high-level executive functions and decision-making (medial frontal gyrus), and reward processing (putamen). Such sequential effects, if they are genuine ones, have not hitherto been demonstrated before and so they are worthy of further scrutiny, not least when we consider the prevalence of music listening as a pre-performance routine (Bishop, Karageorghis, & Loizou, 2007).

In summary, the studies described above all provide evidence for the ease with which visual and auditory stimuli, in isolation and in combination, can be used to manipulate participants' emotional states within an MRI scanner—and, importantly, that there are potential and actual effects on subsequent motor performance.

fMRI Investigation of Head Injury

Another area of research in which fMRI has proven to be a useful and valid technique is the investigation of head injury as a consequence of sport participation—largely in competitive American football, possibly due to the prevalence of brain injuries that have historically been sustained through repeated high-velocity collisions (Vos, Nieuwenhuijsen, & Sluiter, 2018). To address this considerable body of work is beyond the scope of this chapter—even if the consequences of such research may/should ultimately impact on performance practices (e.g., rule changes). Therefore, if you should want to engage in additional reading around this important area of research, then we recommend the article by Eierud et al. (2014), who provide a useful review of the various neuroimaging techniques that have been used to assess mild traumatic brain injury.

Limitations and Methodological Considerations

Limitations of fMRI as a Technique

In their recent analysis of 396 resting-state fMRI datasets, Eklund et al. (2016) ran 1,000 random group analyses and examined the veracity of accepted parametric methods for inferential analyses, at the level of both the voxel and the cluster (using two cluster-defining thresholds, $p = 0.01$ and $p = 0.001$). Although they found that the parametric approach yielded conservative estimates of voxel-wise activations, those for cluster-based inference were spurious, resulting in false positive rates of up to 70%. The authors suggested that their findings called into question the validity of approximately 40,000 studies in which cluster-based analyses were employed. We should take this important finding into consideration when assessing the evidence that we have covered in this book chapter.

This important consideration aside, fMRI does provide good spatial resolution, and enables the concurrent acquisition of data from the entire brain, including both cortical and subcortical regions, which is useful when considered in the context of the complex representations of real-world percepts that we tend to employ in our designs. However, the technique does suffer from poor temporal resolution—which ultimately means that it provides us with a fairly indirect assessment of neural activity. Effectively, the BOLD signal is 'raising the alarm' that something has happened, long after the culprits (i.e., neuronal signals) have fled the scene; this makes it difficult to establish causal connections between external events (such as stimuli we present in the scanner) and brain activations. Because of its dependence on blood flow, the BOLD signal is also prone to influences of non-neural changes in the body; for example, increases in blood flow that might occur as a result of engaging in some form of exercise within the scanner (e.g., Fontes et al., 2013). Thus, researchers are increasingly turning to the use of alternative and complementary techniques (e.g., Mijović, Vanderperren, Van Huffel, & De Vos, 2012); they are complementary in the sense that they can be used both in parallel with fMRI (i.e., in the scanner) and in separate investigations.

Alternative and Complementary Techniques

There have been many developments and refinements to functional neuroimaging techniques in recent years, many of which are ongoing at the time of writing, such as functional connectivity analyses (Riedl et al., 2014), multivoxel pattern analysis (Visser et al., 2016), and real-time fMRI (Lorenz et al., 2016). However, there are other non-invasive methods for recording human brain activity; these include magnetoencephalography (MEG), electroencephalography (EEG), transcranial magnetic stimulation (TMS), and another measure that is dependent on blood flow—near-infrared spectroscopy (NIRS). Each of these techniques has its merits and drawbacks, but they can present useful alternatives or complements to fMRI. Although these techniques may be covered in greater detail elsewhere (e.g., Section III), we provide a brief overview of each below for ease of comparison.

Magnetoencephalography (MEG)

MEG is used to measure the magnetic fields generated by neuronal activity of the brain—fields that come about as the result of electrical current flow in the brain's neural circuitry. The spatial distributions of these fields are analyzed to localize the sources of the activity, and the locations of the sources are superimposed on anatomical images, such as those provided by MRI. But unlike fMRI, MEG is a direct measure of brain function. Moreover, it has a very high temporal resolution—in the order of milliseconds—and still affords the same millimeter precision as fMRI. The magnetic fields pass unhindered through brain tissue and the skull, so they can be easily recorded. Although the magnetic field is extremely small, it can be detected by superconducting sensors. By analyzing the spatial distributions of magnetic fields (lower left), it is possible, by using a model such as a single equivalent current dipole (lower middle), to estimate the intracranial localization of the generator source and superimpose it on an MRI (lower right). The main drawback of MEG is that the signals of interest are extremely small, such that other electromagnetic fields within the immediate environment (e.g., those emanating from other electrical equipment) can obscure the signal. Therefore, specialized shielding, such as that afforded by a Faraday cage, is required to eliminate the magnetic interference found in a typical urban clinical environment.

Electroencephalography (EEG)

EEG technology also offers high temporal resolution, in the order of milliseconds, by capturing fluctuations in the electrical voltage of the brain via electrodes placed on the scalp in accordance with the guidelines of the International 10–20 system (Jasper, 1958). EEG data represent changes in the voltage potential differences between different points on the human scalp and the electric field potentials that arise from excitatory and inhibitory postsynaptic potentials. Diagnostic applications of EEH have historically focused on the spectral content of the resulting EEG waveforms; that is, the neural oscillations, or 'brain waves' that can readily be observed in EEG signals. Other popular forms of EEG include event-related potentials, which refer to averaged EEG responses that are time-locked to complex processing of stimuli (both internal and external). Because of the very high temporal resolution of this technique, it is increasingly being used in cognitive psychology and neuroscientific research—although it should be noted that the sources of the observed signals cannot always be easily determined.

Transcranial Magnetic Stimulation (TMS)

TMS is a technique that relies on the process of electromagnetic induction. When multiple coils of copper wire, housed within a casing (known as 'a coil'), are placed close to an individual's scalp, and then a pulse of electrical current is rapidly discharged through the wires, a brief magnetic field is generated. This magnetic field then induces a current in the nearby conductors—notably cortical (and to a lesser extent) subcortical neurons. The end result is an 'evoked potential', the most common of which is the motor evoked potential (MEP), when primary motor cortex (M1) is the target of TMS pulses. This technique can be used to deliver single, paired, and repetitive (rTMS) pulses. We have learnt a great deal about functional connectivity within the cortex via TMS-induced MEPs; for example, interhemispheric interactions between posterior parietal cortex and the contralateral M1 (Koch et al., 2009). Because TMS can temporarily excite or inhibit specific brain regions, researchers have used it to investigate processes including attention, perception, learning-related plasticity, and consciousness.

Functional Near-Infrared Spectroscopy (fNIRS)

fNIRS is a noninvasive method for functional monitoring and imaging of brain hemodynamics via sensors placed on the forehead. Due to its high temporal resolution and portability, this technique is suitable for examining cognitive processing in dynamic tasks, where other measures such as EEG are impractical (Ferrari & Quaresima, 2012). NIRS technology is a powerful tool for detecting acute changes in blood flow, including in brain regions such as the prefrontal cortex (PFC)—the location of our executive and cognitive functions (Roberts, Robbins, & Weiskrantz, 1998). NIRS studies have shown that the PFC is active during performance of executive tasks such as inhibitory control, cognitive shifting, and working memory in young children (Moriguchi & Hiraki, 2013).

Sampling Considerations

One inconsistency that arguably blights our comparisons of fMRI studies of expertise is the disparity in the makeup of groups designated as 'expert' or 'skilled'. For example, in his review of action anticipation, Smith (2016) noted that expert groups tended to range in competitive level from professional and international competitors (Abreu et al., 2012; Olsson & Lundström, 2013; Wright et al., 2010, 2011) to national, regional, or even local amateurs (Balser, Lorey, Pilgramm, Naumann, et al., 2014; Balser, Lorey, Pilgramm, Stark, et al., 2014; Diersch et al., 2013; Wu et al., 2013). This alone is problematic for meaningful interpretation, issues of design and analyses aside. Irrespective of the classification of experts, for those studies in which the experts' mean years of experience in their respective sports was reported (10 in total), the mean was 15.4 years (± 6.2 yrs)—which seems a reasonable approximation of the time required in order to attain expertise, according to the theory of deliberate practice (Ericsson, Krampe, & Tesch-Römer, 1993) at least, and so may help to restore our faith in the integrity of the data somewhat.

The sampling strategies used were largely consistent, in that, for five fMRI studies (Abreu et al., 2012; Balser, Lorey, Pilgramm, Stark, et al., 2014; Olsson & Lundström, 2013; Wu et al., 2013) a group of expert athletes was typically compared to another group with no discernible experience in the sport—i.e., novices—with further differentiation according to age, in another study (Diersch et al., 2013). In the work of Wright and colleagues (2010, 2011, 2013), there were three experimental groups—an intermediate group was also recruited—largely because such comparisons had hitherto been commonplace in behavioral studies of expertise (e.g., Abernethy, Neal, & Koning, 1994; Farrow, McCrae, Gross, & Abernethy, 2010; Muller, Abernethy, Eid, McBean, & Rose, 2010). Three studies that comprised two expert groups and one novice group were TMS-based, and so they will not be discussed here—although the notion of an 'expert watcher' (Agliotti, Cesari, Romani, & Urgesi, 2008) is noteworthy (see Future Directions). Similarly to Calvo-Merino et al.'s (2005) approach, Balser, Lorey, Pilgramm, Naumann, et al. (2014) recruited experts from two different sports, namely tennis and volleyball. All participants performed an anticipation task for each of the two sports; the authors claimed that each sub-sample served as the novice comparator group when performing the task not related to their sport. However, whilst this approach, and the resultant data, are interesting, this approach does not take into consideration the 'generalized anticipation skill' that interceptive ball sports players will undoubtedly have accrued over years of practice; a skill should arguably exhibit 'positive transfer' (Issurin, 2013).

Although the preferred strategy for studies of anticipation skill has been to recruit people who are highly skilled, preferably expert, in the sport or activity of interest, and then to compare their brain function with that of less-skilled peers, our colleagues and we (Bishop et al., 2013) adopted a different approach. We used an in-task performance criterion (cf. Vaeyens, Lenoir, Mazyn, Williams, & Philippaerts, 2007) to group participants in a post hoc manner, into high-skill: (≥ 60% accuracy), intermediate (51–59% accuracy), and low-skill (≤ 50% accuracy) groups. Smith (2016) suggested that this approach is not recommended—although no reason was proffered as to why. To the contrary, two important considerations for future work are (i) the representativeness of the task design in the MRI scanner, as there is a lack of correspondence between the real-world tasks and those required in the laboratory (see 'Task considerations') and (ii) the potential distinction between motor and perceptual experts. It is possible, through extensive watching, to become an 'expert watcher'(Agliotti et al., 2008)—and therefore to be adept at perceptual decision-making tasks, but with relatively impoverished motor skills; experienced coaches, who have long-since 'hung up their boots' may be good examples of such individuals. Therefore, if we wish to exploit fMRI as a technique for all its worth, then we may need to concede that, with present practical constraints (the portability of NIRS notwithstanding), fMRI protocols are best suited to the investigation of perceptual, not motor, expertise—and the extent of this expertise may best be determined within the scanner.

Task Considerations

The eminent neuroscientist Professor Vincent Walsh (2014) recently called into question the utility of carefully controlled laboratory-based tasks that have been, and still are, used to understand complex behavior, and challenged cognitive neuroscientists to confront the complex, 'messy' real world circumstances of sport performance. This will be no mean feat, not least because of the technological limitations of MRI scanning that restrict us from collecting data in vivo—although there are alternative measures, such as near-infrared spectroscopy (NIRS), which offers suitable portability without compromising data quality too greatly. Walsh also pointed out that we should consider treating elite athletes as in some way 'abnormal', much as neuropsychologists have done in case studies for decades—in our attempts to determine precisely what it is that makes the consistent winners so consistently different. Our concern is that, by taking such an approach, the frequently observed 'halo effect' (Nisbett & Wilson, 1977; Thorndike, 1920) may emerge. This established effect has, in our view, often caused us to look at the development of expertise as being largely the result of extensive and ritualized practice (Crust & Clough, 2011; Weinberg, Butt, & Culp, 2011), rather than something that is also contingent upon more than a smattering of good fortune during that 'journey'. Hence, even a rigorous approach to exploring the Pandora's Box that may constitute the athlete's brain could reveal something disappointingly ordinary.

The concept of 'representative design' (Brunswik, 1956) has been a topic of recent debate in the sport psychology literature—mostly with regard to the design of behavioral studies (Araújo, Davids, & Passos, 2007; Pinder, Davids, Renshaw, & Araújo, 2011; Pinder, Renshaw, Headrick, & Davids, 2014). This refers to the extent to which experiments and studies that are designed to investigate real-world phenomena manage to replicate the environmental conditions under which they occur. In behavioral tasks outside of the scanner, it is easier to approximate (but only approximate) real-world conditions. However, for reasons that are obvious, this is considerably more challenging within the confines of an MRI scanner; requiring participants to lie still cannot possibly come close to replicating the dynamic multivariate context of competitive sport (Mann, Dicks, Cañal-Bruland, & van der Kamp, 2013; Mann, Williams, Ward, & Janelle, 2007). In many of the anticipation studies discussed herein, participants were required to respond at the appropriate time, by pressing a button, clicking a mouse, or directing a joystick, in response to a range of experimental stimuli that included predicting the outcome of basketball free throws (Wu et al., 2013), the flight path of a shuttlecock (Wright et al., 2010, 2013), oncoming soccer opponents' movements (Bishop et al., 2013; Wright et al., 2013), hockey shots (Olsson & Lundström, 2013), tennis ground strokes (Balser, Lorey, Pilgramm, Stark, et al., 2014), and volleyball and tennis serves (Balser, Lorey, Pilgramm, Naumann, et al., 2014). For any one of these tasks, it is clear to see that there is very little 'mapping' of response format onto the requisite response in the real world, but when we consider that the same, or highly similar, responses may be used to encompass such a broad range of real-world actions, the gulf between fMRI research and competitive practices seems even wider.

In his review of sport anticipation studies, Smith (2016) noted that, within the 15 studies he reviewed, some appeared to be more ecologically valid (a misnomer, according to recent discussions; Pinder et al., 2011) than others. For example, eight of the studies used action sequences that were recorded from a first-person perspective, whereas the remaining seven used a third-person perspective. This is clearly a dichotomy that needs to be addressed if fMRI investigations of sport and performance are to move in a suitable direction. Smith also asserted that studies could be more 'ecologically valid' by combining video-based tasks and neuroimaging with active tasks using the same participants—something that may be achieved both within and across studies. He also asserted that longitudinal studies should be developed, in order to examine the relationships between what he termed 'relevant variables'—we would suggest 'neural activation and the development of expertise', for example—intraindividually, i.e. within athletes. In line with Professor Walsh's (2014) suggestion, case studies, or even single-subject multiple-baseline designs, might lend themselves to such investigations.

In apparent contradiction to his earlier assertion, that to use an in-task to determine levels of perceptual expertise is not recommended, Smith (2016) noted that researchers' tendency to attribute experts' superior anticipation performance to their motor expertise was flawed, noting that "it is plausible that some young athletes possess a predisposition to exceptional visual perception and action anticipation, perhaps due to genetics or early experience". We have to agree with this notion: perceptual and motor expertise should be differentiated appropriately, be it at the design, implementation and/or analysis stages.

Smith also rightly pointed out that some, if not all, authors' claims relating to observed activations appeared to be tailored to supporting their original research questions and hypotheses. For example, when the experts in Abreu et al.'s (2012) exhibited stronger visual cortex activation than did their novices, the authors explained this finding as being "probably due to their expert reading of the observed action kinematics". However, in Olsson and Lundstrom's (2013) study, when visual cortex activation was reduced, the authors claimed that a potential explanation "may be because experts do not have to rely on a visual search strategy, instead they can directly extract the information from the motor representations and analyze the interaction much faster using parts of the temporal lobe". From our own experiences of being confronted with the extensive datasets that inevitably emerge from whole-brain fMRI analyses, we can see how researchers might feel compelled to produce a viable explanation for their observations in this way. And ambiguity in the fMRI literature is not confined to sport and performance-based research; for example, with regard to the functions of some brain regions (e.g., posterior cingulate cortex; Leech, Braga, & Sharp, 2012).

Conclusions and Future Directions

The finding that there are multiple activations in diverse brain regions, with similarly broad interpretations as a result, is not uncommon in many fMRI investigations of sport expertise, including our own (Bishop et al., 2013; Wright et al., 2010, 2011, 2013). Typically, complex real-world stimuli are presented to the participants and a whole-brain approach is used, both to postulate hypotheses and to subsequently analyze the resulting data. Then explanations for each of the significant expert-novice differences are proffered, in the context of what is currently known about the regions. Whilst this has been, and possibly still will be, a useful step for us to develop our knowledge base, we should give consideration to experimental designs, in terms of both the behavioral task and the fMRI design (the two are separable but mutually dependent) that enable us to more confidently determine the contributions of specific brain regions to specific elements of a specific task; for example, detection of action observation network [AON] sub-regions that respond to the onset of subtle kinematic changes in an observed action, such as a 'step-over' in soccer. Our hypotheses should be correspondingly specific, and therefore event-related designs may be more appropriate—pursuant to ongoing improvements in the use of the technique (e.g., Liu, 2012)

Some researchers have introduced bespoke equipment into fMRI protocols in order to effectively bring the real world into the scanner (e.g., Fontes et al., 2013). Putting aside our own misgivings about any kind of aerobic exercise inside an MRI scanner, we recommend such innovations, so that our findings may have greater applicability to the real world. MR-compatible transducers, such as accelerometers, are now widely available, and so could be attached to a similarly compatible object that resembles the handle of a tennis racket, for example—maybe one that is weighted so as to approximate the weight of a full racket. Although this is still far removed from the real world—a technique such as NIRS may be more suitable in vivo—this is likely to elicit a more 'situated' mindset in the participant, which would almost certainly be manifested in neural activity. A useful starting point to determine the advantages of such an approach would be to run within-subjects validation studies, using traditional button box or joystick responses as a comparator condition. The main challenges to such innovations are the narrow bore of the scanner, which severely restricts movement, and the movement artefacts that would inevitably arise from engaging in a dynamic task—but such artefacts can be accounted for during data analysis (e.g, Novakova, Mikl, & Jan, 2014; Sun & Hinrichs, 2009).

The notion of motor versus perceptual expertise also warrants further investigation, and fMRI studies are particularly suited to doing so. Motor expertise is something that can readily be quantified. For example, proponents of the theory of deliberate practice (Ericsson et al., 1993) would also support the idea that an individual's years of practice in their sport might also be a good index of proficiency—although recent evidence suggests otherwise (Macnamara, Moreau, & Hambrick,

2016). However, an individual's motor expertise may be categorized in terms of the level at which they compete and/or have competed for an extended period of time. Conversely, 'perceptual experts' are more elusive, as they may comprise individuals who are suitably genetically gifted (e.g., in terms of pattern recognition; Wilmer et al., 2010), but who have not gravitated toward sport participation, let alone serious competition. Hence, a suitable compromise may be to adopt the traditional method of recruiting people of ostensibly varying motor expertise, and then to differentiate them according to their perceptual abilities within the scanner. The use of video stimuli containing difficult (Cross et al., 2010) or even humanly impossible (Leonetti et al., 2015) movements may be useful tools for doing so, as participants' pickup of subtle, almost impercepti-ble, stimulus manipulations might be both detectable and localizable in fMRI data. If perceptual and motor expertise are truly differentiable attributes, then we would expect a zero correlation between the extent of task-relevant activations (e.g., components of the AON during complex action observation) and level of motor expertise.

With regard to action observation studies, fMRI researchers could take the lead from the TMS work of Stefan and colleagues. Following on from an earlier study (Stefan et al., 2005), in which the authors found that action observation of thumb movements brought about a kinemat-ically specific memory trace of the observed motions in primary motor cortex, Stefan, Classen, Celnik and Cohen (2008) investigated the effect of action observation and physical practice in combination for the same thumb movements (i.e., flexion and extension). This combined condi-tion was superior to either of the tasks in isolation. Specifically, the resultant MEPs were larger when participants performed thumb movements that were congruent with the observed direc-tion, suggesting a high degree of specificity in the learning process; specificity, that has been seen in dance action observation (Calvo-Merino et al., 2005, 2006; Cross et al., 2006). fMRI lends itself well to longitudinal studies of changes to structural and functional reorganization, and so would be an appropriate means by which we can investigate the effects of combined ac-tion observation and physical practice on such reorganization—or even the interaction between ventral and dorsal streams during action observation (cf. Leitão, Thielscher, Tünnerhoff, & Noppeney, 2015).

And Finally: A Region of Interest…?

One region of the brain, which is small and hidden away in posterior parietal cortex, and so has tended to escape the attention of researchers, is the precuneus, a component of the default-mode network (Raichle & Snyder, 2007) whose activation may signify introspective thought, includ-ing activities like daydreaming or retrieving memories. Speaking of memory retrieval, we have many memories of seeing precuneus activations in preliminary (i.e., uncorrected) fMRI data analyses; activations that subsequently disappeared when some stringency was applied. In Yang's (2015) analysis, fairly extensive bilateral precuneus activation was recorded for both experts and novices relative to baseline, although this manifested itself more strongly for experts when a comparison was made. Activation that emerged as lateralized and greatly reduced in its extent when experts and novices were compared (experts > novices—right precuneus; novices > experts for prediction—left precuneus). Hence, we tentatively propose that activation of this region may signify engagement with the experimental task—or, more precisely, a lack of it. In other words, participants were 'switching off'. In our view, this is an important consideration for future fMRI studies: We, as researchers, often present participants with incredibly repeti-tive and tedious stimuli, for a prolonged period of time; although we also sometimes assess the participants' engagement with the task, be that objectively or subjectively, the tendency to en-gage in introspection is not something that one can easily control. Hence, the design of fMRI studies to maximize participant engagement, yet still produce usable and informative data, is a very real challenge.

Daniel T. Bishop and Michael J. Wright

References

Abernethy, B., Neal, R. J., & Koning, P. (1994). Visual-perceptual and cognitive differences between expert, intermediate, and novice snooker players. *Applied Cognitive Psychology, 8*, 185–211. doi:10.1002/acp.2350080302

Abreu, A. M., Macaluso, E., Azevedo, R. T., Cesari, P., Urgesi, C., & Aglioti, S. M. (2012). Action anticipation beyond the action observation network: A functional magnetic resonance imaging study in expert basketball players. *European Journal of Neuroscience, 35*(10), 1646–1654. doi:10.1111/j.1460–9568.2012.08104.x

Aglioti, S. M., Cesari, P., Romani, M., & Urgesi, C. (2008). Action anticipation and motor resonance in elite basketball players. *Nature Neuroscience, 11*, 1109–1116. doi:10.1038/nn.2182

Araújo, D., Davids, K., & Passos, P. (2007). Ecological validity, representative design, and correspondence between experimental task constraints and behavioral setting: Comment on Rogers, Kadar, and Costall (2005). *Ecological Psychology, 19*, 69–78.

Babiloni, C., Marzano, N., Infarinato, F., Iacoboni, M., Rizza, G., Aschieri, P., ... Del Percio, C. (2010). 'Neural efficiency' of experts' brain during judgment of actions: A high-resolution EEG study in elite and amateur karate athletes. *Behavioural Brain Research, 207*(2), 466–475. doi:10.1016/j.bbr.2009.10.034

Baeck, J.-S., Kim, Y.-T., Seo, J.-H., Ryeom, H.-K., Lee, J., Choi, S.-M., ... Chang, Y. (2012). Brain activation patterns of motor imagery reflect plastic changes associated with intensive shooting training. *Behavioural Brain Research, 234*, 26–32.

Balser, N., Lorey, B., Pilgramm, S., Naumann, T., Kindermann, S., Stark, R., ... Munzert, J. (2014). The influence of expertise on brain activation of the action observation network during anticipation of tennis and volleyball serves. *Frontiers in Human Neuroscience, 8*, 568–568. doi:10.3389/fnhum.2014.00568

Balser, N., Lorey, B., Pilgramm, S., Stark, R., Bischoff, M., Zentgraf, K., ... Munzert, J. (2014). Prediction of human actions: Expertise and task-related effects on neural activation of the action observation network. *Human Brain Mapping, 35*(8), 4016–4034. doi:10.1002/hbm.22455

Bandura, A. (1986). *Social foundations of thought and action: A social cognitive theory.* Englewood Cliffs, NJ: Prentice-Hall.

Baumann, S., Koeneke, S., Schmidt, C. F., Meyer, M., Lutz, K., & Jancke, L. (2007). A network for audio-motor coordination in skilled pianists and non-musicians. *Brain Research, 1161*, 65–78.

Baumgartner, T., Esslen, M., & Jäncke, L. (2006). From emotion perception to emotion experience: Emotions evoked by pictures and classical music. *International Journal of Psychophysiology, 60*(1), 34–43. doi:10.1016/j.ijpsycho.2005.04.007

Beilock, S. L., & Lyons, I. M. (2009). Expertise and the mental simulation of action. In K. D. Markman, W. M. P. Klein, & J. A. Suhr (Eds.), *Handbook of imagination and mental simulation* (pp. 21–34). New York, NY: Psychology Press.

Beilock, S. L., Lyons, I. M., Mattarella-Micke, A., Nusbaum, H. C., & Small, S. L. (2008). Sports experience changes the neural processing of action language. *Proceedings of the National Academy of Sciences of the United States of America, 105*(36), 13269–13273. doi:10.1073/pnas.0803424105

Berkowitz, A. L., & Ansari, D. (2010). Expertise-related deactivation of the right temporoparietal junction during musical improvisation. *NeuroImage, 49*, 712–719.

Bernardi, G., Cecchetti, L., Handjaras, G., Sani, L., Gaglianese, A., Ceccarelli, R., ... Pietrini, P. (2014). It's not all in your car: Functional and structural correlates of exceptional driving skills in professional racers. *Frontiers in Human Neuroscience, 8*, 888–888. doi:10.3389/fnhum.2014.00888

Bernardi, G., Ricciardi, E., Sani, L., Gaglianese, A., Papasogli, A., Ceccarelli, R., ... Pietrini, P. (2013). How skill expertise shapes the brain functional architecture: An fMRI study of visuo-spatial and motor processing in professional racing-car and naïve drivers. *PLoS ONE, 8*, 1–1.

Bezzola, L., Mérillat, S., & Jäncke, L. (2012). Motor training-induced neuroplasticity. *GeroPsych: The Journal of Gerontopsychology and Geriatric Psychiatry, 25*(4), 189–197. doi:10.1024/1662–9647/a000070

Binkofski, F., Buccino, G., Posse, S., Seitz, R. J., Rizzolatti, G., & Freund, H. (1999). A fronto-parietal circuit for object manipulation in man: Evidence from an fMRI-study. *The European Journal of Neuroscience, 11*(9), 3276–3286.

Bischoff, M., Zentgraf, K., Pilgramm, S., Stark, R., Krüger, B., & Munzert, J. (2014). Anticipating action effects recruits audiovisual movement representations in the ventral premotor cortex. *Brain and Cognition, 92C*, 39–47. doi:10.1016/j.bandc.2014.09.010

Bishop, D. T., Karageorghis, C. I., & Kinrade, N. P. (2009). Effects of musically-induced emotions on choice reaction time performance. *The Sport Psychologist, 23*, 59–76.

Bishop, D. T., Karageorghis, C. I., & Loizou, G. (2007). A grounded theory of young tennis players' use of music to manipulate emotional state. *Journal of Sport & Exercise Psychology, 29*, 584–607.

Bishop, D. T., Wright, M. J., Jackson, R. C., & Abernethy, B. (2013). Neural bases for anticipation skill in soccer: An fMRI study. *Journal of Sport & Exercise Psychology, 35*(1), 98–109.

Bishop, D. T., Wright, M. J., & Karageorghis, C. I. (2014). Tempo and intensity of pre-task music modulate neural activity during reactive task performance. *Psychology of Music, 42*, 714–727. doi:10.1177/0305735613490595

Brown, S., Martinez, M. J., & Parsons, L. M. (2006). The neural basis of human dance. *Cerebral Cortex, 16*(8), 1157–1167. doi:10.1093/cercor/bhj057

Brunswik, E. (1956). *Perception and the representative design of psychological experiments* (2nd ed.). Berkeley, CA: University of California Press.

Calvo-Merino, B., Glaser, D. E., Grèzes, J., Passingham, R. E., & Haggard, P. (2005). Action observation and acquired motor skills: An fMRI study with expert dancers. *Cerebral Cortex, 15*(8), 1243–1249.

Calvo-Merino, B., Grèzes, J., Glaser, D. E., Passingham, R. E., & Haggard, P. (2006). Seeing or doing? Influence of visual and motor familiarity in action observation. *Current Biology, 16*, 1905–1910. doi:10.1016/j.cub.2006.07.065

Calvo-Merino, B., Jola, C., Glaser, D. E., & Haggard, P. (2008). Towards a sensorimotor aesthetics of performing art. *Consciousness and Cognition, 17*, 911–922. doi:10.1016/j.concog.2007.11.003

Chang, Y., Lee, J.-J., Seo, J.-H., Song, H.-J., Kim, Y.-T., Lee, H. J., ... Kim, J. G. (2011). Neural correlates of motor imagery for elite archers. *NMR In Biomedicine, 24*(4), 366–372. doi:10.1002/nbm.1600

Chouinard, P. A., & Paus, T. (2006). The primary motor and premotor cortex areas of the human cerebral cortex. *The Neuroscientist, 12*, 143–152.

Corbetta, M., & Shulman, G. L. (2002). Control of goal-directed and stimulus-driven attention in the brain. *Nature Neuroscience Reviews, 3*, 201–215.

Cross, E. S., Acquah, D., & Ramsey, R. (2014). A review and critical analysis of how cognitive neuroscientific investigations using dance can contribute to sport psychology. *International Review of Sport & Exercise Psychology, 7*(1), 42–71. doi:10.1080/1750984X.2013.862564

Cross, E. S., Hamilton, A. F., & Grafton, S. T. (2006). Building a motor simulation de novo: Observation of dance by dancers [Article]. *NeuroImage, 31*(3), 1257–1267.

Cross, E. S., Hamilton, A. F., Kraemer, D. J., Kelley, W. M., & Grafton, S. T. (2009). Dissociable substrates for body motion and physical experience in the human action observation network. *European Journal of Neuroscience, 30*, 1383–1392. doi:10.1111/j.1460-9568.2009.06941.x

Cross, E. S., Kirsch, L., Ticini, L., & Schütz-Bosbach, S. (2011). The impact of aesthetic appreciation and physical ability on dance perception. *Frontiers in Human Neuroscience, 5*, 102. doi:10.3389/fnhum.2011.00102

Cross, E. S., Kraemer, D. J. M., Hamilton, A. F., Kelley, W. M., & Grafton, S. T. (2009). Sensitivity of the action observation network to physical and observational learning. *Cerebral Cortex, 19*(2), 315–326 (United Kingdom: Oxford University Press).

Cross, E. S., Liepelt, R., Hamilton, A. F., Parkinson, J., Ramsey, R., Stadler, W., & Prinz, W. (2012). Robotic actions preferentially engage the action observation network. *Human Brain Mapping, 33*, 2238–2254.

Cross, E. S., Mackie, E. C., Wolford, G., & Hamilton, A. F. (2010). Contorted and ordinary body postures in the human brain. *Experimental Brain Research, 204*(3), 397–407. doi:10.1007/s00221-009-2093-x

Cross, E. S., Stadler, W., Parkinson, J., Schütz-Bosbach, S., & Prinz, W. (2013). The influence of visual training on predicting complex action sequences. *Human Brain Mapping, 34*(2), 467–486. doi:10.1002/hbm.21450

Crust, L., & Clough, P. J. (2011). Developing mental toughness: From research to practice. *Journal of Sport Psychology in Action, 2*(1), 21–32.

Davis IV, H., Liotti, M., Ngan, E. T., Woodward, T. S., Van Snellenberg, J. X., van Anders, S. M., ... Mayberg, H. S. (2008). fMRI BOLD signal changes in elite swimmers while viewing videos of personal failure. *Brain Imaging and Behavior, 2*, 84–93. Germany: Springer.

Davis IV, H., van Anders, S. M., Ngan, E. T., Woodward, T. S., Van Snellenberg, J. X., Mayberg, H. S., & Liotti, M. (2012). Neural, mood, and endocrine responses in elite athletes relative to successful and failed performance videos. *Journal of Clinical Sport Psychology, 6*(1), 6–21.

Decety, J. (1996). Do imagined and executed actions share the same neural substrate? *Brain Research. Cognitive Brain Research, 3*(2), 87–93.

Decety, J., Perani, D., Jeannerod, M., Bettinardi, V., Tadary, B., Woods, R., ... Fazio, F. (1994). Mapping motor representations with positron emission tomography. *Nature, 371*(6498), 600–602.

Del Percio, C., Babiloni, C., Marzano, N., Iacoboni, M., Infarinato, F., Vecchio, F., ... Eusebi, F. (2009). "Neural efficiency" of athletes' brain for upright standing: A high-resolution EEG study. *Brain Research Bulletin, 79*(3/4), 193–200. doi:10.1016/j.brainresbull.2009.02.001

Del Percio, C., Rossini, P. M., Marzano, N., Iacoboni, M., Infarinato, F., Aschieri, P., ... Eusebi, F. (2008). Is there a "neural efficiency" in athletes? A high-resolution EEG study. *NeuroImage, 42*(4), 1544–1553. doi:10.1016/j.neuroimage.2008.05.061

Diener, E. (2010). Neuroimaging: Voodoo, new phrenology, or scientific breakthrough? Introduction to special section on fMRI. *Perspectives on Psychological Science, 5*(6), 714–715. doi:10.1177/1745691610388773

Diersch, N., Mueller, K., Cross, E. S., Stadler, W., Rieger, M., & Schütz-Bosbach, S. (2013). Action prediction in younger versus older adults: Neural correlates of motor familiarity. *Plos One, 8*(5), e64195–e64195. doi:10.1371/journal.pone.0064195

Eickhoff, S. B., Laird, A. R., Grefkes, C., Wang, L. E., Zilles, K., & Fox, P. T. (2009). Coordinate-based activation likelihood estimation meta-analysis of neuroimaging data: A random-effects approach based on empirical estimates of spatial uncertainty. *Human Brain Mapping, 30*(9), 2907–2926.

Eierud, C., Craddock, R. C., Fletcher, S., Aulakh, M., King-Casas, B., Kuehl, D., & LaConte, S. M. (2014). Neuroimaging after mild traumatic brain injury: Review and meta-analysis. *Neuroimage Clinical, 4*, 283–294. doi:10.1016/j.nicl.2013.12.009

Eklund, A., Nichols, T. E., & Knutsson, H. (2016). Cluster failure: Why fMRI inferences for spatial extent have inflated false-positive rates. *Proceedings of the National Academy of Sciences of the United States of America, 113*(28), 7900–7905. doi:10.1073/pnas.1602413113

Engel, S. A., Rumelhart, D. E., Wandell, B. A., Lee, A. T., Glover, G. H., Chichilnisky, E.-J., & Shadlen, M. N. (1994). fMRI of human visual cortex. *Nature, 369*(6481), 525–525. doi:10.1038/369525a0

Ericsson, K. A., Krampe, R. T., & Tesch-Römer, C. (1993). The role of deliberate practice in the acquisition of expert performance. *Psychological Review, 100*, 363–406.

Farrow, D., McCrae, J., Gross, J., & Abernethy, B. (2010). Revisiting the relationship between pattern recall and anticipatory skill. *International Journal of Sport Psychology, 41*(1), 91–106.

Ferrari, M., & Quaresima, V. (2012). A brief review on the history of human functional near-infrared spectroscopy (fNIRS) development and fields of application. *NeuroImage, 63*(2), 921–935. doi:10.1016/j.neuroimage.2012.03.049

Ferrell, M. D., Beach, R. L., Szeverenyi, N. M., Krch, M., & Fernhall, B. (2006). An fMRI Analysis of neural activity during perceived zone-state performance. *Journal of Sport & Exercise Psychology, 28*(4), 421–433.

Fontes, E. B., Okano, A. H., De Guio, F., Schabort, E. J., Min, L. L., Basset, F. A., … Noakes, T. D. (2013). Brain activity and perceived exertion during cycling exercise: An fMRI study. *British Journal of Sports Medicine, 49*(8), 1–6.

Grèzes, J., & Decety, J. (2002). Does visual perception of object afford action? Evidence from a neuroimaging study. *Neuropsychologia, 40*(2), 212–222.

Hanin, Y. L. (1995). Individual zones of optimal functioning (IZOF) model: An idiographic approach to performance anxiety. In K. Henschen & W. Straub (Eds.), *Sport psychology: An analysis of athlete behavior* (pp. 103–119). Longmeadow, MA: Movement Publications.

Hanin, Y. L. (2000). An individualized approach to emotion in sport. In Y. L. Hanin (Ed.), *Emotions in sport* (pp. 65–90, 157–188). Champaign, IL: Human Kinetics.

Hanin, Y. L. (2003). *Performance related emotional states in sport: A qualitative analysis.* Retrieved from www.qualitative-research.net/fqs-texte/1-03/1-03hanin-e.htm

Harris, R., & de Jong, B. M. (2014). Cerebral activations related to audition-driven performance imagery in professional musicians. *PLoS One, 9*, e93681.

Hasegawa, T., Matsuki, K., Ueno, T., Maeda, Y., Matsue, Y., Konishi, Y., & Sadato, N. (2004). Learned audiovisual cross-modal associations in observed piano playing activate the left planum temporale. An fMRI study. *Cognitive Brain Research, 20*, 510–518.

Haslinger, B., Erhard, P., Altenmüller, E., Hennenlotter, A., Schwaiger, M., Gräfin von Einsiedel, …, & Ceballos-Baumann, A. O. (2004). Reduced recruitment of motor association areas during bimanual coordination in concert pianists. *Human Brain Mapping, 22*, 206–215.

Haslinger, B., Erhard, P., Altenmüller, E., Schroeder, U., Boecker, H., & Ceballos-Baumann, A. O. (2005). Transmodal sensorimotor networks during action observation in professional pianists (Article). MIT Press. doi:10.1162/0898929053124893.

Herholz, S. C., & Zatorre, R. J. (2012). Musical training as a framework for brain plasticity: Behavior, function, and structure. *Neuron, 76*(3), 486–502. doi:10.1016/j.neuron.2012.10.011

Hoshi, E., & Tanji, J. (2007). Distinctions between dorsal and ventral premotor areas: Anatomical connectivity and functional properties. *Current Opinion in Neurobiology, 17*(2), 234–242.

Hye Ju, P., Ren Xi, L., Jingu, K., Sung Woon, K., Doo Hwan, M., Myung Hwa, K., & Woo Jong, K. (2009). Neural correlates of winning and losing while watching soccer matches. *International Journal of Neuroscience, 119*, 76–87.

Issurin, V. (2013). Training transfer: Scientific background and insights for practical application. *Sports Medicine, 43*(8), 675–694.

Jasper, H. H. (1958). The ten-twenty electrode system of the International Federation. *Electroencephalography and Clinical Neurophysiology, 10*, 371–375.

Johnson, P. B., Farraina, S., Bianchi, L., & Caminiti, R. (1996). Cortical networks for visual reaching: Physiological and anatomical organization of frontal and parietal lobe arm regions. *Cerebral Cortex, 6*(2), 102–119. doi:10.1093/cercor/6.2.102

Karageorghis, C. I., & Drew, K. M. (1996). Effects of pretest stimulative and sedative music on grip strength. *Perceptual & Motor Skills, 83*(3), 1347.

Kelly, A. M. C., & Garavan, H. (2005). Human functional neuroimaging of brain changes associated with practice. *Cerebral Cortex, 15*(8), 1089–1102. doi:10.1093/cercor/bhi005

Kim, J., Lee, H. M., Kim, W. J., Park, H. J., Kim, S. W., Moon, D. H., … Tennant, L. K. (2008). Neural correlates of pre-performance routines in expert and novice archers. *Neuroscience Letters, 445*, 236–241.

Kim, W., Chang, Y., Kim, J., Seo, J., Ryu, K., Lee, E., … Janelle, C. M. (2014). An fMRI study of differences in brain activity among elite, expert, and novice archers at the moment of optimal aiming. *Cognitive and Behavioral Neurology, 27*, 173–182. doi:10.1097/wnn.0000000000000042

Kim, Y.-T., Seo, J.-H., Song, H.-J., Yoo, D.-S., Lee, H. J., Lee, J., … Chang, Y. (2011). Neural correlates related to action observation in expert archers. *Behavioural Brain Research, 223*(2), 342–347. doi:10.1016/j.bbr.2011.04.053

Koch, G., Ruge, D., Cheeran, B., Del Olmo, M. F., Pecchioli, C., Marconi, B., … Rothwell, J. C. (2009). TMS activation of interhemispheric pathways between the posterior parietal cortex and the contralateral motor cortex. *The Journal of Physiology, 587*(17), 4281–4292. doi:10.1113/jphysiol.2009.174086

Konen, C. S., Mruczek, R. E. B., Montoya, J. L., & Kastner, S. (2013). Functional organization of human posterior parietal cortex: Grasping- and reaching-related activations relative to topographically organized cortex. *Journal of Neurophysiology, 109*(12), 2897–2908.

Kwong, K. K., Belliveau, J. W., Chesler, D. A., Goldberg, I. E., Weisskoff, R. M., Poncelet, B. P., … Rosen, B. R. (1992). Dynamic magnetic resonance imaging of human brain activity during primary sensory stimulation. *Proceedings of the National Academy of Sciences of the United States of America, 89*(12), 5675–5679.

Lancaster, J. L., Tordesillas-Gutiérrez, D., Martinez, M., Salinas, F., Evans, A., Zilles, K., … Fox, P. T. (2007). Bias between MNI and Talairach coordinates analyzed using the ICBM-152 brain template. *Human Brain Mapping, 28*(11), 1194–1205.

Landau, S. M., & D'Esposito, M. (2006). Sequence learning in pianists and nonpianists: An fMRI study of motor expertise. *Cognitive, Affective & Behavioral Neuroscience, 6*(3), 246–259. doi:10.3758/CABN.6.3.246

Lang, P. J., Bradley, M. M., & Cuthbert, B. N. (2008). International affective picture system (IAPS): Affective ratings of pictures and instruction manual. Technical Report A-8. University of Florida, Gainesville, FL.

Lazarus, R. S. (2000). How emotions influence performance in competitive sports. *Sport Psychologist, 14*(3), 229.

Lee, H., & Noppeney, U. (2011). Long-term music training tunes how the brain temporally binds signals from multiple senses. *Proceedings of the National Academy of Sciences of the United States, 108*, E1441–1450.

Leech, R., Braga, R., & Sharp, D. J. (2012). Echoes of the brain within the posterior cingulate cortex. *The Journal of Neuroscience, 32*(1), 215–222. doi:10.1523/JNEUROSCI.3689-11.2012

Leitão, J., Thielscher, A., Tünnerhoff, J., & Noppeney, U. (2015). Concurrent TMS-fMRI reveals interactions between dorsal and ventral attentional systems. *The Journal of Neuroscience, 35*(32), 11445–11457. doi:10.1523/JNEUROSCI.0939-15.2015

Leonetti, A., Puglisi, G., Siugzdaite, R., Ferrari, C., Cerri, G., & Borroni, P. (2015). What you see is what you get: Motor resonance in peripheral vision. *Experimental Brain Research, 233*, 3013–3022. doi:10.1007/s00221-015-4371-0

Liu, T. T. (2012). The development of event-related fMRI designs. *NeuroImage, 62*(2), 1157–1162. doi:10.1016/j.neuroimage.2011.10.008

Loizou, G., Karageorghis, C. I., & Bishop, D. T. (2014). Interactive effects of video, priming, and music on emotions and the needs underlying intrinsic motivation. *Psychology of Sport and Exercise, 15*(6), 611–619. doi:10.1016/j.psychsport.2014.06.009

Lorenz, R., Monti, R. P., Violante, I. R., Anagnostopoulos, C., Faisal, A. A., Montana, G., & Leech, R. (2016). The automatic neuroscientist: A framework for optimizing experimental design with closed-loop real-time fMRI. *NeuroImage, 129*, 320–334. doi:10.1016/j.neuroimage.2016.01.032

Ludyga, S., Gronwald, T., & Hottenrott, K. (2015). The athlete's brain: Cross-sectional evidence for neural efficiency during cycling exercise. *Neural Plasticity*, 1–7. doi:10.1155/2016/4583674

Lyons, I. M., Mattarella-Micke, A., Cieslak, M., Nusbaum, H. C., Small, S. L., & Beilock, S. L. (2010). The role of personal experience in the neural processing of action-related language. *Brain & Language, 112*(3), 214–222. doi:10.1016/j.bandl.2009.05.006

Lütcke, H., & Frahm, J. (2008). Lateralized anterior cingulate function during error processing and conflict monitoring as revealed by high-resolution fMRI. *Cerebral Cortex, 18*, 508–515. doi:10.1093/cercor/bhm090

Lütcke, H., Gevensleben, H., Albrecht, B., & Frahm, J. (2009). Brain networks involved in early versus late response anticipation and their relation to conflict processing. *Journal of Cognitive Neuroscience, 21*, 2172–2184. doi:10.1162/jocn.2008.21165

Macnamara, B. N., Moreau, D., & Hambrick, D. Z. (2016). The relationship between deliberate practice and performance in sports: A meta-analysis. *Perspectives on Psychological Science, 11*(3), 333–350. doi:10.1177/1745691616635591

Majdandzic, J., Bekkering, H., van Schie, H. T., & Toni, I. (2009). Movement-specific repetition suppression in ventral and dorsal premotor cortex during action observation. *Cerebral Cortex (New York, N.Y.: 1991), 19*(11), 2736–2745. doi:10.1093/cercor/bhp049

Mann, D., Dicks, M., Cañal-Bruland, R., & van der Kamp, J. (2013). Neurophysiological studies may provide a misleading picture of how perceptual-motor interactions are coordinated. *i-Perception, 4*(1). doi:10.1068/i0569ic

Mann, D. T. Y., Williams, A. M., Ward, P., & Janelle, C. M. (2007). Perceptual-cognitive expertise in sport: A meta-analysis. *Journal of Sport & Exercise Psychology, 29*, 457–478.

McLean, J., Brennan, D., Wyper, D., Condon, B., Hadley, D., & Cavanagh, J. (2009). Localisation of regions of intense pleasure response evoked by soccer goals. *Psychiatry Research: Neuroimaging Section, 171*, 33–43.

Meister, I., Krings, T., Foltys, H., Boroojerdi, B., Müller, M., …, & Thron, A. (2005). Effects of long-term practice and task complexity in musicians and nonmusicians performing simple and complex motor tasks: implications for cortical motor organization. *Human Brain Mapping, 25*, 345–352.

Mijović, B., Vanderperren, K., Van Huffel, S., & De Vos, M. (2012). Improving spatiotemporal characterization of cognitive processes with data-driven EEG-fMRI analysis. *Prilozi/Makedonska Akademija Na Naukite I Umetnostite, Oddelenie Za Biološki I Medicinski Nauki, 33*(1), 373–390.

Milner, A. D., & Goodale, M. A. (1995). *The visual brain in action.* New York, NY: Oxford University Press.

Milton, J., Solodkin, A., Hluštík, P., & Small, S. L. (2007). The mind of expert motor performance is cool and focused. *NeuroImage, 35*, 804–813. doi:10.1016/j.neuroimage.2007.01.003

Moran, A., Guillot, A., MacIntyre, T., & Collet, C. (2012). Re-imagining motor imagery: Building bridges between cognitive neuroscience and sport psychology. *British Journal of Psychology, 103*(2), 224–247. doi:10.1111/j.2044–8295.2011.02068.x

Moriguchi, Y., & Hiraki, K. (2013). Prefrontal cortex and executive function in young children: A review of NIRS studies. *Frontiers in Human Neuroscience, 7.* doi:10.3389/fnhum.2013.00867

Muller, S., Abernethy, B., Eid, M., McBean, R., & Rose, M. (2010). Expertise and the spatio-temporal characteristics of anticipatory information pick-up from complex movement patterns. *Perception, 39*(6), 745–760.

Nadel, L., & Peterson, M. A. (2013). The hippocampus: Part of an interactive posterior representational system spanning perceptual and memorial systems. *Journal of Experimental Psychology: General, 142*(4), 1242–1254. doi:10.1037/a0033690

Nakata, H., Yoshie, M., Miura, A., & Kudo, K. (2010). Characteristics of the athletes' brain: Evidence from neurophysiology and neuroimaging. *Brain Research Reviews, 62*, 197–211.

Newman-Norlund, R. D., van Schie, H. T., van Zuijlen, A. M. J., & Bekkering, H. (2007). The mirror neuron system is more active during complementary compared with imitative action. *Nature Neuroscience, 10*(7), 817–818.

Niedenthal, P. M. (2007). Embodying Emotion. *Science, 316*(5827), 1002–1005.

Nisbett, R. E., & Wilson, T. D. (1977). The halo effect: Evidence for unconscious alteration of judgments. *Journal of Personality and Social Psychology, 35*(4), 250–256. doi:10.1037/0022–3514.35.4.250

Novakova, M., Mikl, M., & Jan, J. (2014). 30. Mapping of movement artifacts in fMRI. *Clinical Neurophysiology, 125*(5), e34–e34. doi:10.1016/j.clinph.2013.12.068

O'Craven, K. M., Rosen, B. R., Kwong, K. K., Savoy, R. L., & Treisman, A. (2000). Voluntary attention modulates fMRI activity in human MT-MST. In S. Yantis & S. Yantis (Eds.), *Visual perception: Essential readings.* (pp. 365–373). New York, NY: Psychology Press.

O'Craven, K. M., Rosen, B. R., Kwong, K. K., Treisman, A., & Savoy, R. L. (1997). Voluntary attention modulates fMRI activity in human MT-MST. *Neuron, 18*(4), 591–598.

Olsson, C.-J., & Lundström, P. (2013). Using action observation to study superior motor performance: A pilot fMRI study. *Frontiers in Human Neuroscience, 7*, 819.

Orgs, G., Dombrowski, J.-H., Heil, M., & Jansen-Osmann, P. (2008). Expertise in dance modulates alpha/beta event-related desynchronization during action observation. *European Journal of Neuroscience, 27*(12), 3380–3384. doi:10.1111/j.1460–9568.2008.06271.x

Page, M. P. A. (2006). What can't functional neuroimaging tell the cognitive psychologist? *Cortex; A Journal Devoted To the Study of the Nervous System and Behavior, 42*(3), 428–443.

Panksepp, J. (1998). *Affective neuroscience: The foundations of human and animal emotions.* New York, NY: Oxford University Press.

Pau, S., Jahn, G., Sakreida, K., Domin, M., & Lotze, M. (2013). Encoding and recall of finger sequences in experienced pianists compared with musically naïve controls: A combined behavioral and functional imaging study. *NeuroImage, 64*, 379–387. doi:10.1016/j.neuroimage.2012.09.012

Petrini, K., Pollick, F. E., Dahl, S., McAleer, P., McKay, L., Rocchesso, D., … Puce, A. (2011). Action expertise reduces brain activity for audiovisual matching actions: An fMRI study with expert drummers. *NeuroImage, 56*(3), 1480–1492. doi:10.1016/j.neuroimage.2011.03.009

Pilgramm, S., Lorey, B., Stark, R., Munzert, J., Vaitl, D., & Zentgraf, K. (2010). Differential activation of the lateral premotor cortex during action observation. *BMC Neuroscience, 11,* 89–89. doi:10.1186/1471–2202–11–89

Pinder, R. A., Davids, K., Renshaw, I., & Araújo, D. (2011). Representative learning design and functionality of research and practice in sport. *Journal of Sport & Exercise Psychology, 33*(1), 146–155.

Pinder, R. A., Renshaw, I., Headrick, J., & Davids, K. (2014). Skill acquisition and representative task design. In K. Davids, R. Hristovski, D. Araújo, N. Balagué Serre, C. Button, & P. Passos (Eds.), *Complex systems in sport* (pp. 319–333). New York, NY: Routledge/Taylor & Francis Group.

Raichle, M. E., & Snyder, A. Z. (2007). A default mode of brain function: A brief history of an evolving idea. *Neuroimage, 37*(4), 1083–1090.

Ramnani, N., & Owen, A. M. (2004). Anterior prefrontal cortex: Insights into function from anatomy and neuroimaging. *Nature Reviews Neuroscience, 5*(3), 184–194. doi:10.1038/nrn1343

Raymond, M., Pontier, D., Dufour, A. B., & Møller, A. P. (1996). Frequency-dependent maintenance of left handedness in humans. *Proceedings. Biological Sciences/The Royal Society, 263*(1377), 1627–1633.

Riedl, V., Bienkowska, K., Strobel, C., Tahmasian, M., Grimmer, T., Förster, S., … Drzezga, A. (2014). Local activity determines functional connectivity in the resting human brain: A simultaneous FDG-PET/fMRI study. *The Journal of Neuroscience, 34*(18), 6260–6266. doi:10.1523/JNEUROSCI.0492-14.2014

Rizzolatti, G., Cattaneo, L., Fabbri-Destro, M., & Rozzi, S. (2014). Cortical mechanisms underlying the organization of goal-directed actions and mirror neuron-based action understanding. *Physiological Reviews, 94*(2), 655–706. doi:10.1152/physrev.00009.2013

Rizzolatti, G., & Craighero, L. (2004). The mirror-neuron system. *Annual Review of Neuroscience, 27*(1), 169–192.

Rizzolatti, G., & Maddalena Fabbri, D. (2007). Understanding actions and the intentions of others: The basic neural mechanism. *European Review, 15,* 209–222. doi:10.1017/S1062798707000221

Robazza, C., Pellizzari, M., Bertollo, M., & Hanin, Y. L. (2008). Functional impact of emotions on athletic performance: Comparing the IZOF model and the directional perception approach. *Journal of Sports Sciences, 26*(10), 1033–1047.

Robazza, C., Pellizzari, M., & Hanin, Y. L. (2004). Emotion self-regulation and athletic performance: An application of the IZOF model. *Psychology of Sport and Exercise, 5,* 379–404.

Roberts, A. C., Robbins, T. W., & Weiskrantz, L. (1998). *The prefrontal cortex: Executive and cognitive functions.* New York, NY: Oxford University Press.

Sabbe, B., Hulstijn, W., van Hoof, J., Tuynman-Qua, H. G., & Zitman, F. (1999). Retardation in depression: Assessment by means of simple motor tasks. *Journal of Affective Disorders, 55*(1), 39–44. doi:10.1016/S0165–0327(98)00087-1

Schultz, W. (2016). Reward functions of the basal ganglia. *Journal of Neural Transmission.* doi:10.1007/s00702-016-1510-0

Sekiguchi, A., Yokoyama, S., Kasahara, S., Yomogida, Y., Takeuchi, H., Ogawa, T., … Kawashima, R. (2011). Neural bases of a specific strategy for visuospatial processing in rugby players. *Medicine & Science in Sports & Exercise, 43*(10), 1857–1862.

Seo, J., Kim, Y.-T., Song, H.-J., Lee, H. J., Lee, J., Jung, T.-D., … Chang, Y. (2012). Stronger activation and deactivation in archery experts for differential cognitive strategy in visuospatial working memory processing. *Behavioural Brain Research, 229*(1), 185–193. doi:10.1016/j.bbr.2012.01.019

Smith, D. M. (2016). Neurophysiology of action anticipation in athletes: A systematic review. *Neuroscience and Biobehavioral Reviews, 60,* 115–120. doi:10.1016/j.neubiorev.2015.11.007

Sparing, R., Mottaghy, F. M., Ganis, G., Thompson, W. L., Töpper, R., Kosslyn, S. M., & Pascual-Leone, A. (2002). Visual cortex excitability increases during visual mental imagery—A TMS study in healthy human subjects. *Brain Research, 938*(1–2), 92–97. doi:10.1016/S0006–8993(02)02478-2

Stefan, K., Classen, J., Celnik, P., & Cohen, L. G. (2008). Concurrent action observation modulates practice-induced motor memory formation. *European Journal of Neuroscience, 27*(3), 730–738.

Stefan, K., Cohen, L. G., Duque, J., Mazzocchio, R., Celnik, P., Sawaki, L., … Classen, J. (2005). Formation of a motor memory by action observation. *Journal of Neuroscience, 25*(41), 9339–9346. doi:10.1523/jneurosci.2282–05.2005

Stout, D., Passingham, R., Frith, C., Apel, J., & Chaminade, T. (2011). Technology, expertise and social cognition in human evolution. *European Journal of Neuroscience, 33*(7), 1328–1338. doi:10.1111/j.1460–9568.2011.07619.x

Sun, L., & Hinrichs, H. (2009). Simultaneously recorded EEG-fMRI: Removal of gradient artifacts by subtraction of head movement related average artifact waveforms. *Human Brain Mapping, 30*(10), 3361–3377. doi:10.1002/hbm.20758

Talairach, J., & Tournoux, P. (1988). *Co-planar stereotaxis atlas of the human brain.* New York, NY: Thieme.

Thorndike, E. L. (1920). A constant error in psychological ratings. *Journal of Applied Psychology, 4*(1), 25–29. doi:10.1037/h0071663

Tomasino, B., Maieron, M., Guatto, E., Fabbro, F., & Rumiati, R. I. (2013). How are the motor system activity and functional connectivity between the cognitive and sensorimotor systems modulated by athletic expertise? *Brain Research, 1540*, 21–41.

Vaeyens, R., Lenoir, M., Mazyn, L., Williams, A. M., & Philippaerts, R. M. (2007). The effects of task constraints on visual search behavior and decision-making skill in youth soccer players. *Journal of Sport & Exercise Psychology, 29*, 156–175.

Vingerhoets, G. (2014). Contribution of the posterior parietal cortex in reaching, grasping, and using objects and tools. *Frontiers in Psychology, 5*, 151.

Visser, R. M., de Haan, M. I. C., Beemsterboer, T., Haver, P., Kindt, M., & Scholte, H. S. (2016). Quantifying learning-dependent changes in the brain: Single-trial multivoxel pattern analysis requires slow event-related fMRI. *Psychophysiology, 53*(8), 1117–1127.

Vogt, B. A., Berger, G. R., & Derbyshire, S. W. G. (2003). Structural and functional dichotomy of human midcingulate cortex. *The European Journal of Neuroscience, 18*(11), 3134–3144.

Vos, B. C., Nieuwenhuijsen, K., & Sluiter, J. K. (2018). Consequences of traumatic brain injury in professional American football players: A systematic review of the literature. *Clinical Journal Of Sport Medicine, 28*(2), 91-99.

Walsh, V. (2014). Is sport the brain's biggest challenge? *Current Biology: CB, 24*(18), R859-R860. doi:10.1016/j.cub.2014.08.003

Wei, G., & Luo, J. (2010). Sport expert's motor imagery: Functional imaging of professional motor skills and simple motor skills. *Brain Research, 1341*, 52–62. doi:10.1016/j.brainres.2009.08.014

Weinberg, R., Butt, J., & Culp, B. (2011). Coaches' views of mental toughness and how it is built. *International Journal of Sport & Exercise Psychology, 9*(2), 156–172.

Wilmer, J. B., Germine, L., Chabris, C. F., Chatterjee, G., Williams, M., Loken, E., … Duchaine, B. (2010). Human face recognition ability is specific and highly heritable. *Proceedings of the National Academy of Sciences of the United States of America, 107*(11), 5238–5241. doi:10.1073/pnas.0913053107

Wilson, K. D., & Farah, M. J. (2006). Distinct patterns of viewpoint-dependent BOLD activity during common-object recognition and mental rotation. *Perception, 35*(10), 1351–1366. doi:10.1068/p5571

Wong, C., & Gallate, J. (2012). The function of the anterior temporal lobe: A review of the empirical evidence. *Brain Research, 1449*, 94–116. doi:10.1016/j.brainres.2012.02.017

Wright, M. J., Bishop, D. T., Jackson, R. C., & Abernethy, B. (2010). Functional MRI reveals expert-novice differences in brain activation during sport-related anticipation. *NeuroReport, 21*, 94–98. doi:10.1097/WNR.0b013e328333dff2

Wright, M. J., Bishop, D. T., Jackson, R. C., & Abernethy, B. (2011). Cortical fMRI activation to opponents' body kinematics in sport-related anticipation: Expert-novice differences with normal and point-light video. *Neuroscience Letters, 500*, 216–221. doi:10.1016/j.neulet.2011.06.045

Wright, M. J., Bishop, D., Jackson, R. C., & Abernethy, B. (2013). Brain regions concerned with the identification of deceptive soccer moves by high-skilled and low-skilled players. *Frontiers in Human Neuroscience.* doi:10.3389/fnhum.2013.00851

Wright, M. J., & Jackson, R. C. (2007). Brain regions concerned with perceptual skills in tennis: An fMRI study. *International Journal of Psychophysiology, 63*, 214–220. doi:10.1016/j.ijpsycho.2006.03.018

Wu, Y., Zeng, Y., Zhang, L., Wang, S., Wang, D., Tan, X., … Zhang, J. (2013). The role of visual perception in action anticipation in basketball athletes. *Neuroscience, 237*, 29–41.

Yang, J. (2015). The influence of motor expertise on the brain activity of motor task performance: A meta-analysis of functional magnetic resonance imaging studies. *Cognitive, Affective & Behavioral Neuroscience, 15*(2), 381–394. doi:10.3758/s13415-014-0329-0

Yarrow, K., Brown, P., & Krakauer, J. W. (2009). Inside the brain of an elite athlete: The neural processes that support high achievement in sports. *Nature Neuroscience Reviews, 10*, 585–596. doi:10.1038/nrn2672

Zhu, F. F., Poolton, J. M., Wilson, M. R., Hu, Y., Maxwell, J. P., & Masters, R. S. W. (2011). Implicit motor learning promotes neural efficiency during laparoscopy. *Surgical Endoscopy, 25*(9), 2950–2955. doi:10.1007/s00464-011-1647-8

From Investigation to Intervention
Biofeedback and Neurofeedback Biomarkers in Sport

Michela Balconi, Francesca Pala, Davide Crivelli, and Valeria Milone

Sport neuroscience, lying at the intersection of applied neuroscience and sport psychology, includes among its hot topics the cognitive and affective processes and mechanisms that accompany the athletic performance.

This chapter focuses on present applications of psychophysiological and electrophysiological techniques, such as biofeedback and neurofeedback, to support or empower performance in sports. In particular, you will find an introduction to the mechanisms of action of most relevant techniques in the field, neural-bodily-behavioral modulations that are targeted by different intervention opportunities, and technical application notes.

We will discuss the value of self-awareness and of the ability to properly recognize bodily feedbacks, especially when athletes have to face competition, and the relevance of robust self-regulation skills to achieve maximum performance. Further, we will report a critical comparison between the efficacy and strong/weak points of bio/neurofeedback techniques and more traditional mental training techniques within the field of sport science. Finally, we will present and discuss different protocols applied to specific sports, such as baseball, golf, soccer, and gymnastics.

Biofeedback and Neurofeedback: Principles and Mechanisms of Action

The biofeedback technique aims at making practicers able to intentionally modulate their physiological activity and responses thanks based on real-time recording of such biosignals via noninvasive electronic sensors, in order to better their health status or to improve neurocognitive performance (Gilbert & Moss, 2003; Schwartz & Andrasik, 2003; Shaffer & Moss, 2006). Biometric sensors included in biofeedback devices are used to collect data about ongoing physiological processes and modulation of bodily activity and then provide a real-time feedback mirroring such modulations, thus helping the individual to increase awareness of such processes and to strengthen voluntary control over body and mind. Biofeedback applications are usually grounded on the measurement of muscle activity, electrodermal activity (commonly quantified as skin conductance), blood pressure, and cardiac activity. Because of that, the biofeedback technique has been described as a "psychophysiological mirror", which allows practicers to adaptively monitor and learn from physiological signals produced by their bodies (Peper, Harvey, & Takabayashi, 2009). On the other hand, neurofeedback is a technique that helps practicers to develop the ability to intentionally modulate their brain waves based on the accurate recording of patterns of cortical oscillatory activity via electroencephalography (Marzbani, Marateb, & Mansourian, 2016). Such information flow is used to reinforce and model neural behavior and, then, to increase awareness and to achieve self-regulation goals. Biofeedback and neurofeedback are now deemed as valuable intervention tools, which are able to provide the kind of evidence-based practice the health care establishment is demanding (Geyman, Deyo, & Ramsey, 2000; Sackett, Strauss, Richardson, Rosenberg, & Haynes, 2000).

Both biofeedback and neurofeedback techniques have their roots deep into the operant conditioning paradigm, in which reinforcement and punishment are used to implicitly promote learning and to shape behavior, and apply its principles and techniques to help people to build a stronger bodily awareness and to learn how to influence the responses of their bodies and brains.

In general, the goal of biofeedback and neurofeedback protocols is to increase the voluntary control over physiological processes that otherwise lie outside awareness by translating information on their development and modification into external and easily-accessible feedbacks (Balconi & Crivelli, in press; Balconi, Fronda, Venturella, & Crivelli, 2017; Pop-Jordanova & Demerdzieva, 2010). At the beginning, biofeedback was developed as a research-based approach. Indeed, it directly stem from laboratory research on psychophysiology and behavior therapy, which forsook further understanding of neurophysiological mechanisms underlying psychological disorders. In particular, biofeedback therapies were born as non-pharmacologic treatments that use psychophysiological instruments to measure, amplify, and feedback physiological information to the patient being monitored. Psychophysiological self-regulation was – and currently is – a primary goal of biofeedback therapies. Feedbacks are provided to foster self- and bodily-control, just as they are used to facilitate learning of other skills in different training situations. Such real-time external feedback, which are typically visual and/or acoustic, guides the practicer during the training by making them learn, for example, to warm specific portions of their skin, to relax specific muscles, or to reduce blood pressure.

It has been proposed that these non-invasive intervention techniques also share further specific goals: (1) to give individuals a more active role in taking care of themselves and of their health; (2) to promote a holistic emphasis on body, mind, and spirit; and (3) to elicit the body's own healing and empowerment resources (Gilbert & Moss, 2003; Jonas & Levin, 1999).

Biofeedback and neurofeedback techniques have been widely used to intervene on many diseases and disorders, such as schizophrenia, autistic spectrum disorder, insomnia, drug addiction, attention disorders, altered stress response, and anxiety-related disturbances. Again, biofeedback and neurofeedback are used in a variety of applied settings:

1   assessment and treatment of clinical pictures, such as headache, attention-deficit hyperactivity disorder (ADHD), epilepsy, stress/anxiety, respiratory and sleep problems, pain, and many others;
2   empowerment and promotion of learning in education settings, e.g. reduction of learning anxiety, improvement of focusing skills, assessment of the learning processes;
3   enhancement of performance and optimal functioning for sports, business, and military activities;
4   promotion of self-exploration and self-enhancement, e.g. evaluation of the impact of life events on physiology, improvement of imagination and creativity, etc.

The use of peripheral biofeedback and central neurofeedback techniques is rapidly growing and, given the strong relationship between mental and physical performance in sport practice, sport neuroscience is a notably representative field with respect to novel applications of such techniques.

Brain Correlates of Bio/Neurofeedback Applications

Biofeedback and neurofeedback are procedures for self-regulation that, starting from the detection of peripheral biological signals, are intended to better the psychophysiological state of the practicer and thus foster the best level of performance. The scientific bases of those instruments are to be found in neuroscience, a discipline that has highlighted the strict mutual bond between changes of the physiological and the mental status.

The relevance of biofeedback in athletes' training and sport interventions can be traced back to the very same "psychophysiological principle" that determines how every physiological change is associated to a parallel change in mind processes and emotional states (Green, Green, & Walters, 1970). Equally, every conscious or unconscious change of such processes and emotional states can be associated to a corresponding change of physiological states.

The process supporting bio/neurofeedback practice involves three methodological elements:

1   information about the physiological modifications, obtained by using sensing electrodes that collect specific signals;
2   amplification and transcription of those signals into easily-perceivable feedbacks by the bio/neurofeedback system;
3   feedbacks, advices, and instructions from the trainer or therapist, used by the practicer to try and increase (or decrease) the target physiological signal.

Specifically, the neurofeedback process involves training and learning self-regulation of brain activity associated to altered cognitive-affective states and central control of bodily responses. Such potential outcome has been deemed as a valuable help even in sports since, for example, the ability to develop a new adaptive response to situational stressors might change the life course of athletes and facilitate much more favorable athletic outcomes.

That, however, requires a gradual learning process. Neurofeedback training may be applied to any aspect of brain functioning that can be measured. Based on Skinner's theory of operant conditioning (1954), neurofeedback training grounds on the idea that learning is a function of change in overt behavior. Changes of conducts are the result of an individual's response to events (stimuli) that occur in the environment. The distinctive characteristic of operant conditioning with respect to previous behaviorist models of conditioning and learning is that the organism can actively produce responses instead of only generating elicited responses consequent to external stimuli. Reinforcements linked to such active responses are then the key element in Skinner's Stimulus-Response (S-R) theory. A reinforcer is anything that strengthens the desired response, i.e. the adaptive response that is intended to be trained. It could be a verbal praise, a good grade, or a feeling of increased accomplishment or satisfaction. The theory also covers negative reinforcers, defined as any stimulus that results in an increase of the frequency of a desired response when it is withdrawn. A great deal of attention was given to the investigation of schedules of reinforcement and of their effects on the promotion and maintenance of the desired behavior. The same principles are applied during a typical bio/neurofeedback training session. First, sensors are placed in correspondence to specific locations on the scalp or the body. Then, the sensors measure the pattern of autonomic responses or electrical activity generated by the neurons and such data are filtered and relayed to the computer and recorded. Finally, by using cutting edge technology, the practicer receives real-time visual and audio feedbacks about his/her bodily or brainwave activity, which are especially designed to reinforce the physiological activity that is intended to be trained.

Behavioral Correlates of Bio/Neurofeedback Applications

It's important, especially for athletes, to be able to recognize all the signs their body provides during exercise, and particularly to know how to control them adequately. Learning to maintain a specific balance between activation and relaxation supports the achievement of optimal performance, so that the athlete might be able to answer competition requests more effectively.

During the last decades, the analysis of the psychological, physiological, kinematic, and behavioral mechanisms underlying the performance of élite athletes has received increasing attention, especially in precision sports (Goodman, Haufler, Shim, & Hatfield, 2009; Hatfield & Landers, 1983). At present, the measurement of performance-related emotional experiences is also taken in great consideration and it is evaluated by multimodal and multidimensional assessment procedures derived from the integration of different fields of investigation – such as motor behavior, sport psychology, and affective psychophysiology. Monitoring the entire spectrum of psychophysiological and behavioral correlates related to the athletic performance is important in order to develop and implement biofeedback and neurofeedback protocols for sports. The principal aims of such protocols are, indeed, to support athletes in identifying their subjective zones of optimal functioning, in enhancing their performance, and in strengthening their ability to self-regulate and regulate emotions, so to prevent choking under competitive pressure.

Furthermore, besides improving subjective control of central and autonomic nervous system, stress responses, and affective reactions to trying situations, biofeedback and, in particular, neurofeedback practice leads to additional advantages including:

1   improved depth and quality of sleep, which is known to directly correlate to performance;
2   increased neural plasticity, which helps the central nervous system to learn more efficiently and to better cope with stress due to pressure on performance;
3   greater focusing and attention skills, which are essential for athletes;
4   maintenance of clarity of mind and cognitive efficiency over time and in spite of fatigue;
5   helping to avert one-way, negative thinking, athletes are indeed subject to downturns in sports not only because of potential inefficiency of their bodies, but also because of what is happening into their brains and minds.

What's New in Sport Neuroscience? Bio/Neurofeedback as Biological Markers of Physical and Mental Activity

The integration of neurosciences and sport psychology fueled the study of cognitive and emotional mechanisms for the achievement of peak athletic performance. In high-performance sports, in fact, many cognitive functions are concurrently involved in modulating athletic outcomes, such as the information-processing speed and readiness to respond to stimuli, the storage capacity in short and long term memory, the ability to conceive and implement effective strategies, and the ability to quickly change mindset and action plans on the basis of environmental changes and needs.

Biofeedback and neurofeedback can be used to support the learning process during training of such cognitive and psychomotor skills. Indeed, in the field of applied sport research, biofeedback and neurofeedback already have a quite well-established tradition with regard to three primary practical implications (Zaichkowsky & Fuchs, 1988):

1   as techniques for teaching athletes to deal with general and specific anxiety;
2   as a mean of restoring function after muscle injury;
3   as a mean for providing biomechanical and muscle feedback to athletes so that they could perfect highly-skilled movements and enhance performance.

The efficacy of different training protocols designed to foster cognitive and emotional self-regulation and to improve athlete performance with regard to sport-specific tasks has been tested in many studies. Additionally, sport-specific performance measures proved to be enhanced following bio/neurofeedback interventions. For example, it was shown that, by using the skills learned during bio/neurofeedback training, athletes may become able to regulate their breathing and arousal levels so to increase their performance in their sport (Perry, Shaw, & Zaichkowsky, 2011).

A Comparison Between Visual, Kinesthetic and Mental Imagery Performance and Psychophysiological Techniques (Biofeedback and Neurofeedback)

There are several techniques used in sports for the evaluation of the processes that allow us to mentally simulate a sequence of movements and actions to be implemented in a context that, consequently, may help to achieve a deeper knowledge about the functional organization of the cognitive engine system and the use of this potential. In particular, among the various approaches, visual imagination, kinesthetic motor imagery, and mental images have also been used in combination with psychophysiological techniques.

Conditions that promote the formation of mental images are: vividness and controllability, practice, attitude and expectations of athletes, influence of past experience, attention, and a relaxed stance (Corbin, 1972). A vivid image is one in which the imagined events are as realistic as possible and involve connected sensory and emotional experiences. The more realistic the image is, the more the current task will be facilitated in its execution. The principle of specificity of the formation of mental images is based on the assumption that individuals can benefit from imagination in so far as such condition is similar to a past experience, and that such similarity contributes to better learning.

In addition to the visual imagery, kinesthetic images – e.g. the mental focusing on the bodily correlates of a sequence of complex movements – are also often used. Instructions that are typically given when using that kind of imagery technique – namely, kinesthetic imagery or sensorimotor imagination – initially include the actual repetition of a target movement several times and then require the practicer to keep repeating it internally via mental simulation while focusing on its kinesthetic correlates. The rationale underlying the use of such mental images is that focusing on kinesthetic aspects of a gesture, after the actual experience of the target movement, allows for developing a greater awareness of the motor act and of specific movements that was initially carried out unconsciously (Jeannerod, 1995).

Compared to the effect of the mere kinesthetic image formation, it has been shown that mental practice improves the performance of athletes with regard to learning motor skills in a variety of situations (Driskell, Copper, & Moran, 1994). Motor imagery is indeed an active process, in which an action is represented and mentally reproduced, taking into account even specific cognitive components such as attention and working memory. Those internal representations of motor acts are centrally organized and, just as any other representation, they are stored, can be modified by practice, and can be retrieved through specific cognitive processes.

A quite long tradition of experimental studies suggests that there are limited differences between neural and functional correlates of actual execution of an action and of its mental simulation. In fact, the areas that are activated within the planning and execution sensorimotor networks (medial supplementary motor area, the premotor cortex, dorsolateral prefrontal cortex, and posterior parietal cortex) are often the same (see Balconi, Cortesi, & Crivelli, 2017; Balconi, Crivelli, & Cortesi, 2017; Balconi, Crivelli, & Bove, 2018). Furthermore, mental images that are used in sport-related training do not necessarily involve just a motor, somatosensory, auditory, or visual experience, but can be an integration of all these elements (Balconi & Caldiroli, 2011; Balconi, Caldiroli & Vitaloni, 2011; Balconi & Cortesi, 2016). Given that such shared physiological modulations, though not easily-accessible by the consciousness, are directly associated with executed and imagined movements, the use of psychophysiological techniques is a valuable opportunity to help athletes to access such internal source of information even in combination to imagery techniques and to monitor and control the variations observed in autonomic parameters, such as heart rate, respiratory rate, and skin conductance responses (Decety, Jeannerod, Germain, & Pastene, 1991; Guillot & Collet, 2008).

The Contribution of Mental Training and Biofeedback

The contribution of both the peripheral and the central nervous system to the coordination of movement, as well as its efficiency, are mediated in various ways by psychological factors. Since mental training can help to build attention towards psychological processes involved in sport practice and, in particular, to build awareness of how they influence athletic outcomes, it is an opportunity for all athletes who want to improve their sports performance. Through mental training and the use of related techniques, the athlete can increase self-knowledge, become more aware of his/her resources, improve self-confidence, and understand how his/her body and mind interact, thus allowing the realization of his/her potential.

The main techniques that are traditionally included among mental training practices are relaxation, self-talk, and biofeedback.

Relaxation refers to a physiological status characterized by the reduction of the overall level of activation of the organism, which corresponds to calmness, harmony, and minimized anxiety and tension. In sports, relaxation techniques are used to become aware of muscle tension at rest and to manage anxiety or stressful situations that can adversely affect the performance.

Another important mental training technique is self-talk. This technique consists in an "internal" dialogue that the athlete sustains with him/herself, through which it is possible to act upon concentration, to arouse positive emotions, and to increase self-confidence. Thoughts that do often automatically show up into the athlete's mind can affect performance both positively and negatively. A typical internal dialogue of an athlete can be constituted by statements like "I can do it!", "Hang in there a few more minutes!", and "It happens to everyone to make a mistake, and then it can happen to me!". On the one side, positive thoughts promote feelings of adequacy to the task and facilitate therefore a good performance. On the other, inappropriate and negative thoughts of inadequacy arouse apprehension and adversely affect the outcome of the performance.

Again, in sport psychology, biofeedback is one of the most effective techniques to facilitate the learning of self-regulation of the level of arousal. Indeed, biofeedback is advisable for the promotion of relaxation even in those individuals who have difficulty with other techniques such as hypnosis or mental imagery. In fact, the immediate feedback regarding physiological states allows the athlete for more easily perceiving and modulating his/her level of activation than alternative techniques. To train such skills is peculiarly important since, when we are faced with a trying challenge (affecting, for example our social or working life) or, even more specifically, with a sport competition, our mind-body system prepares to deal with it through a complex set of responses that support psychophysiological activation. A series of relevant processes and mechanisms are then set in motion, including increase of vigilance and attention (activation of the central nervous system), preparation of the muscles to endure the expected amount of effort (activation of the musculoskeletal system), and increase of cardiovascular and respiratory activity to optimize the distribution of resources (sympathetic autonomic system). Research in sport psychology has shown that there is a very close relationship between psychophysiological activation and psychomotor performance, and that learning to optimize such form of activation positively influences performance outcomes. When the mind-body system presents a low level of activation (under-activation), the athlete may feel detached and may find it hard to concentrate and enter the race because of a lack of motivation and because he/she feels not challenged enough. As the activation grows, the performance improves, until reaching its optimal maximum corresponding to the vertex of an inverted U curve (such point is often related to the state of flow). Then, if activation grows too much (hyperactivation), the athlete may experience feelings of excessive fatigue, anxiety, and helplessness that undermine performance outcomes.

Biofeedback, unlike other mental training techniques, provides an immediate feedback on the achievement of training goals, allowing the athlete for real-time continuous monitoring of his/her psychophysiological state. Therefore, the integration of such approach with adequate mental preparation techniques offers the athlete the opportunity to make more appropriate interpretations of his/her bodily sensations and affective reactions, to gain deeper knowledge of his/her self-regulation skills, and to strengthen such self-acquired abilities. Since biofeedback practice is actually devised as a training process (as opposed to a passive treatment), individuals undergoing biofeedback training must take an active role, self-experiment, and keep practicing in order to develop the desired skills and to reach the goals that have been planned. As is the case with other mental training techniques, the practicer is an active learner rather than a passive beneficiary of some kind of treatment. However, unlike other mental training technique, biofeedback also directly informs practicers on how their bodily systems react to mental tasks and particularly stressful situations and, thus, adds a relevant source of information to the learning process. Trainers and therapists can indeed pause the recording and show to the athlete the correlates of his/her physiological reactivity, as well as the extent to which and the speed with which his/her physiological activity returns to baseline values. Then, trainers and therapists may use those pieces of evidence to explain what the optimal values for each of the physiological variables being measured are, as well as how they relate to the athlete's health. Another important aspect of biofeedback practice is the reinforcement given by the trainer/therapist to the practicer with regard to his/her advancements, to the goals that he/she has achieved, to his/her increased awareness and control, and to the benefits in terms of mental and physical wellness (Frank, Khorshid, Kiffer, Moravec, & McKee, 2010).

The Contribution of Mental Training and Neurofeedback

Recently, there has been a relevant increase of interest and awareness of the potential of neurofeedback training for the improvement of sports performance (Hammond, 2007). The latest research suggests that opportunities to modulate brain activity can have a positive impact on performance. Nonetheless, despite the potential of the technique, systematic investigations of the effect of neurofeedback training on objective measures of performance are still very limited.

Through an integrated approach to mental training and neurofeedback, it may be possible to increase awareness of specific central correlates of athletic performance and sport practice. Further, an athlete undergoing neurofeedback training might learn to optimize brain activity and central control over athletic gestures, by strengthening neural connections, improving coherence across the activity of neural structures, and empowering core cognitive abilities, such as focusing, attention, and memory.

Among the advantages of integrating mental training practice with specific neuroscience techniques, there might be the possibility to reach desired training goals in a much shorter time due to the opportunity to more directly work on inherent plasticity of the brain. Neurofeedback training may act as a compass, showing the way into physical and mental states that are difficult to reach without guidance and then, after some practice, allowing the practicer to get there autonomously. You might think of neurofeedback as a personal training session for the brain, where the brain eventually becomes its own trainer. Training the brain to function at its maximum potential is conceptually similar to the way the body is trained, toned, and maintained. Namely, brain training uses repeated practice to exercise the neural networks supporting core cognitive functions such as concentration and focusing, just as muscle training uses exercise to strengthen and optimize the functioning of effectors enacting a movement.

With respect to mental preparation in sports, neurofeedback practice has also been combined with the goal setting, or training objectives, approach. As for the goal setting approach, it has been shown that a good understanding of what you want to achieve, with which strategy you may get there, and how long will it take increases performance more than having no goals or simply setting the aspecific goal to give the best of ourselves. If implemented in the right way, goal setting allows you to avoid some typical mistakes, like defining goals that are too ambitious or too uninspiring with respect to our resources and skills. Helping an athlete to set achievable and challenging goals affects his/her cognitive performance and attention, and increases his/her motivation. Integrating such practice with neurofeedback training fosters the optimization of neural responses to environmental requests, may improve neurocognitive efficiency, and helps the athlete to define adaptive individual strategies to manage stress and workload.

Furthermore, recent technological innovations lead to the development of a novel integrated approach that combines mindfulness-based mental training and wearable neurofeedback devices for the empowerment of stress management, neurocognitive efficiency, and mental focus skills (Balconi & Crivelli, *in press*; Balconi et al., 2017). First available efficacy data depict such novel technology-supported mindfulness-based protocol as a promising training approach (Crivelli, Fronda, Venturella, & Balconi, 2018); nonetheless its potential still needs to be further tested in different applied contexts.

Investigating the Efficacy of Neurofeedback and Biofeedback Training for Expertise and Excellence in Sport

Neurofeedback is a tool by which the athlete learns to change the amplitude, frequency, and coherence of the electrophysiological correlates of brain activity, thus allowing him/her to achieve a specific improvement of associated mental states. Neurofeedback practice may train athletes to be aware of their own mental states under different conditions and to modify them adaptively so to face performance requests. Indeed, while practicing neurofeedback, athletes can picture their mindset and its modulations by using visual and acoustic feedbacks provided by a computer on the basis of recorded transient patterns of neural activity, and can then identify specific states that are mostly functional with regard to their training goals and the needs of their sport specialty. In this way, it is possible to train to achieve the individual "optimal zone" for performance.

Currently, no universally-recognized and standardized practice exists for training athletes with neurofeedback. Further, it is still unclear whether there are particular athletes that respond better to that kind of training, which training protocol is the best to achieve optimal performance goals, or which is the minimum number of training sessions for improvement to occur.

Neurofeedback and Biofeedback Training for Peak Performance

Peak experience in sport is defined as a state of exceptional functioning of an athlete's psychological and physical systems, which determines optimal performance (Berger & Tobar, 2007).

Csikszentmihalyi (1975) has conceptualized the term flow as the subjective psychological state of maximum optimism and gratification that can be experienced when carrying out activities for which our resources optimally meet the requests and challenges posed by the activity and that corresponds to a complete immersion in the task. The state of flow is not a stable condition, but a transient experience that depends on the continuous adaptation to external (opponent unanticipated move, weather changes, etc.) and internal (increase of lactic acid, variation of heartbeats, etc.) conditions. One of the methods that are commonly used in sport psychology to work on the flow and on the ability to voluntarily enter in such state is mental imagery, which can be used to mentally evoke an athletic episode that went particularly well together with the associated mindset and affective states.

In order to improve the ability to experience flow and to reach peak performance, it is however important also to recognize and be aware of bodily functioning before, during, and after training or competition (brain activity, heart rate, respiration, muscle tension, and many other quantifiable measures of human performance). By recording, analyzing, and identifying individual ideal levels of bodily functions, it is possible to help an athlete to reach his/her peak in terms of performance, to improve stress management, to contain performance anxiety, and to decrease pre-competition tension. The pressure associated to sport performance can be generated by both internal and external factors but, whatever the cause, it may have harmful effects on the athlete and on the team as a whole. Often, athletes can be their worst enemies. Indeed, focusing on past failures undermines athletes' confidence, making easier for them to fail again as long as they remain unfocused and self-critical (Wilson et al, 2006).

Specifically, by practicing neurofeedback, an athlete can reach a deeper understanding of his/her own mind-brain activity and, above all, to modify it by developing individual mental strategies with the help of experts. Besides relieving psychological symptoms (e.g. anxiety, depression) and supporting the recovery from sport-related injuries (e.g. concussion, headache, muscle tension) that may interfere with sports performance, neurofeedback training may aim at improving different abilities that are necessary to maximize performance, such as relaxation, focusing, agility, and timing, as well as the maintenance or increase of motivation (Wilson, Peper, & Moss, 2006). The most frequently-cited benefits of bio\neurofeedback training for sport practice are: better concentration, better attention, optimized decision-making processes, reduced number of errors, shorter response times, enhanced creativity, more efficient memory, accelerated learning, increased resilience to stress, increased productivity, lowered susceptibility to burn-out, quicker and deeper relaxation, better mind/body integration, enhanced well-being, reduced anxiety and stage fright, increased self-confidence and assertiveness, enhanced self-control and self-awareness, and improved emotional intelligence.

Brain-Training for Physical Performance, Neurofeedback Applications and Relaxation Training in Athletes

In recent years, the integration of EEG-based neurofeedback and relaxation techniques have been more and more used to optimize athletes' brain functioning and performance, as a valuable training opportunity for coach and trainers in professional sports training centers.

EEG investigations within the field of sport research largely focused on the alpha rhythm (8–12.5 Hz). The alpha rhythm is easily distinguishable from other brain rhythms (for example, theta 4–7.5 Hz, and beta at 13–30 Hz). Alpha is a dominant frequency band in the EEG of adults and it is also the most widely studied neural oscillatory activity. A wealth of contemporary studies supports the view that alpha plays an active role in cognitive processing and that it modulation marks the shift between cortical idling, relaxed wakefulness, and active information-processing (Cooper, Croft, Dominey, Burgess, & Gruzelier, 2003; Klimesch, Sauseng, & Hanslmayr, 2007).

Alpha oscillations are thought to mirror active inhibition of unnecessary cortical activity and control mechanisms that prevent processing of information that is not relevant for the task (Klimesch, Doppelmayr, Schwaiger, Winkler, & Gruber, 2000; Pfurtscheller & Da Silva, 1999). Thus, the modification of alpha activity can be detected in a wide range of tasks and can be considered as a marker of the modulation of information-processing linked to a number of different functions. Support for this view comes from empirical findings that show how distinct sub-alpha bands are associated with multiple operations – many of which are very important for sport practice – including the modulation of global arousal and attention processes (Pfurtscheller & Da Silva, 1999; Thut, Nietzel, Brandt, & Pascual-Leone, 2006), processing of sensorimotor and semantic information (Klimesch, Doppelmayr, Pachinger, & Ripper, 1997; Klimesch, Doppelmayr, Pachinger, & Russegger, 1997), maintenance of pieces of information within the working memory buffers (Jensen & Tesche, 2002; Tuladhar et al., 2007), inhibition of motor programs (Hummel, Andres, Altenmüller, Dichgans, & Gerloff, 2002), and motor learning (Koeneke, Lutz, Herwig, Ziemann, & Jäncke, 2006).

For example, in the EEG literature on sports correlates, variations of alpha power during a task or an exercise with respect to resting-state baseline levels (often measures during eye-closed idling conditions) are often used as a marker of task-related or exercise-related cortical activation/

deactivation. Because alpha frequency components are always present in the cortical activity to a certain extent, the choice of the baseline has a significant impact on the pattern of brain activation that can be reported. Variations of the power of EEG frequency bands reflect the presence or the release of cortical inhibition. The constructs of inhibition and neural efficiency are pervasive in the sport literature based on EEG investigations and they are consistent with different models of learning and motor skills proficiency that have been very influential in the field of sports science.

As an example, Mikicin and colleagues (2015) devised a study to specifically test the impact of neurofeedback training for physical performance on physiological (EEG) and behavioral measures in a sample of semi-professional athletes. The neurofeedback protocol was designed to increase the amplitude of the sensorimotor rhythm (12–15 Hz, a set of frequency components encompassing the highest portion of the alpha band) and of the lower beta frequency components (13–20 Hz), and to concurrently reduce the amplitude of the theta band (4–7.5 Hz) and of the highest beta frequency components (20–30 Hz). The training program increased alpha and beta power in trained participants when measured at rest with eyes-closed. In addition, during eyes-open recording, trained participants presented similar levels of activity across all frequency bands in contrast to control subjects, who showed a decrease of the power of the lower portion of the beta band. Again, with respect to the control group, the trained group improved the response time during a visual attention test and showed an improvement in the speed, efficiency, and accuracy of performance. These results hint at the potential of neurofeedback training for sports training.

Biofeedback and Neurofeedback and Sport Disciplines

The advancement of biofeedback and neurofeedback applications holds great promise for sport psychology and specifically for psychological skills training. Sport achievement is the result of well-planned hard training with progressively growing demands and challenges over a long time period. The main goal of the training process is to increase the athlete's work capacity, skill, and capabilities as well as to develop strong psychological qualities for successful performance (Bompa & Carrera, 2003; Bompa & Haff, 2009).

As above noted, one of the applications of the neurofeedback methodology is the achievement of peak performance in sport. Neurofeedback holds potential for retraining brainwave activity to enhance optimal performance in athletes in various sports (Hammond, 2007). It has been shown to have the potential for quieting the mind and improving performance in archery, for example. It can also be used to improve concentration and focus, cognitive functions, and emotional control following concussions and mild head injuries. Furthermore, it has untapped potential for increasing physical balance in gymnastics, ice skating, skiing, and other areas of performance (Ziólkowski et al., 2014).

The integration of biofeedback and neurofeedback into the common training routine of athletes can support assessment and can teach the athletes to maintain appropriate breathing, relaxed muscles, coherent heart rhythms, and dominant alpha brain states even under pressure.

Neurofeedback Training in Soccer Athletes

Soccer performance depends on several basic skills. Achieving optimal performance is not an easy or automatic process, since lots of environmental disturbances and contextual factors may induce dysfunctional stress in the player. Athletes need to deal with many aspects, such as their emotional stability and focus of attention notwithstanding adverse environmental conditions.

People's ability to influence their own psychological states mostly rely on cognitive-emotional control (Wegner & Pennebaker, 1993), which involves the deliberate use of strategies to change or maintain thoughts, feelings, or actions (Totterdell, 2000). Coping with stressful competitive situations is deemed as a natural ability of the players, yet without effective stress management skills the effect of stress on emotional response and performance for the player may be severe (Eubank & Gilbourne, 2003). Many of the psychological techniques used with athletes require them to intentionally regulate their moods or emotions, in order to check out the counterproductive emotions such as tension (Totterdell, 2000). For that purpose, neurofeedback training can help to regulate heightened emotionality. The rationale underlying the use of emotion regulation techniques to empower athletes is that there is a relationship between emotion and performance, which can then be enhanced by them via adaptive control of their mood states. More specifically, emotional regulation is thought to influence performance because it enables people to get into the sort of positive mood that facilitates certain cognitive processes (Matthews, 1992), which in turn increase effort and persistence on tasks (George & Brief, 1996).

A recent study on the Italian soccer team, which won the World Championship in 2006, describes the use of neurofeedback as a "secret weapon" to achieve that success. In fact, they attributed their win in part to that very training. This result shows that biofeedback and neurofeedback training in professional soccer players reflects the increasing acceptance and application of such training with professionals whose performance must be optimal during times of extreme stress (Wilson et al., 2006).

Building Performance: Brain Training for Baseball Players

The idea behind the application of neurofeedback training with baseball players is that it can be used to increase attention orientation and focusing, thus helping athletes to force their focus only on the most relevant anticipatory cues and to identify the signs in body position and movements that anticipate which action will be enacted next.

A study with a Major League baseball team has evaluated the feasibility of conducting a brain training and neurofeedback protocol within a professional organization and the effects of such training on quantitative EEG (qEEG) and qualitative self-report data (Sherlin, Larson, & Sherlin, 2013). The brain training protocol proved to be able to significantly change physiological levels and to reduce commission errors at a specific performance test. The significant reduction of commission errors likely mirrors the improvement of executive functions and impulse control. Future investigation should examine to what extent this improvement can be transferred to other domains and affect actual athletic performance in baseball. Again, participants reported increased attention and ability to focus, and they noted that those improvements may be critical for their sport. Baseball players who were training to decrease excessive cortical activity linked to the generation of intrusive thoughts (by enhancing slower EEG frequency bands and inhibiting faster ones) have shown a significant modulation of related EEG indices. Although it was not a primary target of the training, many participants also noted improvements in sleep quality. That outcome is rather valuable because it is well-known that sleep is especially important for the recovery period of a high performance athlete.

Sensorimotor Rhythm Neurofeedback and Golf Performance

Efficient and well-balanced mental processes can differentiate standard and superior performance in precision sports, such as golf. For example, "pitch & putt" is a particular part of golf practice that favors skill and clarity of mind in the short game on the greens and that is one of the most important elements of the game (Pelz & Frank, 2000).

Such part of the game is the most stressful one, since it put precision skills under strong test while relying on automatized athletic gestures. The complexity of such situations, which combines controlled and automated processes, is well represented by neuroimaging evidence. Indeed, it was shown that players who are involved in an automated process present altered activity within bilateral cerebellum, motor areas, and pre-supplementary, premotor, parietal, and prefrontal cortices (Wu, Chan, & Hallett, 2008). Again, it has been shown that high-frequency alpha power in correspondence to those cortical areas reflects attention processes related to the task (Klimesch, Doppelmayr, Pachinger, & Ripper, 1997). In parallel, frontal midline theta power seems to mirror top-down sustained attention (Sauseng, Hoppe, Klimesch, Gerloff, & Hummel, 2007). Thus, it is possible to hypothesize that these findings support the value of training specialized task-related attention mechanisms so to achieve superior motor performance.

Even facilitating a sense of control and confidence proved to positively influence the performance after a neurofeedback treatment targeting the sensorimotor rhythm (Gruzelier, Inoue, Smart, Steed, & Steffert, 2010). The sensorimotor rhythm is associated to the maintenance of a relaxed but ready mindset, to focusing and concentration, and to a reduction of the information-processing within the sensorimotor network (Vernon et al., 2003). This interpretation is similar to the mental characteristics of peak performance in trained athletes (Krane & Williams, 2006), and it is in agreement with the concept of automaticity proposed by Fitts and Posner (1967). So, sensorimotor rhythm power not only may be a sensitive marker of activity within sensorimotor cortex (Mann, Sterman, & Kaiser, 1996) but it also shows a potential for empowerment interventions with precision sports athletes. Indeed, neurofeedback-induced enhancement of sensorimotor rhythm seemed to results in better visuomotor performance and, then, in superior putting skill.

Even biofeedback appears to improve golf performance, specifically as a consequence of the reduction of performance anxiety in competitions. In particular, a detailed understanding of the psychological and physiological state of the participant and a continuous monitoring of heart rate variability during the sport performance may improve the player's ability to cope with stress by increasing the ability to achieve optimal performance. As such, that technique might help to induce substantial improvements of practicers' state of mind and confidence, to reduce the stress experienced during golf competitions, and to improve athletic outcomes.

Using Biofeedback and Neurofeedback with Gymnasts

Goal setting in biofeedback and neurofeedback training begins with identifying potential suboptimal physiological responses and with defining whether these suboptimal states occur during specific situations or contexts, such as competition.

Following neurofeedback training, gymnasts showed improved self-regulatory skills during competitive periods with respect to their initial ability. Furthermore, neurofeedback training proved to promote the rapidity of complex coordinated motion learning, to improve vestibular stability, and to fine-tune self-estimation of functional condition (Svyatogor, 2000). Since they aim at encouraging athletes to maximize their potential in the race, bio/neurofeedback techniques can also be used to strengthen gymnasts' mental components that often affect the outcome of a sport performance. Namely, a coach who wants to improve mental training of athletes can use such techniques to work on their coping strategies and to enhance a sense of inner confidence.

Recent studies have tested the effectiveness of a bio/neurofeedback training program to foster optimal pre-performance mind-body status so to improve balance beam performance in competition for gymnasts. Shaw and colleagues (2012) specifically investigated the effectiveness of a combined bio/neurofeedback training program designed to foster an optimal pre-performance mindset and the related neural state so to improve balance beam skills of gymnasts. Since previous studies acknowledged, among their limitations, that physiological patterns were partly different between training and competition contexts, the authors devised the training so that it could be applied both in the laboratory and at the gym, in an attempt to facilitate the transfer of skills. The training included exercises to improve heart rate variability (HRV) and sensorimotor rhythm. The assessment included baseline measures, psychophysiological evaluation by an independent judge, balance beam performance during competition, and subjective experience reported by the gymnasts. Gradual improvement of balance performance across the training sessions suggested that participants experienced some benefit associated with training. Yet, after the end of the training, those benefits did not remain. It is further worth noting that the withdrawal of training had a negative effect on mood and performance of athletes.

Technical and Practical Notes

Even if there still is no universally valid gold standard protocol for the improvement of athletes' performance, we will briefly describe a couple of protocols exemplifying neurofeedback applications in the field of sport science.

- Alpha training: this protocol mainly focuses on relaxation in order to achieve a calm state of mind. The montage includes one or two recording channels used to collect EEG data and thus compute the real-time feedback on the presence, power, and maintenance of alpha activity (8–12 Hz). Usually, the athlete is asked to keep his/her eyes closed during training, so to help relaxation and to allow the rewarding feedback to start. Feedbacks are usually provided in the form of pleasant acoustic stimuli, e.g. flutes, cellos, violas, natural sounds, etc. Training is designed to facilitate entering an alpha-wave state and concurrently to signal the potential increase of prevalence of lower frequency components (theta and delta oscillations) that are associated to deep inner connection, drowsiness, and lowering of consciousness. Achieving and maintaining that relaxed but aware state is useful for reducing dysfunctional stress and its associated effects, and it also helps to minimize the effect of anxiety, anger, disappointment, and other negative emotions that may arise in the course of a competition. Alpha training may alternatively be focused on the coherence of the activity of right and left hemispheres. Such specific practice aims is thought to promote emotion-regulation, creativity, and sense of well-being, and, as a consequence, to increase the ability to keep the mind clear and play effectively.
- Sensorimotor rhythm (SMR) training: this protocol is mainly aimed at enhancing the ability to focus. The montage typically includes one or two EEG sensors placed in correspondence to sensorimotor areas, so to record SMR fluctuations in the 12-to-15 Hz range. Sessions can be done with the eyes open so to mimic real-life situations. Acoustic and/or visual feedbacks are used to foster the amplification of SMR oscillations while inhibiting theta and high-frequency EEG activities. The SMR collected over central scalp regions has been associated to mental focus and motor readiness.

Neurofeedback protocols aimed at training athletes to voluntarily produce a specific brain activity pattern (specific waveforms in correspondence to specific locations) and to be aware of whether they are entering specific mind-brain states or not can be supported by recording additional physiological parameters (such as skin conductance level or muscle tension) to control for potential side effects due to discomfort during practice.

Setup, Recording and Data Processing

Measurements that are typically used in biofeedback training are:

- electrocardiography: electrical activity generated by the heart muscle is usually recorded by placing sensors in correspondence to the wrists and the ankle;
- electrodermography: a pair of electrodes are usually placed on the palm or on the fingers of the non-dominant hand so to collect data on the tonic and phasic components of skin conductance;

- pneumography: breathing patterns and respiratory activity at rest and under stressful conditions is collected via mechanical sensors;
- peripheral thermography: changes of peripheral skin temperature are collected via highly sensitive sensors placed in correspondence to the hands, feet, or the temples;
- electromyography: tension and sensitivity to fatigue of skeletal muscles is usually assessed and trained by using surface sensors.

Some examples of biosignal analysis approaches used to compute indices and biomarkers for assessment and training are spectrum analysis, trend analysis, analysis of peak activity and variability of responses over time, and rectification and analysis of the root mean square values.

A typical biofeedback setup uses data collected by sensors placed on the skin to detect both electrical and non-electrical peripheral biosignal, to distinguish between relevant physiological activity and noise, and to convert such relevant activity into easily-perceivable acoustic and/or visual feedbacks provided to the practicer (Prentice, 2003). Usually, sensor montages that are used to collect electrical biosignals include active sensors and a reference sensor, which is typically placed in-between the active ones, so to create a "differential amplifier" (Prentice & Voight, 2001).

Differently, neurofeedback practice grounds on recording brain activity via EEG sensors that are placed on the scalp and ear lobes. The placement of sensors can be determined on the basis of previous quantitative EEG assessments or it can be set a priori following standard electrode placement systems on the basis of available evidence on anatomical-functional correspondence. Brain biosignals are then processed by a computer program, which typically analyzes the collected data in the frequency-domain. Neurofeedback training does not include any kind of electrical stimulation of the brain. It simply relies on the collection of electrical neural activity, which is used to provide the practices with real-time feedbacks on such activity. The opportunity to see correlates of brain activity on a computer screen or to hear their modulations allows the practicer to build the ability to consciously monitor such activity and to modulate it, according to operant conditioning principles. Reinforcements and punishments are given to the practicer while he/she trains to develop the ability to voluntarily control his/her brain responses. Typical reinforcing tasks are brain-controlled videogames and video clips (Hammond, 2007). With the progression of practice – after a sufficient number of training sessions – brainwaves and related mindsets can be modeled so to try and achieve the desired self-regulation goals. At first, induced changes are short-lived, but they gradually become more consistent thanks to continuous feedback, coaching, and practice. Depending on the conditions that are being addressed and on individual needs, target frequencies and training protocols are usually personalized.

Ethical and Safety Guidelines

Bio/neurofeedback systems are used both in clinical settings to support functional recovery and treatment of clinical pictures and in training settings to empower individual performance, self-awareness, and self-regulation skills. The devices that are commonly used are typically designated as low-risk equipment, but must conform to special controls such as labeling requirements, post-marketing surveillance, and performance standards.

When used to treat a diagnosed condition, bio/neurofeedback training must be prescribed by a duly authorized dealer, such as a physician or a psychologist. Before the training, the trainer/therapists should collect initial data to properly test the effectiveness of the intervention. Further, he/she has to obtain the patient's written informed consent, which has to clearly state some key issue concerning the treatment/training:

- any risks related to bio/neurofeedback practice and associated techniques (allergic reactions to sensors or materials used to preparation the skin);
- relative risk-to-benefit ratios of bio/neurofeedback techniques;
- reference to potential alternative interventions (e.g. progressive muscle relaxation training without biofeedback to intervene on tension headaches);
- the client's rights and privacy norms.

The trainer/therapist must work with the client to establish mutually-agreed goals for the training. The client must be informed not only on the proposed therapeutic approach but also on the possibility that the intervention may not achieve the desired goals. The client needs to be informed on and to demonstrate proper understanding of the importance of informing the trainer/therapist of any changes in his/her medications, symptoms, and behaviors.

With regard to the client's privacy and dignity issues, country-specific guidelines usually include the consent for physical contact between client and professional. In many cases, however, the trainer/therapist can instruct the client in appropriate sensor placement without the need to touch him/her. While it may be easier for the trainer/therapist to directly place sensors, especially during applied intervention with athletes, touch should never involve areas of the body that would be considered as sensitive. Some therapists mistake their comfort with a client for the client's comfort with them. Clients, in fact, can be very uncomfortable in many situations but not be willing to verbalize their feeling.

Finally, especially in sport domain, training can also be provided at distance via web-based communication channels. Even in such cases, however, clients cannot be left to themselves during practice, since they cannot learn to control their bodily activity by merely observing a bio/neurofeedback display. Rather, clients must be properly coached throughout the bio/neurofeedback session by using the principles of operant conditioning and other training techniques. Athletes must not be left alone to attempt changes for significant periods of time unless this is a specific goal for the client (National Commission for the Protection of Human Subjects of Biomedical and Behavioral Research & Department of Health, Education, and Welfare, 1988).

References

Balconi, M., & Caldiroli, C. L. (2011). Semantic violation effect on object-related action comprehension. N400-like event-related potentials for unusual and incorrect use. *Neuroscience, 197*, 191–199. doi:10.1016/j.neuroscience.2011.09.026

Balconi, M., Caldiroli, C. L., & Vitaloni, S. (2011). tDCS effect on EEG profile in response to semantic motor anomaly detection. *Neurorehabilitation and Neural Repair, 26*(4), 426.

Balconi, M., & Cortesi, L. (2016). Brain activity (fNIRS) in control state differs from the execution and observation of object-related and object-unrelated actions. *Journal of Motor Behavior, 48*(4), 289–296. doi:10.1080/00222895.2015.1092936

Balconi, M., Cortesi, L., & Crivelli, D. (2017). Motor planning and performance in transitive and intransitive gesture execution and imagination: Does EEG (RP) activity predict hemodynamic (fNIRS) response? *Neuroscience Letters, 648*, 59–65. doi:10.1016/j.neulet.2017.03.049

Balconi, M., & Crivelli, D. (in press). Wearable devices for self-enhancement and improvement of plasticity: effects on neurocognitive efficiency. In A. Esposito & G. Cordasco (Eds.), *Quantifying and Processing Biomedical and Behavioral Signals. Smart Innovation, Systems and Technologies.* Heidelberg: Springer. Doi:10.1007/978-3-319-95095-2

Balconi, M., Crivelli, D., & Bove, M. (2018). 'Eppur si move': The association between electrophysiological and psychophysical signatures of perceived movement illusions. *Journal of Motor Behavior, 50*(1), 37–50. doi:10.1080/00222895.2016.1271305

Balconi, M., Crivelli, D., & Cortesi, L. (2017). Transitive versus intransitive complex gesture representation: A comparison between execution, observation and imagination by fNIRS. *Applied Psychophysiology and Biofeedback, 42*(3), 179–191. doi:10.1007/s10484-017-9365-1

Balconi, M., Fronda, G., Venturella, I., & Crivelli, D. (2017). Conscious, pre-conscious and unconscious mechanisms in emotional behaviour. Some applications to the mindfulness approach with wearable devices. *Applied Sciences*, 7(12), 1280. doi:10.3390/app7121280

Berger, B. G., & Tobar, D. A. (2007). Physical activity and quality of life: Key Considerations. In G. Tenenbaum & R. C. Eklund (Eds.), *Handbook of Sport Psychology* (3rd Ed., pp. 598–620). Hoboken, NJ: John Wiley & Sons. doi:10.1002/9781118270011.ch27

Bompa, T. O., & Carrera, M. C. (2003). Peak conditioning for volleyball. In J. C. Reeser & R. Bahr (Eds.), *Handbook of Sports Medicine and Science: Volleyball* (pp. 29–44). Oxford, UK: Blackwell Science Ltd. doi:10.1002/9780470693902.ch4

Bompa, T. O., & Haff, G. G. (2009). *Periodization: Theory and methodology of training*. Champaign, IL: Human Kinetics Publishers.

Cooper, N. R., Croft, R. J., Dominey, S. J., Burgess, A. P., & Gruzelier, J. H. (2003). Paradox lost? Exploring the role of alpha oscillations during externally vs. internally directed attention and the implications for idling and inhibition hypotheses. *International Journal of Psychophysiology*, 47(1), 65–74. doi:10.1016/S0167-8760(02)00107-1

Corbin, C. B. (1972). Mental practice. In W. P. Morgan (Ed.), *Ergogenic aids and muscular performance* (pp. 93–118). San Diego, CA: Academic Press.

Crivelli, D., Fronda, G., Venturella, I., & Balconi, M. (2018). Supporting mindfulness practices with brain-sensing devices. Cognitive and electrophysiological evidences. *Mindfulness*, Advance Online Publication. doi:10.1007/s12671-018-0975-3

Csikszentmihalyi, M. (1975). *Beyond boredom and anxiety*. San Francisco, CA: Jossey-Bass Publishers.

Decety, J., Jeannerod, M., Germain, M., & Pastene, J. (1991). Vegetative response during imagined movement is proportional to mental effort. *Behavioural Brain Research*, 42(1), 1–5. doi:10.1016/S0166-4328(05)80033-6

Driskell, J. E., Copper, C., & Moran, A. (1994). Does mental practice enhance performance? *Journal of Applied Psychology*, 79(4), 481–492. doi:10.1037/0021-9010.79.4.481

Eubank, M., & Gilbourne, D. (2003). Stress, performance and motivation theory. In T. Reilly & A. M. Williams (Eds.), *Science and Soccer* (2nd Ed., pp. 214–229). London: Routledge.

Fitts, P. M., & Posner, M. I. (1967). *Human performance*. Belmont, CA: Brooks/Cole.

Frank, D. L., Khorshid, L., Kiffer, J. F., Moravec, C. S., & McKee, M. G. (2010). Biofeedback in medicine: who, when, why and how? *Mental Health in Family Medicine*, 7(2), 85–91.

George, J. M., & Brief, A. P. (1996). Motivational agendas in the workplace: The effects of feelings on focus of attention and work motivation. *Research in Organizational Behavior, 18*, 75–109.

Geyman, J. P., Deyo, R. A., & Ramsey, S. D. (Eds.). (2000). *Evidence-based clinical practice : Concepts and approaches*. Boston, MA: Butterworth-Heinemann.

Gilbert, C., & Moss, D. (2003). Biofeedback and Biological Monitoring. In D. Moss, A. McGrady, T. C. Davies, & I. Wickramasekera (Eds.), *Handbook of Mind-Body Medicine for Primary Care* (pp. 109–122). Thousand Oaks, CA: SAGE Publications, Inc. doi:10.4135/9781452232607.n8

Goodman, S., Haufler, A., Shim, J. K., & Hatfield, B. (2009). Regular and random components in aiming-point trajectory during rifle aiming and shooting. *Journal of Motor Behavior, 41*(4), 367–382. doi:10.3200/JMBR.41.4.367–384

Green, E. E., Green, A. M., & Walters, E. D. (1970). Voluntary control of internal states: psychological and physiological. *The Journal of Transpersonal Psychology*, 2(1), 1–26.

Gruzelier, J., Inoue, A., Smart, R., Steed, A., & Steffert, T. (2010). Acting performance and flow state enhanced with sensory-motor rhythm neurofeedback comparing ecologically valid immersive VR and training screen scenarios. *Neuroscience Letters, 480*(2), 112–116. doi:10.1016/j.neulet.2010.06.019

Guillot, A., & Collet, C. (2008). Construction of the motor imagery integrative model in sport: A review and theoretical investigation of motor imagery use. *International Review of Sport and Exercise Psychology*, 1(1), 31–44. doi:10.1080/17509840701823139

Hammond, D. C. (2007). What is neurofeedback? *Journal of Neurotherapy*, 10(4), 25–36. doi:10.1300/J184v10n04_04

Hatfield, B. D., & Landers, D. M. (1983). Psychophysiology: a new direction for sport psychology. *Journal of Sport Psychology*, 5(3), 243–259.

Hummel, F., Andres, F., Altenmüller, E., Dichgans, J., & Gerloff, C. (2002). Inhibitory control of acquired motor programmes in the human brain. *Brain*, 125(2), 404–420. doi:10.1093/brain/awf030

Jeannerod, M. (1995). Mental imagery in the motor context. *Neuropsychologia*, 33(11), 1419–1432. doi:10.1016/0028-3932(95)00073-C

Jensen, O., & Tesche, C. D. (2002). Frontal theta activity in humans increases with memory load in a working memory task. *European Journal of Neuroscience*, 15(8), 1395–1399. doi:10.1046/j.1460-9568.2002.01975.x

Jonas, W. B., & Levin, J. S. (Eds.). (1999). *Essentials of complementary and alternative medicine*. Philadelphia, PA: Lippincott Williams & Wilkins.

Klimesch, W., Doppelmayr, M., Pachinger, T., & Ripper, B. (1997). Brain oscillations and human memory: EEG correlates in the upper alpha and theta band. *Neuroscience Letters, 238*(1–2), 9–12. doi:10.1016/S0304-3940(97)00771-4

Klimesch, W., Doppelmayr, M., Pachinger, T., & Russegger, H. (1997). Event-related desynchronization in the alpha band and the processing of semantic information. *Cognitive Brain Research, 6*(2), 83–94. doi:10.1016/S0926-6410(97)00018-9

Klimesch, W., Doppelmayr, M., Schwaiger, J., Winkler, T., & Gruber, W. (2000). Theta oscillations and the ERP old/new effect: Independent phenomena? *Clinical Neurophysiology, 111*(5), 781–793. doi:10.1016/S1388-2457(00)00254-6

Klimesch, W., Sauseng, P., & Hanslmayr, S. (2007). EEG alpha oscillations: the inhibition–timing hypothesis. *Brain Research Reviews, 53*(1), 63–88. doi:10.1016/j.brainresrev.2006.06.003

Koeneke, S., Lutz, K., Herwig, U., Ziemann, U., & Jäncke, L. (2006). Extensive training of elementary finger tapping movements changes the pattern of motor cortex excitability. *Experimental Brain Research, 174*(2), 199–209. doi:10.1007/s00221-006-0440-8

Krane, V., & Williams, J. M. (2006). Psychological characteristics of peak performance. In J. M. Williams (Ed.), *Applied Sport Psychology: Personal Growth to Peak Performance* (5th Ed., pp. 204–224). New York, NY: McGraw-Hill.

Mann, C. A., Sterman, M. B., & Kaiser, D. A. (1996). Suppression of EEG rhythmic frequencies during somato-motor and visuo-motor behavior. *International Journal of Psychophysiology, 23*(1–2), 1–7. doi:10.1016/0167-8760(96)00036-0

Marzbani, H., Marateb, H. R., & Mansourian, M. (2016). Neurofeedback: A comprehensive review on system design, methodology and clinical applications. *Basic and Clinical Neuroscience, 7*(2), 143–158. doi:10.15412/J.BCN.03070208

Matthews, G. (1992). Mood. In A. P. Smith & D. M. Jones (Eds.), *Handbook of Human Performance* (pp. 161–193). San Diego, CA: Academic Press.

Mikicin, M., Orzechowski, G., Jurewicz, K., Paluch, K., Kowalczyk, M., & Wróbel, A. (2015). Brain-training for physical performance: A study of EEG-neurofeedback and alpha relaxation training in athletes. *Acta Neurobiologiae Experimentalis, 75*(4), 434–445.

National Commission for the Protection of Human Subjects of Biomedical and Behavioral Research, & Department of Health, Education, and Welfare. (1988). *The Belmont report: Ethical principles and guidelines for the protection of human subjects of research.* Washington, D.C: Department of Health, Education and Welfare, Office of the Secretary.

Pelz, D., & Frank, J. A. (2000). *Dave Pelz's putting bible: The complete guide to mastering the green.* New York, NY: Doubleday.

Peper, E., Harvey, R., & Takabayashi, N. (2009). Biofeedback an evidence based approach in clinical practice. *Japanese Journal of Biofeedback Research, 36*(1), 3–10.

Perry, F. D., Shaw, L., & Zaichkowsky, L. (2011). Biofeedback and neurofeedback in sports. *Biofeedback, 39*(3), 95–100. doi:10.5298/1081-5937-39.3.10

Pfurtscheller, G., & Lopes da Silva, F. H. (1999). Event-related EEG/MEG synchronization and desynchronization: basic principles. *Clinical Neurophysiology, 110*(11), 1842–1857. doi:10.1016/S1388-2457(99)00141-8

Pop-Jordanova, N., & Demerdzieva, A. (2010). Biofeedback training for peak performance in sport – Case study. *Macedonian Journal of Medical Sciences, 3*(2), 113–118. doi10.3889/MJMS.1857–5773.2010.0098

Prentice, W. E. (2003). *Therapeutic Modalities for Sports Medicine and Athletic Training* (5th Ed.). New York, NY: McGraw-Hill.

Prentice, W. E., & Voight, M. L. (2001). *Techniques in Musculoskeletal Rehabilitation.* New York, NY: McGraw-Hill.

Sackett, D. L., Strauss, S. E., Richardson, W. S., Rosenberg, W., & Haynes, R. B. (2000). *Evidence-Based Medicine: How to Practice and Teach EBM* (2nd Ed.). Edinburgh: Churchill Livingstone.

Sauseng, P., Hoppe, J., Klimesch, W., Gerloff, C., & Hummel, F. C. (2007). Dissociation of sustained attention from central executive functions: local activity and interregional connectivity in the theta range. *The European Journal of Neuroscience, 25*(2), 587–593. doi:10.1111/j.1460–9568.2006.05286.x

Schwartz, M. S., & Andrasik, F. (Eds.). (2003). *Biofeedback: A practitioner's guide* (3rd Ed.). New York, NY: Guilford Press.

Shaffer, F., & Moss, D. (2006). Biofeedback. In C.-S. Yuan, E. J. Bieber, & B. A. Bauer (Eds.), *Textbook of Complementary and Alternative Medicine* (2nd Ed., pp. 291–312). Abingdon, UK: Informa Healtcare.

Shaw, L., Zaichkowsky, L., & Wilson, V. (2012). Setting the balance: using biofeedback and neurofeedback with gymnasts. *Journal of Clinical Sport Psychology, 6*(1), 47–66.

Sherlin, L. H., Larson, N. C., & Sherlin, R. M. (2013). Developing a Performance Brain Training™ approach for baseball: A process analysis with descriptive data. *Applied Psychophysiology and Biofeedback, 38*(1), 29–44. doi:10.1007/s10484-012-9205-2

Skinner, B. F. (1954). The science of learning and the art of teaching. *Harvard Educational Review, 24*(2), 86–97.

Svyatogor, I. A. (2000). The method of cerebrum potential biofeedback and clinical using of it. *Biological, 1*, 5–7.

Thut, G., Nietzel, A., Brandt, S. A., & Pascual-Leone, A. (2006). α-band electroencephalographic activity over occipital cortex indexes visuospatial attention bias and predicts visual target detection. *The Journal of Neuroscience, 26*(37), 9494–9502. doi:10.1523/JNEUROSCI.0875–06.2006

Totterdell, P. (2000). Catching moods and hitting runs: Mood linkage and subjective performance in professional sport teams. *Journal of Applied Psychology, 85*(6), 848–859. doi:10.1037/0021-9010.85.6.848

Tuladhar, A. M., Huurne, N. T., Schoffelen, J. M., Maris, E., Oostenveld, R., & Jensen, O. (2007). Parieto-occipital sources account for the increase in alpha activity with working memory load. *Human Brain Mapping, 28*(8), 785–792. doi:10.1002/hbm.20306

Vernon, D., Egner, T., Cooper, N., Compton, T., Neilands, C., Sheri, A., & Gruzelier, J. (2003). The effect of training distinct neurofeedback protocols on aspects of cognitive performance. *International Journal of Psychophysiology, 47*(1), 75–85. doi:10.1016/S0167-8760(02)00091-0

Wegner, D. M., & Pennebaker, J. W. (1993). Changing our minds: An introduction to mental control. In D. M. Wegner & J. W. Pennebaker (Eds.), *Handbook of Mental Control* (pp. 1–12). Englewood Cliffs, NJ: Prentice-Hall.

Wilson, V. E., Peper, E., & Moss, D. (2006). "The Mind Room" in Italian soccer training: The use of biofeedback and neurofeedback for optimum performance. *Biofeedback, 34*(3), 79–81.

Wu, T., Chan, P., & Hallett, M. (2008). Modifications of the interactions in the motor networks when a movement becomes automatic. *The Journal of Physiology, 586*(17), 4295–4304. doi:10.1113/jphysiol.2008.153445

Zaichkowsky, L. D., & Fuchs, C. Z. (1988). Biofeedback applications in exercise and athletic performance. *Exercise and Sport Sciences Reviews, 16*(1), 381–422.

Ziółkowski, A., Gorkovenko, A., Pasek, M., Włodarczyk, P., Zarańska, B., Dornowski, M., & Graczyk, M. (2014). EEG correlates of attention concentration in successful amateur boxers. *Neurophysiology, 46*(5), 422–427. doi:10.1007/s11062-015-9468-3

Understanding Neural Mechanisms of Memory in Rapid Recognition of Football Formations

Kyle K. Morgan, Don M. Tucker, and Phan Luu

Introduction

The transition from high school to college football brings a multitude of challenges that a young athlete needs to overcome within the timeframe of a single summer. Commonly, we emphasize the magnitude of the physical demands that come with making this transition, and overlook the substantial mental adjustment that must occur simultaneously to ensure success. This chapter addresses the neural mechanisms of the cognitive processes that take place when a new quarterback is taught how to analyze defensive formations to make play decisions. Through the training process, this information must be consolidated to the point where the athlete is game-ready in the fall. We focus on the stages of learning, the brain mechanisms involved in each, and the human neuroscience technologies that allow us to study these brain mechanisms. Finally, we highlight important challenges, including the effects of stress and the lack of sleep, which must be considered to maximize health and performance.

Learning to Read the Defense

The quarterback lines up and faces a specific defensive formation that will immediately shape how the play unfolds. To understand how one learns to make the necessary split-second decisions in reading the defense, we can break down the learning process into two stages using the classic dual-stage learning model: (1) early/deliberate and (2) automatic (Shiffrin & Schneider, 1977). The deliberate stage always precedes the automatic stage, and is where we would traditionally consider most of the "learning" is taking place. The deliberate stage is defined as a period where the quarterback must exert a high level of concentration to recognize a defensive formation and relies more heavily on consciously holding information in mind (i.e. working memory). In this deliberate stage, the athlete is slow to make the analysis, and commonly makes mistakes. The time a quarterback spends in the deliberate stage is very sensitive as the brain is working hard to consolidate the concepts they are learning, and even the slightest variations in how these skills are taught or how the player takes care of themselves during this period can have a considerable impact on how the athlete performs in a game situation, as we will discuss later in the chapter.

The end-goal of every coach is to get their player to the automatic stage. As the name implies, this stage is defined as a shift towards a more automatic or *unconscious* mode of operation (Shiffrin & Schneider, 1977). The quarterbacks that reach this stage do not need to focus all their attention to read a defense, do not need to rely as heavily on working memory, and can make their analysis quickly and accurately. When competing in high-level athletics, it is important for a player to operate unconsciously. Cognition is not only fast, but they can focus their attention on multiple aspects of the game at once. Attention and working memory are finite resources, and by practicing a skill to the point of automaticity the player is effectively shrinking the amount of mental and neural real-estate it takes to perform that skill.

Measuring the Neural Mechanisms of Becoming Unconscious

A player's progress through the learning stages can be tracked by monitoring distinct changes in the brain that occur in each stage (Chein & Schneider, 2005). Specifically, it is important to measure and understand the neural mechanisms of memory consolidation as it allows us to evaluate healthy versus insufficient learning. Several advances in human neurophysiology allow us to measure the neural mechanisms of learning and memory as they unfold.

Brain activity is commonly measured using two noninvasive neuroimaging methods: Electroencephalography (EEG) and functional Magnetic Resonance Imaging (fMRI). EEG measures the electrical activity of brain cells by placing a network of electrodes on the scalp. With enough (256) channels, we call this dense array or "high density" EEG (dEEG) (Tucker, 1993). When EEG is recorded during a task, small changes in voltage can correlate with specific operations within the task, called an Event Related Potential (ERP) (Figure 8.1).

Small experimental manipulations or changes in behavior can have a measurable impact on ERPs and, as we will soon discuss, can allow us to track learning. The pros of recording EEG is that it picks up brain activity with high temporal resolution, down to one millisecond. However, EEG can be non-specific and records the activity of tens of thousands of brain cells at once. Moreover, due to differences in cell structure in different brain parts, EEG can only record activity from the cerebral cortex (the wrinkled, outer-most layer of the brain). Some of the spatial shortcomings of EEG are made-up for using MRI. Standard MRI (not to be confused with functional MRI) uses a strong magnet combined with radio frequencies (RF) to measure the presence of hydrogen atoms in soft tissue. The brain is made-up of several different types of tissue with very reliable differences in hydrogen, and thus we can tune an MRI to give us a grayscale image of the brain and its tissues (Figure 8.2).

Using some of the same techniques as standard MRI, we can tune the machine to measure oxygen levels in blood vessels after a neuronal event occurs. The brain is constantly being fed oxygen through its matrix of vasculature, and when neurons fire oxygen is stripped from hemoglobin (a protein in red blood cells that carries oxygen) until subsequent cardiac events occur to resupply the brain with oxygenated hemoglobin. fMRI can detect the subtle difference between oxygenated and de-oxygenated hemoglobin while a subject preforms a task, and when we superimpose the map of where oxygen exchange is occurring over a structural image of the brain, we get the

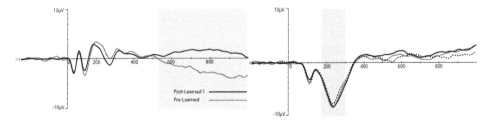

Figure 8.1 Example of Event Related Potentials (ERPs) showing progression of the P300 (left, in red) versus the MFN (right, in blue) over one day of formation analysis training. P300 amplitude significantly increased as learning progressed, whereas the MFN significantly decreased as learning progressed. The amplitude of the MFN is measured in reference to the amplitude of the preceding positive wave (P2).

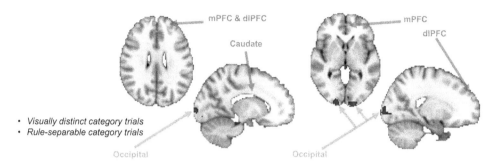

Figure 8.2 Example of functional MRI data (red and blue areas) superimposed on top of structural MRI (grayscale brain images) displaying preferential engagement of multiple memory systems during defensive formation analysis. Visually distinct blitz and goal-line defenses recruited a memory system centered on lateral occipital cortex (blue), whereas visually similar defenses (4-3 and 3-4 formations) relied on a rule-based system that involves several frontal areas and caudate nucleus (red).

classic map of brain activity we are mostly familiar with (Figure 8.2). This map is only limited by the presence of blood vessels, which is luckily very dense, and can image activity in deeper brain regions than EEG. However, blood flow in the brain is substantially slower than the electrical events happening between neurons, and fMRI is stuck measuring activity five to 10 seconds after a neural event has occurred. This makes it difficult for fMRI to tease-apart brain activity that occurs below the approximately seven-second timescale in multifaceted tasks: e.g. if visual analysis of an image, response selection, and feedback evaluation all happen within one second, it can be difficult to analyze activity for each specific subtask. Due to the complimentary shortcomings of both popular neuroimaging methods, our laboratory, like many others, employs both to get the spatial (fMRI) and temporal (EEG) benefits from each modality.

Dual Neural Systems of Memory Consolidation

By looking at how the structures that support memory interact with one another, we can gain insight into how the brain forms, organizes, and retrieves memories within the context of defensive formation analysis. Information about objects and events, and the context or location under which they occurred are processed in two streams in the cerebral cortex (Schneider, 1969). Within this model, the sensory pathways (e.g. primary visual cortex) take information in from the outside world and help us form an initial identification of an event or object, and then send this information up to the parietal lobe (Ungerleider & Mishkin, 1982; Keele, Ivry, Mayr, Hazeltine, & Heuer, 2003). We refer to this stream as the dorsal, or "where" pathway. This pathway specializes in the spatial analysis of stimuli, such as how players are configured on the line of scrimmage, and organizes holistic attention that eventually leads to impulsive actions. There is also a second pathway that is responsible for the identification of "what" event or object is being presented, and this information is processed by the ventral limbic system—parahippocampal gyrus, piriform, and entorhinal cortex (with the addition of the amygdala, in humans)—and is referred to as the ventral processing stream (Ungerleider & Mishkin, 1982; Keele, Ivry, Mayr, Hazeltine, & Heuer, 2003). Information from both streams converge at the hippocampus, which is a structure situated in the medial temporal lobe (MTL) that plays a key role in organizing input to link memories by their contextual representation (Luu et al., 2011). Once processing commences within the hippocampus, the output returns to the cortical areas from which the inputs originated (dorsal or ventral). In the dorsal pathway an additional structure, the medial prefrontal cortex (mPFC), selects the memory from the hippocampal feedback, whereas the striatum aids in memory selection for the ventral pathway. This feedback structure allows the hippocampus to organize memory retrieval based off "what" occurred or "where" something occurred, and makes it an essential mechanism for memory retrieval. We can now use this model of memory system dynamics/organization as a guide to understand how our athlete's memories are formed throughout the learning process.

Simulating Game Decisions in the dEEG Laboratory

When a new quarterback is working on formation recognition, it is becoming common practice to train them in a classroom environment. This affords coaches the opportunity to control the speed of the game, the formations they are viewing, and record their performance. Luckily for researchers, this environment is easily replicated in an experimental setting. Recently, our lab took 20 novice football players and ran them through a training program that taught them how to identify formations (Morgan, Luu, & Tucker, 2016). Players were shown an array of formations from the quarterback perspective one at a time (Figure 8.3).

On every trial, the participant was asked to either hit a button on a keypad or take no action (Go vs. No Go), which corresponded to a game-time scenario where a player may need to call an audible to switch a play after analyzing the defense (Go) or take no action if a desirable defense is shown (No Go). The participants were given corrective feedback which helped guide their actions or inactions toward each formation. Over three days, we recorded EEG from each participant as their abilities improved, and found two ERPs that accurately reflect the transition from the early/deliberate to the automatic stages of learning. The Medial Frontal Negativity is an ERP that reflects activity from the Anterior Cingulate Cortex (ACC), which is a region that is commonly thought of as the control center of the frontal lobe (Figure 8.1). Frontal brain regions are responsible for higher-level evaluations of a stimulus such as attention, effortful control, performance monitoring, and working memory—all aspects of the deliberate stage. In our study, we found that the MFN was largest when subjects performed poorly on formation recognition in the first day, but as performance increased with practice, the MFN reduced in size. As the MFN was shrinking, we witnessed a sizeable increase in a more posterior ERP termed the P300 (Figure 8.1). The

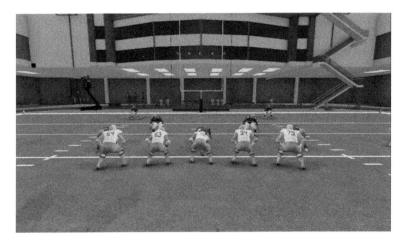

Figure 8.3 Example defensive formation. The players in white (offense) are held constant in our dEEG study, whereas the players in red (defense) change position from trial to trial. The subject in our study is tasked with learning how defensive formations map onto responses on a keypad.

P300 is an ERP which indexes the updating or confirmation of the context under which an action was learned and performed, and is estimated to reflect activity in the posterior cingulate cortex (PCC) and areas surrounding the hippocampus—two regions responsible for the consolidation of memories—amongst several others (Polich, 2007; Luu et al., 2011; Halgren et al., 1995). By combining the dual-stage model of learning with the dual-processing model discussed earlier for memory organization, we can get a clear picture as to why this happens. The early/deliberate stage is responsible for forming the context under which a quarterback learns to recognize a formation and requires controlled processing from frontal regions, whereas the automatic phase marks a reduction in frontal engagement (reflected as a reduction in the need for controlled attention) and an increase in activity from more posterior regions where the context is simply monitored. Put more clearly, the early stage is a time where the brain requires more attentional resources to build-up the contextual blueprint that binds inputs and outputs—where we know the hippocampus plays a large role in associating the two. The lack of context in the early stage leaves little work for the hippocampus to do, but as that context forms with practice, the role of the hippocampus becomes increasingly important to the point where controlled processes are no longer needed and the brain can rely on the object/event recognition system (the ventral processing stream) (Donchin & Coles, 1988; Polich, 2007; Luu et al., 2011). This allows the player to perform the learned action without a substantial cognitive load, and can focus their attention on other aspects of the game.

Implications for Quarterback Training

Within the context of formation analysis, quarterbacks in the early stages of learning are relying heavily on attention and working memory when viewing a defense. They will typically take a considerable amount of time to scan the entire formation and consciously think about the play that counters what is shown. Corrective feedback is given to the quarterback in the form of yards gained or lost as a result of their play calling, and this feedback is critical during the early stages of learning. At the neural level, the anterior brain regions are focusing attention on the most relevant aspects of a scene that lead to success or failure (e.g. how far apart are the players?), and with every trial and error it is interfacing with the hippocampus to generate a small bank of this spatially important data. When a quarterback has had sufficient training, we see that the player no longer needs to scan the entire defense. Instead, they can filter-out the irrelevant aspects of the scene (reducing cognitive load), and quickly peak at the relevant features that garner success and failure. This is measured behaviorally by significantly faster and less variable reaction times than the early stages, along with error reduction. In the brain, our results show that activity has shifted away from anterior regions, and towards the posterior. All the trial and error committed in the early stages of learning has formed an easily accessible database of inputs (formations) and outputs (audible plays). This shift is important as it can be used as a metric during training. Players who report a need to focus attention on a defense could benefit from more analysis drills, whereas a player who reports being unconscious during accurate decision making will only see incremental improvements from the same training.

The anterior-posterior shift observed in our study reflects a well-known phenomenon when a task involves mapping inputs (formations in our example) to a set of corresponding outputs (play selection or button presses) (Shiffrin & Schneider, 1977). In fact, this reliable input/output format is a prerequisite for a skill to reach automaticity, and is an important concept for coaches to understand as they take their athletes through training. Practice sessions must have a concrete set of inputs (with little variation at first) that map onto outputs so that the relay of information from the control processing system (ACC and frontal cortical brain areas) to areas associated with automatic processing (such as the hippocampus or other memory systems) is stable. Unreliable input/output mappings can delay the transition to automaticity, or worse, can contaminate the information that gets into the automatic stream which is the premise for forming bad habits that need to be retrained (Chein & Schneider, 2005). To emphasize this point even more, the introduction of stress into the equation forces athletes to rely on their instincts—that is, they rely on information that comes automatically (Schwabe et al., 2007; Schwabe, Schachinger, de Kloet, & Oitzl, 2010). This is due in part to the modulation of attention, where peripheral attention is incapacitated by stress, and attention becomes more focused (a phenomenon known as "tunnel vision"). This supports the concept of attention being a finite resource.

Recall that a main proponent of the deliberate learning stage is attention, but not for the automatic stage. If a player's ability to focus on multiple aspects of the game is hindered, then they run the risk of stripping attention away from a skill that requires it (in the case that the skill has not be practiced to the point of automaticity). Doing so will certainly lead to errors if the information available to the automatic processing stream is unreliable. In addition, overly focused attention limits the amount of spatial information required by the dorsal ("where") processing stream, and we see disengagement from the dorsal processing stream under stress and a reliance upon the more primitive ventral stream. The brain defaults to relying on actions that are associated with object recognition because this information is readily available. This is the premise for why it is important to practice performing under pressure, as it exposes gaps in a player's current state of training. Quality training regimens will ensure that what comes automatically to a player is the correct action when the pressure of a game-time situation occurs, and that they do not default to an undesirable habit (Schwabe et al., 2007).

Mapping the Appropriate Memory System with Functional MRI

Stress is not the only thing that leads to errors or slow performance during training. As discussed earlier, memories can be broken down into multiple processing streams or memory systems that specialize in different types of memories. Failure to recruit the optimal memory system for processing an incoming stimulus can be detrimental to learning (Maddox, Ashby, Ing, & Pickering, 2004; Zeithamova & Maddox, 2007). In our laboratory, we used fMRI to understand if various types of defensive formations recruit the same or different memory systems. Like our EEG study, 13 participants were trained on how to recognize different defensive formations by pressing a button that corresponds to a play that exploits the defense. However, in this study, we shortened the training to one session, and the different formations were grouped into predetermined categories that reflect some of the most popular formations used in college and professional football. One category of formations corresponded to a goal-line defense (six players on the line of scrimmage and one player in the background, 6-1) and was visually distinct from the other two categories. The two remaining categories were visually similar to each other, with one category having four players on the line of scrimmage and three players in the backfield (4-3), and the other having three players on the line of scrimmage and four players in the backfield (3-4). Twelve total formations were used, resulting in four examples per category (Figure 8.4).

Subjects were instructed to figure out how to place each formation shown into one of the three categories, but they were not given any hints about how to do so. We hypothesized that the goal-line defense would recruit a memory system in visual brain regions that is optimal for making similarity judgments, whereas the two visually alike formations would rely on a rule-based system in the striatum (Figure 8.4) (Kemler-Nelson, 1984; Nosofsky 1986; Smith & Sloman, 1994). In support of our hypothesis, we found that subjects reliably recruited a memory system that is similar to the dorsal processing stream with support from the lateral occipital region (LO). In contrast, subjects relied more on a system similar to the ventral processing stream with engagement from a structure within the dorsal striatum called caudate nucleus, a sub-cortical region that plays a role in rule-application, and mPFC (Figure 8.2). A key takeaway from this study is that training football players to recognize defensive formations should not be treated as a unitary phenomenon—the formations simply are not all processed in the

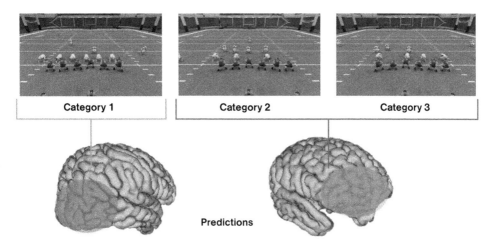

Figure 8.4 [Production: Fix color descriptions] Illustration of predictions in a categorization fMRI experiment. Blue: A visually distinct category should recruit the similarity-based categorization system, centered over the posterior visual regions. Red: Two visually similar categories should recruit the rule-based categorization system, centered over the frontal regions and caudate nucleus (not shown).

same way. In fact, the two memory systems engaged in our study differ in their speed of acquisition, reaction time dependent upon which phase of the learning process they are in, and their flexibility to make accurate responses when shown formations that only partially look like members of a category (Medin & Shaffer, 1978; Smith & Sloman, 1994). Although a person can still accurately categorize a formation with a suboptimal memory system, preliminary results from this study suggest that a mismatch between the formation category and memory system recruited on a single trial (measured by total signal present in each system) results in a higher error rate. These initial results are backed by other research that suggests category/memory system mismatches led to errors, impaired learning, and slow performance (Maddox Ashby, Ing, & Pickering, 2004). Thus, it is important to not only monitor where an athlete is in the learning process, but also where the learning is taking place and whether that system is the one that is going to maximize performance.

The preferential engagement of multiple memory systems has large implications for a quarterback's performance. The two memory systems discussed in our fMRI study are behaviorally expressed in the form of strategies a player uses to identify a formation (Smith & Sloman, 1994). The rule-based memory system is engaged when a player looks at a defense and uses a rule to recognize the formation. In our example, counting the number of players on the line of scrimmage and in the backfield, suffices as a rule. By contrast, the visual similarity system works through a general scanning of a formation and relies on comparing the formation shown to a general idea or exemplar of that formation to determine membership. Although the strategies are similar, using the wrong system can slow them down. To illustrate the point: if a quarterback is presented with a blitz, it will take much longer for the quarterback to count the large number of players on the line versus generally scanning the formation and comparing it to a general concept for a blitzing defense: e.g. "I should count the number of players on the line: 1, 2, 3... 6, that looks like a blitz is coming" vs "I generally see lots of players on the line of scrimmage and I should call an audible to get rid of the ball quickly". However, if the defense has been using two different formations that look visually similar but with different coverages, the quarterback will need to execute the counting rule to detect the subtle visual difference. Relying on a similarity system which works best when between-category variance is high will result in errors when between-category variance is low. Monitoring which system is recruited on a single trial basis can help coaches facilitate the appropriate analysis strategy to maximize performance.

Consolidating Memory with a Good Night's Sleep

If monitoring the brain during training doesn't seem feasible, perhaps the best way to maximize memory efficiency is to ensure that each athlete gets a full eight hours of sleep, because one of the best ways to disrupt memory consolidation and performance is sleep deprivation. Sleep research over the past century has established that memories of a day's experience are temporarily stored in a short-term center during waking hours, and only when someone sleeps does this information get transferred to long-term storage (Jenkins & Dallenbach, 1924; Morris, Williams, & Lubin, 1960; Harrison & Horne, 2000). However, it is not as simple as just falling asleep. Sleep happens in stages where, throughout the night, we oscillate between these different stages (Hobson & Pace-Schott, 2002). The sleep stages are most easily monitored using EEG as they have distinct oscillatory patterns than govern their classification. Perhaps the most widely recognized sleep stage is the period of Rapid Eye Movement (REM) sleep. However, there are also four stages of non-REM (nREM) that are equally important to understand. Stage I nREM is a period of light sleep where one can be awakened easily. Stage II nREM is classified as a time where eye movement stops and body temperature begins to drop. Stage III nREM, or deep sleep, is marked by a slowing heart rate, a further body temperate drop, and the presence of very slow brain waves called delta waves. Interspersed between the delta waves are periods of very fast, but smaller brain waves. Stage IV is commonly referred to as Slow Wave Sleep (SWS), where the brain produces delta waves almost exclusively. After Stage IV, the body enters REM sleep, where the eyes dart back and forth, but the brain activity reflects that of being awake. Sensory input during REM is no longer relayed to the sensory processing centers of the brain by the thalamus, and the body is paralyzed. The clear majority of dreaming happens during REM sleep. A healthy person will spend more time in Stage IV nREM during the early hours of the night, but as the night goes on the amount of REM increases and Stage IV nREM decreases (Figure 8.5). This means that, if an athlete (or anyone, for that matter) is deprived of as little as 2 hours of sleep, they can effectively cut off as much as 40–60% of their time spent in REM. This will become important as we discuss the significance of the sleep stages.

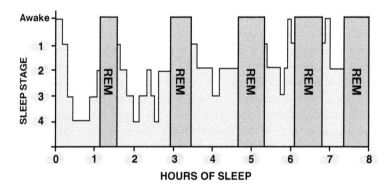

Figure 8.5   Illustration of sleep stages during an eight-hour night. Throughout the night, the body oscillates through four nREM sleep stages and a single REM stage. In the later hours, the amount of time spent in REM sleep increases, while the time spent in deep sleep (stages III and IV nREM) decreases.

A growing body of evidence suggests that slow-wave sleep (SWS) (stages III and IV nREM) is responsible for the consolidation of declarative memories, which is the type of memory we associate with things such as explicit facts (Plihal & Born, 1997; Harris & Horne, 2000). Studies have shown that time spent in SWS can predict learning outcomes on a memory task the next day. More recently, the literature further specifies that not only is the time spent in SWS important, but the phase alignment of the slow oscillations and sleep spindles within this stage can also predict performance (Molle & Born, 2011). This means that, even if an athlete is getting a full eight hours of sleep, it is the brain activity during those hours that have an important role in subsequent performance the next day.

Perhaps even more jarring, Stage II nREM sleep spindles in the last two hours of sleep (hours seven and eight) are closely tied to motor memory consolidation (Laventure et al., 2016). This has profound implications for the sports domain, as motor memory is a key aspect of any formal sport, and if an athlete is woken up early to go to practice (cutting their sleep to six hours), the coach could be inadvertently hindering their brains ability to form connections in motor memory pathways.

The significance of REM sleep and its vivid dreams has long been debated. Several findings suggest that REM is important to emotional integration (van der Helm et al., 2011). This would imply that fully integrating the emotional significance of training and performance challenges may be impaired if sleep is limited, because REM is the main stage that suffers from too little sleep. Furthermore, other evidence suggests that creativity in problem-solving is impaired if REM is disrupted (Cai, Mednick, Harrison, Kanady, & Mednick, 2009). Is creativity important to the quarterback's effective gameplay decisions? On the one hand, we might think that with adequate automaticity the quarterback's decisions are already made, and no creative problem solving is required. On the other hand, the creative mental skill of many quarterbacks is impressive, as they not only understand the intentions of the defense, but they select play options and executions that cause those intentions to be lead the defense in the wrong directions. In any sense, it is clear to see why, perhaps above and beyond any monitoring of memory system function during training, we allow them to sleep for as long as the body requires.

Future Directions

Future research in our lab will focus on using the information discussed in this chapter to improve the learning process. By using fMRI and dEEG, we will continue to classify neural signatures to track the learning process, along with the preferential engagement of multiple memory systems to consolidate and recall these memories efficiently. Our work will move toward understanding how memories are consolidated through sleep, and whether there is a way to enhance an athlete's time spent in the stage(s) of sleep most conducive to transferring relevant information to long-term memory. In addition, we will begin to develop tools (such as brain stimulation devices) to facilitate activity in the optimal memory system for categorizing a specific formation to prevent memory system/stimulus mismatches that lead to poor performance. Our long-term goal is to provide teams with an avenue to augment their training by measuring how their players are progressing through the program at the neural level, and use that information to develop tailored interventions to bring all players up to the desired skill level. This could give teams a competitive edge in a domain where it is common to see several teams in a division utilizing the same or similar strength training programs. Importantly, bridging sports and neuroscience represents a prime example of how brain research can have a positive impact beyond the traditional laboratory experiment.

References

Cai, D. J., Mednick, S. A., Harrison, E. M., Kanady, J. C., & Mednick, S. C., (2009). REM, not incubation, improves creativity by priming associative networks. *PNAS, 106*(25), 10130–10134.

Chein, J. M., & Schneider, W. (2005). Neuroimaging studies of practice-related change: fMRI and meta-analytic evidence of a domain general control network for learning. *Cognitive Brain Research, 25*, 607–623.

Donchin, E., & Coles, M. G. H. (1988). Is the p300 component a manifestation of context updating? *Behavioral and Brain Sciences, 11,* 357–374.

Halgren, E., Baudena, P., Heit, G., Clarke, J. M., Marinkovic, K., Chauvel, P., et al. (1995). Intracerebral potential to rare target and distractor auditory and visual stimuli. I. Superior temporal plane and parietal lobe. *Electroencephalography and Clinical Neurophysiology, 94,* 191–220.

Harrison, Y., & Horne, J. A. (2000). Sleep loss and temporal memory. The *Quarterly Journal of Experimental Psychology, 53,* 271–279.

Hobson, J. A., & Pace-Schott E. F. (2002). The cognitive neuroscience of sleep: neuronal systems, consciousness and learning. *Nature Reviews Neuroscience, 3,* 679–693.

Jenkins, J. G., & Dallenbach, K. M. (1924). Obliviscence during sleep and waking. *The American Journal of Psychology, 35,* 605–612.

Keele, S., Ivry, R. Mayr, U., Hazeltine, E., & Heuer, H. (2003). The cognitive and neural architecture of sequence learning. *Psychology Review, 110*(2), 316–339.

Kemler-Nelson, D. (1984). The effect of intention on what concepts are acquired. *Journal of Verbal Learning and Verbal Behavior, 23,* 734–759.

Laventure, S., Fogel, S., Lungu, O., Albouy, G., Sevigny-Dupont, P., Vien, C., et al. (2016). NREM2 and sleep spindles are instrumental to the consolidation of motor sequence memories. *PLoS Biology, 14*(3), e1002429.

Luu, P., Jiang, Z., Poulsen, C., Mattson, C., Smith, A., & Tucker, D. M. (2011). Learning and the development of contexts for action. *Frontiers in Human Neuroscience, 5,* 1–12.

Maddox, W. T., Ashby, F. G., Ing, A. D., & Pickering, A. D. (2004). Disrupting feedback processing interfere with rule-based but not information-integration category learning. *Memory & Cognition, 32,* 582–591.

Medin, D. L., & Shaffer, M. M. (1978). Context theory of classification learning. *Psychological Review, 85*(3), 207–238.

Molle, M., & Born, J. (2011). Slow oscillations orchestrating fast oscillations and memory consolidation. *Progress in Brain Research, 193,* 93–110.

Morgan, K. K., Luu, P., & Tucker, D. M. (2016). Changes in p3b latency and amplitude reflect expertise acquisition in a football visuomotor learning task. *PLoS ONE, 11*(4), e0154021.

Morris, G. O., Williams, H. L., & Lubin, A. (1960). Misperception and disorientation during sleep. *Archives of General Psychiatry, 2,* 247–254.

Nosofsky, R. M. (1986). Attention, similarity, and the identification-categorization relationship. *Journal of Experimental Psychology: general, 115*(1), 39–57.

Plihal, W., & Born, J. (1997). Effects of early and late nocturnal sleep on declarative and procedural memory. *Journal of Cognitive Neuroscience, 9*(4), 534–547.

Polich, J. (2007). Updating p300: An integrative theory of p3a and p3b. *Clinical Neurophysiology, 118,* 2128–2148.

Schneider, W. (1969). Two visual systems. *Science, 163*(3870), 895–902.

Schwabe, L., Oitzl, M. S., Philippsen, C., Richter, S., Bohringer, A., & Wippich, W. (2007). Stress modulates the use of spatial and stimulus-response learning strategies in human. *Learning & Memory, 14,* 109–116.

Schwabe, L., Schachinger, H., de Kloet, E. R., & Oitzl, M. S. (2010). Corticosteroids operate as a switch between memory systems. *Journal of Cognitive Neuroscience, 22,* 1362–1372.

Shiffrin, R. M., & Schneider, W. (1977). Controlled and automatic human information processing: II. Perceptual learning, automatic attending and a general theory. *Psychological Review, 84,* 127–190.

Smith, E. E., & Sloman, S. A. (1994). Similarity—versus rule-based categorization. *Memory and Cognition, 22*(4), 377–386.

Tucker, D. M. (1993). Spatial sampling of head electrical fields: the geodesic sensor net. *Electroencephalography and Clinical Neurophysiology, 87*(3), 154–163.

van der Helm, E., Yao, J., Dutt, S., Rao, V., Saletin, J. M., & Walker, M. P. (2011). REM sleep deteriorates amygdala activity to previous emotional experience. *Current Biology, 21*(23), 2029–2032.

Ungerleider, M., & Mishkin, M. (1982). Object vision and spatial vision: two cortical pathways. In D. J. Ingle, M. A. Goodale, & R. J. W. Mansfield (Eds.), *Analysis of visual behavior* (pp. 549–586). Cambridge, MA: MIT Press.

Zeithamova, D., & Maddox, W. T. (2007). The role of visuospatial and verbal working memory in perceptual category learning. *Memory & Cognition, 35*(6), 1380–1398.

Psychologically Mediated Heart Rate Variability during Official Competition

Ambulatory, Ecological Investigations of the Heart Rate Deceleration Response with Implications for Quantifying Flow

Roland A. Carlstedt

Ambulatory sport psychophysiology involves the continuous instrument-based monitoring, observation, and analysis of mind-body-technical performance of athletes during real training and competition. It is particularly important to the study of athletes where research findings should have a high degree of ecological validity, meaning acquired data must be procured from and reflect conditions encountered in the context of sport-specific situations and actions (Fahrenberg & Myrtek, 1996; Carlstedt, 2012). For example, it is not sufficient to assume that shifts in relative brain hemispheric activation that were observed in an experimental situation will transfer to the playing field without measuring brain functioning during real competition. Or, it cannot be assumed that an analysis of heart rate variability (HRV) in vitro will be predictive of an athlete's autonomic balance during real competition (de Geus & van Doornen, 1996; van Doornen, Knol, Willemsen, & de Geus, 1994; Carlstedt, 2012). Ultimately, replicable and predictive psychophysiological response tendencies that are observed during real competition will help better explain the role or impact of mind-body variables in the peak performance equation.

While the value of ambulatory psychophysiological assessment has been recognized, it is still a relatively unexplored and underused procedure in Sport Psychology, despite the fact that many of the central constructs and theories of sport performance have physiological and psychophysiological components (Heil & Henschen, 1996; Taylor, 1996). For example, Yerkes and Dodson's (1908) Inverted-U Theory proposes that a curvilinear relationship exists between physiological reactivity and performance, whereby increases in reactivity results in incremental improvement in performance, but only to a certain point, after which excessive reactivity disrupts performance. The psychophysiological concomitants of the Inverted-U-Theory are delineated in Duffy's (1972) description of activation theory and include increasing levels of HR, BP, muscle tension, skin conductance, and desynchronization of EEG alpha activity. In extending the Inverted-U Theory to account for individual differences in physiological reactivity, Hanin's (1980) Zone of Optimal Functioning theory is also based on similar physiological markers of activation or intensity. Catastrophe Theory, the most recent postulate of intensity, similarly alludes to physiological processes (Hardy & Fazey, 1987). This theory advances the idea that cognitive anxiety mediates the effects of physiological arousal on performance (Hardy & Fazey, 1987).

Unfortunately, many of the physiological measures these theories allude to have not been operationalized beyond the theoretical. Little is known about the psychophysiological functioning of athletes during actual competition. Attempts to delineate physiological functioning during real competitive are rare with the field of Sport Psychology still relying on imprecise operationalizations of key physiological components of sport performance. This is illustrated in Taylor's (1996) view of intensity, which he refers to as

> the most critical factor prior to competitive performance because, no matter how confident, motivated, or technically or physically prepared athletes are to perform, they will simply not be able to perform their best if their bodies are not at an optimal level of intensity, accompanied by the requisite physiological and psychological changes.
>
> *(p. 75)*

In viewing Taylor's notion of intensity, one must ask, what do "confident" and "motivated" mean? Also, what is an "optimal level of intensity," and what are "requisite physiological" and "psychological changes" that accompany intensity?

These questions have yet to be answered. Without studying the effects and impact of physiological and psychophysiological processes on performance, assumptions about intensity or states of activation and performance remain speculative.

The ultimate goal of ambulatory psychophysiology in sports is to establish performance relationships that have a high degree of ecological validity as well as to establish ways of testing the efficacy of interventions and replicating laboratory data that have implications for performance. To date, the use of ambulatory psychophysiology in studying performance has been neglected, despite the potential it holds for deriving data that may be vital to the credibility of many of the theories and interventions in sport psychology. In the following study, relationships between psychological factors (for traits and behaviors comprising the Athlete's Profile [AP] model of peak performance, see Carlstedt, 2012), and psychophysiology (using heart rate variability as predictor and outcome measures) and performance were investigated using methods in ambulatory, ecological assessment.

Background and Review of the Literature

Heart Activity: An Ideal Measure of Psychological Performance

Research has revealed significant interactions between the cardiovascular, the central nervous system, and the somatic nervous system (Andreassi, 1995). One line of research has established relationships between cardiac activity and reaction time (RT), with Lacey and Lacey (1964); Obrist, Webb, and Sutterer (1969); and Webb and Obrist (1970) reporting decreased heart rate (HRD) during the fixed foreperiod of simple RT experiments. It has also been shown that greater magnitudes of HRD are related to faster RTs (Lacey, 1967). It has been suggested that HRD represents a preparation to respond when an individual expects a significant stimulus (Andreassi, 1995). Another line of research has focused on power spectral density analysis (PSD) or spectrum analysis of heart rate variability (HRV) to assess sympathetic versus parasympathetic influence on the heart (i.e., autonomic balance; Akselrod et al., 1981; Jorna, 1992; McCraty & Watkins,1996; Porges & Byrne,1992). As a sensitive, noninvasive test of autonomic nervous system (ANS) function, spectrum analysis of HRV has been used in clinical settings to investigate stress-related disorders, such as hypertension and cardiovascular disease (McCraty & Watkins, 1996). Clinical research has found that lowered HRV is associated with aging, depressed hormonal responses, and increased incidence of sudden death (Malik & Camm, 1995). In addition, spectrum analysis of HRV has shown that depression, panic disorders, anxiety, and worry affect autonomic function, and can reduce the protective influence parasympathetic activity exerts on the heart (Malik & Camm, 1995).

The Theory of Critical Moments (see, Carlstedt, 2012) predicts that negative constellations of AP factors (hypnotic susceptibility/absorption/subliminal attention, neuroticism/subliminal reactivity, and repressive coping/subliminal coping) that have been shown to drive physiological hyper-reactivity and resulting clinical complaints in patients can disrupt motor/technical and psychological performance in athletes (Taylor, 1996; Wickramasekera, 1988). By contrast, it is predicted that athletes who possess ideal constellations of AP factors are more likely to reach their zone of optimal functioning and maintain peak performance, especially during critical moments of competition. Since both physiological reactivity and autonomic balance are reflected in spectrum analyses of HRV, and HRD, cardiac activity is a valuable measure of physiological reactivity (intensity), emotions, attention, and mediator of outcome in athletes (Akselrod et al., 1981; Tiller, McCraty, & Atkinson, 1996; McCraty, Atkinson, Tiller, Rein, & Watkins, 1995; Carlstedt, 2012).

HRV can be viewed as the window into mind-body interactions. In addition to reflecting physiological reactivity and emotions, heart activity has also been found to be an important measure of attention and cognitive activity (Sandman, Walker, & Berka, 1982). In reviewing the literature, Sandman et al. (1982) concluded that heart rate (HR) and blood pressure (BP) were the physiological parameters that best differentiated the cognitive-perceptual process. Their observation was based on the Lacey's (1964; 1967) investigations that discovered that HR decreased during tasks demanding attention to the environment and increased during tasks requiring mental concentration (or, rejection of the environment). This phenomenon has been explained on the basis of brain-heart interactions whereby HRD has been found to release the cortex from the inhibitory control of the baro-receptors, as reflected in fast-frequency (i.e., beta waves in the 23–38+ Hz range) electroencephalographic (EEG) activity (23–38+ Hz EEG activity has been associated with vigilant or attentive behavior; Lindsley, 1969; Sandman et al., 1982). Conversely, heart rate acceleration (HRA) has been shown to stimulate baro-receptor activity and thereby inhibit cortical activity. This is reflected in slower wave EEG (8–12 Hz) that has been associated with decreased perceptual processing (Sandman et al., 1982; Wolk & Velden, 1987).

Galin (1974) maintains that heart activity is more useful than EEG for analyzing attentional processes, because EEG represents only activity at the dorsal convexity of the brain but does not reflect activity in deep medial brain areas such as the hippocampus and the amygdala. Pribam and McGuiness (1975) have proposed that the hippocampus and amygdala (deep, medial brain areas) play an important role in attentional processes.

Not surprisingly, attention and cognitive activity play central roles in the anecdotal literature and research of sports performance (Gallwey, 1974; Waller, 1988). As might be expected, attention (e.g., focusing on the ball) is considered a desirable psychological state, whereas cognitive activity (e.g., thinking about winning during a point) is thought to disrupt sport performance. For instance, Gallwey (1974), in his classic book *The Inner Game of Tennis*, advocates letting things flow, or happen naturally, by focusing on the ball and warns of thinking too much about the consequences of hitting the ball. These notions appear to have found acceptance, with Ravizza (1977) reporting that 95% of the athletes he surveyed believed that thinking hinders performance. In addition, Waller (1988) reported that reduced levels of cognitive activity were experienced by athletes during peak performance episodes.

Since HRV has been shown to reflect many psychological states (e.g., attention & cognition), its importance to externally validating predictions from the TCM is highlighted. It is an ideal measure for operationalizing psychological constructs that have yet to be defined beyond anecdotal conjecture in sports (e.g., attention, cognitive activity, physiological reactivity, or intensity).

Given that there have been no studies on psychologically mediated HRV during real competition, research exploring the dynamics of AP-brain-heart interactions and their effects on performance is presented here. In extending research on HRD and HRV to the field, this study investigates some cardiovascular concomitants of constellations of AP factors during actual competition, in this case, official tennis tournament matches.

Roland A. Carlstedt

Heart Rate Variability/Heart Rate Deceleration: A Primer

In order to understand how HRV can reflect psychological processes (e.g., AP factors) and performance, it is necessary to review how the heart responds to autonomic nervous system activity.

HRV represents the net effect of parasympathetic (vagus) nerves, which slows HR, and the sympathetic nerves which accelerate it (Porges & Byrne, 1992). At rest, both parasympathetic and sympathetic nerves remain tonically active, with vagal effects being dominant (McCraty & Watkins, 1996; Obrist, 1981). Stimulation of the vagus nerves slows the heart. This slowing occurs almost immediately, within one or two heart beats after its onset. After vagal stimulation ceases, HR quickly returns to its previous level. An increase in HR can result from a reduction in vagal activity. Therefore, sudden changes in HR are initiated by parasympathetic activity (Lacey & Lacey, 1978). Increases in sympathetic activity cause HR to rise above the intrinsic HR level produced by the sinoatrial node. After sympathetic stimulation begins, there is a delay of up to five seconds before a progressive increase in HR occurs, which reaches a steady level in 20–30 seconds (McCraty & Watkins, 1996). The slowness of HR response to sympathetic stimulation is contrasted to vagal stimulation that produces immediate HR deceleration (McCraty & Watkins, 1996).

Blood Pressure, Baro-receptors, and HRV

Blood pressure (BP) regulation is of primary importance to cardiovascular function. The factors that control BP also regulate HRV (McCraty & Watkins, 1996; Obrist, 1981). Short-term regulation of BP is achieved through an intricate system of pressure-sensitive baro-receptors located throughout the heart, aortic arch, and the carotid artery (Lacey & Lacey, 1978; Obrist, 1981). Afferent impulses (i.e., signals transmitted to the brain) from the baro-receptors travel via the glosso-pharyngeal and vagal nerves to the vasomotor centers in the medulla oblongata where they regulate sympathetic nervous system (SNS) transmissions to the heart and blood vessels. Some modulation of parasympathetic nervous system (PNS) transmission also occurs in the medulla oblongata (Obrist, 1981; Porges & Byrne, 1992). Baro-receptors regulate HR, vasoconstriction, venoconstriction, and cardiac contractility to maintain BP (Obrist, 1981).

The regulation of BP by baro-receptors is hypothesized to differentially facilitate or inhibit cortical activity and attentional efficiency (Lacey & Lacey, 1978). Specifically, elevated HR and BP are thought to inhibit cortical activity, thereby decreasing attention, whereas HR deceleration and lowered BP are thought to facilitate attentional processes (Lacey & Lacey, 1978; Sandman et al., 1982).

In summary, ANS (sympathetic and parasympathetic) activity along with afferent signals from the baro-receptor produce the beat-to-beat changes that characterize HRV (Obrist, 1981; Porges & Byrne, 1992).

Measures of HRV

Time and frequency domain measures are used to analyze HRV (Leiderman & Shapiro, 1962; Akselrod et al., 1981). The most common method for obtaining these measures is to plot the sequence of time intervals between the R-waves of the heart period (HP; such data can be obtained using ambulatory HR monitoring equipment, e.g., Holter & Polar systems). The resulting graph of heart rate changes (i.e., HRV) is called a tachogram (Andreassi, 1995). The tachogram reflects the ANS mediated HRV signal and beat-to-beat changes in HR (Andreassi, 1995; McCraty & Watkins, 1996).

With both methods, the time intervals between consecutive R-waves of the HP are first calculated (Andreassi, 1995). Thereafter, HRV measures of interest are delineated and analyzed accordingly (e.g., HR deceleration or PSD analysis).

Time Domain Measures

Time Domain Measures of HRV reflect changes in heart activity that occur within a single cardiac cycle (i.e., HP, or inter-beat interval [IBI], and are expressed in milliseconds; [ms] Andreassi, 1995). Time domain measures of interest include heart rate deceleration (HRD) and, to a lesser extent, heart rate acceleration (HRA). HRD is the progressive slowing of one or more successive IBIs (i.e., HR slowing from R-wave to R-wave of the HP). For example, IBI ms values of 555, 560, 570, 575, and 580 reflect HRD between four IBIs (increasing values reflect a longer HP, or slowing of the heart; Andreassi, 1995). By contrast, IBI values of 580, 575, 570, and 565 reflect HRA between three consecutive IBIs (decreasing IBI values indicate a shorter HP or acceleration of the heart).

Time domain measures of HRV have been used to study RT, task performance, complex motor activity, perception, mental imagery, attention, motivation, emotion, and operant conditioning of HR (Carriero & Fite, 1977; Elliott, 1974; Elliott, Bankert & Light, 1970; Hahn, 1973; Jennings & Wood, 1977; Lacey & Lacey, 1974; Lang, Levin, Miller, & Kozak, 1983; McCanne & Sandman, 1976; Obrist, Howard, Sutterer, Hennis, & Murrell, 1973; Schell & Catina, 1975).

Frequency Domain Measures

Frequency domain measures refer to power spectral density (PSD) or spectrum analysis measures of HRV (McCraty & Watkins, 1996). PSD shows how the power of heart activity is distributed as a function of frequency (McCraty & Watkins, 1996). The PSD of HRV is obtained by filtering and extracting the different frequency components of HRV that are discernible in the tachogram. The HRV power spectrum contains three main frequency ranges: (1) very low frequency (VLF, 0.033–0.04 Hz); (2) low frequency (LF, 0.04–0.15 Hz); and high frequency (HF, 0.15–0.4 Hz; Akselrod et al., 1981; Malik & Camm, 1995). The HF range reflects rapid changes in beat-to-beat variability (i.e., HRV) that are caused by parasympathetic or vagal stimulation (Akselrod et al., 1981; Malik & Camm, 1995). The VLF range is thought to reflect predominantly sympathetic stimulation (Akselrod et al., 1981; Malik & Camm, 1995). The LF range reflects both a mixture of sympathetic and parasympathetic stimulation of the heart (Akselrod et al., 1981; Malik & Camm, 1995). The LF/HF ratio is used to quantify the overall balance between the sympathetic and parasympathetic systems and is a measure of special interest in this study (Malik & Camm, 1995).

Frequency domain analysis of HRV (i.e., PSD or spectrum analysis) provides reliable measures of the effects stress and emotions exert on autonomic function. To date, PSD analysis of HRV research has been limited mostly to clinical and organizational settings (McCraty & Watkins, 1996; Jorna, 1992; Myrtek, Bruegner, & Mueller, 1996). It has not been used to analyze continuous psychologically mediated HRV during official sports competition (Carlstedt, 2012).

Heart Rate Variability Research

The presented study is based on two lines of research. The first is traced to Lacey & Lacey's (1964; 1978) seminal investigations of cardiac deceleration (HRD) in the simple reaction time paradigm. The second line can be traced to Akselrod's et al. (1981) mathematical quantification of the physiologic mechanisms of beat-to-beat HR fluctuations, or spectrum analysis of HRV. Research of HRD and spectrum analysis has been numerous, although interest in HRD has waned over the years (due to time consuming methods and analytics that are required to accurately isolate HRD trends over time), while interest in spectrum analysis of HRV has been increasing. This is also attributable to the fact that psychologically mediated HRD is no longer disputable, and spectrum analysis, which is more relevant to clinical, educational, and work place issues and can be derived and analyzed using user-friendly hard-and software (Andreassi, 1995; Sandman et al., 1982).

Although there is literature on HRD research in sports, it has been limited to static, non-action types of sports such as shooting, archery, and golf (Hatfield, Landers, & Ray, 1984, 1987;

Boutcher & Zinsser, 1990). Other than this author's long line of HRD investigations (Carlstedt, 2012) this cardiac response has not been studied ecologically, during real competition or in action sports where little is known about the effects of cardiac deceleration, especially during critical moments. Furthermore, no studies of have investigated HRD in athletes as a function of AP factors and other psychological measures. There also, are no previous studies on spectrum analysis of psychologically mediated HRV in athletes during official competition.

HRD Research

HRD research falls into two categories. (1) Mechanistic studies are investigations that have detailed the properties of HRD within experimental variations of the simple RT paradigm. These studies have demonstrated the existence of HRD. Simple RT time and choice RT paradigms are presented in some detail to illuminate components of the simple RT model that have been adapted to the presented study and other investigations of HRD in sports. (2) Performance studies have investigated the effects of HRD on performance. These studies have associated HRD with differential RT and task performance, both in the laboratory and structured sport experiments.

Mechanistic Studies of HRD

HRD has been demonstrated in a variety of studies, with Lacey and Lacey (1964) being the first to show that HR decreased in response to an imperative (i.e., imminent or impending) stimulus. The Laceys' work introduced the simple RT paradigm in which subjects were required to press a key after the appearance of a ready signal (a green circle in a display box), hold the key down until the imperative signal (a white cross) was superimposed on the green circle, and respond as quickly as possible to the white cross, by releasing the key. The so-called fixed foreperiod, or time offset, between the time of initial key depression and the presentation of the imperative signal lasted four seconds. Results of this study showed a progressive slowing of the heart (i.e., HRD), from the time of the ready signal (i.e., pressing the key) to when the imperative signal was presented (as reflected in the lengthening of successive IBIs prior to the imperative signal).

In an extension of their original research, the Laceys (1978) measured HP as a function of time in which the imperative stimulus was presented in the cardiac cycle. They found that the magnitude of HR deceleration during the fixed foreperiod depended on where in the cardiac cycle the imperative stimulus was presented. If it occurred early (4th decile) in the cycle, deceleration was significantly greater than if the imperative signal came late (10th decile) in the cycle.

The Laceys (1970) also reported anticipatory slowing (i.e., HRD) in experiments requiring self-initiated responses (choice RT paradigm). For example, subjects having a prior knowledge of the onset of a significant stimulus tended to exhibit increasingly greater heart rate slowing (HRD) as the time of voluntary motor response approached.

The simple RT paradigm and variations thereof (e.g., choice RT paradigm) lend themselves well to studying HRD in settings where persons are waiting to respond to a stimulus including prior to certain sport-specific tasks (Edwards & Alsip, 1966; Heslegrave, Ogilvie, & Furedy, 1979; Nowlin, Eisdorfer, Whalen, & Troyer, 1970; Surwillo, 1971; Walter & Porges, 1976). For example, in measuring heart activity as a function of task demand, the Laceys (1968) measured HRD during a six second interval prior to the foreperiod, for six seconds of the foreperiod, and for six seconds after the response. In tennis this would amount to a player waiting six seconds prior to entering the ready position to receive serve, after which six more seconds pass before the ball is served (stimulus presentation-response), followed by action lasting six seconds (time period from when the serve was returned to when the point ends). Similar intervals occur in golf, baseball, softball, and basketball, sports that were investigated in Study 1 (below). The Laceys' original mechanistic studies of HR deceleration have been replicated numerous times (e.g., Webb & Obrist, 1970). In essence, replication investigations support the hypothesis that HRD is a species-wide response, in anticipation of an imperative stimulus.

Performance Studies of HRD

The mere fact that HRD has been empirically validated as a species-wide response is of minor importance to athletes if HRD cannot be linked to within- or between-subject differences in performance. Thus, if HRD does not distinguish good from poor performance, why should it be studied? This question is in part answered by performance studies of HRD which suggest that within- and between-subject differences in HRD are associated with differential task performance and level of skill. For example, Wang and Landers (as cited in Boutcher & Zinsser, 1990; original source unavailable), Landers et al. (1994) and Salazar et al. (1990) comparing highly and moderately skilled archers, reported HRD in both subject groups prior to shooting (i.e., in the preparation phase before arrow release). In addition, they found differences in HRD between groups. Although both groups exhibited HRD patterns, highly skilled archers demonstrated significantly greater HRD in comparison to lesser skilled archers, during the aiming phase.

In a similar study involving golf, Boutcher and Zinsser (1990) replicated the basic findings of Wang and Landers. In a comparison of elite and beginning golfers during putting, they also reported individual differences in HRD-performance effects. Specifically, they showed that both elite and beginning golfers exhibited significant HRD compared to baseline HR, prior to putting. In addition, elite golfers were found to experience significantly slower HR than beginning golfers immediately before, during, and after the ball was putted. Hatfield et al. (1984) also reported that elite rifle shooters exhibited HRD prior to shooting. Although this study did not differentiate performance proficiency, it did provide evidence in support of previous electrophysiological and neurocardiologic explanations of psychologically mediated HRV (e.g., Armour, 1994; Lacey & Lacey, 1978; McCraty & Watkins, 1996; Sandman et al., 1982). These researchers reported that increased right hemispheric EEG activity was concomitant to HRD prior to shooting. This finding is in line with previous research associating HRD with increased cortical activity (as observed in increased EEG alpha activity (Lacey & Lacey, 1978; Sandman et al., 1982). The authors proposed that elite marksmen have developed attentional focus to the extent that they are unconsciously capable of reducing cognitive activity in the left hemisphere (i.e., left half of the brain). Left hemisphere cognitive activity has been associated with the disruption of motor performance (Hatfield et al., 1984; Langer & Imber, 1979).

The above studies are important because they clearly establish that the magnitude of HRD during self-paced sports is associated with a performer's level of skill. They provide evidence that HRD is not only a species-wide physiological response, but that it also reflects individual differences in athletic ability. However, they did not investigate within- or between-subject differences in HRD as a function of personality traits or behavioral measures (e.g., AP factors/constellations). Recent research by Hassmen and Koivula (2001) showing that anxiety can disrupt HRD trends supports the TCM hypothesis that personality and behavioral factors can affect physiological responding and should be considered in all psychophysiological research.

HRD I: A Case Study of HRD during Official Tennis Matches: Hypotheses

Hypothesis 1: Total HRD

Hypothesis 1 predicted that HRD patterns during tennis matches would resemble deceleration trends observed in previous research of self-paced sports. For example, it was hypothesized that during the pre-action phases of matches, IBIs would progressively lengthen (i.e., become slower) up to the point when action commences.

Hypothesis 2: HRD and Successful Performance

Hypothesis 2 predicted that more and greater magnitudes of HRD would occur in a match that was won compared to a match that was lost.

Roland A. Carlstedt

Spectrum Analysis of HRV

A spectrum analysis of HRV was performed for exploratory purposes to determine if differences in heart rate variability existed between matches.

Participant

This study involved a 16-year-old male who was a nationally ranked tennis Player. He was assessed on AP factors and found to have the constellation High Absorption, Medium Neuroticism, and Low Repressive Coping. It should be noted that this is considered a relatively negative constellation in the context of critical moments of competition (TCM).

Research Design

The study used a single-case/repeated measures design and was carried out during an official USTA tennis tournament. The player's heart activity was monitored using ambulatory cardiac monitoring instrumentation during his first, second, and third round matches. Since the goal of this study was to establish differences in HRD and HRV between matches that were won and lost, Match 1 (won) was compared with Match 3 (lost). Match 2, which was won, was not analyzed since it was played on the same day as Match 1. All the matches were videotaped in their entirety. Performance measures in the matches were obtained using qualitative and quantitative methods of content analysis. The exploratory nature of this field study precluded the manipulation of variables.

Instrumentation

Heart activity was recorded using a Polar Heart Rate Monitoring system consisting of a noninvasive wireless and telemetry system to transmit heart signals from a chest strap (housing electrodes) to a wrist-watch for data storage. Data is then transferred to a computer by an interface for analysis. IBIs of each HP were extracted using Polar HR analysis software. HRD and HRA epochs were delineated in the context of downtime before and between points, pre-action preparation, and action using a special developed application that synchronized the match time line video with the Polar derived HRV/HRD-IBI (Figure 9.1).

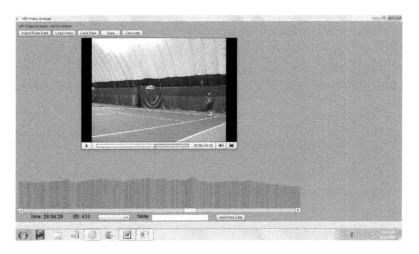

Figure 9.1 Heart rate deceleration analysis app.

Video Analysis

Matches were video-taped using a Sony camcorder. Tapes of the matches were time coded using a Sony video-editing system to establish a timeline between match events and heart activity.

Procedure

This study was carried out at an official USTA men's tennis tournament in central California. Prior to the tournament the subject was familiarized with the Polar equipment. This involved learning how to start the receiver (wristwatch) and how to read its data display. A practice session was also carried out in which it was established that the equipment would not hinder the player's stroking ability and mobility. Upon arriving at the tournament venue, preparation to carry out the study commenced. The Sony camcorder was placed on a platform overlooking the court on which the player's matches would be played. A computer station for receiving data was set up in the club house. Approximately 10 minutes before the beginning of the first match, the subject was fitted with the Polar chest strap. The wristwatch was attached to the player's left arm. The player was instructed to start the watch immediately prior to the first point. The camcorder was started just prior to the end of the warm-up session before the match. These procedures were repeated prior to both matches.

Methods and Analysis of Data

The heart activity-performance time line was calibrated from the time on the videotape when the watch was started. That time was compared with the heart activity time-line of the watch to discern HRD trends prior to, during, and after action. Videotapes of the two matches were analyzed to obtain performance data. HRD and HRV data were extracted using computer generated data sheets that sequentially listed all IBIs stored in the watch. A questionnaire was used to debrief the subject. The purpose of this questionnaire was to obtain self-report feedback on the player's perceived psychological state during the matches.

Statistics

T tests were used to analyze the HRD data. They were performed on pre-action interbeat intervals within and between matches. The exploratory spectrum analysis generated descriptive data on HRV between matches. Tests for the difference between two proportions were carried out to examine between match differences in HRV.

Results

Match Outcome

The player won Match 1 by a score of 6-4, 6-1. He lost Match 3 6-0, 6-1 (the score of Match 3 is the second worst score possible in a best of three set match).

Self-Report of Psychological State during Matches

The player reported that he was very attentive in Match 1 (5 on a 5-point Likert like scale) and not very nervous (2 on a 5-point scale). He further described himself as very motivated, and confident of winning every point in the match (4 on a 5-point scale). The player also mentioned not having "much respect for the game of his opponent." During changeovers, the player stated that he visualized how he would play the upcoming game, something a player who is high in the AP factor absorption would be likely to do and benefit from. In general, the player reported highly positive emotions and cognitive activity in Match 1.

As would be expected, the player described vastly different emotions prior to and during Match 3. He reported a high degree of nervousness (4 on a 5-point scale) and a low level of attention (2 on a 5-point scale) during Match 3. He also stated that after being unable to make his best shots throughout the match, "negative thoughts" tended to dominate. He frequently thought about losing, lost motivation (1 on a 5-point scale), and eventually resigned himself to being defeated.

This feedback is highly consistent with what would be expected to occur in an athlete having an AP factor constellation of high absorption, medium to high neuroticism, and low repressive coping, especially once performance becomes disrupted during competition.

Qualitative Observations

The first match was won easily. At no time was the player in danger of losing control of the match and appeared motivated as well as psychologically stable throughout. Besides remaining both calm and attentive (high absorption) from beginning to end, the player conveyed the impression that he had confidence in his technical abilities and was not afraid to attempt difficult or risky shots. The first match was routine in nature and he was obviously better than his opponent from a technical standpoint. Critical moments did not emerge in this match, with the average criticality level for all points being between 1 and 2 (lowest rating on a 1–5 criticality scale). Consequently, potential negative manifestations of his AP factor constellation did not emerge. The player appeared to benefit from his high intrinsic level of absorption since the overall level of stress associated with this match was low. This facilitated focus on the task at hand as opposed to internal cognitions that might have emerged to disrupt performance during a more demanding match. Essentially, potential manifestation of the player's neuroticism remained dormant, allowing for full absorption in the tasks at hand.

The player's behavior and performance in the third match visibly contrasted with that of the first. In facing the number one seeded player, a 31-year-old veteran of the professional tennis tour, he appeared nervous from the beginning of the match. His agitation was reflected in poor movement and technique, which resulted in numerous unforced errors. The player also displayed displeasure with his performance by frequently chiding himself. These emotional displays stood in stark contrast to the calmness he exhibited in the first match. However, after it became apparent that the match would be very difficult to win, the player reverted to a state of emotional indifference, indicative of an athlete who is resigned to losing.

Although points in Match 3 only averaged about 3 points on the criticality scale, it should be noted that the player lost all criticality level 5 points. This was to be expected on the basis of his constellation of AP factors whereby it appeared that the player's medium level of neuroticism emerged under the stress associated with Match 3 to drive excessive physiological reactivity. The heightened stress and resulting physiological hyper-reactivity in Match 3 (as reflected in decreased HRD) coincided with the player's self-report of negative intrusive thoughts. In the presence of high level of neuroticism, such cognitions are the kind that people high in absorption tend to ruminate on during times of increased stress. Consequently, the player's increased ability to focus on tasks at hand, an ability associated with high absorption (which was exhibited in Match 1) shifted from sport-specific tasks to internal negative thoughts in Match 3, leading to poor performance. The fact that the player was low in repressive coping allowed for the unmitigated interaction of absorption-neuroticism. In accord with predictions from the TCM, the player's low level of repressive coping and high absorption made him especially vulnerable to negative intrusive thoughts associated with neuroticism that are more likely to occur during critical moments of competition.

Match Statistics

The subject committed 10 unforced errors, 16 forced errors, and hit 16 winners in the first match. Forced errors are considered unavoidable and a result of an opponent's forcing shot. Thus, a winners-to-unforced errors ratio of 16:10 is consistent with matches that are well played and won. By contrast, the subject committed 28 unforced errors, three forced errors, and hit four winners in Match 3. The low winners-to unforced errors ratio of 1:7 reflects a match that was poorly played and lost, and underscores the above qualitative observations. Conversely, statistics from the first match support the contention that the player was psychologically in control of his game in Match 1.

HRD and HRA Phases

There were 51 usable (for HRD analysis) pre-action phases in Match 1 and 27 in Match 3. Pre-action phases were identified in the videotapes of the matches. These phases corresponded with clean heart activity data extracted from the computer analysis data read-out (with in artifact tolerance range). Pre-action phase with excessive artifact were eliminated from the analysis. It should be noted that although artifact corrections can be made, doing so can also impact the ability to isolate HRD trends accurately.

In contrast to previously cited laboratory research, in which a pre-specified number of IBIs were studied prior to action, a field study cannot predict in advance how many IBIs will occur prior to action. Thus, the number of IBIs prior to each action phase was variable. In Match 1 there were 283 decelerating IBIs prior to the 51 action phases, or a mean of 5.55 IBIs per pre-action phase. There were 112 decelerating IBIs prior to 27 action phases in Match 3, or a mean of 4.15 IBIs per pre-action phase.

Hypothesis 1

An examination of all pre-action IBIs in Match 1 and Match 3 revealed HRD in all IBIs prior to action. The presence of HRD in the IBIs prior to action supported the hypothesis that HRD trends during tournament tennis would resemble HRD that was observed in previous laboratory and field studies (Figure 9.2).

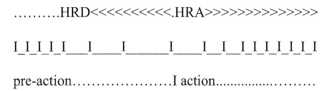

Figure 9.2 Sample selection of pre-action, action, and post-action IBIs in Match 1. Notice that the IBIs become progressively longer, leading up the response IBI. Thereafter the IBIs become progressively shorter during the action phase. After action ceases, the IBIs again become longer in the post-action recovery phase. Longer IBIs indicate a slowing of the heart. Shorter IBIs indicate an acceleration of the heart or a shorter and faster heart period.

Roland A. Carlstedt

Hypothesis 2

Hypothesis 2 was tested by comparing various combinations of IBIs in pre-action phases of Match 1 and 3. The following IBI combinations were examined to determine if greater magnitudes of HRD would be evident in a match that was won compared to a match that was lost: (1) the difference in the rate of HRD between all IBIs prior to action in Match 1 compared to Match 3 (Figure 9.2); (2) the difference in the rate of HRD between the last IBI prior to action in Match 1 compared to Match 3; Figure 9.3; (3) the difference in HRD between the 2nd to last IBI and the next to last IBI, compared to the difference between the next-to-last IBI and last IBI prior to action, in Match 1, compared to Match 3.

The following significant effects in support of Hypotheses 2 were found: (1) total IBIs prior to action in Match 1 compared to Match 3 revealed more pre-action HRD in Match 1 than in Match 3 (mean IBI = 6.79 vs. 5.57; p = 0.05; (2) HRD in IBIs prior to the last IBI before action in Match 1 compared to Match 3, revealed more HRD in match 1 (mean IBI = 6.37 vs. 5.42; p = 0.085); (3) the next to last IBI, compared to the last IBI prior to action in Match 1, revealed significant HRD between the last 2 IBIs (mean = 11.67; p = 0.008); (4) the next to last IBI, compared to the last IBI prior to action in Match 3, also revealed significant HRD between the last two IBIs (mean = 8.67; p = 0.079; Figure 9.3); and (5) the IBI decelerative trend between the 2nd to last IBI and the next to last IBI, and the next-to-last IBI and the last IBI prior to action in Match 1, compared to Match 3, revealed more HRD in Match 1 (mean = 3.86 vs. −1.67; p = 0.037)

Although a comparison of the next-to-last IBI with the last IBI prior to action in Match 1 with Match 3 did not reveal significant differences (mean= 11.67 vs. 8.67; p = 0.16) more HRD did

Match 1

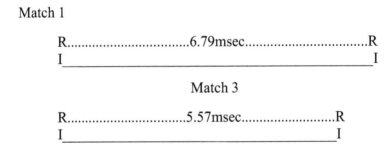

Figure 9.3 Mean rate of heart rate deceleration for all IBIs prior to action in Match 1 compared to Match 3 (p < 0.045).

Match 1

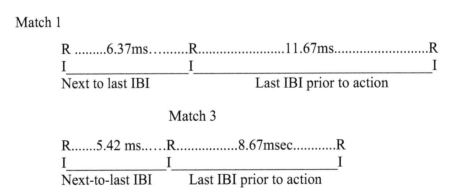

Figure 9.4 Mean difference of the rate of heart rate deceleration between the last IBI prior to action compared to the next-to-last IBI in Match 1 (p < 0.008) and mean difference of the rate of heart rate deceleration between the last IBI prior to action compared to the next-to-last IBI in match 3 (p < 0.079).

occur in the last IBI prior to action in Match 1. This is important in the context of within-match performance, where significant HRD in the last IBI prior to action was demonstrated (Figure 9.4).

Spectrum Analysis of HRV: Exploratory Data

A spectrum analysis was performed to determine if matches could be distinguished on the basis of autonomic nervous system activity.

The spectrum analysis of Match 1 revealed the following values: (1) 5-minute total power = 1573.4 (power in the band <0.40 Hz); (2) 5-minute VLF = 1378.6 (power spectrum range from 0.0033 to 0.04 Hz); (3) 5-minute LF = 180.6 (power spectrum range from 0.04 to 0.15 Hz); and (4) 5-minute HF = 14.3 (power spectrum range from 0.15–0.4 Hz; (5) LF/HF = 12.7). Spectrum analysis of Match 3 revealed the following values: (1) 5 minute total power = 2288.7; (2) 5-minute VLF = 2094.5; (3) 5-minute LF= 174.6; (4) 5-minute HF = 19.6; and (5) LF/HF= 8.9.

Discussion

The results of this study showed that varying magnitudes of HRD preceded action phases during both tennis matches. These findings were the first to demonstrate HRD during official action-sport competition. Moreover, the general hypothesis of this study, which predicted more HRD would occur prior to action phases in a match that was won compared to a match that was lost, was supported. Although both matches were marked by progressive HRD leading up to action, Match 1 showed significantly greater HRD in all configurations of IBIs prior to action. A particularly noteworthy finding was that the last IBI prior to the action response was significantly longer than the IBI preceding the action response (i.e., more HRD) in Match 1 compared to Match 3. This finding is consistent with studies by Lacey and Lacey (1978) and Jennings and Wood (1977) that reported the greatest amount of HRD in the last IBI prior to the presentation of a stimulus. In addition, when comparing the last the IBIs prior to action in Match 1 with those of Match 3, it was found that HR slowing was significantly greater between IBI 2 and IBI 1(last IBI prior to action) in Match 1 than between IBI 3 and IBI 2 in Match 3. These data also replicate studies reporting that successive IBIs, prior to the imperative stimulus, become progressively slower as the time of response nears (Jennings & Wood, 1977; Lacey & Lacey, 1978).

It should be noted that significant HRD occurred both within matches and between matches. However, this study marks the first time that significant within-subject differences between HRD and performance outcome have been reported. Previous research has focused either on between-subject differences in performance, or did not report significant within-subject results as a function of performance (Boutcher & Zinsser, 1990; Nowlin, Eisdorfer, Surwillo, 1971; Whalen, & Troyer, 1971).

This study also marks the first time that HRD has been demonstrated at higher HR levels. For example, in previous research, HRD was observed in the 70–90 bpm range, whereas in this study, HRD occurred at levels as high as 150 bpm (Boutcher & Zinsser, 1990). This is noteworthy since experiments of operant conditioning of HR have only been successful in slowing HR below resting baseline or slightly elevated HR (McCanne & Sandman, 1976). Although the HRD observed at higher HRs in this study could be attributed to the exercise recovery response, this is only a partial explanation since HRD here resembled HRD trends in other laboratory and field studies (Obrist, 1981; Boutcher & Zinsser, 1990). These trends were thought to be mediated by constellations of AP psychological factors.

The results of the spectrum analysis indicate that, in general, there was more sympathetic activity in Match 1 and more parasympathetic activity in Match 3. This is reflected in the LF/HF ratio of each match (LF/HF ratio = 12.7, in Match 1, vs. 8.9, in Match 3). Although parasympathetic predominance was evident in Match 3, it is pointed out that VLF, which is also thought to reflect sympathetic activity, was higher in Match 3 than in Match 1. Since there are no norms for, or studies of, spectrum analysis during tennis or any sport, there is much room for interpretation and speculation when analyzing these results. Thus, the results of spectrum analysis can only be addressed in the context of the comprehensive data of this study.

The results of this study become more meaningful when interpreted in relationship to the diametrically opposed performance and outcome of the two matches. These extreme differences are reflected in quantitative performance data (e.g., match score and statistics) and qualitative impressions of the match (i.e., psychological performance) and are consistent with the player's constellation of AP factors. The player's self-report of experiencing major differences in attention, emotions, self-confidence, cognitive activity, and reactivity between matches suggest that his AP factors impacted the above measures, HRD, and performance.

Of these factors, attention is considered by many to be the most central to performance since it is directly related to observing and processing environmental stimuli (Boutcher & Zinsser, 1990). Relative to the findings of this study, it was hypothesized that this player's level of attention was mediated by his constellation of AP factors negatively exerting their effects on cognitive activity and disrupting HRD in the match he lost.

In Match 1, AP factors may have potentiated vagal activity and resultant greater HRD prior to action. This could have increased attention by limiting competing sensory feedback such as negative intrusive cognitions from reaching the left-frontal lobes of the brain (seat of rumination; Sandman et al., 1982; Carlstedt, 2012). In essence, limiting superfluous and disruptive feedback to the left-frontal lobes prevents sensory flooding from diverting attentional resources away from a significant stimulus (Klemm, 1996). Consequently, heart-brain feedback loops marked by increases in HRD may have facilitated attention in Match 1 by efficiently taking in stimuli that was significant, and excluding stimuli that was potentially disruptive (intake-rejection hypothesis; Lacey & Lacey, 1964). These dynamics were thought to occur because of the positive influences of high absorption in Match 1 that allowed for optimum focusing.

Paradoxically, although HRD was significantly greater in Match 1, this match was marked by less total parasympathetic activity. This may be attributable to an overall higher level of sympathetic activation during action phases of the match, indicative of motivated performance and greater intensity. Thus, levels of sympathetic activity associated with greater motivation, activation, and energy expenditure in Match 1 may have skewed the spectrum analysis data to under-reflect the parasympathetic activity associated with increased HRD and attention (Jorna, 1992; McCraty, Barrios-Choplin, Rozman, Atkinson, & Watkins, 1996; Porges & Byrne, 1992).

Match 3 was marked by a major decrease in overall performance and HRD. Self-report indicated that the player was more nervous, less motivated, and less attentive in this match. In addition, the player reported a loss of confidence and a sense of helplessness as the match progressed. He also admitted to frequent negative cognitions. Thus, it was hypothesized that negative intrusive thoughts associated with the player's increased levels of neuroticism interfered with attention during pre-action phases of Match 3 by diverting focus away from (external) sport-specific tasks toward disruptive (internal) cognitions. Since negative cognitive activity has been associated with decreased attention, it was posited that focus on internal thoughts prior to action disrupted the priming of neuronal networks responsible for initiating motor responses and HRD, leading to more errors in Match 3 (Klemm, 1996; Ravizza, 1977; Waller, 1988). The player's tendency to fixate on negative intrusive thoughts was believed to have been facilitated by his high level of absorption.

Match 3 was marked by more parasympathetic than sympathetic activity. Since it was believed that losing a match would be marked by greater emotion, stress, and hyper-reactivity, the data on spectrum analysis from Match 3 were surprising. However, since the player revealed that after recognizing that the match could not be won he became more relaxed, it was to be expected that parasympathetic activity would increase. Thus, it was hypothesized that the stress and effort associated with a difficult match was attenuated once the subject gave up hope of winning, leading to increased parasympathetic activity in Match 3.

The fact that performance and outcome between matches were highly incongruous suggests that HRD is not only a species-wide physiological response to an impending stimulus, but that it also varies as a function of specific tasks, performance demands, and psychological factors (e.g., AP factors). This contention is based on a comprehensive evaluation of the data. Although initial p values were set at <0.10 for this exploratory study, most HRD effects were demonstrated to be significant at $p < 0.05$, with the most important effect being significant at $p < 0.008$ (next to-last IBI, compared to last IBI in Match 1), and $p < 0.038$ (comparing last three IBIs in Match 1 to Match 3). Even though statistical procedures and their results can be broadly interpreted to suit a particular hypothesis, the quantitative results of this study lend additional support by extreme differences in match scores, performance statistics, data on content analysis, and self-report feedback (Denzin & Lincoln, 1994; Gall et al., 1996). Consequently, there was a high degree of qualitative certainty that HRV effects in this study were not random.

It can be argued that, since an athlete's constellation of AP factors does not change over time (i.e., it is stable and trait-like), it should have the same impact on performance regardless of match outcome. However, one is again reminded that AP factors are not static. Constellations of AP factors are dynamic and predicted to impact performance the most during critical moments of competition by mediating physiological responses and subsequent motor performance. Since HRD has been shown to reflect physiological reactivity, attention, and cognitive activity, the changes in HRD that were observed between matches having highly incongruent performance and outcome may have been mediated by AP factors. The player's self-report between matches supports this interpretation since it was consistent with theoretical conceptualizations of AP factors and how they can impact performance and physiology. These dynamics were also quasi-validated in the context of the observed HRD trends.

Although this investigation involved only one athlete, single case studies have an important advantage in that a person serves as his or her own control. Such control is particularly important in psychophysiological studies. Consequently, changes in physiological response tendencies across diverse conditions in the same individual may very likely reflect psychological influences. Single-subject ambulatory psychophysiological field studies such as this one also can have a higher degree of ecological validity than laboratory studies involving a larger population (Gall et al. 1996; Myrtek et al., 1996) making them more useful for exploratory and validation purposes.

HRD II: Toward a Global Physiological Biomarker of Psychological Performance during Critical Moments of Competition: Assessing Zone or Flow States

Since the psychophysiological approach to the assessment of critical moments can be laborious, a quick, efficient, and reliable method for assessing global psychological performance is needed. An emerging method that I am developing involves monitoring and analyzing heart activity over the course of an entire competition since it appears to be the physiological measure that best illuminates mind-body interactions. It is also the only measure that can be reliably monitored during actual competition in a relatively non-intrusive manner, making it ideal for assessing psychological performance during critical moments of competition.

While it has been established that HRD reflects heightened attention during competitive moments that are preceded by a mental preparation phase, it has yet to be determined to what extent HRD occurs over the course of an entire competition independent of mental preparation phases (i.e., during action phases). Consequently, in this exploratory study, a tennis player's heart activity was monitored during an actual match to not only isolate HRD trends prior to action, but also delineate global heart activity over an entire competition.

Roland A. Carlstedt

Participant and Procedure

A German amateur Men's 35 division ranked tournament tennis player's heart activity was monitored during the first round of tournament competition using a Polar cardiac monitoring system. The player was assessed for AP factors and cerebral laterality prior to the match and found to be high in absorption, high in neuroticism, and low in repressive coping. He was also shown to be relative right brain hemisphere predominant on the basis a line-bisecting test. His cerebral laterality score was consistent with high neuroticism and low repressive coping (relative left hemispheric hypo-activation and increased right hemisphere's activation). The player's constellation of AP factors made him psychologically vulnerable during critical moments of competition.

The player's heart activity was monitored continuously but not synchronized to specific competitive events. Set statistics included points played, pre-action points, and action moments. Afterward, the match data were transferred from the Polar device into HRV and HRD software for analysis.

Analysis of the Data

Previous research (Carlstedt, 1998) indicates that "true" heart rate deceleration, as distinguished from heart rate slowing due to diminishing metabolic demands, consists of an uninterrupted linear progression of at least four but less than 15 inter-beat-intervals (e.g., 468, 473, 480, 487). A HRD trend is considered to be over whenever its linearity is broken by an accelerating IBI (e.g., 468, 473, 465). Linear HRD trends of four or more IBIs were isolated and interpreted in the context of previous research, the TCM and set statistics (post-hoc).

Match Result and Set Statistics

The player lost his first round match 4-6, 7-6, 6-1. For the purpose of this analysis, Set 1 was compared with Set 3, which were highly incongruous in outcome and HRD trends. Set 1 consisted of 60 points, 60 pre-action preparation moments and 360 action moments (X = 6 strokes per point). Action moments are defined as strokes (hitting the ball) occurring during the course of a point including the serve or return of serve. Set 3 consisted of 35 points, 35 pre-action moments, 175 action moments (X = 5 strokes/pt).

These results were blind to me (not known) until after the heart activity data were analyzed.

Heart Rate Deceleration Trends

The Y axis of the histogram depicts the number of HRD trends listed on the X axis. Considering that both sets consisted of only 95 points it is obvious that HRD occurred in excess of actual pre-action moments (preparing to serve or return serve). However, when one considers the amount of strokes (action moments) that correspond to each point (competitive moment) most of the HRD trends can be accounted for (Figure 9.5).

In Set 1 there was an average of six strokes per point or a total of 360 action moments within the 60 points. In Set 3 there were 175 action moments within the 35 points played. When analyzing HRD trends without being able to precisely synchronize them with competitive events, it is important to rely on previous investigations for guidance. Since most studies of HRD in sports and in the laboratory have revealed HRD trends of at least four IBIs, trends of 3 IBIs were eliminated from the analysis. Very short HRD trends (≤3 IBIs) were considered random, superfluous, or irrelevant to performance and thought to occur mostly during phases of movement not having a direct effect on preparation or sport-specific task (e.g., walking to get into position, walking to the bench).

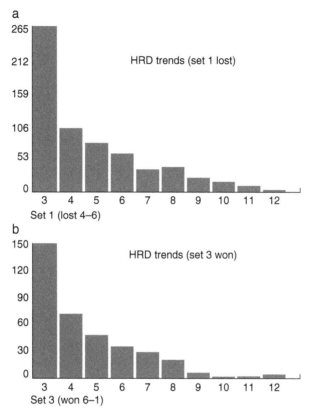

Figure 9.5 Set 1 (lost 4–6) Set 3 (Won 6-1).

HRD trends of 4, 5, and 6 IBIs were considered relevant to performance, leading to a preliminary theory attempting to explain their presence during action, something that has not previously been considered or thought possible. Because of their high prevalence and inability to explain HRD during action on the basis of 2 and 3 and 8 or more linear IBI sequences, I hypothesized that HRD trends of 4, 5, and 6 IBIs had to have occurred primarily during action moments in which technical, tactical or physical performance was consistent with or exceeded normative performance standards. These magnitudes of HRD trends are thought most likely to occur during action moments when an athlete does not experience negative psychological influences (e.g., AP mediated negative intrusive thoughts). Instead, they are hypothesized to reflect psychophysiological micro-events during action phases in which baro-receptor activity regulates flow of blood to the brain to facilitate task performance. I predict that athletes who are in control of mind-body processes (free from negative intrusive thoughts) will exhibit HRD not only prior to the initiation a sport-specific task (e.g., preparing to putt) but during action moments as well (e.g., shooting at a goal while moving). By contrast, athletes who experience negative intrusive thoughts during action will exhibit excessive or extra HR (heart rate acceleration; Blix, Stromme, & Unsinn, 1974) exceeding metabolic demands that can disrupt motor performance or technical skills. When this occurs, baro-receptor activity permits more blood flow to the brain, activating cortical areas that should normally remain dormant during motor performance.

When comparing HRD trends of 4, 5, or 6 IBIs between sets, we observe that Set 1 contained 240 such trends out of 360 action moments. This suggests that 120 action moments were devoid of HRD. In Set 3 there were 155 HRD trends of 4, 5, or 6 IBIs and 175 action moments. Although we cannot be certain that these HRD trends corresponded to action moments it is highly probable that they did, since lower and higher magnitude HRD trends are most likely to occur during other competitive and non-competitive moments. As previously noted, HRD trends of 2 or 3 IBIs are most likely to occur in a random fashion, accompanying walking, slight movements or resting, whereas HRD trends of 7, 8, 9, and 10 IBIs have been shown to occur when preparing for action. Since it is unlikely that a linear trend of 4, 5, or 6 progressively slowing IBIs will occur randomly, action moments can be best accounted for on the basis of HRD trends of these magnitudes, with the ratio of HRD trends of 4–6 IBIs to total action moments being a potential index of psychological performance during action moments of competition (action moments/HRD trends = PPPQ-Phrd [Psychological Performance Proficiency Quotient-Psychophysiological Index/HRD]) in this study.

Using this formula, the player's PPPQ-Phrd was 0.667 in Set 1 and 0.889 in Set 3. This means that in Set 1 it is probable that 120 action moments were not accompanied by HRD, suggesting compromised technical, tactical and/or physical performance when HRD did not occur. By contrast, in Set 3 it is probable that this player experienced HRD during action moments approximately 89% of the time or 155 out of 175 action moments. A PPPQ of 0.889 is very high and may reflect a level of psychophysiological functioning associated with a zone or flow-like state.

Pre-action moments were also analyzed on the basis of HRD trends. In Set 1 there were 75 HRD trends of 8, 9, or 10 IBIs, 15 more than actual pre-action moments. In Set 3 there were 40 HRD trends in this range, five more than there were points or competitive moments (pre-action phases). In the context of my preliminary TCM-HRD-action theory, whenever a range of HRD trends associated with a specific type of competitive moment exceeds the amount of actual pre-action competitive moments or action moments, one can assume that technical, tactical, and physical performance were relatively free from negative psychological influences (intrusive thoughts) during those periods. Conceptually consistent occurring HRD during any competitive moment is thought to increase the probability that motor performance will not be disrupted. Thus, in this match the player appeared to be psychologically in control during all preparation or pre-action phases as reflected in a 1:1 or greater ratio of competitive moments to HRD trends (8, 9, or 10 IBIs) in both sets.

Toward the Quantification of Zone or Flow States using HRD

As previously mentioned, to date, most research has only documented HRD during non-action phases of laboratory experiments where it has been observed that HRD occurs prior to the initiation of an action response. Since it also has been observed that any movement occurring prior to responding disrupts the linear trend of consecutive slowing IBIs (HRD), few if any attempts have been made to study HRD in the context of action or during movement, as one would expect movement to disrupt HRD during sport-specific action tasks. The effects of movement on HRD was elucidated by Obrist (1968), leading to the cardiac-somatic concept which essentially contends that HRD is more a function of heart-muscle than heart-brain interactions. However, Lacey (1964) took exception to the cardiac-somatic concept, attributing HRD more to attention and the orienting response as opposed to somatic quieting.

Thus, when interpreting HRD in the context of the TCM and sports, I hypothesize that HRD can occur during action moments of competition regardless of level of heart rate, metabolic demands, and muscular/motor activity during a sport-specific task, since attentional and other cognitive components of focusing and orientation toward a stimuli during action, very likely involve similar cortical and cardiovascular processes and interactions observed when focusing or orienting in a more static or non-action situation. For example, when a tennis player is involved in an intense rally or a basketball player is trying to get open to shoot a jump-shot, although having to maintain cardiac-output associated with high metabolic demands, he or she is still expected to experience a brief episode of HRD (micro-HRD) when positive psychological processes involved in the initiation of a sport-specific action are manifested (e.g., attention, strategic planning).

Since it has clearly been demonstrated that HRD occurs prior to action when focusing on a stimulus (hole in golf, ball toss in tennis, hoop in basketball), it is reasonable to expect that HRD will occur even at high levels of heart rate. Such a micro-psychophysiological moment is hypothesized to occur unconsciously or subliminally. If this moment is of the positive kind, free from negative psychological influences (e.g., intrusive thoughts), the linear heart rate acceleration that normally occurs with increased metabolic demands during intense action will briefly be interrupted precisely prior to the commencement of action (hitting a tennis shot while on the run, or kicking a soccer ball, etc.). This temporary "freeze" in heart rate acceleration is thought to facilitate neurophysiological processes underlying optimum motor control, including the baro-receptors and ensembles of neuronal units that function to block other "intrusive" neurons from interfering with performance (functional disconnection syndrome associated with high repressive coping). Relative to the TCM, the probability of achieving such a homeostatic peak performance state is more likely during innocuous routine action moments when psychological stress is minimal. However, once critical moments occur, depending on an athlete's constellation of AP factors, an athlete will be more or less likely to experience a disruption of the delicate balance between the heart and brain.

Athletes possessing an ideal constellation of AP factors (high or low hypnotic susceptibility/subliminal attention [HS/SA], neuroticism/subliminal reactivity [N/SR], and high repressive coping/subliminal coping [RC/SC]are less likely to be affected by negative intrusive thoughts during critical moments as reflected in HRD, even during action phases of competition). By contrast, athletes possessing less than ideal constellations of AP factors (high HS/SA, high N/SR and low RC/SC) are more likely exhibit increases in HRA that exceed metabolic demands and that will disrupt motor performance during critical moments.

Anecdotal notions such as "loss of concentration," "just do it," and being "in the Zone" can be explained on the basis of and are hypothesized to be reflected in HRD trends, whereby remaining focused and free from intrusive thoughts is associated with micro-HRD trends of 4–6 IBIs during action phases and greater magnitude HRD trends (six or more IBIs) during preparation phases prior to action. It is hypothesized that so-called zone or flow states can be quantified on the basis of HRD trends, whereby consecutive HRD trends proportionate and appropriate to a specific competitive moment (action phase = 4–6 IBIs, preparation phase, six or more IBIs) will be an objective physiological marker of peak psychological or flow performance. Being in the zone or a flow state would be determined on the basis of a physiological measure (HRD) that correlates highly with successful technical and statistical performance outcome measures as well as self-report.

A Zone or Flow experience might look like this:

Return of serve: 450 ms, 455, 468, 475, 488, 492, 495 (HRD), action phase: 467, 460, 445, 430, 423, 410, 400, 390, 378 (HRA), 385, 399, 403, 410 (micro-HRD prior to stroke), 391, 380, 370, 360, 345 (HRA), 366, 378, 382, 390, 399 (micro-HRD prior to stroke), 376, 369, 360, 355, 345 (HRA), 362, 366, 376, 384, 390 (micro-HRD), point ends.

In this point, we observe one pre-action preparation phase marked by a linear HRD trend of 6 IBIs (remember, increasing value reflects longer heart period or cardiac cycle, i.e., HRD) followed by an action phase. The action phase is delineated on the basis of commencement of a HRA trend (decreasing values, shorter heart period/cardiac cycle) consisting of nine linear accelerating IBIs. HRA occurs as a function of increasing metabolic demands associated with running to the ball. After the 378 IBI, notice that there is a one decelerating IBI (385) followed by three more slowing IBIs. Another HRD trend starts with IBI 366 and 362. These are micro-HRD trends that are thought to reflect psychological influences involving strategic planning, priming of neuronal ensembles responsible for technical-motor action occurring at the millisecond level, long enough to maintain focus on the task at hand, but short enough so as not to disrupt cardiac output necessary to fulfill metabolic demands. Thereafter, HRA resumes until the next shot of the point occurring at IBI 366 and again at 362. This heart activity sequence depicts the hypothesized order of HRD and HRA acceleration trends during competitive moments of a tennis match. The observed trends are consistent with what research has revealed regarding HRD trends during preparation phases prior to the initiation of action and what is hypothesized to occur during actual action phases of competition. Approximations or variations of the above cycle are hypothesized to occur repeatedly whenever an athlete is in a zone or flow state.

Competitive moments and episodes consisting of appropriate HRD and HRA trends, like the above, that are sustained over the course of longer periods of time during competition are hypothesized to reflect optimum psychological performance or being "in the Zone." It is expected that greater technical and physical performance will occur during phases of ideal heart rate variability (HRD-HRA) along with subjective feelings of well-being and mastery, and in many instances will coincide with a winning performance. Once a series of ideal HRD trends comes to an end, it is predicted that a zone or flow state will also cease.

TCM-AP factors play an important role in the HRD-Zone/Flow equation. Consistent with the TCM, it is expected that HRD trends are more likely to be disrupted during critical moments of competition in athletes possessing less than ideal constellations of AP factors and vice versa.

Although the HRD-Zone/Flow model needs to be further investigated, a preliminary analysis of heart activity data from this match is promising and suggests that HRD may indeed be the marker of psychological performance.

The TCM-HRD-action theory evolved from observing HRD trends in athletes, mostly tennis players over the course of actual tournament competition and practice. Repeatedly, an analysis of heart activity revealed trends of HRD that could not be explained merely on the basis of metabolic demands or in the context of the cardiac-somatic concept, especially since many of these trends were observed to occur at high heart rate during action phases of competition, something that was not thought possible.

An fMRI study of golfers by Ross et al. (2003) suggests that cortical "quieting" occurs more frequently in skilled golfers compared to less skilled golfers. Fattaposta et al. (1996) also found more cortical effort expenditure in non-athletes attempting to learn a task never previously engaged in compared to expert marksmen. I hypothesize that reductions in cortical activity is marked by less blood perfusion in ensembles of neurons associated with specific motor activity and preparatory cognitions in expert or successful athletes. This reduction in cellular blood flow to specific neurons is regulated by baro-receptors that also induce concomitant heart rate deceleration that is seen in peak performance. By contrast, in novices or even skilled athletes who are disrupted by intrusive thoughts, more cellular blood profusion is predicted to occur as a function of less baro-receptor control over regional cerebral blood flow (rCBF) resulting in heart rate acceleration or lessened heart rate deceleration.

Directions for Future Research

Future research must delineate the general HRD observed during competition more precisely. Should it be determined that HRD is unequivocally associated with performance and affected by psychological factors (AP factors), interventions can be designed to help athletes manipulate their HR in the desired direction. Since HR biofeedback has been successfully demonstrated both in the field and in laboratory studies, it is plausible that this mental training method could be used to enhance the psychological performance of athletes (Fahrenberg & Myrtek, 1996; Ludwick-Rosenfeld & Neufeld, 1985; Weiss & Engel, 1971). Since this study also demonstrated that within subject HRD varied situationally, individualized norms for HRD should be derived through future research. A large-scale study should be implemented to determine if HRD can be used to distinguish and assess level of ability, attention, motivation, and activation in athletes and equivocally determine to what extent AP factors affect this cardiovascular response.

Although the results of the spectrum analyses in this chapters first study were only revealing at the macro-level, spectrum analysis of HRV still holds much potential for assessing states of activation in athletes. Spectrum analysis could be used to establish individual norms for activation and reactivity in athletes and to establish parameters of physiological reactivity beyond the hypothetical (Hanin, 1980; Hardy & Fazey, 1987; Taylor, 1996). Doing so would have major implications with regard to preparing athletes for competition. In addition, spectrum analysis could be used to better discern to what extent specific psychophysiological processes are active during certain phases of competition (e.g., levels of attention, cognitive activity, autonomic nervous system activity). Such research could lead to a better understanding of how cognitive activity, and hence psychological variables, facilitates or disrupts motor performance during action phases of competition.

References

Akselrod, S., Gordon, D., Ubel, F. A., Shannon, D. C., Barger, A. C., & Cohen, R. J. (1981). Power spectrum analysis of heart rate fluctuation: A quantitative probe of beat-to-beat cardiovascular control. *Science, 213,* 220–222.

Andreassi, J. L. (1995). *Psychophysiology: Human behavior and physiological response* (3rd ed.). Hillsdale, NJ: Erlbaum.

Armour, J. A. (1994). *Neurocardiology.* New York: Oxford University Press.

Blix, A. S., Stromme, S. B., & Ursinn, H. (1974). Additional heart rate: An indicator of psychological activation. *Aerospace Medicine, 14,* 1219–1222.

Boutcher, S. H., & Zinsser, N. W. (1990). Cardiac deceleration of elite and beginning golfers during putting. *Journal of Sport and Exercise Psychology, 12,* 37–47.

Carlstedt, R. A. (1998). *Psychologically mediated heart rate variability: A single case study of heart rate deceleration and a spectrum analysis of autonomic function during tournament tennis.* Unpublished master's thesis, Saybrook Graduate School, San Francisco.

Carlstedt, R. A. (2012). Evidence-based applied sport psychology: A practitioner's manual. New York, NY: Springer Publishing Company.

Carriero, N. J., & Fite, J. (1977). Cardiac deceleration as an indicator of correct performance. *Perceptual and Motor Skills, 44,* 275–282.

Denzin, N. K., & Lincoln, Y. S. (1994). *Handbook of qualitative research.* Thousand Oaks, CA: Sage.

de Geus, E. J. C., & van Doornen, L. J. P. (1996). Ambulatory assessment of parasympathetic/sympathetic balance by impedence cardiography. In J. Fahrenberg & M. Myrtek (Eds.), *Ambulatory assessment: Computer assisted psychological and psychophysiological methods in monitoring and field studies* (pp. 141–164). Goettingen, Germany: Hogrefe & Huber.

Duffy, E. (1972). Activation. In N. S. Greenfield & R. A. Sternbach (Eds.). *Handbook of psychophysiology* (pp. 572–622). New York: Holt, Rinehart & Winston.

Edwards, D. C., & Alsip, J. E. (1969). Stimulus detection during periods of high and low heart rate. *Psychophysiology, 19,* 431–434.

Elliott, R. (1974). The motivational significance of heart rate. In P.A. Obrist, A.H. Black, J. Brener, & L. V. DiCara (Eds.). *Cardiovascular psychophysiology* (pp. 505–537). Chicago: Aldine.

Fahrenberg J., & Myrtek, M. (1996). *Ambulatory psychophysiology: computer assisted psychological and psychophysiological methods in monitoring and field studies.* Seattle, WA: Hogrefe & Huber.

Fattapposta, F., Amabile, G., Cordischi, M. V., di Venanzio, D., Foti, A., Pierelli, F., et al. (1996). Long-term practice effects on a new skilled motor learning: An electrophysiological study. *Electroencephalography and Clinical Neurophysiology, 99,* 495–507.

Galin, D. (1974). Implications for psychiatry of left and right cerebral specialization. *Archives of General Psychiatry, 31,* 572–581.

Gallwey, T. (1974). *The inner game of tennis.* New York, NY: Random House.

Gall, M. D., Borg, W. R., & Gall, J. P. (1996). *Educational research: An introduction.* White Plains, New York: Longman.

Hahn, W. W. (1973). Attention and heart rate: A critical appraisal of the hypothesis of Lacey and Lacey. *Psychological Bulletin, 79*(1), 59–70.

Roland A. Carlstedt

Hanin, Y. L. (1980). *A study of anxiety in sports*. In W. F. Straub (Ed.), *Sport psychology: An analysis of athletic behavior* (pp. 81–106). Chichester, England: Wiley.

Hardy, L., & Fazey, J. (1987). *The inverted-U hypothesis: A catastrophe for sport psychology*. Paper presented at the annual meetings of the North American Society of Sport and Physical Activity, Vancouver, British Columbia, Canada.

Hassmen, P., & Koivula, N. (2001). Cardiac deceleration in elite golfers as modified by noise and anxiety during putting. *Perceptual and Motor Skills*, *92*, 947–957.

Hatfield, B. D., Landers, D. L., & Ray, W. J. (1984). Cognitive processes during self paced motor performance: An electroencephalographic profile of skilled marksman. *Journal of Sport Psychology*, *6*, 42–59.

Hatfield, B. D., Landers, D. L., & Ray, W. J. (1987). Cardiovascular-CNS interactions during a self-paced, intentional attentive state: Elite marksmanship performance. *Psychophysiology*, *24*, 542–549.

Heil, J., & Henschen, K. (1996). Assessment in sport and exercise psychology. In J. L. Van Raalte & B. W. Brewer (Eds.), *Exploring sport and exercise psychology* (pp. 229–256). Washington, DC: American Psychological Association.

Heslegrave, R. J., Olgilvie, J. C., & Furedy, J. J. (1979). Measuring baseline treatment differences in heart rate variability: Variance versus successive differences mean square and beats per minute versus interbeat interval. *Psychophysiology*, *16*, 151–157.

Jennings, J. R., & Wood, C. C. (1977). Cardiac cycle time effects on performance, phasic cardiac responses, and their intercorrelation in cardiac reaction time. *Psychophysiology*, *14*(3), 297–307.

Jorna, P. G. A. M. (1992). Spectral analysis of heart rate and psychological state: A review of its validity as a work load index. *Biological Psychology*, *34*, 237–257.

Klemm, W. R. (1996). *Understanding neuroscience*. St. Louis, MO: Mosby.

Lacey, J. I. (1967). Somatic response patterning and stress: Some revisions of activation theory. In M. H. Appley & R. Trumbell (Eds.), *Psychological stress: Issues in research* (pp. 14–42). New York: Appleton-Century-Crofts.

Lacey, J. I., & Lacey, B. C. (1964). *Cardiac deceleration and simple visual reaction in a fixed foreperiod experiment*. Paper presented at the meeting of the Society for Psychophysiological Research, Washington, D.C.

Lacey, J. I., & Lacey, B. C. (1966). Changes in cardiac response and reaction time as a function of motivation. Paper presented at the meeting of the Society for *Psychophysiological Research*, Denver, Colorado.

Lacey, J. I., & Lacey, B. C. (1970). Some autonomic-central nervous system interreltionships. In P. Black (Ed.), *Physiological correlates of emotions* (pp. 205–227). New York: Academic Press.

Lacey, J. I., & Lacey, B. C. (1974). On heart rate response and behavior: A reply to Elliott. *Journal of Personality and Social Psychology*, *30*(1), 1–18.

Lacey, J. I., & Lacey, B. C. (1978). Two-way communication between the heart and the brain: Significance of time within the cardiac cycle. *American Psychologist*, *33*(2), 99–113.

Landers, D., Han, M., Salazar, W., Petruzzello, S., Kubitz, K., & Gannon, T. (1994). Effects of learning on electroencephalographic and electrocardiographic patterns in novice archers. *International Journal of Sport Psychology*, *25*, 56–70.

Lang, P. J., Levin, D. N., Miller, G. A., & Kozak, J. J. (1983). Fear behavior, fear imagery, and the psychophysiology of emotion: The problem of affective response integration. *Journal of Abnormal Psychology*, *92*, 276–306.

Leiderman, P. H., & Shapiro, D. (1962). Application of a time series statistic to physiology and psychology. *Science*, *138*(6), 141–142.

Ludwick-Rosenthal, R., & Neufeld, R. W. J. (1985). Heart rate interoception: A study of individual differences. *International Journal of Psychophysiology*, *3*, 57–65.

Malik, M. & Camm, A. J. (Eds.) (1995). *Heart rate variability*. Armonk, NY: Futura.

McCanne, T. R., & Sandman, C. A. (1976). Human operant heart rate conditioning: The importance of individual differences. *Psychological Bulletin*, *83*, 587–601.

McCraty, R., Atkinson, M., Tiller, W. A., Rein, G., & Watkins, A. D. (1995). The effects of emotions on short-term power spectrum analysis of heart rate variability. *The American Journal of Cardiology*, *76*(14), 1089–1093.McCraty, R., Tiller, W. A. & Atkinson, M. (1996). *Head heart entrainment: A preliminary survey*. (Technical Report from the Institute of HeartMath), Boulder Creek, CA: Institute of HeartMath.

McCraty, R., & Watkins, A. D. (1996). *Autonomic assessment report: A comprehensive heart rate variability analysis*. Boulder Creek, CA: Institute of HeartMath.

Myrtek, M., Bruegner, G., & Mueller, W. (1996). Interactive monitoring and contingency analysis of emotionally induced ECG changes: Methodology and applications. In J. Fahrenberg & M. Myrtek (Eds.), *Ambulatory assessment: Computer assisted psychological and psychophysiological methods in monitoring and field studies* (pp. 115–128). Goettingen: Hogrefe & Huber.

Nowlin, B., Eisdorfer, C., Whalen, R., & Troyer, W. G. (1970). The effect of exogenous changes in heart rate and rhythm upon reaction time performance. *Psychophysiology*, *7*, 186–193.

Obrist, P. A. (1981). *Cardiovascular psychophysiology: A perspective*. New York, NY: Plennum.

Obrist, P. A., Howard, J. L., Sutterer, J. R., Hennis, R. S., & Murrell, D. J. (1973). Cardiac-somatic changes during a simple reaction time task: A developmental study. *Journal of Experimental Child Psychology, 16*, 346–362.

Obrist, P. A., Webb, R. A., & Sutterer, J. R. (1969). Heart rate and somatic changes during aversive conditioning and a simple reaction time task. *Psychophysiology, 5*, 696–723.

Porges, S. W., & Byrne, E. A. (1992). Research methods for measurement of heart rate and respiration. *Biological Psychology, 34*, 93–130.

Pribam, K. H., & McGuinness, D. (1975). Arousal, activation, and effort in the control of attention. *Psychological Review, 82*, 116–149.

Ravizza, K. (1977). Peak experiences in sports. *Journal of Humanistic Psychology, 4*, 35–40.

Ross, J. S., Tkach, J., Ruggieri, P. M., Lieber, M. & Lapresto, E. (2003) The mind's eye: Functional MR imaging evaluation of golf motor imagery. *American Journal of Neuroradiology, 24*(6), 1036–1044.

Salazar, W., Landers, D. M., Petruzzello, S. J., Han, M., Crews, D. J., & Kubitz, K. A. (1990). Hemispheric asymmetry, cardiac response, and performance in elite archers. *Research Quarterly for Exercise and Sport, 61*(4), 351–359.

Sandman, C. A., Walker, B. B., & Berka, C. (1982). *Influence of afferent cardiovascular feedback on behavior and the cortical evoked potential.* In J. T. Cacioppo, & R. E. Petty (Eds.), *Perspectives in cardiovascular psychophysiology* (pp. 189–222). New York, NY: Guilford.

Schell, A. M., & Catania, J. (1975). The relationship between cardiac activity and sensory acuity. *Psychophysiology, 12*, 147–151.

Surwillo, W. W. (1971). Human reaction time and endogenous heart rate changes in normal subjects. *Psychophysiology, 8*, 680–682.

Taylor, J. (1996). Intensity regulation and athletic performance. In J. L. Van Raalte & B. W. Brewer (Eds.). *Exploring sport and exercise psychology* (pp. 75–106). Washington DC: American Psychological Association.

Tiller, W. A., McCraty, R., & Atkinson, M. (1996). Cardiac coherence: A new noninvasive measure of autonomic nervous system order. *Alternative Therapies, 2*(1), 52–65.

van Doornen, L. J. P., Knol, D. L., Willemsen, G., & de Geus, E. J. C. (1994). The relationship between stress reactivity in the laboratory and in real-life: Is reliability the limiting factor? *Journal of Psychophysiology, 8*, 297–304.

Waller, S. (1988). *Alterations of consciousness in peak sports performance.* Unpublished doctoral dissertation. San Francisco, CA: Saybrook Graduate School.

Walter, G. F., & Porges, S. W. (1976). Heart rate and respiratory responses as a function of task difficulty: The use of discrimination analysis in the selection of psychologically sensitive physiological responses. *Psychophysiology, 13*, 563–571.

Webb, R. A., & Obrist, P. A. (1970). The physiological concomitants of reaction time performance as a function of prepatory interval and prepatory interval series. *Psychophysiology, 22*, 342–352.

Weiss, T. & Engel, B. T. (1971). Operant conditioning of heart rate in patients with pre-mature ventricular contractions. *Psychosomatic Medicine, 33*, 301–322.

Wickramasekera, I. E. (1988). *Clinical behavioral medicine.* New York, NY: Plennum.

Wolk, C., & Velden, M. (1987). Detection variability within the cardiac cycle: Toward a revision of the "baroreceptor hypothesis." *Journal of Psychophysiology, 1*, 61–65.

Yerkes, R. M., & Dodson, J. D. (1908). The relation of strength of stimulus to rapidity of habit formation. *Journal of Comparative Neurology and Psychology, 18*, 459–482.

This chapter was adapted in part from the Author's book: *Critical Moments During Competition: A Mind-Body Model of Sport Performance when it Counts the Most.* Psychology Press 2004.

Section II

Applied Sport Neuroscience and Psychophysiology

Intervention and Mental Training

Ecological, Volitional Induce-ment of Heart Rate Deceleration in Athletes during Competition

A Mental Training Protocol

Roland A. Carlstedt

Heart rate deceleration biofeedback (HRD BF) is a relatively unknown intervention whose origin can be traced to an extensive body of research on pre-stimulus or pre-action cardiac activity (e.g., Hatfield, Landers, & Ray, 1984, 1987; Boutcher & Zinsser, 1990; Carlstedt, 2001). It is a potent, conceptually well-grounded mental training (MT) modality that is designed to mechanistically set-off a cascade of mind-body-motor responses that have been shown to reflect optimum pre-action preparation and the transition to action and motor/technical responding.

It is a validated intervention whose effects can be documented independent of speculative interpretive components associated with more cognitively-based interventions such as mental imagery, mindfulness, and other related approaches to mental-control in sports (see Chapter 7 for more on HRD).

This chapter presents a HRD-BF mental training protocol method and an intervention efficiency and efficacy testing experiment. It is strongly recommended that practitioners and athletes who want to apply this MT procedure undergo intensive training relative to all components of this HRD protocol, especially analytics that are critical to evidence-based practice.

The HRD Response

HRD occurs automatically (subliminally) when an individual anticipates the appearance of a stimulus that must be responded to or in the context of mentally preparing to self-induce a response in both non-performance and performance situations (Lacey & Lacey, 1964, 1978). It can also be volitionally shaped and conditioned and is associated with a distinct inter-beat-interval (IBI) signature.

The manifestation of HRD has been shown to precede a cascade of performance facilitative mind-body-motor/technical responses. It predominates in the pre-action phase of competition in the absence of perceived competitive pressure/stress (a developed response). It can also be consciously generated in athletes whose mental state prior action is not optimal (and devoid of pre-action HRD) by using a specifically timed-breathing MT procedure. Whereas MT methods, including mental imagery, are nebulous processes that, at best, can only be indirectly linked to peak performance responses (e.g. mental imagery as a mediator of HRD) if at all, HRD is a validated peak-performance response biomarker that is associated with faster reaction times and motor priming and subsequent control and successful outcomes. As such, it should be considered as the go-to primary MT intervention for in-the-moment facilitation of optimum responding especially during critical moments of competition.

Roland A. Carlstedt

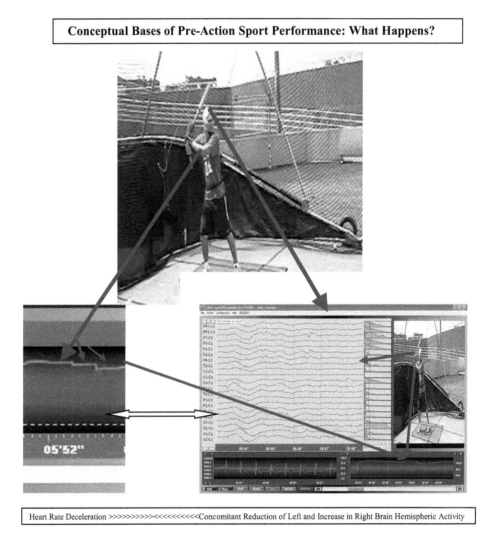

Figure 10.1   Pre-action brain-heart dynamics.

(start of HRD trend) > R_R____R_____R_____R_____**R_R** < (end of HRD trend)

Figure 10.2   HRD: each R-R cycle (IBI) becomes longer (slower), marked by linear lengthening.

Conceptual Rationale

HRD can be considered a valid and reliable biomarker of pre-action psychological and psycho-physiological readiness. It can be seen as the "Zone" mind-body measure that reflects optimum pre-action strategic planning, intensity, and mind-body-motor control (technical and motor priming). Ultimately, all interventions should lead to the HRD response in pre-action phases of competition, a response that is hypothesized to also occur throughout an entire competitive, sport-specific action (e.g., throughout an entire tennis point or from the point of getting off the mark and driving past an opponent to make a lay-up in basketball). HRD has been shown to occur in virtually all athletes in numerous sports that have pre-action phases in which an athlete must either respond to an impending stimulus (like a ball being pitched or served) or initiate a response

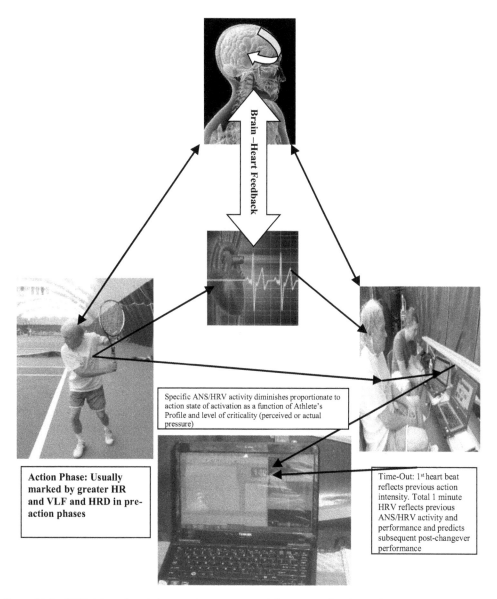

Specific ANS/HRV activity diminishes proportionate to action state of activation as a function of Athlete's Profile and level of criticality (perceived or actual pressure)

Action Phase: Usually marked by greater HR and VLF and HRD in pre-action phases

Time-Out: 1st heart beat reflects previous action intensity. Total 1 minute HRV reflects previous ANS/HRV activity and performance and predicts subsequent post-changeover performance

Figure 10.3 HRD Mental training-performance model: temporally discordant version/temporally remote paradigm (TRP; above).

(e.g. a free throw). HRD can be disrupted or not manifested during critical moments of competition when an athlete consciously or subliminally experiences competitive stress (as reflected in mind-body responses [e.g. specific HRV measures] that are incongruent with previously documented performance facilitative HRV baseline or pre-action HRD readings).

The non-appearance of HRD prior to action when an athlete is under stress is more likely to occur in athletes who possess the "worst" AP (high level of Hypnotic Susceptibility/Subliminal Attention [HS], high level of Neuroticism/Subliminal Reactivity [N], and low level of Repressive Coping/Subliminal Coping [SC] see, Carlstedt, 2004, 2012). Athletes who are known to have a more maladaptive AP tend to be aware of their performance-related psychological frailties. They are an athlete-subset most likely to seek MT services. Nevertheless, all athletes, regardless of their AP should be educated about pre-action HRD dynamics and their relevance to peak performance. They should also be taught how to volitionally set-off the brain-heart-mind-body cascade that leads to the onset of HRD.

How Does Biofeedback Work?

Biofeedback attempts to induce or shape mind-body responses by first showing baseline autonomic (ANS) and/or central nervous system (CNS) activity as reflected in waveform oscillations or other representations that are observable on a computer screen (e.g., bar graphs) and then reinforcing prescribed performance or wellness-related target psychophysiological responses with feedback. The successful self-induced response is shaped subliminally over time through operant conditioning in an attempt to entrain optimum situation self-regulation, attention, or physiological reactivity. ANS/CNS changes are shaped by visual scenarios and/or audio feedback on a computer screen incrementally. For example, if a practitioner prescribes the generation of more parasympathetic (PNS) activity via controlled breathing to reduce sympathetic nervous system (SNS) associated with panic attacks, a patient will know if he or she is generating more or less or an ideal amount of PNS activity on the basis of feedback in the form of a rising bar and audio signal when a wellness facilitative PNS activity threshold is reached. Parallel to this process, over time, the patient will feel the difference between extreme, panic-like SNS predominant mind-body state and a PNS predominant relaxation psychophysiological state, first in context of doing biofeedback and receiving reinforcement for manifesting prescribed adaptive responses and then later without biofeedback, in the real world and in the presence of an actual panic attack that a patient is then capable of volitionally shutting down (Andreassi, 1995; Wickramasekera, 1988; Carlstedt, 2009).

Essentially, well consolidated adaptive and/or health or performance facilitative mind-body responses that were shaped in the clinic, in theory, can then be self-induced in the presence of actual or perceived environmental or internal stressors to restore psychophysiological homeostasis.

Description of HRD BF Procedure I: ABSP-CP BioCom Paradigm

Initially, athletes should be educated regarding the cardiovascular mechanisms associated with HRD, commencing with inhalation/inspiration and exhalation/expiration breathing mediated cardiac responses both in static/naturalistic and HRD BF in sport training and competition contexts using research grade cardiologic monitoring instrumentation such as the BioCom Heart Scanner (BHS) system.

HRD Mental Training Procedures

1 The athlete is attached to computer via an ear-based sensor. A two-minute HRV baseline is established using the BHS program.
2 Thereafter, while running the BHS program the athlete is instructed to just look at the screen and observe the tachogram progression that shows each heartbeat, noticing how cardiac activity is influenced by "normal" breathing. The athlete should be made aware that inspiration (inhalation-SNS response) leads to increasing heart rate (heart rate acceleration-HRA) and expiration (exhalation-PNS response) leads to decreases in heart rate (heart rate deceleration-HRD).
3 After about two minutes of observing heart activity stop the initial session, save the data and run a two-minute HRV analysis using the BHS program.

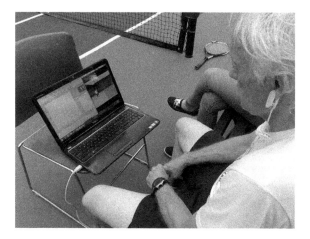

Figure 10.4 Initial HRD education, familiarization and observation session.

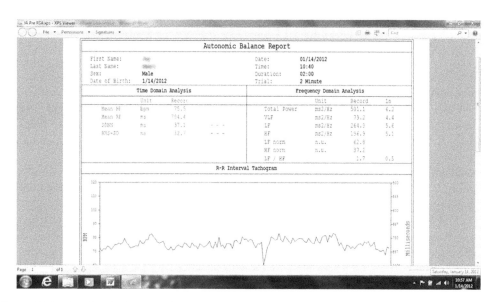

Figure 10.5 Baseline HRV report (note: consent given to not mask identity, disregard Date-of-Birth info).

4 Compare the two generated HRV reports (baseline with no mental engagement compared to the initial observation condition). The above screen shot (Figure 10.4.) depicts the initial two-minute baseline reading (familiarization and observation session). Notice the heart rate (HR), SDNN and LF/HF readings. These are important measures in the RSA-HRD BF equation. They are very sensitive to subliminal/unconscious changes in breathing as well as volitional manipulation of breathing as was attempted after this initial baseline session.

5 Review inhalation-exhalation principles and their relevance to HRD before using HT to introduce athlete to manipulated paced breathing.

6 Start with classic respiratory sinus arrhythmia (RSA) training at a pace of eight breaths per minute, instructing the athlete synchronize his or her inhalation(s) with the rising pacer bar; do the same when exhaling (synched with the falling pacer bar). Continue this procedure for

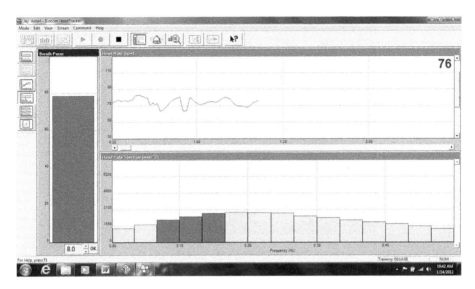

Figure 10.6 Screen shot of pacer guided (eight breaths per minute) inhalation cycle of an RSA training session.

two minutes. Be sure to teach the athlete to inhale by gently compressing the stomach inward and simultaneously lifting the chest or diaphragm and taking in air through the nostrils (not the mouth) being sure to complete the inspiration cycle by the time the pacer reaches its apex and then gently expel the inhaled air through the nostrils, allowing the chest to drop and belly to protrude (relax controlling muscles), being sure to fully complete the expiration cycle by the time that the pacer reaches bottom.

7 Immediately run a two-minute HRV scan using BioCom HS for comparison purposes (determine differences in HRV measures across the baseline, observation, and manipulation conditions).

Figure 10.7 depicts a spectrum analysis of HRV measures after a two-minute paced breathing RSA training session. Note the changes compared to baseline. HR was almost the same. This is very illustrative and points to the need to take other more sensitive HRV markers of psychophysiological influences into account in the context of athlete assessment and intervention. HR is an overused and publicized cardiologic measure that in of itself can be very misleading. A more sensitive performance relevant biomarker, SDNN (the HRV index) increased significantly in the RSA training session, from 37 to 51 milliseconds. In addition, another important indicator of autonomic nervous system (ANS) balance, the low frequency-high frequency (LF/HF) ratio increased from 1.7 to 2.5 in the training condition, revealing significant more low frequency activity (a mixture of sympathetic [SNS] and parasympathetic nervous [PNS] nervous system activity) in the paced breathing condition. Breathing was paced to elicit 8 breaths per minute in the RSA condition that can later be reduced to six per minute in an attempt to facilitate greater ANS balance for health and wellness purposes. Note again though, RSA training in this scenario was used to help the athlete gain awareness of the impact breathing has on HR and HRV as a precursor to temporally-guided, sport-specific pre-action HRD, that is not based on RSA inhalation-exhalation dynamics.

8 After analyzing and discussing the HRV reports, being sure to focus on HR, SDNN, and L/H ratio as a function of a select measuring condition, proceed to the playing field to introduce and operationalize HRD in the context of the pre-action temporal dynamics of a specific sport (in this case tennis).

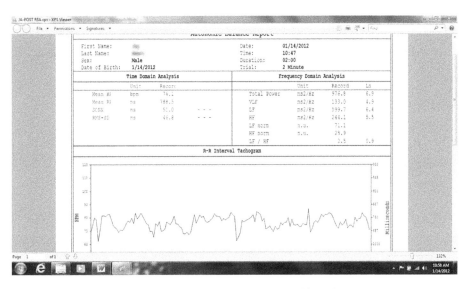

Figure 10.7 Spectrum analysis of HRV after two-minute paced breathing session.

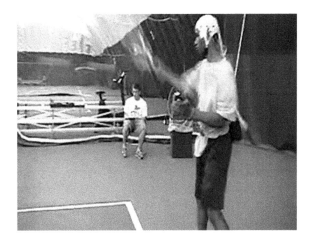

Figure 10.8 Tennis player's heart and brain responses being monitored using the Nexus 32 EEG/ HRV telemetry system to determine heart rate deceleration-brain response relationships and heart rate deceleration temporal zone (can also be done without EEG brain wave acquisition instrumentation).

Once the athlete's individual heart rate deceleration temporal zone (HRDtz = sport-specific pre-action HRD trends) has been established commence with sport-specific breathing induced HRD BF that can then be practiced in accord with practitioner instructions. HRD training should always be documented and analyzed for efficiency and efficacy.

9 Sport-specific HRD BF training requires calibrating the HT breathing pacer with the length and duration of pre-action epochs in which HRD should occur. Pre-action HRD can be induced by consciously manipulating the inhale/exhale cycles. In tennis, when returning, inhalation should commence in conjunction with the rise of the server's arm (e.g. the pacer bar of the HT program can be thought of or visualized as a server's arm) with exhalation occurring immediately and progressively until the oncoming tennis ball is struck. Athletes

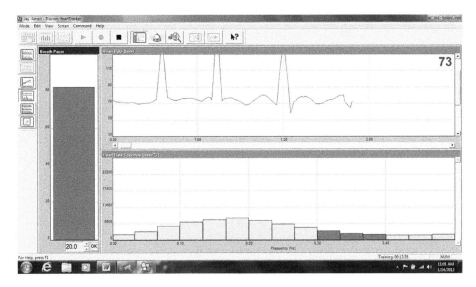

Figure 10.9   Calibration of paced breathing for sport-specific HRD-BF.

can use a tactile learning method to "feel" the inhalation-exhalation cycles; by letting their cheeks fully expand with incoming air and then blowing it out, with all air being expelled by the time the ball is struck (this is associated with grunting that spectators often hear when tennis players hit the ball). Once the HRDtz parameters of a specific sport have been set for an individual athlete, HT can be calibrated to allow for practicing paced-breathing induced HRD, prior to competition.

10   Once it has been determined that an athlete has learned the basics of HRD and its inducement, he or she should be tested for intervention efficacy on-the-playing field in the context of both experimental and competition paradigms. If using the BioCom system (that cannot be applied during actual action phases of competition, but can be during change-overs or time-outs during practice and official competition) indirect assessment of the manifestation of HRD and its impact can be employed using the *temporally distant* method. In this paradigm, an athlete is taught and then instructed to engage in breathing-induced HRD cycles during change-overs/time-outs and between action phases on-the-playing field during competition; usually within an A-B design (HRD on for one time-out cycle and non-action phase and off for the next time-out/non-action phase, etc.). This analytic approach to assessing HRD efficiency – efficacy will be elaborated in the documentation – accountability section below.

Post HRD and HRDtz Training On-the-Playing Field: ABSP-BioCom HS Procedure

In contrast, to pervasive approaches to biofeedback that are almost exclusively carried out in office or lab settings, the ABSP-CP BF protocols are designed to be administered and engaged in on-the-playing field during practice games/matches and real-official competition The BioCom system can be used within a time-out or change over paradigm whereby an athlete goes to a computer station on the sideline, dugout, bench, or other area to practice HRD and HRDtz BF prior to the initiation or continuation of a game/match or performance task. The temporal parameters of time-out and/or pre-action HRD BF should be established on the basis of pilot testing that determines the best time for MT onset (i.e. how soon or how close to game time should MT commence) and duration (i.e. how long should MT last). Recommendations regarding temporal parameters are made on the basis of variance explained metrics that are derived from a longitudinal repeated measures design during intervention training periods leading up to official or real competition using sport-specific outcome measures to determine intervention efficacy[1]. Once competition has started, MT or intervention duration is usually determined by the progression of the game/match or event. In a sport like tennis, interventions are engaged during change-overs and limited to one minute. In baseball, players do mental training prior to each at bat within a three-phased paradigm. In basketball or other sports with similar time-out structures, players are instructed to engage in HRD or related HRV BF within one to five minutes of being made aware that they will return to the game; this requires coordination and communication with coaches to ensure that sport psychology practitioners and players alike know when to start and finish MT.

Step-by-Step HRD BF Procedures: Ecologically-Based MT-Official Competition

1   Athletes in all sports engage in a sport-specific customized pre-action oriented HRD BF mental training session ranging from two to five minutes in duration within 10 minutes of competition onset or in accord with pilot testing established temporal guidelines. Pre-competition MT timeframes can be modified as a function of ongoing intervention efficacy data. If initial intervention temporal properties before and/or during a match are associated with negative or minimal to no gain outcome, MT timelines can be modified, as can the intervention modality itself be tweaked. For example, Multi-modal approaches that integrate HRD BF and HRV monitoring that will be presented later in this chapter can be used and tested for efficacy.

2   The HRD BF session should be based on HRDtz parameters for sport-specific tasks or actions; for example, in tennis, the serve or return of serve and pre-shot pre-action timeframe. In baseball, a batter's HRDtz is based on a pitcher's pre-action routine, with the inhale cycle coinciding with the wind-up and exhale cycle with the release of the ball.

   In sports, having self-initiation components that are not opponent dependent or based on an on-coming stimulus, time to initiate action can be highly variable, even open-ended unless time to commence rules mandate the maximum amount of time allowed before action must start. Golf, downhill skiing, marksmanship, and even free-throw shooting in basketball or penalty shots in soccer and ice-hockey are examples of sports and sport-specific actions that are self-initiated.

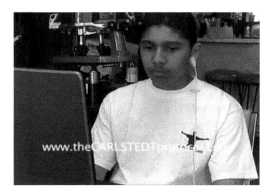

Figure 10.10   Tennis player engaging in pre-competition HRD BF.

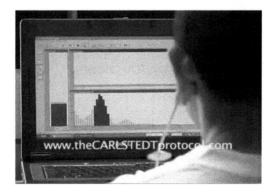

Figure 10.11 Tennis player engaging in pre-competition HRD BF.

3   A MT-intervention computer station should be set up in a private area on the side-line or in the dug-out in baseball or bench in tennis. Golfers can use a golf-cart in which to engage in HRD MT as they are driven to where their ball lies.

4   The players are called to the intervention-station to start HRD MT in accord with sport-specific timelines and/or time restrictions by the sport psychology practitioner or independently in certain situations (when an athlete does not have a coach or assistant).

5   The player looks at the monitor (HS screen; the HS program is used as a first step in weaning an athlete from the breathing pacer in the HT program; it is possible though and can be beneficial in the initial phase of HRD BF intervention training, to use the HT program with a practitioner [see Figures 10.9 & 10.10 above] to guide the pacing of the inhalation-exhalation cycles until the athlete has mastered the procedure). In multi-modal HRD BF, video and visualization components are integrated into the MT process (see below). In the absence of video-augmented HRD BF, the athlete is told to focus intensely on the temporal dynamics of his or her HRDtz. Doing so is hypothesized to subliminally prime an athlete to carry out a sport-specific task independent of seeing or generating internal images of an impending sport-specific action since time-locked pre- action HRD that has been consolidated through extensive pre-competition MT is expected to set-off a precise cascade of brain-heart-mind-motor responses once an athlete steps on to the playing field[2]. The goal of direct HRD BF is to shut-down or shut-out visual and other mechanisms (e.g. negative intrusive thoughts) that cannot be controlled by directly manipulating and inducing brain-heart-mind-body responses that have been directly linked to optimum attention, reaction time, and technical control. Thus, if HRD occurs naturally, or is self-induced via BF facilitated manipulation of time-locked breathing, superfluous and negative intrusive thoughts and images (even when supposed positive visualization scenarios are thought to be active) can be prevented from ever being manifested and hindering peak performance.

The primary task when engaging in HRD BF is to practice one's HRDtz cycle up to four times per minute. This is done by inhaling in synchrony with the sport specific pre-action routine of the task at hand. The inhale cycle is always longer or more protracted than the exhale cycle, which is usually short or quick in duration and forceful, especially in sports that have fast reaction time and strength demands of varying magnitude such as tennis, golf, baseball, and football, to name a few. When inhaling, the goal is to progressively drive the digital HR reading that can be seen in the upper right hand corner of the HS screen as high as possible (highest reading should occur at the apex of the inhalation cycle). For example, in this scene the athlete after having his inhale cycle guided upwards by the practitioner using the HT program exhales quickly and forcefully (HR decreases linearly to 82 bpm, Figures 10.12 & 10.13).

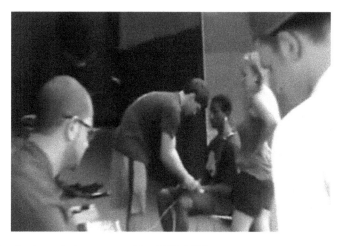

Figure 10.12   Tennis player being prepped for HRD-HRV scan.

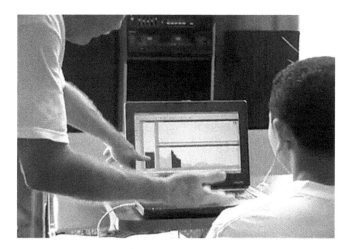

Figure 10.13   Practitioner guided HRD BF.

6   After the sport-specific time-out has expired, either on the basis of rules stipulating its maximum duration, the progression of the game and its impact on time of performance (e.g. waiting to get up to bat in baseball or cricket), or being called into a game by the coach, the athlete must now perform. The previously practiced HRD BF and HT or HS guided, induced, and reinforced mind-body procedures and responses (HRD), if strongly consolidated in procedural memory, should be accessible and used once the task-specific technical or sporting action is encountered during actual competition, especially if and when an athlete faces critical moments or feels competitive stress anytime during the course of a game or match. While conscious efforts to engage in mental training constantly throughout an entire competition can have a paradoxical effect and negatively impact technical performance, eventually (must be documented) hypothetically, it is expected that athletes will, upon reaching a to be determined MT consolidation threshold, eventually engage in intervention routines subliminally or automatically. Thus, one can expect in the initial phases of learning, applying, and consolidating HRD BF and subsequent, non-instrument aided attempts to induce

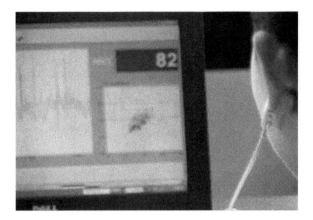

Figure 10.14 Practitioner guided HRD BF.

HRD responses during competition, that more susceptible athletes (AP of high-high-low) will regress before making progress (note though that this observation and associated MT Onset Performance Decrement Hypothesis [MTOPDH]) must be tested empirically on all athletes individually). Readers are reminded that mind-body responses including pre-action HRD and mediated heightened attention, faster reaction time, and enhanced motor control tend to occur in all athletes during routine moments of competition. As such, one might ask why risk disrupting phases of competition when an athlete feels comfortable and in control by coaching or prompting them to engage in MT of any kind, especially when it is obvious that an athlete is playing up to peak potential? Practitioners need to consider an athlete's schedule and the availability of sufficient amounts of time in which to intensively and systematically practice an intervention or risk failing to reach consolidation thresholds and paradoxically disrupting performance due to thinking about how to do an MT procedure instead of it just happening. As with technical training, ultimately, engaging in a MT technique should occur automatically without conscious effort. Extensive MT should lead to the neuronal consolidation of MT facilitated mind-body-motor responses that can be switched on or off as needed, subliminally. Subliminal MT activation thresholds must be documented before one can be certain that an athlete is actually engaging in an intervention procedure independent of conscious efforts to do so, something that is much easier to do with direct MT procedures like HRD-BF, since HRD is a known performance facilitative response that routinely occurs during pre-action phases of many sports, in the absence of situational or perceived competitive pressure.

The photos below (Figures 10.15–10.21) depict a tennis player engaging in post change-over HRD BF training on-the-court volitional breathing induced pre-action HRD extending from the moment his opponent makes contact with the ball to the onset of returning the oncoming ball. Note the protrusion of the cheeks showing the effect of the inhale cycle in the first photo and the subsequent exhalation of inhaled air in the second and third photos. This player was trained to transfer the paced breathing cycles associated with the inducement of sport-task-specific HRD BF off-the-tennis court in front of a computer monitor to the court without the aid of instrumentation, the goal of BF (weaning an athlete off instrumentation under the assumption that lab-based BF shaped mind-body responses will generalize to the playing field and critical situations that require optimum attention, physiological reactivity, and motor control).

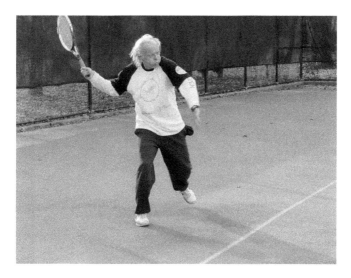

Figure 10.15   End of pre-action inhale cycle inhalation cycle apex.

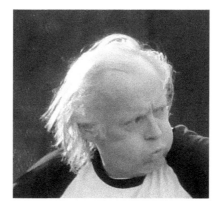

Figure 10.16   Heart rate acceleration.

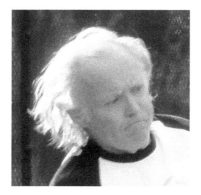

Figure 10.17   Exhale induced HRD.

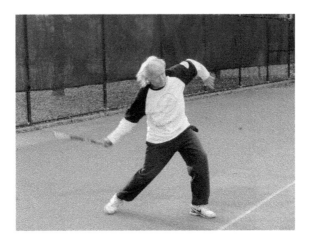

Figure 10.18   Exhale cycle and HRD in progress.

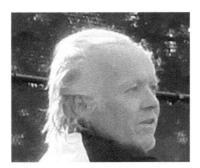

Figure 10.19   Close-up-end of exhalation

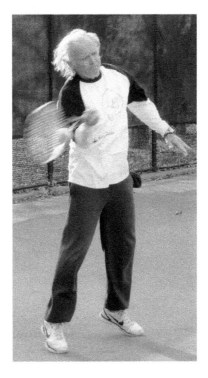

Figure 10.20   Exhale continues.

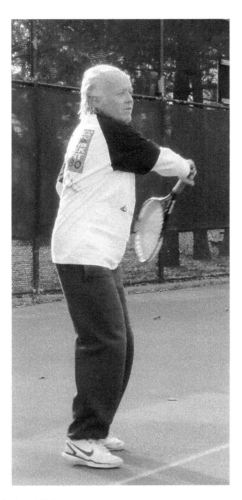

Figure 10.21   End of exhalation HRD.

HRD BF Efficiency and Efficacy Testing

High evidentiary analytic methodologies must be used to determine to what extent responses that are assumed to have occurred at specific times really did and if they are associated with better outcomes. With the BioCom system HRV/HRD, responses can only be analyzed within the *Temporally Discordant Paradigm* (TDP; non-real time monitoring), since heart activity can only be monitored before and after competition and during time-outs. Hence, in order to establish intervention efficiency and efficacy for HRD BF it must be determined if time-out/change-over, paced-breathing guided HRD BF, and resulting HRV measures are different from HRV measures that are derived during time-outs in which no HRD BF is administered. On a more ecologically valid level, one can also test for intervention efficacy using a structured experimental paradigm in which an athlete is instructed to engage in the previously practiced HRD-BF (off-the-playing field), on-the-playing prior to every competitive event, like the service return that is depicted in the above photos. After "x" amount of returns in which self-induced BF shaped HRD is attempted by a player prior to action (pre-action phase of the service return), a HRV scan of the player's heart activity is administered. Thereafter, in a no-intervention phase of the same paradigm with same amount of service returns, another scan is obtained. The resultant intervention/no intervention

HRV measures are then compared. Conceptually, if HRD exerts an enduring temporal effect on post time-out, pre-action HRV that is significantly different from HRV occurring in the post time-out-no intervention condition, intervention efficiency has been established. Then, if HRD BF associated HRV measures predict specific macro and/or micro level outcome (e.g. level 5 critical moment success or points won vs. lost), intervention efficacy will have been established. Again, intervention efficacy can exist on a continuum from very low to very high; as such, merely establishing intervention efficacy, while necessary, is not sufficient to unabashedly advocate for the universal application of a particular MT method. Nevertheless, minute performance gains that can be attributed to an intervention may have major practical significance, for example, winning one additional game or match that impacts an athlete's world or national ranking.

HRD BF Intervention Efficiency and Efficacy Testing: Intervention vs. No Intervention

In the context of the TDP, conceptually, intervention efficiency has been shown to exist if one or more HRV measures obtained during time-outs of the intervention (HRD BF) phase immediately after the last in a series of points have been played (during which HRD BF was also engaged in after each point) significantly differ from HRV measures obtained during time-outs of the no-intervention phase (also no intervention between points in this condition). In addition, the greater the conceptual consistency of such differences, the greater the intervention efficiency.

The following data emanates from an advanced senior level tennis player engaging in an experimental paradigm to determine if on-the-bench HRD-BF, subsequent to self-initiated HRD using paced breathing after each point played between time-out HRV scans, would be associated with conceptually relevant changes in HRV (as would be predicted) compared to HRV measures obtained during no-intervention time-outs subsequent to points played after which HRD BF was not self-initiated. Each phase (no-intervention vs. intervention HRD-BF) consisted of about 17 or 18 games, 11 in which each player attempts to win the point after two free "hits" (ball is introduced using a bounce-stroke and no winner can be hit on the first ball). A one-minute HRV scan using BioCom Heart Scanner was immediately administered after the 11th game ended (first player to win 11 points by a margin of at least two wins the game). The obtained data spanned three sessions over the course of one week.

Intervention Efficiency

Two statistically significant, including one highly conceptually consistent findings emerged. In the HRD-BF, intervention condition SDNN (the HRV index) was significantly different than in the no-intervention condition. Since volitionally-breathing induced HRD (or attempts to induce HRD) via paced inhalation and exhalation cycles are associated with greater HRV (as reflected in intervention associated HRD BF here) one can infer that the exhibited differences did not happen by chance, at least, the probability is high (see Figure 10.20. $p = .023$) that this was not a random effect. SDNN is one of two most conceptually, HRD relevant HRV measures (along with L/H ratio). As such, HRD-BF intervention efficiency was established for the specific athlete over the course of one week of testing trials. A second, borderline finding revealed less Very Low frequency activity in the intervention phase. This finding is also conceptually consistent, since paced breathing and resulting HRD has a strong parasympathetic nervous system (PNS) component (VL frequency is a measure of sympathetic nervous system activation).

This pilot investigation was undertaken in an attempt to preliminarily validate the temporally remote-HRD and HRD BF no-versus-intervention paradigms by documenting changes in HRV across divergent and distant measurement occasions.

Independent Samples Test

		Levene's Test for Equality of Variances		t-test for Equality of Means						
									95% Confidence Interval of the Difference	
		F	Sig.	t	df	Sig. (2-tailed)	Mean Difference	Std. Error Difference	Lower	Upper
MEASURE	Equal variances assumed	5.884	.019	-2.348	49	.023	-13.4785	5.7404	-25.0143	-1.9427
	Equal variances not assumed			-2.383	32.480	.023	-13.4785	5.6558	-24.9923	-1.9646

Figure 10.22 SDNN frequency HRV No HRD BF vs. HRD BF.

Independent Samples Test

		Levene's Test for Equality of Variances		t-test for Equality of Means						
									95% Confidence Interval of the Difference	
		F	Sig.	t	df	Sig. (2-tailed)	Mean Difference	Std. Error Difference	Lower	Upper
MEASURE	Equal variances assumed	5.515	.023	-1.888	49	.065	-106.5754	56.4441	-220.0041	6.8533
	Equal variances not assumed			-1.923	27.496	.065	-106.5754	55.4281	-220.2086	7.0578

Figure 10.23 Very Low frequency No HRD BF vs. HRD BF.

Intervention Efficacy

In terms of intervention efficacy, the tested player won more and lost less games in the HRD BF compared to the no-intervention condition (PTS11W 7.9 vs. 5.5 and 6.3 vs. 8.1 PTS11L). These macro-level outcome findings, while encouraging, would have to be replicated across about 60 trials for statistical significance to be established. On the other hand, practical significance, a potentially important efficacy metric in some sports in which small differences in an outcome measure are associated with global outcome measures such as games won or lost. This particular athlete, who previously lost about 80% of all 11 games against the same player who served as his opponent in this study, won close of 40% of all 11 games in the HRD-BF intervention condition, a 20% increase over his norm performance. His self-report was also supportive. He maintained that he felt more focused and less nervous during critical moments during the 11 games (e.g. when being close to arriving at game point). Although self-report has little to any empirical stature, if it is consistent with actual performance and likely not be high Athlete's Profile (AP, see Carlstedt, 2004, 2012) driven or placebo-mediated (this player's AP was M-L-M, a more ambiguous AP), then it can serve an investigative/diagnostic purpose.

Overall, intervention efficacy was established for HRD-BF in this athlete. His provisional Global Intervention Efficacy Quotient (GIEQ) for the 11s competition paradigm was .400 or 40%.

Intervention efficacy can also be investigated in the context of conceptually relevant mind-body measure; in this case HRD-BF based intervention. The following SPSS correlational outcome data (Figures 10.24 & 10.25) depict no-intervention and HRD-BF intervention HRV measures and their relationship with point and streak outcome (an ancillary continuous performance statistic [number of consecutive shots during an 11s point). There were no significant associations between HRV and outcome measures in the no-intervention condition.

By contrast, in the HRD-BF intervention condition (Figure 10.26 & 10.27), the HRV L/H frequency ratio (LHIGHHRD) was negatively correlated with points won ($r = -.47$, $p = .04$; PTS11WHD). This is another conceptually consistent finding attesting to intervention efficiency

Descriptive Statistics

	Mean	Std. Deviation	N
STRKNOIN	20.5294	5.5240	17
PTS11W	5.4706	3.6076	17
PTS11L	8.1176	3.6722	17
HR	125.1111	9.2093	18
SDNN	34.0000	5.7701	18
VL	31.1111	26.2205	18
L	47.4444	43.5947	18
H	63.5000	72.7819	18
LH	2.6556	3.8933	18
HHR	138.4444	8.3611	18
LHR	116.7778	9.5150	18

Figure 10.24   HRD BF No intervention: points and HRV.

Descriptive Statistics

	Mean	Std. Deviation	N
STRKHRD	20.1579	8.1531	19
PTS11WHD	7.8421	3.4523	19
PTS11LHD	6.2632	2.8644	19
HRHD	119.7368	13.8156	19
SDNHRD	49.1053	30.8399	19
VLOWHRD	139.5263	298.7220	19
LOWHRD	608.6316	2221.1748	19
HIGHHRD	343.0526	1074.7273	19
LHIGHHRD	2.2000	2.1736	19
HIGHHRHD	133.2632	11.7324	19
LOWHRHD	113.7368	13.0973	19

Figure 10.25   HRD BF intervention: points and HRV.

mediated intervention efficacy. Since a smaller L/H ratio usually contains more PNS related HF activity, and greater HF activity is mediated by the exhalation phase of the HRD breathing cycle, (brain–heart responses that have been associated with peak performance components), it could be expected that lower levels of L/H frequency activity would result in better performance (lesser L/H frequency ratio = more points won).

Summary: Temporally Remote HRD-BF Intervention Paradigm

The presented pilot investigation of the BHS-based TDP was validated in this tennis player. Clear, conceptually consistent intervention efficiency an efficacy findings support its utility as an athlete assessment and intervention approach. Nevertheless, this paradigm is limited by its lack of real time monitoring of HRV and pre-action epoch-specific HRD analysis capabilities. These limitations along with more advanced approaches to HRD BF are addressed in the next section.

Correlations

		STRKNOIN	PTS11W	PTS11L	HR	SDNN	VL	L	H	LH	HHR	LHR
STRKNOIN	Pearson Correlation	1.000	-.095	-.237	-.110	.269	-.254	-.172	.174	-.195	-.028	-.046
	Sig. (2-tailed)		.717	.359	.675	.297	.326	.509	.504	.454	.914	.862
	N	17	17	17	17	17	17	17	17	17	17	17
PTS11W	Pearson Correlation	-.095	1.000	.585*	.240	.126	.203	.221	-.105	.351	.153	.139
	Sig. (2-tailed)	.717		.014	.354	.631	.435	.394	.687	.167	.557	.595
	N	17	17	17	17	17	17	17	17	17	17	17
PTS11L	Pearson Correlation	-.237	.585*	1.000	.092	.171	-.097	.266	-.053	.304	.030	.058
	Sig. (2-tailed)	.359	.014		.724	.512	.712	.302	.840	.235	.909	.824
	N	17	17	17	17	17	17	17	17	17	17	17
HR	Pearson Correlation	-.110	.240	.092	1.000	-.194	.242	.093	.222	-.171	.869**	.925**
	Sig. (2-tailed)	.675	.354	.724		.441	.333	.713	.376	.498	.000	.000
	N	17	17	17	18	18	18	18	18	18	18	18
SDNN	Pearson Correlation	.269	.126	.171	-.194	1.000	.101	.352	.297	-.110	-.200	-.255
	Sig. (2-tailed)	.297	.631	.512	.441		.691	.152	.232	.664	.426	.307
	N	17	17	17	18	18	18	18	18	18	18	18
VL	Pearson Correlation	-.254	.203	-.097	.242	.101	1.000	.558*	.605**	-.167	.251	.269
	Sig. (2-tailed)	.326	.435	.712	.333	.691		.016	.008	.509	.316	.281
	N	17	17	17	18	18	18	18	18	18	18	18
L	Pearson Correlation	-.172	.221	.266	.093	.352	.558*	1.000	.665**	-.191	-.061	.165
	Sig. (2-tailed)	.509	.394	.302	.713	.152	.016		.003	.447	.811	.513
	N	17	17	17	18	18	18	18	18	18	18	18
H	Pearson Correlation	.174	-.105	-.053	.222	.297	.605**	.665**	1.000	-.447	.192	.361
	Sig. (2-tailed)	.504	.687	.840	.376	.232	.008	.003		.063	.446	.141
	N	17	17	17	18	18	18	18	18	18	18	18
LH	Pearson Correlation	-.195	.351	.304	-.171	-.110	-.167	-.191	-.447	1.000	-.142	-.176
	Sig. (2-tailed)	.454	.167	.235	.498	.664	.509	.447	.063		.575	.484
	N	17	17	17	18	18	18	18	18	18	18	18
HHR	Pearson Correlation	-.028	.153	.030	.869**	-.200	.251	-.061	.192	-.142	1.000	.811**
	Sig. (2-tailed)	.914	.557	.909	.000	.426	.316	.811	.446	.575		.000
	N	17	17	17	18	18	18	18	18	18	18	18
LHR	Pearson Correlation	-.046	.139	.058	.925**	-.255	.269	.165	.361	-.176	.811**	1.000
	Sig. (2-tailed)	.862	.595	.824	.000	.307	.281	.513	.141	.484	.000	
	N	17	17	17	18	18	18	18	18	18	18	18

*. Correlation is significant at the 0.05 level (2-tailed).

**. Correlation is significant at the 0 01 level (2-tailed).

Figure 10.26 HRD BF-No intervention condition, macro-outcome (points and streaks) and HRV.

Correlations

		STRKHRD	PTS11WHD	PTS11LHD	HRHD	SDNHRD	VLOWHRD	LOWHRD	HIGHHRD	LHIGHHRD	HIGHHRHD	LOWHRHD
STRKHRD	Pearson Correlation	1.000	-.080	.127	-.254	-.266	-.329	-.389	-.381	.015	-.146	-.204
	Sig. (2-tailed)		.745	.606	.295	.271	.170	.100	.108	.951	.552	.403
	N	19	19	19	19	19	19	19	19	19	19	19
PTS11WHD	Pearson Correlation	-.080	1.000	.763**	.286	.019	.171	.211	.228	-.471*	.214	.316
	Sig. (2-tailed)	.745		.000	.236	.939	.485	.387	.348	.042	.380	.187
	N	19	19	19	19	19	19	19	19	19	19	19
PTS11LHD	Pearson Correlation	.127	.763**	1.000	.146	.089	.246	.224	.232	-.242	-.025	.237
	Sig. (2-tailed)	.606	.000		.550	.717	.309	.356	.339	.319	.918	.328
	N	19	19	19	19	19	19	19	19	19	19	19
HRHD	Pearson Correlation	-.254	.286	.146	1.000	-.239	-.220	-.084	-.040	-.696**	.911**	.968**
	Sig. (2-tailed)	.295	.236	.550		.324	.366	.732	.870	.001	.000	.000
	N	19	19	19	19	19	19	19	19	19	19	19
SDNHRD	Pearson Correlation	-.266	.019	.089	-.239	1.000	.885**	.885**	.883**	.143	-.285	-.178
	Sig. (2-tailed)	.271	.939	.717	.324		.000	.000	.000	.559	.237	.467
	N	19	19	19	19	19	19	19	19	19	19	19
VLOWHRD	Pearson Correlation	-.329	.171	.246	-.220	.885**	1.000	.977**	.969**	.049	-.345	-.157
	Sig. (2-tailed)	.170	.485	.309	.366	.000		.000	.000	.844	.148	.520
	N	19	19	19	19	19	19	19	19	19	19	19
LOWHRD	Pearson Correlation	-.389	.211	.224	-.084	.885**	.977**	1.000	.998**	-.023	-.173	-.032
	Sig. (2-tailed)	.100	.387	.356	.732	.000	.000		.000	.926	.480	.898
	N	19	19	19	19	19	19	19	19	19	19	19
HIGHHRD	Pearson Correlation	-.381	.228	.232	-.040	.883**	.969**	.998**	1.000	-.071	-.132	.015
	Sig. (2-tailed)	.108	.348	.339	.870	.000	.000	.000		.772	.589	.952
	N	19	19	19	19	19	19	19	19	19	19	19
LHIGHHRD	Pearson Correlation	.015	-.471*	-.242	-.696**	.143	.049	-.023	-.071	1.000	-.543*	-.694**
	Sig. (2-tailed)	.951	.042	.319	.001	.559	.844	.926	.772		.016	.001
	N	19	19	19	19	19	19	19	19	19	19	19
HIGHHRHD	Pearson Correlation	-.146	.214	-.025	.911**	-.285	-.345	-.173	-.132	-.543*	1.000	.848**
	Sig. (2-tailed)	.552	.380	.918	.000	.237	.148	.480	.589	.016		.000
	N	19	19	19	19	19	19	19	19	19	19	19
LOWHRHD	Pearson Correlation	-.204	.316	.237	.968**	-.178	-.157	-.032	.015	-.694**	.848**	1.000
	Sig. (2-tailed)	.403	.187	.328	.000	.467	.520	.898	.952	.001	.000	
	N	19	19	19	19	19	19	19	19	19	19	19

**. Correlation is significant at the 0.01 level (2-tailed).

*. Correlation is significant at the 0.05 level (2-tailed).

Figure 10.27 HRD BF-intervention condition, macro-outcome (points and streaks) and HRV.

Ecological Real-Time HRD MT: Polar Wireless System

In terms of HRD BF efficacy testing, because of limitations associated with HRV monitoring systems that use wired as opposed to telemetry-based wireless data acquisition methods, this MT modality and the HRD response that it is supposed to shape, could only be analyzed in the context of more static paradigms in which responses could not be isolated or time-locked to competitive situations-epochs of interest (as with the previously described BioCom Heart Scanner system).

This limitation has been overcome with the advent of wireless cardiac monitoring instrumentation.

While the BHS is excellent for educating and training athletes in HRD BF and can be reliably adapted for real competition-based efficiency and efficacy checks, ideally, one would want to observe and know when and to what extent HRD has occurred and whether the manifestation of HRD in a specific athlete is associated with better outcome than when it is not manifested. Telemetry systems allow for such time-locked analyses of HRD during competition as well as in-the-moment pre-action HRV biofeedback on the playing field. Being able to engage in instrument-guided BF during official competition is a major breakthrough since to date practitioners primarily work on the premise that a BF shaped response in the lab or office or on the sideline had to be well engrained or consolidated to reliably generalize to the playing-field. Yet, practitioners and researchers alike have been unable to consistently demonstrate, if at all, that lab-based BF generated and shaped mind-body responses could be reproduced by an athlete on command when necessary, and importantly, if such responses were actually associated with optimum performance and/or successful outcome. Such ambiguity and the equivocal generalizability of lab-based BF shaped psychophysiological responses to the playing field calls into question the utility and viability of BF as a reliable intervention despite claims to the contrary by stakeholders in BF. Consequently, wireless HRV/HRD assessment has leaped to the forefront since data can now be reliably obtained in real time and time locked to all important competitive epochs, ranging from pre-action to specific moments during an action phase (e.g., the precise moment when a field-goal kicker's foot makes contact with the football). Importantly, since specific cardiac responses are strongly correlated with performance relevant cortical (brain) responses it is an ideal ersatz measure for criterion-referencing in-the-lab induced and shaped EEG-neurofeedback responses with HRV/HRD, a response that can reliably induced, manipulated, and documented on-the-playing field.

The ABSP-CP Polar paradigm offers cross-validation capabilities (lab-based with in-the-field during real competition data comparisons) because of the robustness of this system's instrumentation during extreme movement (resistance to motion artifact) another important methodological issue.

HRD Biofeedback On-the-Playing Field during Competition: Ecological Mental Training

The following photos depict step-by-step HRD BF procedures using the Polar RS800CX heart activity monitoring system. This instrumentation is emerging as the primary monitoring system for all ABSP-CP interventions and MT since HRV and HRD trends can be isolated throughout competition in virtually all sports, in real time and as MT is being engaged in by the athlete, wirelessly. The ability to obtain time locked mind-body response data during real competition offers unprecedented insight into comprehensive sport-specific psychophysiological response dynamics.

1 The photo below (Figure 10.28) shows the Polar chest strap and heart activity receiver/ transmitter.
2 The chest strap is attached so that the receiver/transmitter is tightly secured over the breastbone (Figure 10.28). Wearing a chest strap is a non-issue for the vast majority of athletes who quickly adapt to wearing it.

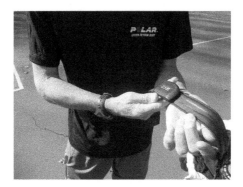

Figure 10.28   Preparing to use the polar instrumentation.

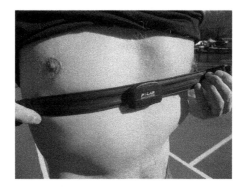

Figure 10.29   Polar chest strap with receiver.

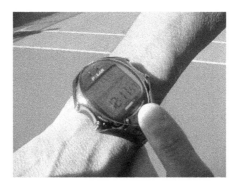

Figure 10.30   Polar computer-watch-receiver.

3   Once the chest strap is in place, the watch, which functions as a data receiver and storage as well as a BF device, is started by the athlete (Figure 10.29). When engaging in HRD/HRV assessment and BF it is necessary to videotape training and competition sessions from beginning to end. The video recorder should be started concomitant to the Polar watch/data receiver.

4   Here, the player has just returned a serve (Figure 10.30). Heart activity signals are transmitted from the chest monitoring/receiver unit to the watch/computer receiver and stored over the course of entire training or competition.

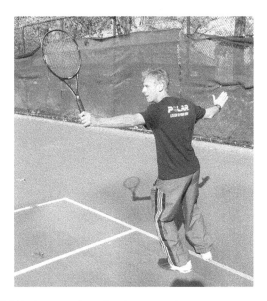

Figure 10.31 Player's HRV being monitored as he competes.

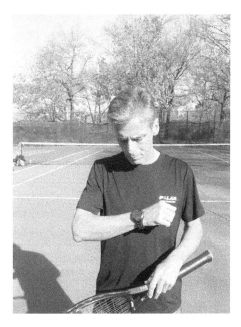

Figure 10.32 Post point HRD BF.

5   Player checks his post-action/post point heart rate (Figures 10.32 & 10.33). The watch can also be used as a BF device. Here we see at 2′ 23″of this tennis set a heart rate of 106 bpm (Figure 10.32). The depicted tennis player was previously trained in HRD BF and conditioned to check his heart rate by looking at the watch immediately after a point, in this case a service return that resulted in no further action, hence the relatively low heart rate.

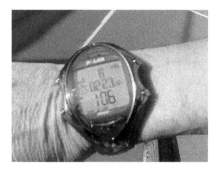

Figure 10.33   Heart rate at HRD BF onset (106).

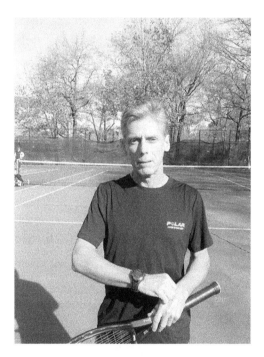

Figure 10.34   Start of Inhale-Exhale cycles.

6   Thereafter the player commences breathing-based HRD BF prior to the next point (Figure 10.34.). In tennis, players have about 20–25 seconds between points. This down time or part of this time is used, as necessary, to "practice" HRD and HRD BF for the purpose of priming automatic mind-body responses that a player then synchronizes to the task demands and temporal parameters of a specific-sport, in this case, either the serve or return of serve. In this photo, the player is in his exhalation/expiration breathing phase. His goal is to induce HRD through a continuous, quick, and forceful exhale cycle that is time locked to the impending onset of action; either the start of the upward racquet swing when serving or swing of the racquet when returning serve. Exhalation should be timed to be fully completed by the time contact is made with the ball.

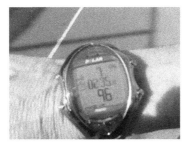

Figure 10.35   Heart rate after HRD BF (from 106 to 96).

7   The above HRD BF epoch lasted 12 seconds, from 2′ 23″ to 2′ 35 (Figure 10.35) resulting in a linear reduction in heart rate from 106 to 96 bpm.[3] The player successfully self- generated HRD through timed breathing that was initially learned and consolidated in the lab. The watch provides on-the-playing field feedback and reinforcement by showing HRV changes over a prescribed amount of time in which an intervention is engaged in. It should be noted that 12 seconds, although possibly seeming to be a too lengthy timeframe, was the mean time that the player's opponent took from the onset of the service ready position to when the ball was struck. Consequently, the player was instructed to engage in a pre-return HRD BF routine for 12 seconds and then get into his service return position, do one more HRD BF cycle if possible (dependent on whether the server who per rule can dictate the pace of play so long as the maximum between point time allowed [25 seconds] is not exceeded), and then, initially, on a conscious level, pace and time his inhalation-exhalation cycles to his opponent's 12″ service cycle. Over time, it is expected that a player will initiate pre-action HRD automatically as most athletes do during non-stressful routine phases of competition, a performance facilitative response that hopefully will be so well conditioned and consolidated that an athlete can depend upon it occurring naturally without self-or external prompting by a coach or volitionally "tell" oneself to do the HRD BF routine whenever he or she feels competitive stress or is aware of the importance or heightened criticality of a certain point or competitive situation.

HRD Mental Training Efficiency and Efficacy Testing: Case Study Observations

A former professional tennis player's (CR: AP of L-M-M) heart activity was monitored during a practice match to determine whether pre-action phases of competition would be marked by volitionally induced HRD trends. A HRD trend is considered to have occurred when the following or similar configuration of IBIs can be isolated during the pre-action phase of a point, from the moment a player commences his or her pre-action ritual and inhale/exhale cycle: *one or more linearly slowing cardiac cycles leading up to the start of action (start of service windup when serving or start of the return split-step when returning), for example: 100 bpm, 98 bpm, 95 bpm **action***. This would be a HRD trend of 3 (HRDt3). Since minute movements, such as even wiping one's face can disrupt a linear HRD trend and lead to a brief acceleratory IBI as follows (same sample IBIs): 100 bpm, **102 bpm**, 98 bpm, **99 bpm**, 95 bpm, one can consider these accelerations as superfluous

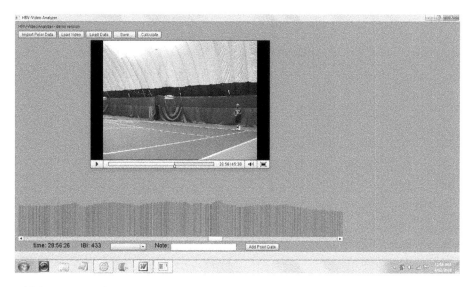

Figure 10.36   HRD analysis app.

IBIs and of a metabolic nature and not psychologically mediated. Consequently, so long as the last IBI prior to action is a decelerating IBI one can assume that pre-action HRD has occurred. Thus, in terms of how to analyze pre-action HRD the following is recommended: 1) count all decelerating IBIs within the pre-action epoch commencing with the IBI corresponding with the video-synchronized/identified pre-action ritual onset and ending with the last HRD IBI prior to action to derive the total HRD IBIs in a pre-action epoch; 2) delineate the longest HRD IBI trend, that is, the number of consecutive (without interruption) linearly slowing cardiac cycles (IBIs; if using the above example 100, 98 and 95 it would be a HRDt3, the longest of this pre-action epoch); and 3) finally determine how many pre-action epochs end with a decelerating IBI. The same procedure is used to identify HRA trends. Thereafter, comparisons are made between HRD and HRA in the context of numerous outcome measures including level of criticality (CM), points won or lost and points won or lost when serving or returning. Since tennis outcome can be strongly influenced by opponent factors the mere manifestation of HRD does not guarantee successful performance or outcome, but at minimum, is expected to prime an athlete to perform up to peak potential by helping set off a cascade of mind-body-motor responses that have been associated with enhanced attention (focus), faster reaction time and motor (technical) preparation, thereby reducing the possibility that an athlete will falter because of psychological factors. An athlete might lose a point immediately after pre-action HRD, but when this occurs opponent factors and not "choking" could have contributed to negative outcome. Note: HRD appears to be a species-wide response to an impending stimulus or when expecting to respond to a stimulus like an approaching ball. This phenomena (HRD) is pervasive across almost all athletes in pre-action phases of most sports. However, once level of criticality reaches or exceeds an athlete's mental toughness or "choke" threshold, psychologically mediated competitive anxiety is expected to disrupt pre-action performance preparatory HRD; instead HRA predominates, an ANS response that is associated with left-frontal lobe-based rumination, the generation of intrusive thoughts, and a failure to become technically primed to react. Vulnerability to HRA along with a lower "choke" threshold has been strongly linked to most performance detrimental AP PHO constellations (e.g. H-H-L).

Findings: Action Phase HRV

Each action epoch was isolated on the basis of the video timeline. The Polar software allows for the delineation of any epoch of interest and the subsequent automatic generation of HRV time and frequency domain measures for a specified epoch. CR's mean bpm (Mbpm) during action epochs was correlated with points won (r =.30) as was his low frequency activity (r =.27). This finding suggests that greater HR during action epochs, a marker of greater effort or intensity, facilitated performance during points in this match. The LF activity and outcome finding is more ambiguous, since this HRV measure can reflect ANS balance, a mind-body response that may be associated with greater F-C-C in certain athletes (a specific IZOF biomarker response). However, this would need to be determined with greater statistical certainty over the course of additional matches. The fact that maximum bpm during action phases explained 11% of the variance in points won supports the above interpretation of the Mbpm finding, namely, that greater action phase HR and associated higher levels of psychologically mediated intensity enhanced performance in this player. While this may make intuitive sense, this finding too must be validated across additional matches. In addition, data modeling of action epochs should be undertaken to determine whether relationships between HRV and outcome are influenced by a number of variables including action epoch duration, number of shots during action phases, as well as the type of shots that were engaged in and how a point was won or lost.

Heart Rate Deceleration (HRD) and Heart Acceleration (HRA) Action Trends

Of major conceptual importance is to what extent HRD is present immediately prior to action. In this match's first set (for CR) consisting of 65 action epochs, HRD occurred 44 times prior to action (in which at least one or more decelerating IBI(s) preceded the onset of action).

Subsequent to these 44 HRD trends, 24 points were won and 20 were lost resulting in a global HRD-win index (HRDgwi) of .545 (55%) and a global HRD-index (HRDgi) of .676 (68%). While the win index may seem relatively low, it should be noted that the global win index encompasses all points including opponent serve initiated points. The serve in tennis, as with pitching in baseball, can be very dominating to the extent of neutralizing any advantage pre-action HRD may bring in the moment. Thus, on one hand, HRD and the HRDgi while hypothesized to reflect an in-the-moment peak performance state that is marked by optimum attention (focus), physiological reactivity (comfortable level of intensity), and technical/motor priming (control), opponent factors like a big serve or overpowering ground strokes can render HRD moot at times. This reality, however, does not diminish the importance of HRD as a potent performance biomarker (mind-body correlate of peak pre-action psychological readiness).

By contrast, HRA immediately prior to action may reflect a lack of pre-action F-C-C with the HRA global index (HRAgi) serving to quantify a lack of mind-body preparedness. CR exhibited 21 HRA trends prior to action (HRAgi of .477 [47%]) and a HRA global loss index (HRAgli) of .619 (62%). Norms for HRD and HRA trends (both group and individual averages) are being developed by the ABSP research consortium of board certified practitioner/researchers, student certification final project research, summer fellowship program, and other client/team athlete organization research. Nevertheless, irrespective of not yet having comprehensive HRD/HRA norms, intuitively, the higher the HRDgi and its converse (the lower the HRAgi), the more in control of mind-body performance processes an athlete is thought to be. Furthermore, relative to technical and physical ability, with all things being about equal in terms of player/athlete match-ups, ultimately, especially in the context of increasing criticality (competitive pressure), an athlete who manifests more HRD trends prior to action can be expected to win most games/matches and or perform better than an opponent who exhibits a greater HRAgi (a greater HRAgi always indicated a lower HRDgi).

There was also one ancillary finding from this pilot HRD investigation, namely, HF HRV activity was correlated with total pre-action HRD IBIs (r =.30). This has conceptual significance in that HRD is PNS mediated and HF reflects, exclusively, PNS activity.

When possible, micro-analyses and modeling of HRD trends should be performed, especially global win and loss indexes to determine to what extent opponent or other factors that may be beyond the control of an athlete mitigate his or her HRDgwi. In addition, secondary operationalizations of HRD trends, including total HRD IBIs and the longest HRD trend within a pre-action epoch, irrespective of whether the last IBI prior to action is a decelerating IBI, should be analyzed in the context of multiple sport-specific performance outcome measures.

These HRD findings are encouraging and are consistent with the first study of HRD-BF during official tennis tournament matches that was carried out in 1997 using the first generation Polar system (Carlstedt, 1998, 2001). They underscore the potential utility of using HRD trends to quantify in-the-moment comprehensive psychologically mediated mind-body-motor performance and HRD-MT efficacy.

An Experimental Efficacy Analysis of HRD Mental Training

An advanced tennis player ("PP"; male with AP of H-L-M) wearing the Polar chest strap and attached data collection and transmission component was linked to a telemetry enabled computer for real time cardiac signal processing, display, and analysis of his heart activity. He was stationed in the service return area of a tennis court and was told to prepare for an impending serve (60 return trials), being sure to engage in the preparatory HRD-BF that he was trained in. A participating player (the server) was instructed to serve first serves (associated with more speed) into the deuce court service box/area. PP was told to focus on the service motion of the server and transition from timed inhalation to forceful exhalation once the server commenced his upward swing from the backscratcher position toward the ball.

The purpose of this experiment was to document all IBIs in the pre-action phase of the service return and analyze their properties after the experiment was completed. The lead researcher (a sport psychologist, pro-tour level tennis coach, and former professional tennis player) rated the quality of the return (QoS) on a zero to five scale (from worst to best outcome) after each shot (return). The experiment consisted of 51 valid trials out of 60 that were attempted. Ten trials were rejected due to motion artifact.

Sixty trials is the approximate number of repetitions that is recommended when investigating single individuals in the context of a repeated-measures design and is methodologically comparable to having 60 subjects doing one trial each. Sixty trials are associated with a level of statistical power between .80-.90 that balances the probability of making a Type I or Type II error during hypothesis testing. This type of design allows a researcher/practitioner to reach more empirically informed conclusions about the psychophysiological responding and performance of an individual athlete. Findings pertaining to individual mind-body responses should always supersede group findings in terms of athlete assessment or evaluation and the interpretation of data/results provided by a repeated measures study's methodology/procedures replicate those of a group investigation (same study, but with a single case vs. multiple subjects).

Since group study findings and interpretations, for the most part, are based on mean scores/results and are usually marked by wide variability relative to outcome or distribution of scores, in the context of applied sport psychological consulting, each individual athlete subject who participated in a group study should be analyzed separately or independently, irrespective of a group study's consolidated findings and interpretations. Decisions or expectations about athletes' performance should not be made on the basis of assumptions that are influenced by group findings no matter how compelling the results may be. Group findings need to be replicated at the intraindividual level, cognizant of methodological and analytic issues including statistical power. The 60 trial guideline is an important rule of thumb, and, as previously mentioned, provides a methodological framework that can render individual longitudinal investigations more meaningful and sensitive to predictor-criterion variable relationships, especially for the select athlete of interest and his or her coach and other stakeholders.

Findings

This experiment was interested in determining whether, and to what extent, volitional HRD-BF would be associated with a greater QoS (better return).

The following was found:

1   In 31 (61%) of 51 trials, HRD was documented immediately prior to action. By contrast, 20 of 51 trials were marked by HRA (39%).

Interpretation: conceptually, it would be expected that during routine moments of competition volitional HRD-BF will result in HRD prior to all action phases. Hence, questions that must be asked include why did HRD not occur prior to action every trial (service return) and what interfered with this well-established pre-action HRD that is expected to always occur in response to an impending/anticipated sport-specific stimulus (the ball when returning serve) or in conjunction with preparation to initiate action (e.g., when serving). In addition to measurement error (a methodological issue since it can be difficult to exactly synchronize heart beats at the millisecond level with the onset of action), psychological and physical factors, even during routine moments of a MT training experiment like this one (or during competition), can influence performance. For example, it is conceivable that peak levels of attention (focus) could not be maintained across 60 consecutive trials that were carried out consecutively without a break. Visual and cognitive fatigue could have led to a breakdown of the expected left to right cortical shift and concomitant HRD that has been associated with pre-action readiness, quicker reaction time, and successful outcome. Since PP's AP of H-L-M is on the cusp of being the ideal PHO constellation, one would not expect him to "choke" in the context of a routine performance experiment that was not designed to test or assess his mental toughness, per se. However, it is plausible that he (an athlete with a near ideal AP) was not challenged enough by an innocuous "performance" drill" to the extent that his superior potential to focus intently through all trials was activated, leading to mental lapses and associated HRA across select pre-action epochs (39% of all trials). Additional assessment of PP should be undertaken to test the above possibility.

Nevertheless, irrespective of these interpretations pre-action HRD occurred 61% of the time, a finding that tends to support and partially replicate the pre-action HRD hypothesis. In terms of global focus-comfort-control (F-C-C), PP's HRDgi of .61 is line with CR's match play HRDgi of .68. HRDgi is an exploratory/hypothetical emerging indicator of level of attention/focus (F) situational comfort/intensity/physiological reactivity (C) and coping/pre-action strategic planning/motor-technical priming and can be used to compare F-C-C at the intraindividual level across competitions and in relationship to other athletes.

2   Relative to QoS outcome at threshold level I (QoS of 3, 4 or 5), HRD was associated with a QoS I in 26 out of 31 trials (83%), whereas HRA was associated with a QoS of I 15 out of 20 trials (75%).

Interpretation: this is a critical outcome measure domain in that, conceptually, one would expect, predict and want performance subsequent to pre-action HRD to be significantly better than performance after pre-action HRA. After all, if post pre-action HRD responses are not associated with better performance that distinguishes HRD from HRA, then both measures are rendered relatively meaningless in terms of predicting or distinguishing performance. However, it should be cautioned that, even in instances where HRA and not HRD is associated with better performance, numerous performance related extraneous variables can possibly be implicated in driving poor performance after pre-action HRD, such as opponent variables including personal skill level, technical weaknesses, and subliminal mind-body processes that are associated with specific AP constellations, as well as perceived stress or competitive anxiety, even in the absence of higher levels of criticality. Thus, in order to better illuminate the etiology of HRD-HRA performance outcome discrepancies or paradoxical outcome, group studies are necessary (hundreds of athletes who are assessed across similar controlled experimental HRD paradigms and real competition) as well as extensive modeling of HRV (HRD/HRA) in the context of as many relevant performance outcome mediating or moderating variables as can be derived/extracted from a dataset in individual athletes (e.g. HRD and criticality level 4 or 5; HRD and forehand returns [e.g., whether a return's quality is influenced by the type of stroke] or HRD and time of epoch's outcome [e.g. HRA occurring to a greater extent at the end of a series of trials to assess fatigue and attention decrement or boredom, lack of motivation]; all of these as well as other factors could undermine the HRD-enhanced performance hypothesis and even call into question the omnipresence of HRD as a pre-action biomarker).

The finding that HRD and Level I performance outcome only exceeded the HRA-Level I performance by 8% highlights the above concerns and issues. Conceptually, one would expect, predict, and, ideally, want pre-action HRD to result in greater Level I performance and performance decrement to be associated with HRA. It appears that individual difference factors that drive performance outcome can be capable of neutralizing the performance enhancing mind-body-motor mechanisms associated with pre-action HRD. For example, even though an athlete may be highly focused, mentally prepared, and in control of his or her motor response system (F-F-C) and as such, manifest pre-action HRD and concomitant brain responses that lead to peak reaction time and an initial stellar response (e.g., a great service return), the positive cascade of brain-heart mediated responses associated with HRD may not be sufficient to counter what is to come in the impending action phase (e.g. an opponent's backhand winner down the line; or a baseball pitcher's 95 miles per hour fastball). Ultimately, a psychophysiological response, even if initially associated with optimal focus, comfort and control can at most foster initial peak performance responses, but it will not necessarily always lead to successful performance through-out a subsequent action epoch. Individual variability in psychologically mediated pre-action HRV (HRD & HRA) and later action phase motor, technical, and strategic responses are likely to impact performance in both directions. Moreover, mind-body responses within the pre-action-action equation are expected to be influenced, to a large extent, by an athlete's AP constellation, especially during critical moments during competition.

3   HRD occurred 13 out of 31 times (42%) and HRA occurred 7 out of 20 times (35%) prior to QoS Level II outcome (QoS of 4 or 5).

Interpretation: This finding can be interpreted similarly to the previous outcome analysis. Essentially, even in a controlled experiment in which the task is to try and return a serve as proficiently as possible (as determined by placement and power criteria that is assessed by an expert rater), variation in speed and direction of the oncoming serve, coupled with an athlete's technical strengths, weaknesses, and limitations are potential extraneous variables that are capable of neutralizing the performance facilitative HRD response. Relative to HRA during pre-action, while its manifestation and subsequent association with positive outcome (Level 4 or 5 QoS) would not have been predicted, it is possible that most serves in an HRA occurring pre-action epoch were very easy to return. As such, even a non-performance facilitative pre-action response like HRA may not have a negative influence on *actual performance*.

For example, further analysis and statistical modeling might determine that most HRA successes and HRD failures were associated with serves to this player's strength and weakness respectively, increasingly the likelihood that the impact of pre-action HRV would be differentially lessened or increased when interpreted in the context of technically mediated, post, pre-action phase outcome Statistical modeling requires more repeated measures to ensure adequate sample size relating to each variable of interest. As a result, an in-depth multi-factorial micro-analyses can only be done after additional entire experimental trials (multiple 60+ serve return experiments; circa 10 additional trials per additional predictor/criterion variable).

4   Finally, worst performance (Qos level 1 or 2) was associated with HRA in five out of 20 trials (25%) and in five of 31 (16%) trials with HRD.

Interpretation: This finding is more in line with expectations with the difference between HRD and HRA being slightly greater than with the previous performance outcome categories 11% vs. 8% and 7% in favor of HRD). However, even this finding reveals far less outcome separation than one would have liked. Directional discrepant performance differences, as with the previous findings may be attributable to numerous other psychological and technical factors, some that were mentioned.

These findings attest to the need to meticulously engage or practice HRD-MT to reach a high level of intervention efficiency. The entire MT process should be well documented and analyzed. For further information on the ABSP-CP HRD analytics and MT, contact the author.

Notes

1   About 50–65 MT trials in which HRV measures are analyzed in the context of sport-specific macro and micro outcome measures including situational criticality (level of critical moment); an A-B-A design can also be used, with or without concurrent HRV monitoring [100-120 trials] to determine no-intervention/intervention differences as a function of temporal lag (time of intervention prior to start of competition).

2   This process can be viewed as an inverse or reverse visualization dynamic in which technical-performance related neuronal ensembles are primed for activation directly via motor pathways, independent of visual priming, that can be contaminated, perceptually (how an athlete see, perceives or imagines his or her technique may be incongruent with how it should be) or by an inability to exploit potential performance facilitative aspects of mental imagery because of an athlete's low level of HS/SA, rendering him or her unable to engage in structured visualization.

3   It should be noted that reduction in HR also occurs as a function of decreasing metabolic demands. Consequently, it is important to observe HRD trends in the pre-intervention training phase in the context of natural metabolic mediated HRD and breathing-mediated HRD as well as orienting-response mediated HRD. Volitional breathing-based HRD and HRD BF should be distinct from metabolic mediated HRD and marked by less of a linear HR slowing trend, whereas self-induced and stimulus-oriented HRD should exhibit linear trends consisting of two or more linearly slowing inter-beat-intervals.

References

Andreassi, J. L. (1995). *Psychophysiology: Human behavior and physiological response* (3rd ed.). Hillsdale, NJ: Erlbaum.

Boutcher, S. H., & Zinsser, N. W. (1990). Cardiac deceleration of elite and beginning golfers during putting. *Journal of Sport and Exercise Psychology, 12*, 37–47.

Carlstedt, R.A. (2001). Line bisecting test reveals relative left brain hemispheric predominance in highly skilled athletes: Relationships among cerebral laterality, personality, and sport performance. *Doctoral dissertation*, Saybrook Graduate School, San Francisco.

Carlstedt, R. A. (2012). *Evidence-based applied sport psychology: A practitioner's manual*. New York, NY: Springer Publishing Company

Hatfield, B. D., Landers, D. L., & Ray, W. J. (1984). Cognitive processes during self paced motor performance: An electroencephalographic profile of skilled marksman. *Journal of Sport Psychology, 6*, 42–59.

Roland A. Carlstedt

Hatfield, B. D., Landers, D. L., & Ray, W. J. (1987). Cardiovascular–CNS interactions during a self-paced, intentional attentive state: Elite marksmanship performance. *Psychophysiology, 24,* 542–549.

Lacey, J. I., & Lacey, B. C. (1964). Cardiac deceleration and simple visual reaction in a fixed foreperiod experiment. Paper presented at the meeting of the Society for Psychophysiological Research, Washington, D.C.

Lacey, J. I., & Lacey, B. C. (1978). Two-way communication between the heart and the brain: Significance of time within the cardiac cycle. *American Psychologist, 33*(2), 99–113.

Wickramasekera, I. (1988). Clinical behavioral medicine. NY: Plenum.

This chapter was adapted in part from the Author's book: *Critical Moments During Competition: A Mind-Body Model of Sport Performance when it Counts the Most.* Psychology Press 2004.

The Use of Gaze Training to Expedite Motor Skill Acquisition

Mark R. Wilson and Samuel J. Vine

Setting the Scene: The Strategic Role of Eye Movements

Vision is the dominant sensory system underpinning human function. Gaze changes and the resultant fixations that orchestrate the sequential acquisition of information from the visual environment are central features of the human visual system (Land, 2009). With experience and through training, experts learn to conserve limited cognitive resources and strategically direct their gaze control system to optimise information acquisition and guide accurate goal-directed *motor control (perceptual motor)* and *decision-making (perceptual cognitive)* performance. Studies of gaze selection in natural environments point to a consistent set of principles underlying eye guidance, involving (1) behavioral relevance (based on reward mechanisms), (2) uncertainty about the state of the environment, and (3) learned models of the environment (prior experience). These factors control the decision mechanisms that govern what we should attend to on the basis of where we will gain information for fulfilling the current behavioural goals (Tatler, Hayhoe, Land, & Ballard, 2011).

In relation to motor control, researchers have demonstrated that fixations are tightly coupled, temporally and spatially, to the motor actions of well-learned tasks (see Land 2009 for a review). Specifically, gaze tends to move to the target in advance of movement initiation and remains stable as the movement unfolds. Novices, still exploring their visuomotor environment and the consequences of their actions within it, do not display this tight coupling (Sailer, Flanagan, & Johansson, 2005). As such, benefits may arise from the co-alignment of functional neural structures related to the control of eye and limb movements. For example, not only are there strong links between attention and eye movements within frontal and parietal lobes (Corbetta et al., 1998), but frontoparietal networks are also involved in the integration of signals related to eye and limb movements (van Donkelaar & Staub, 2000).

The quiet eye (QE; Vickers, 1996) is a specific measure reflecting this anchored gaze strategy and has been the subject of much research attention in sport over the last 20 years (Vickers, 2016). The QE is defined as the final fixation towards a relevant target that has an onset prior to the initiation of a critical movement and an offset that can occur during or after the movement's completion. The QE is postulated to represent a critical period of cognitive processing during which the parameters of the movement such as force, direction, and velocity are fine-tuned and programmed (Vickers, 2007), and can be considered as a critical period when sensory information is synthesized with the mechanisms necessary to both plan (pre-programme) and control (online) the appropriate motor response (Vine, Moore, & Wilson, 2014). There is a robust relationship between superior task performance and longer QE durations in studies adopting a range of different paradigms, including expert-novice comparisons; examinations of intra-individual performance variability (hits v misses); anxiety manipulations; and manipulations of task difficulty (see Rienhoff, Tirp, Strauss, Baker, & Schorer, 2015; Wilson, Causer, & Vickers, 2015 for recent reviews).

Given that expert-novice differences have been determined in gaze behaviour across a wide range of performance domains (Gegenfurtner, Lehtinen, & Säljö, 2011), it is not surprising that psychologists have sought to investigate training programmes to improve perceptual-cognitive skills like visual search, decision-making and problem solving (Litchfield & Ball, 2011). In such cases, it is felt that cueing participants' attention towards task relevant areas of a display may increase the likelihood of task success. In tasks involving movement control, additional benefits may arise from the co-alignment of functional neural structures related to the control of eye and limb movements. Taken together, the premise behind gaze training is that novices can benefit from learning the precise eye movements and gaze strategies that experts use to decide, plan, and control a course of action for a given task. Indeed, such video-based instruction has been shown to help novices attain both a higher level of proficiency and superior performance under stressful conditions (compared to current 'best practice' instructions) in tasks as varied as laparoscopic surgery (Wilson, Vine, Bright, Masters, Defriend, & McGrath, 2011); machine gun shooting (Moore, Vine, Smith, Smith, & Wilson, 2014); and sport (Moore, Vine, Cooke, Ring, & Wilson, 2012; Vine & Wilson, 2010, 2011).

The following section discusses the main forms of gaze training that have been applied to the acquisition of motor skill, and outlines some of their commonalities and differences.

Gaze Training Introduction

Gaze training sits within a larger umbrella term, feed forward eye movement training (FFEMT), which has been applied successfully to cognitive tasks. FFEMT refers to the viewing of an expert 'prototype' of the correct and most efficient way to move the eyes to obtain the visual information and focus of attention needed to complete a task. In cognitive or judgement tasks, it is proposed that cueing participants' attention towards task relevant areas of a display will increase the likelihood of task success (e.g., Gegenfurtner, Lehtinen, & Säljö, 2011). The stimulus through which this demonstration occurs can vary, but typically trainees will see a view of the task (video or static image) with a cursor displaying the location of fixations and the transition of eye movements between locations. FFEMT has been operationalized in a number of different ways within the literature including Quiet eye training (Vickers, 2007), gaze training (Wilson, Vine, et al., 2011), perceptual skills training (Broadbent, Causer, Williams, & Ford, 2015), eye movement modelling (Jarodzka, van Gog, Dorr, Scheiter, & Gerjets, 2013), and collaborative eye tracking (Chetwood et al., 2012).

A gaze training intervention for motor skills is typically carried out in two main steps. First, it is necessary to determine the specific gaze characteristics of experts (e.g., the QE) as they perform the motor skill of interest, and identify how these differ from those of non-expert performers. Second, novice performers are then taught to follow this 'expert model' while they perform training repetitions of the to-be-learned task. In some studies, the performer is provided with feedback of their own eye movements after they have performed the task (feedback; FBEMT) as well as the expert model to replicate (feedforward; FFEMT; e.g., Wilson et al., 2011). This may provide the performer with information that is not necessarily open to introspection (it is often hard to determine what you are paying attention to), and also provides them with evidence of lapses in focus of attention. The objective is for performers to be able to detect differences in where they are currently with the expert model and work on 'closing the gap'.

The Practicalities

In order to perform a gaze training intervention it is necessary to create a first person video recording of the expert performing the task using a mobile eye tracker (e.g. Figure 11.1). Tracking the movements of the eye in space is a non-invasive technique that is commonly used by

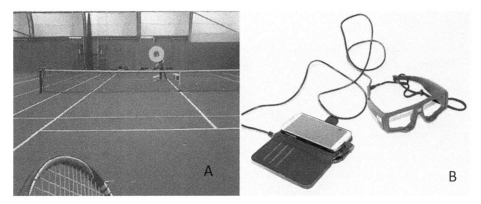

Figure 11.1   A still image from the eye tracking video that is produced by combining the eye camera (location of gaze; the grey circle) and the scene camera (A); and a mobile eye tracker, displaying the head mounted goggles, and the digital recording device (worn by the subject) that stores the eye and scene video data, connected by a USB cable (B).

researchers to understand human behaviour and movement. Technological advancements have allowed for the development of mobile head mounted eye trackers, that allow for the assessment of eye movements in natural environments, and therefore a more representative assessment of the functionality of these eye movements (see Panchuk, Vine, & Vickers, 2015). The mobile eye tracker captures both the scene in front (with a head mounted camera) and the eye movements (with either monocular or binocular eye recording cameras). Software automatically combines these two videos to provide a vision-in-action video. The point of gaze is depicted as a 'cursor' (a dot, a circle or a crosshair), which is then viewed in the video Figure 11.1).

In many examples of FFEMT, the visual display of eye movements is accompanied by verbal instructions. These instructions act to verbalise what is being displayed in the video to further clarify what trainees need to mimic. For example, for FFEMT of motor skills, gaze videos are accompanied by a list of bullet points summarising the critical learning points from the video (Moore, Vine, Cooke, Ring, & Wilson, 2012), or a training video may have an audio commentary (Miles, Wood, Vine, Vickers, & Wilson, 2015).

Vickers (2016) discusses a specific seven-step program that she proposes should be used for QE training:

1   *Define expert QE prototype.* The first step is to isolate the QE of elite performers in the task during successful and unsuccessful trials.
2   *Test trainees in the same task.* The trainee is tested in the same task using a mobile eye tracker and a motion analysis system in conditions similar to those used in step 1.
3   *Provide instruction of QE characteristics.* The trainee should be shown the QE video data of an elite QE prototype (derived from step 1) and taught the importance of the QE using the frame- by-frame video controls.
4   *Provide QE feedback.* Video feedback is used to show the trainee his/her own QE as collected in step 2, in comparison to the elite prototype using side-by-side QE videos. The key is to cognitively probe how much the athletes understand about the control of their attentional focus as they perform.
5   *Decision training.* The trainee decides how he/she wants to work on improving QE. This is an important step as it passes control to the athletes in terms of learning how to master their attention. Re-test often using the eye tracker and plot improvements.

6   *Blocked and random training.* Blocked training drills are designed to promote the desired QE focus in repetitive trials with little variation. Variable and random drills are designed to help master the gaze strategy in more game-like situations (Vickers, 2007).

7   *Assess competitive QE.* Performance in competition should be assessed and follow-up QE tests carried out, as needed, designed to improve the athlete's performance in a variety of real-world competitive situations.

Training Perceptual-Motor Tasks

There has been increasing interest in the use of gaze training interventions to support efficient and effective visuomotor skill acquisition in a range of environments (including, surgical, military, aviation, and clinical populations). The research has followed three main lines of enquiry: (1) training expert performers to fine-tune skills, (2) training novices to acquire new skills, and (3) in both cases, trying to determine if the learning is more resilient to relevant transfer conditions (e.g., multi-tasking, pressure, etc.). This chapter will focus on (2) and (3). In terms of task types, these tend to be broken down into those requiring accurate aiming to a far target (e.g., golf putting); those requiring the interception of an object (e.g. catching, shotgun shooting); and those requiring the manipulation and fine control of objects (e.g., surgery).

Far Aiming Tasks

The most studied far aiming task in the gaze training literature is the golf putt. The visuomotor control involved in the golf putt was first explored in Vickers' (1992) seminal paper. This study found that experts and near experts differed in the extent to which they maintained a focused, steady gaze on the back of the ball prior to and during the putting stroke and held this until just after contact. Experts initiated their gaze earlier and held it for longer; a strategy that was later defined as the quiet eye (QE; Vickers, 1996). Vine and Wilson (2010) were the first to apply this knowledge to the training of novice golfers, and found that the QE-trained participants performed better than a control group (receiving putting instructions from a well-known coaching book) after training. Similar positive effects have also been found in the skill of basketball free throw shooting. Vine and Wilson (2011) replicated their findings for golf putting by revealing benefits of QE training for basketball free throw. As with Vine and Wilson (2010), the benefits of QE training transferred to a highly pressurised condition in which performers were cognitively anxious. The QE trained group managed to maintain their performance, despite the anxiety, likely due to the effective maintenance of their attentional control.

Interestingly, Vine, Moore, & Wilson (2011) revealed similar benefits for a brief (one hour) QE training intervention with already skilled golfers. Relative increases in QE and performance in a laboratory-based putting task were found, compared with a control group. The benefits also transferred to the competition environment with the QE trained golfers revealing a relative improvement in golf putting performance on the course; taking 1.92 fewer putts per round and holing 5% more putts from six to 10 feet following the training. Again, the control group revealed no significant changes in on-course putting performance.

Moore et al. (2012) extended Vine and Wilson's (2010) study to examine some of the processes that might underlie the performance advantage of QE-training. These authors found that not only did the QE-trained performers reveal the accuracy and QE advantage from the earlier study (see Figure 11.2), but also, that they also revealed more efficient putting kinematics, left arm extensor carpi radialis muscle activation, and cardiac deceleration. In effect, QE-training resulted in changes to the mechanics of the putting stroke and the general psychophysiological state of the performer without these being explicitly taught. Importantly, these differences were most pronounced under

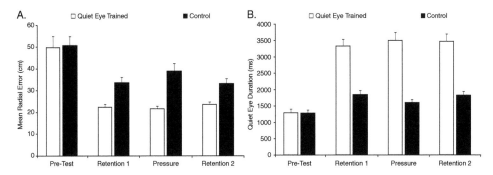

Figure 11.2 Moore et al. (2012) found significant interaction effects for both radial error (A) and QE duration (B) across the test conditions. The QE-trained group had generally longer QE durations and better performance after training, but this effect was most pronounced under pressure. The control group revealed drops in performance and QE when under pressure whereas the QE-trained group were insulated against these deficits.

pressure, suggesting that QE-training not only expedites the skill acquisition process, but also helps to ensure that the skills are resilient when performed under competitive conditions.

Harle and Vickers (2001) performed one of the first QET interventions in sport in an attempt to improve the free throw accuracy of a Canadian Women's basketball team. One team (team A) took part in a QE training regime and two other teams (B and C) acted as control groups. The QE of each member of team A was recorded and viewed relative to an elite prototype in a feedback session using vision-in-action data (Vickers, 1996). Participants were then taught a three step QE training regime aimed at improving their visuo-motor control. In the laboratory, team A showed a significant increase in QE from pre (783 ms) to post (981 ms) and this was accompanied by a significant improvement in free throw accuracy (12%). Results also showed that training transferred to match performance: after two seasons of competitive play, team A had improved their free throw percentage by 23%, whereas the free-throw performance of teams B and C remained relatively constant.

Interception Tasks

Causer, Holmes, & Williams (2011) examined QE training in shotgun shooting. Twenty international level skeet shooters were assigned to either a QE trained or control group and tested before and after an eight-week intervention. The QE trained group were shown video feedback of their eye movements and taught a pre-shot routine aimed at lengthening their QE. After training, the QE trained group had a significantly earlier onset of QE on the clay, tracked it for longer and demonstrated significantly improved performance, while the control group revealed no significant changes in QE or performance.

Also in a shooting task Moore, Vine, Smith, Smith, & Wilson (2014) examined the benefits of QE training in a simulated maritime marksmanship task. The task required novice gunners to shot at fast approaching moving targets with a decommissioned general-purpose machine gun. Twenty participants were randomly assigned to a quiet eye trained (QET) or technical trained (TT) group and completed two baseline, 20 training, and two retention trials on the moving-target task. Compared to their TT counterparts, the QET group displayed more effective gaze control (longer quiet eye durations and greater target locking) and more accurate performance (smaller radial error of both the initial shot and average of all shots) at retention. These findings highlight the potential for quiet eye training to be used to support the training of marksmanship skills in military settings.

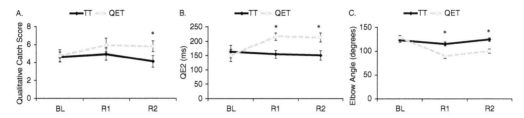

Figure 11.3 Data from Miles et al. (2015). The qualitative catching performance score (a), QE2 duration (b), and elbow angle at catch (c) for technique-trained (TT) and Quiet eye trained (QET) groups across baseline (pre-training), immediately post training (R1, retention 1), and four weeks post training (R2, retention 2) conditions. (Error bars represent s.e.m.).

Until recently, QE-based training interventions had not been applied to children or to clinical groups. Developmental Coordination Disorder (DCD) affects approximately 6% of children (depending on the stringency of diagnostic criteria; Hendrix, Prins, & Dekkers, 2014). Wilson, Miles, Vine, & Vickers (2013) examined gaze behaviour in eight- to ten-year-old children as they performed a throw and catch task, and were able to determine QE periods for both the throw and catch attempt that mediated performance differences between high and low coordinated participants. This information was used to develop a video-based QE training protocol that was piloted on typically developing children (Miles, Vine, Wood, Vickers, & Wilson, 2014) before being applied to children with DCD (Miles, Wood et al., 2015). Compared to a group taught to focus on their catching technique (technique-training), the QE-trained group improved their catching success (Figure 11.3a), by lengthening the time they tracked the ball into their hands (QE2; Figure 11.3b) and by implicitly changing their catching technique (reducing their elbow angle thereby catching the ball closer to their chests; Figure 11.3c).

Manual Dextrous Control

An important goal of surgical education research is to better understand the psychomotor mechanisms that underpin surgery, and to predict how these are influenced by directed training. This is particularly important given the perceptual-motor demands of performing laparoscopic surgery, where additional constraints are placed on the operator due to the use of long stemmed surgical tools and a 2-dimensional screen. Wilson and colleagues found systematic differences in the gaze strategies of experienced laparoscopic surgeons compared to novices as they completed training tasks in a virtual reality learning environment (Wilson, McGrath, Vine, Brewer, Defriend, & Masters, 2010; 2011). As predicted by the sensorimotor mapping model of Sailer et al. (2005), experts tended to lock their gaze on the target, whereas novices had more scattered gaze control, frequently switching between the instruments they were controlling and the target.

Wilson, Vine et al. (2011) used video-based training instructions to assess the benefits of gaze-focused information compared to information about the movements of tools (technique-focused information), using the same task as adopted in their previous expert-novice study (Wilson et al., 2010). A video of a representative trial from one of the experts was used to create training videos. In the gaze-focused video, the gaze cursor revealing the eye movements was visible and participants were instructed to adopt these same eye movements (feed *forward* eye movement training). Participants were shown their own videos after each of their 10 learning trials and were asked to compare their gaze behaviour to the expert model (feed*back* eye movement training). In the movement-focused video, the gaze cursor was removed and participants were instructed to

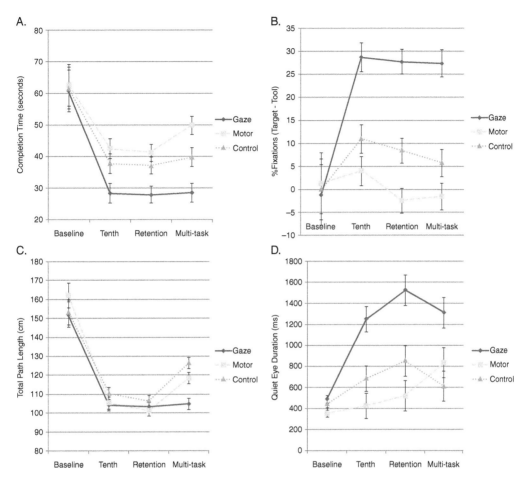

Figure 11.4   Mean (± s.e.m.) completion time (A), target locking gaze strategy (B), tool path length (C) and quiet eye duration (D) for gaze, motor and control groups across baseline, tenth training trial, retention and multi-tasking trials. After training, the gaze-trained group revealed significantly more expert-like performance and process measures than the other comparative groups (Wilson, Vine et al., 2011).

adopt the smooth tool movements of the expert. As with the gaze-trained group, they were provided with video feedback after each learning trial. A third group received no video instruction but completed the same number of training repetitions on the task. Not only did the gaze-trained group reveal more expert-like gaze behaviour, but they also used a more efficient technique (as indexed by tool path metrics) and completed the task more quickly than either of the other two groups. Importantly, this performance advantage was even greater under multi-tasking conditions (a tone counting task), designed to replicate the more complex environment inherent in the operating theatre (see Figure 11.4).

How Does Gaze Training 'Work'?

One of the limitations with the gaze training literature is that it is not always clear as to *why* it provides a performance advantage. There are several potential explanations, but differences in the nature of the task, the delivery of the training and the findings of each study make it very difficult to draw clear conclusions. Below are some of the explanations posed:

Gaze Training as a Form of Implicit Learning

It is possible that gaze training, by directing gaze via visualisation of an expert model, limits the accrual of explicit (declarative) knowledge about the rules governing task performance. Eye movement training has been found to limit declarative knowledge in perceptual motor tasks when used with novices (e.g., Vine, Moore, Cooke, Ring, & Wilson, 2013). Therefore, gaze training may help individuals to learn in an implicit manner, acquire skills/tasks more quickly, and perform better under pressure. Thomas and Lleras (2009) provide support for the suggestion that explicit attention guidance may be less beneficial than implicit attention guidance. Often, the guiding of eye movements is not viewed by participants as overt "hints" at the problem's solution or the correct decision, but rather as distracting and interfering (Thomas & lleras, 2007). As such, this provides further evidence for an implicit link between eye movement patterns and spatial cognition.

Attentional Control

Joint Attention

Gaze training may act to mimic mechanisms of learning seen in early childhood. Young children obtain information about what is important in their environment by mimicking the focus of attention of others (*joint attention*). Children will follow the eye movements of elders/carers to develop an understanding of the task they are engaged in and the relative importance of the objects in the environment (Tomasello, 1995). This form of learning is maintained to some extent in adulthood, as other people's gaze behaviour provides a salient example of where others are allocating their attention and directing their resources (Friesen & Kingstone, 1998). Individuals seem to instinctively assess the value of a location of a scene based on the gaze of others (Bayliss, Paul, Cannon, & Tipper, 2006). As such, in gaze training the trainee is seeing a visualisation of the expert's eye movements. This perhaps acts to enhance or augment the information obtained from joint attention. This idea is encapsulated nicely by the work of Argyle and Cook (1976) who discuss the dual function of gaze: *"whenever organisms use vision, the eyes become signals as well as channels"* (p. xi). In other words, the eyes both gather information (i.e., act as a channel) and communicate information to others (i.e., act as a signal).

Focusing on Relevant Information

Gaze training may help trainees simply to focus on the information within the scene that is most important to task performance. Visualising, as opposed to verbalising this information may make it more salient and easily 'digested' by the learner. This is in keeping with the observational learning literature (Fryling, Johnston, & Hayes, 2011). Experts, through learning, have developed excellent knowledge of the spatial and temporal (sequence) nature in which information needs to be extracted from a scene in order to make good decisions and perform well; visualising this for novices provides an insight into these processes and helps them to acquire appropriate attentional control. This 'development of attention' viewpoint suggests that we are highly sensitive to ostensive cues that direct attention and guide cognition in ways that are vital for learning (e.g., Csibra & Gergely, 2009).

Visuomotor Control

Specifically related to perceptual motor tasks, Vine et al. (2014) outlined three proposed causal mechanisms for gaze training related to improved attentional, visuomotor, and psychological control. Most researchers have linked attentional and visuomotor explanations to the importance of extracting the most relevant and timely visual information to support response planning (while ignoring distractions). Learners are guided to coordinate the gaze and motor systems in an effective way that simplifies the problem of visually guided movement for the central nervous system. This benefit is supported by the motor control literature that shows that early and accurate fixations pass visually acquired goal position information to the motor control systems, ensuring accurate movements (Land, 2009; Sailer et al., 2005). However, some evidence has been presented which suggests that the simplicity of the intervention (focus on one external cue) helps individuals to maintain a sense of psychological control (Wood & Wilson, 2012) and a 'challenge' mentality (Moore, Vine, Freeman, & Wilson, 2013) when faced with a pressurised situation. The benefits are therefore likely to be multi-factorial.

Embodied Perception

Some researchers offer an embodied cognition explanation of gaze training. It is possible that task-related attentional shifts that are spatially and temporarily matched with a solution or appropriate decision could assist learning and performance. Although it may often seem that attention and eye movements are the result of cognitive processing, it may be that sometimes cognitive processing is the result of attention and eye movements. Attentional shifts provide an embodied physical mechanism that triggers a perceptual simulation of an insightful solution (e.g., Barsalou, 1999). Growing evidence is showing just how intertwined the interactions among the visual environment, attention, and mental operations are (e.g., Ballard, Hayhoe, Pook, & Rao, 1997). Gaze training may exploit this relationship and enable trainees to develop cognitive solutions to problems.

Caveats

While there is research supporting the efficacy of gaze training, the specific mechanisms supporting its benefits are not as well clarified. For example, it is unlikely that the same mechanisms that help QET-trained children with DCD improve their throw and catch performance (Miles et al., 2015), are the same that help QE-trained, single handicap golfers improve their putting statistics (Vine et al., 2011). Wilson et al. (2016) suggested that in order to improve our understanding of QET mechanisms there is a need to consider; appropriate control groups (not just technical-training) and transfer tasks (are there any cross-over benefits?); the exploration of QE dose-response relationships (is an optimal threshold duration enough?); the manipulation of the timing and location of the QE period (what degree of variability can be withstood before performance disruption occurs?); and the role of different phases of the QE (is early or late information more important?).

There are also practical issues surrounding exactly how long training should last to be optimal; whether verbal instructions are enough or whether the video model is critical; and when in the 'learning' curve training will have most impact. These questions are harder to answer due to the variations in research methodologies used. For example, some studies use a single training session with absolute novices (Vine & Wilson, 2010) and some will use multiple session with elite athletes (Causer et al., 2011).

Conclusion

To conclude, the objective of gaze training is to guide a performer's judgement as to where and when to fixate their gaze when executing a motor skill in order to process the most relevant information guiding the planning and control of the action (Vine et al., 2014). While there is increasing support for the efficacy of gaze training in a variety of environments, the underpinning processes supporting its utility are less clear. It is likely that a combination of factors is at play and that the benefits may be task specific. Future research is needed to explore the attentional, neural, physiological, mechanical, and psychological mechanisms by which gaze training delivers its benefits (Wilson, Wood, & Vine, 2016).

References

Argyle, M., & Cook, M. (1976). *Gaze and mutual gaze*. Cambridge, England, UK: Cambridge University Press.

Ballard, D. H., Hayhoe, M. M., Pook, P. K., & Rao, R. P. N. (1997). Deictic codes for the embodiment of cognition. *Behavioral and Brain Sciences, 20*, 723–767.

Barsalou, L. W. (1999). Perceptual symbol systems. *Behavioral and Brain Sciences, 22*, 577–660.

Bayliss, A. P., Paul, M. A., Cannon, P. R., & Tipper, S. P. (2006). Gaze cuing and affective judgments of objects: I like what you look at. *Psychonomic Bulletin & Review, 13*, 1061–1066.

Broadbent, D. P., Causer, J. A., Williams, M., & Ford, P. R. (2014). Perceptual-cognitive skill training and its transfer to expert performance in the field: Future research directions. *European Journal of Sport Science*, doi: 10.1080/17461391.2014.957727.

Causer, J., Holmes, P. S., & Williams, A. M. (2011). Quiet eye training in a visuomotor control task. *Medicine & Science in Sports & Exercise, 43*, 1042–1049. doi:10.1249/Mss.0b013e3 182035de6

Chetwood, A. S. A., Kwok, K. W., Sun, L. W., Mylonas, G. P., Clark, J, Darzi, A., & Yang, G. Z. (2012). Collaborative eye tracking: a potential training tool in laparoscopic surgery. *Surgical Endoscopy, 26*, 2003–2009.

Corbetta, M., Akbudak, E., Conturo, T. E., Snyder, A. Z., Ollinger, J. M., Drury, H. A., & Shulman, G. L. (1998). A common network of functional areas for attention and eye movements. *Neuron, 21*(4), 761–773.

Csibra, G., & Gergely, G. (2009). Natural pedagogy. *Trends in Cognitive Sciences, 13*, 148–153.

Friesen, C. K., & Kingstone, A. (1998). The eyes have it! Reflexive orienting is triggered by nonpredictive gaze. *Psychonomic Bulletin & Review, 5*, 490–495.

Fryling, M. J., Johnston, C., & Hayes, L. J. (2011). Understanding observational learning: An interbehavioral approach. *The Analysis of Verbal Behavior, 27*(1), 191–203.

Gegenfurtner, A., Lehtinen, E., & Säljö, R. (2011). Expertise differences in the comprehension of Visualizations: A meta-analysis of eye-tracking research in professional domains. *Educational Psychology Review, 23*, 523–552. doi: 10.1007/s10648-011-9174-7.

Harle, S., & Vickers, J. N. (2001). Training quiet eye improves accuracy in the basketball free-throw. *The Sport Psychologist, 15*, 289–305.

Hendrix, C. G., Prins, M. R., & Dekkers, H. (2014). Developmental coordination disorder and overweight and obesity in children: A systematic review. *Obesity Reviews, 15*(5), 408–423. doi: 10.1111/obr.12137.

Jarodzka, H., van Gog, T. A. J. M., Dorr, M., Scheiter, K., & Gerjets, P. (2013). Learning to see: Guiding students' attention via a Model's eye movements fosters learning. *Learning and Instruction, 25*, 62–70. doi:10.1016/j.learninstruc.2012.11.004.

Land, M. F. (2009). Vision, eye movements, and natural behavior. *Visual Neuroscience, 26*(1), 51–62. doi: 10.1017/s0952523808080899.

Litchfield, D., & Ball, L. J. (2011). Using another's gaze as an explicit aid to insight problem solving. *The Quarterly Journal of Experimental Psychology, 64*(4), 649–656. doi: 10.1080/17470218.2011.558628.

Miles, C. A. L., Vine, S. J., Wood, G., Vickers, J. N., & Wilson, M. R. (2014). Quiet eye training improves throw and catch performance in children. *Psychology of Sport & Exercise, 15*(5), 511–515. doi: 10.1016/j.psychsport.2014.04.009.

Miles, C. A. L., Wood, G., Vine, S. J., Vickers, J. N., & Wilson, M. R. (2015). Quiet Eye Training facilitates visuomotor coordination in children with developmental coordination disorder. *Research in Developmental Disabilities, 40*, 31–41. doi: 10.1016/j.ridd.2015.01.005.

Moore, L. J., Vine, S. J., Cooke, A., Ring, C., & Wilson, M. R. (2012). Quiet eye training expedites motor learning and aids performance under heightened anxiety: The roles of response programming and external attention. *Psychophysiology, 49*(7), 1005–1015. doi: 10.1111/j.1469–8986.2012.01379.x.

Moore, L. J., Vine, S. J., Freeman, P., & Wilson, M. R. (2013). Quiet eye training promotes challenge appraisals and aids performance under elevated anxiety. *International Journal of Sport & Exercise Psychology, 11*(2), 169–183. doi: 10.1080/1612197X.2013.773688.

Moore, L. J., Vine, S. J., Smith, A., Smith, S. J., & Wilson, M. R. (2014). Quiet eye training improves small arms maritime marksmanship. *Military Psychology, 26*, 355–365, doi: 10.1037/mil0000039.

Panchuk, D., Vine, S. J., & Vickers, J. (2015). *Eye Tracking Methods in Sport Expertise*. In J. Baker & D. Farrow (Eds.), *Routledge Handbook of Sport Expertise* (pp. 176–186). London, UK: Routledge.

Rienhoff, R., Tirp, J., Strauss, B., Baker, J., & Schorer, J. (2015). The "Quiet Eye" and motor performance: A systematic review based on Newell's constraints-led model. *Sports Medicine*, Epub ahead of print. doi: 10.1007/s40279-015-0442-4.

Roads, B., Mozer, M. C., & Busey, T. A. (2016). Using Highlighting to Train Attentional Expertise. *PLoS One, 11*(1), e0146266. doi:10.1371/journal.pone.0146266.

Sailer, U., Flanagan, J. R., & Johansson, R. S. (2005). Eye-hand coordination during learning of a novel visuomotor task. *Journal of Neuroscience, 25*, 8833–8842.

Tatler, B. W., Hayhoe, M. M., Land, M. F., & Ballard, D. H. (2011). Eye guidance in natural vision: Reinterpreting salience. *Journal of Vision, 11*(5), 5, 1–23. doi: 10.1167/11.5.5.

Thomas, L. E., & Lleras, A. (2007). Moving eyes and moving thought: On the spatial compatibility between eye movements and cognition. *Psychonomic Bulletin & Review, 14*, 663–668.

Thomas, L. E., & Lleras, A. (2009). Covert shifts of attention function as an implicit aid to insight. *Cognition, 111*, 168–174.

Tomasello, M. (1995). Joint attention as social cognition. In C. Moore & P. Dunham (Eds.), *Joint Attention: Its Origins and Role in Development*. Mahwah, NJ: Lawrence Erlbaum Associates.

van Donkelaar, P., & Staub, J. (2000). Eye-hand coordination to visual versus remembered targets. *Experimental Brain Research, 133*(3), 414–418.

Vickers, J. N. (1992). Gaze control in putting. *Perception, 21,* 117–132.

Vickers, J. N. (1996). Visual control when aiming at a far target. *Journal of Experimental Psychology-Human Perception and Performance, 22*(2), 342–354. doi: 10.1037/0096–1523.22.2.342.

Vickers, J. N. (2007). *Perception, cognition & decision training: The Quiet Eye in action*. Champaign, IL: Human Kinetics.

Vickers, J. N. (2016). Origins and current issues in quiet eye research. *Current Issues in Sport Science, 1*, 101. doi: 10.15203/CISS_2016.101.

Vine, S. J., & Wilson, M. R. (2010). Quiet eye training: effects on learning and performance under pressure. *Journal of Applied Sport Psychology, 22*(4), 361–376. doi: 10.1080/10413200.2010.495106.

Vine, S. J., & Wilson, M. R. (2011). The influence of quiet eye training and pressure on attention and visuo-motor control. *Acta Psychologica, 136*(3), 340–346. doi: 10.1016/j.actpsy.2010.12.008.

Vine, S. J., Moore, L. J., Cooke, A., Ring, C., & Wilson, M. R. (2013). Quiet eye training: A means to implicit motor learning. *International Journal of Sport Psychology, 44*(4), 367–386. doi: 10.7352/ijsp2013.44.367.

Vine, S. J., Moore, L. J., & Wilson, M. R. (2014). Quiet eye training: The acquisition, refinement and resilient performance of targeting skills. *European Journal of Sport Science, 14*, S235–S242. doi: 10.1080/17461391.2012.683815.

Wang, M. J., Lin, S., & Drury, C. G. (1997). Training for strategy in visual search. *International Journal of Industrial Ergonomics, 20*(2), 101–108. doi:10.1016/S0169-8141(96)00043-1.

Wilson, M. R., Causer, J., & Vickers, J. N. (2015). Aiming for excellence: The quiet eye as a characteristic of expert visuomotor performance. In J. Baker & D. Farrow (eds.) *The Routledge handbook of sport expertise* (pp. 22–37). London, UK: Routledge.

Wilson, M. R., McGrath, J., Vine, S. J., Brewer, J., Defriend, D, & Masters, R. S. W. (2010). Psychomotor control in a virtual laparoscopic surgery training environment: Gaze control parameters differentiate novices from experts. *Surgical Endoscopy, 24*, 2458–2464.

Wilson, M. R., McGrath, J. S., Vine, S. J., Brewer, J., Defriend, D., & Masters, R. S. W. (2011). Perceptual impairment and psychomotor control in virtual laparoscopic surgery. *Surgical Endoscopy and Other Interventional Techniques, 25*(7), 2268–2274. doi: 10.1007/s00464-010-1546-4.

Wilson, M. R., Miles, C. A. L., Vine, S. J., & Vickers, J. N. (2013). Quiet eye distinguishes children of high and low motor coordination abilities. *Medicine and Science in Sports and Exercise, 45*(6), 1144–1151. doi: 10.1249/MSS.0b013e31828288f1.

Wilson, M. R., Vine, S. J., Bright, E., Masters, R. S. W., Defriend, D., & McGrath, J. S. (2011). Gaze training enhances laparoscopic technical skill acquisition and multi-tasking performance: A randomized controlled study. *Surgical Endoscopy, 25*, 3731–3739.

Wilson, M. R., Wood, G., & Vine, S. J. (2016). Say it quietly, but we still do not know how Quiet Eye training works – comment on Vickers. *Current Issues in Sport Science, 1*, 117. doi: 10.15203/CISS_2016.117.

Wood, G., & Wilson, M. R. (2012). Quiet-eye training, perceived control and performing under pressure. *Psychology of Sport and Exercise, 13*, 721–728. doi: 10.1016/j.psychsport.2012.05.003.

Cognitive Strategies to Enhance Motor Performance

Examples of Applying Action Observation, Motor Imagery and Psyching-up Techniques

Ambra Bisio and Marco Bove

This chapter will focus on different aspects of motor cognition and on the possibility of stimulating the motor system and improving motor performance by acting at central level. Although a lot of interesting research has been done in the rehabilitation field, this chapter will present studies on healthy subjects, with particular emphasis on athletes and sport science. In the first part, a definition of motor resonance, and its role in movement planning and execution, will be discussed. The second part will present the motor imagery technique and why it might be considered an "offline operation" of the motor system. The possibility of learning new motor abilities by means of motor resonance, in particular via action observation and motor imagery, will be the topic of the third part. The fourth part will describe the most recent findings on the application of these techniques in sport science. Finally, in the fifth part cognitive strategies, known as psyching-up techniques, and their application in sport domains will be introduced.

Motor Resonance: How Action Perception Is Involved in Movement Planning and Execution

Humans live in a word full of stimuli coming from other humans, animals, inanimate objects, sounds, and motions. How do people interpret these stimuli? How do they react to moving objects or actions performed by other humans? At the end of the 20th century, the discovery of the mirror neuron system (MNS) opened up a new field of research that provided the possibility of explaining the unexplored connection between perception of visual and auditory stimuli, movement, action understanding, and motor learning. All these processes seem to be connected to each other by a resonance mechanism that is evoked during action perception, namely *motor resonance*. Motor resonance is a phenomenon consisting of a significant increase of the activity of the brain's cortical areas during the observation of actions performed by other individuals and while listening to action sounds (Rizzolatti, Fadiga, Fogassi, & Gallese, 1999). The discovery of motor resonance gave rise to the *direct matching hypothesis*, which states that "we understand actions when we map the visual representation of the observed action onto our motor representation of the same action" (p. 661) (Rizzolatti, Fogassi, & Gallese, 2001). This means that the motor knowledge of the observer "resonates" with the observed action and that "we understand an action because the motor representation of that action is activated in our brain" (p. 661) (Rizzolatti et al., 2001). Due to its peculiar features, the activation of the MNS was also advanced as a prerequisite for imitation (Craighero, Bello, Fadiga, & Rizzolatti, 2002; Marco Iacoboni, 2009; Rizzolatti et al., 2001), social/cognitive behaviors (Vittorio Gallese & Goldman, 1998), and speech/language processing (Fadiga, Craighero, Buccino, & Rizzolatti, 2002). In order to understand the principle of motor resonance and how it is involved in action understanding and motor imitation, it is useful to make a brief digression on the mirror neuron system and on its properties.

The Neurophysiological Basis of Motor Resonance: The Mirror Neuron System

In the 1990s, a group of Italian neuroscientists working on macaque monkeys discovered a particular set of visuomotor neurons located in the premotor area of the animal's brain (area F5), which discharged both during the monkey's active movements and when the monkey observed meaningful hand movements made by the experimenter (di Pellegrino, Fadiga, Fogassi, Gallese, & Rizzolatti, 1992; Gallese, Fadiga, Fogassi, & Rizzolatti, 1996; Rizzolatti, Fadiga, Gallese, & Fogassi, 1996). These neurons, subsequently called *mirror neurons*, because they discharge in the same way when non-human and human subjects recreate the observed action, together with neurons discovered in the rostral part of the inferior parietal lobule (area 7b) that have the same properties (Gallese, Fadiga, Fogassi, & Rizzolatti, 2002), represent the core of the MNS.

A huge amount of data from neurophysiological and brain imaging experiments provided strong clues on the existence of an MNS in humans also (Rizzolatti & Craighero, 2004). The first evidence goes back to the studies on the reactivity of cerebral rhythms during movement observation performed by Gastaut and Bert (1954), who showed a modification of the electroencephalographic (EEG) mu rhythm typical of movement execution during movement observation. But it took 40 years for the terms mirror neuron and motor resonance to be associated with humans.

Initial evidence came from studies using transcranial magnetic stimulation (TMS). TMS is a non-invasive technique using a magnetic field to activate neurons located a few centimeters under the coil. A brief stimulation over the cortical representation of a body part in the primary motor cortex (M1) activates the corticospinal tract and evokes a response called motor evoked potential (MEP) in the corresponding contralateral muscle. By means of TMS, Fadiga and colleagues (1995) showed an increase of MEP amplitude when volunteers observed a grasping action or a meaningless arm gesture. This effect was only seen in the muscles that participants used for producing the observed movement. Motor facilitation was explained as the result of the increase activity of M1 due to the mirror activity of the premotor areas from which M1 receives input. This result was confirmed by Maeda and colleagues (2002), who found that this motor resonance effect was evoked during the observation of intransitive, not goal-oriented movement, differently from what was observed in monkeys. Furthermore, another TMS study showed that the time course of cortical facilitation followed the phases of the observed action (Gangitano, Mottaghy, & Pascual-Leone, 2001). Therefore, the results of TMS studies indirectly pointed out the existence of a human MNS, responsible for motor resonance mechanisms.

Brain imaging studies enabled identifying the brain's regions which form the core of the human MNS, namely the rostral part of the inferior parietal lobule and the lower part of the precentral gyrus, together with the posterior part of the inferior frontal gyrus (Buccino et al., 2001; Iacoboni et al., 1999; Iacoboni, 2009). The former codes mostly for the goal of observing motor acts (Rizzolatti, Fogassi, & Gallese, 2002), and the second one is thought to be involved in mirroring others' emotions (Gallese, Keysers, & Rizzolatti, 2004; Singer, 2006).

The first direct proof of the existence of neurons with mirror properties in humans came from a study in 2010 (Mukamel, Ekstrom, & Kaplan, 2010). In this study, researchers realized single neuron recordings from epileptic patients implanted with intracranial depth electrodes and identified neurons with mirror properties in the supplementary motor cortex (SMA), hippocampus, and entorhinal cortex.

Therefore, once the existence of such neurons in humans has been demonstrated (although some controversies persist, see Hickok, 2009), it is important to present the experimental evidence that helps to understand how they are involved in action perception and movement planning.

Motor Resonance during Action Observation

Motor resonance is the coupling between action and perception that causes the automatic activation of the perceiver's motor system during action perception (Rizzolatti et al., 1999). As mentioned before, after Fadiga *et al*.'s study (1995), several works confirmed that observing movement activates the motor system.

Motor resonance can also be evoked during the observation of moving visual stimulus whose pictorial image is not a human form but is degraded, as in the case of *point-light display*. Point-light displays are made by image sequences deriving from a human actor with point-light attached to their body. Contrary to when static images are presented, when starting to move, these images are recognized as human body in motion (Johansson, 1973), even if lacking other visual cues such as colors, shading, and contours.

In a study by Saygin and his colleagues (2004), participants' brain activity was monitored by means of functional magnetic resonance imaging (fMRI) technique during the observation of point-light biological motion and scrambled animations (the latter created by randomizing the starting position of the point-light while keeping the trajectories intact). The results showed that actions characterized by solely motor cues activate the frontal part of the MNS. In particular, frontal areas showed selective increased responsivity to biological motion compared with scrambled stimuli, supporting the hypothesis that motion information can drive inferior frontal and premotor areas involved in action perception.

The relevance of biological motion in activating motor resonance mechanisms was also shown in behavioral studies on automatic imitation. *Imitation* is a motor response that can be interpreted as the behavioral consequence of the matching between perception and action at central level (Wohlschläger, Gattis, & Bekkering, 2003), and it has been suggested that it plays a central role in human development and learning of motor, communicative, and social skills (Piaget, 1952; Tomasello, Kruger, & Ratner, 1993). *Automatic imitation* is an unconscious phenomenon occurring when people react to moving stimuli (Heyes, 2011). From a general perspective, automatic imitation might be considered a combination of two mechanisms: motor priming and motor contagion (Sciutti et al., 2012). Motor priming is responsible for the initial motion facilitation that is present when the observer reacts to stimuli moving in the same way the observer has to move, and consists in a decrease of the reaction time when starting a movement (Heyes, Bird, Johnson, & Haggard, 2005). Motor contagion is the implicit reproduction of some features of the observed action and can be evaluated by comparing the movement kinematics of the observer with that of the stimulus (Blakemore & Frith, 2005). The occurrence of automatic imitation could thus be considered as a sign of the activation of motor resonance mechanisms.

An example of motor priming comes from Brass *et al*.'s study (2001). Participants were engaged in several versions of simple reaction time tasks, during which they have to lift their index finger in response to the observation of a compatible or an incompatible movement. They found that index finger movements were executed faster in response to observed compatible movements than in response to observed incompatible movements. This result was subsequently extended to the observation of robotic movement (Press, Gillmeister, & Heyes, 2006), and depends on the experience participants have with the observed stimulus (Press, Gillmeister, & Heyes, 2007).

Concerning motor contagion, Bove *et al*.'s study (2009) considered the concept of spontaneous movement tempo (SMT), namely the spontaneous and preferred rate for self-paced movements (Bove et al., 2007), that in normal subjects is about 2 Hz. In that behavioral study, Bove tested whether the frequency of self-paced finger movements was modified by prior observation of motion performed at different rates. Participants performed a sequence of finger opposition movements after observing a video showing the same movements at a lower, similar, and higher rate than the SMT. Their findings showed that mere action observation influenced participants' SMT; indeed, after observing movements at a lower/higher rate than their SMT, they moved slower/

faster with respect to a baseline condition. Accordingly, Bisio and colleagues (2010) showed that the automatic tendency to imitate the velocity of the observed movement was present when looking at movements performed by a human demonstrator. This study went further showing that automatic imitation persisted when the visual stimulus was not a human but a white dot displayed on a black screen and whose motion originated from a human agent moving his arm. This result is in line with the results of an fMRI study by Saygin and colleagues (2004) showing the occurrence of motor resonance phenomena when looking at point-light display in motion, but with kinematics that belonged to the biological motor repertoire. These findings suggest that these artificial stimuli, despite totally lacking visual cues, conveyed sufficient information about movements to activate sensorimotor processes similar to those typically evoked by human AO. Furthermore, Bisio *et al.* (2010) also showed that automatic imitation disappeared when a uniformly accelerated motion, not belonging to the motor repertoire of a biological agent, moved the dot, suggesting that the possibility of mapping the observed kinematics onto the internal motor repertoire is a requisite to evoking motor resonance. Similar results were obtained when the visual stimulus was a humanoid robot (Bisio et al., 2014). Namely, automatic imitation was equally evoked by the observation of a human demonstrator and by the observation of a humanoid robot, but only when it moved according to the biological laws of motion.

That the motor system discriminates between biological and non-biological movement has been demonstrated, and its response seems to be modulated by the similarity between the motor repertoire of the observer and that of the observed stimulus. In fact, a recent TMS study showed that the excitability of M1 increased more when participants observed a sequence of finger opposition movements at a rate similar to their own SMT rather than when looking at faster movements (Avanzino et al., 2015). SMT recognition also seems to play a role in judging movement duration when involved in a temporal reproduction task (Gavazzi, Bisio, & Pozzo, 2013), during which participants demonstrated higher temporal accuracy when the observed movement duration was similar to their own SMT.

Some criticisms of these findings come from the neurophysiological results presented in Romani *et al.*'s (2005) and Craighero *et al.*'s (2016) studies. Romani and colleagues conducted a series of experiments examining the effects of observing biologically possible compared to biologically impossible movements (i.e., digits moving in an impossible range of movement) and showed that facilitation occurred in both conditions (Romani et al., 2005). In Craighero *et al.*'s study (2016), participants observed a point-light display moving according to a biological and a non-biological law of motion and failed to find differences in M1 excitability between the two conditions. These findings, which might be difficult to reconcile with previous behavioral results, pointed out that this line of research still needs further experimental evidence to clarify what is at the basis of action recognition.

Most of the studies presented here reveal the occurrence of motor resonance during the observation of movements whose properties are similar to the observer's motor knowledge. But motor knowledge can evolve through motor training leading to changes in subjects' motor repertoire (motor learning), and several studies have shown that motor resonance evolves with the internal motor repertoire of the observer.

Motor Expertise and Action Observation

The previous part described examples of studies providing convincing evidence that, when looking at movement whose features are similar to our own movements, the neural circuits involved in movement planning and execution are activated. It has been shown that this activation might be modulated by motor experience, meaning that the motor resonance is constrained to the acquired skills that person has learned. A particular action may figure in the motor repertoire of a trained expert but not in the motor repertoire of someone who has not been so trained.

Calvo-Merino and colleagues (2005) used an fMRI paradigm to study groups of people with different acquired motor skills to investigate whether the brain's system for action observation is precisely tuned to the individual's acquired motor knowledge. Expert ballet and capoeira dancers watched videos of ballet and capoeira movements. Thus, both groups saw identical stimuli, but only had motor experience of the actions in their own dance style. Comparing the brain's activity when dancers watched their own dance style versus the other style revealed the influence of motor expertise on action observation, namely, an increased bilateral activation in the MNS regions when expert dancers viewed movements that they had been trained to perform compared to movements they had not. This result was attributable to the motor and not the visual familiarity, as suggested by the results of a following study by the same group of researchers, in which male and female dancers watched gender and non-gender-specific videos (Calvo-Merino, Grèzes, Glaser, Passingham, & Haggard, 2006). Indeed, the visual familiarity was the same, but some ballets were performed by only one gender. Authors found greater premotor, parietal, and cerebellar activity when dancers viewed moves from their own motor repertoire, compared to opposite-gender movements that they frequently saw but did not perform, confirming the role of the motor rather than the visual knowledge in activating motor resonance mechanisms. These findings were subsequently confirmed by several fMRI studies that tackled the role of motor expertise during different kinds of tasks involving the observation of sport-related actions (Abreu et al., 2012; Bishop, Wright, Jackson, & Abernathy 2013; Balser et al., 2014a, 2014b; Wright et al., 2010, 2011).

Another body of evidence in support of this hypothesis comes from behavioral and neurophysiological research by Aglioti and colleagues (2008) on action anticipation in basketball players. In a first psychophysical experiment using a temporal occlusion paradigm, authors asked the subjects (elite basketball players, expert watchers, and novices) to predict the outcome of basketball shots observed in a movie. The results showed that basketball players predicted the outcome of free shots earlier and more accurately than people who have similar visual expertise but no direct motor experience with basketball, namely expert watchers and novices. In a neurophysiological experiment of the same study, they also showed an increase of motor excitability in athletes and expert watchers when they observed a basket action (shots in or out of the basket), rather than a soccer action or a static image. However, a specific increase of motor facilitation for the hand muscle more directly involved in controlling the ball trajectory, and for the instant at which the ball left the hand was only found when basketball players observed out shots. The results indicate that "although mere visual expertise may trigger motor activation during the observation of domain-specific actions, a fine-tuned motor resonance system subtending elite performance develops only as a consequence of extensive motor practice" (p. 1114) (Aglioti et al., 2008).

Motor Imagery: A Cognitive Technique to Promote the Activity of the Sensorimotor System

Motor imagery (MI) is the cognitive process of imagining movements without an overt motor output (Jeannerod, 2001). Richardson provided the standard definition of motor imagery as "the symbolic rehearsal of a physical activity in the absence of any gross muscular movements" (p. 95) (Richardson, 1967). Grèzes and Decety proposed that "the concept of mental representation of action corresponds both to the mental content related to the goal and to the consequences of the given action and to the neural operations supposed to occur before an action begins" (p. 15) (Grèzes & Decety, 2001). The literature describes different types of motor imagery. MI can be *implicit*, as in the case of mental rotation tasks (i.e., the cognitive processes of comparing or identifying objects or body parts in differing or non-canonical orientations; Kosslyn, Digirolamo, Thompson, & Alpert, 1998; Parsons, 1987), or *explicit*, namely when a person is voluntarily engaged in the mental simulation of an action (Jeannerod, 1994). Motor imagery modalities can be various. When a person focuses on the sensory information generated during actual action execution (including force and effort), one can refer to *kinesthetic MI* (Callow & Hardy, 2004). Differently, *visual MI* requires self-visualization of a movement from a first- (internal, i.e., to imagine himself or herself self as if he/she is looking out through his own eyes while performing the action) or third-person (external, i.e., to imagine watching himself or herself performing the action from an observer's position) perspective (Guillot et al., 2009). Finally, auditory MI (Landry et al., 2014) and haptic MI (Klatzky, Lederman, & Matula, 1991) need to be mentioned.

Neuroimaging and Neurophysiological Evidence of Motor Imagery

MI can be "considered a special form of motor behavior, intermediate in the continuum extending from motor preparation to movement execution" (p. 117) (Di Rienzo, Collet, Hoyek, & Guillot, 2014). For this reason, it has been suggested that MI shares the same neural mechanisms as movement execution. Several neurophysiological and neuroimaging studies have provided convincing evidence regarding this hypothesis (for a detailed description see also Hétu et al., 2013; Guillot, Di Rienzo, & Collet, 2014; Ruffino et al., 2017).

Since the 1980s, fMRI and positive emission tomography (PET) have been the most used techniques in MI-related brain imaging research, showing the involvement of both cortical and subcortical brain areas during MI. In their meta-analysis, Grèzes and Decety (2001) evaluated to what extent the brain regions activated during movement execution overlapped with those activated during MI and AO. The primary motor cortex, pre-supplementary and supplementary motor areas (pre-SMA and SMA), the premotor cortex, as well as different regions in the parietal lobules were found to be active during these forms of action.

Although currently debated, M1 was identified as part of the neural network activated during imagined actions (Leonardo et al., 1995; Lotze et al., 1999; Porro et al., 1996; Roth et al., 1996). In a seminal paper Ehrsson and colleagues (2003) found that MI of hand, foot, and tongue movements specifically activated the corresponding brain sections of the contralateral M1, showing that cortical activation during MI follows the same functional and anatomical specificity of movement execution. However, M1 activation was not systematically observed in each participant involved in a MI task, and once active, the activation was usually weaker compared to real movement execution (Munzert, Lorey, & Zentgraf, 2009).

SMA is a region involved in action planning and, in particular, in planning internally-generated movements. Its involvement during MI is now well-accepted (Guillot et al., 2008, 2009; Hanakawa et al., 2003; Lotze et al., 1999; Munzert et al., 2009). It has also been suggested that it is implicated in the inhibition of movement execution during MI (Kasess et al., 2008). Pre-SMA is known to be involved in learning and planning spatio-temporal features of actions, and updating motor plans, and seems to provide proper movement sequencing and timing during MI (Malouin, Richards, Jackson, Dumas, & Doyon, 2003). The premotor cortex, involved in the preparation and control of movement, was also found to be active during several MI investigations (Lotze et al., 1999; Martin Lotze & Halsband, 2006; Munzert et al., 2009).

Also parietal regions, including somatosensory cortex, were significantly activated during MI tasks. Consistent evidence has shown the activation of the inferior and superior parietal lobules and the precuneus (Binkofski et al., 2000; Gao, Duan, & Chen, 2011; Gerardin et al., 2000; Guillot et al., 2009; Hanakawa et al., 2003), suggesting their role in the formation of mental images.

Finally, cerebellum and basal ganglia, structures known to be involved in predicting movement outcomes/adjusting movements on the basis of sensorimotor feedback and in motor preparation, respectively, are also constantly reported during MI (Gerardin et al., 2000; Munzert et al., 2009). Nevertheless, one might take into account that cerebral activations during MI change during the day. Indeed, a recent study by Bonzano and colleagues (2016) that compared cerebral activity during actual and imagined movements, revealed that imagined movements in the morning significantly activated the parietal association cortices bilaterally, the left supplementary and premotor areas, and the right orbitofrontal cortex and cerebellum, whilst in the afternoon, the frontal lobe was significantly activated together with the right cerebellum. Contrast analysis showed increased activity in the left parietal lobe in the morning compared to the afternoon, suggesting that motor performance is continuously updated on a daily basis with a predominant role for the frontoparietal cortex and cerebellum. Altogether, these findings supported the existence of shared motor representations (Gallese & Goldman, 1998) between movement execution and motor imagery.

Neurophysiological measurements performed with TMS provided further evidence of the involvement of sensorimotor circuits during MI. Most of the studies in this field used the single-pulse TMS over M1 during motor imagery or before and after mental training via MI to test for modifications of corticospinal excitability. Increase in the amplitude of MEP is interpreted as a motor facilitation due to a decrease in the cortical motor threshold and/or a greater number of recruited motor neurons (Kasai, Kawai, Kawanishi, & Yahagi, 1997; Yahagi & Kasai, 1998). Since the mid-1990s, several authors have reported an increased MEP amplitude during explicit motor imagery that was (1) specific for the muscle involved in the imagined action (muscle-specific) (Fadiga et al., 1998; Rossini, 1999; Stinear & Byblow, 2004; Stinear & Byblow, 2003; Tremblay, Tremblay, & Colcer, 2001; Yahagi & Kasai, 1999), (2) modulated according to the different phases of action (time-specific) (Fadiga et al., 1998; Hashimoto & Rothwell, 1999; Stinear & Byblow, 2004; Stinear & Byblow, 2003; Stinear, Fleming, & Byblow, 2006), and (3) by the action context (content-specific) (Li, Latash, & Zatsiorsky, 2004; Stinear, Byblow, Steyvers, Levin, & Swinnen, 2006). Among the different imagery modalities, a TMS study showed that *kinesthetic* MI activated M1 to a greater extent with respect to the *visual* MI modality (Stinear, Byblow, et al., 2006), which is consistent with other studies using different neurophysiological techniques (Guillot et al., 2009; Stecklow, Infantosi, & Cagy, 2010).

In light of this neuroimaging and neurophysiological evidence showing neural similarities between imagined and executed movements, it could be surmised that these kinds of movement could also be similar when assessed with behavioral techniques. This is the focus of the next part.

Functional Equivalence between Imagined and Executed Movements

Several studies have shown the existence of functional equivalence between imagined and executed movements. To do that, most of them applied the *mental chronometry paradigm* with the aim to correlate the temporal content of real and imagined actions (for an extensive review see Guillot & Collet, 2005; Guillot, Hoyek, Louis, & Collet, 2012). It was postulated that during MI, as during movement execution (Miall & Wolpert, 1996), feedforward models predict the future state of the body and simulate the sensory consequences of a movement on the basis of the efferent copy of the motor command (Gueugneau, Mauvieux, & Papaxanthis, 2009). For this reason, the imagined time would be a replication of the duration of the actual movement. This temporal congruence has been termed *isochrony* and its presence provides information about the individual ability to preserve the temporal organization of the actual movement during MI (Decety & Michel, 1989; Decety, Jeannerod, & Prablanc, 1989). In one study, Decety and colleagues (1989) tested whether the walking time over visual targets placed at different distances (located at 5, 10, or 15 m from the subjects) corresponded to that of the imagined movement. Subjects were instructed to build up a mental representation of the target. Then they had to either actually walk or imagine themselves walking to the target. Walking time measured in the actual and the mental performance was almost the same. The same result was found in a second study (Decety & Michel, 1989) when participants were asked to perform or to imagine two tasks, writing a sentence and drawing a cube, with either the right or the left hand, and with either a small or a large tracing amplitude.

The result showed that in the same subject, for the same hand, mental and actual movement times corresponded, regardless of the tracing amplitude.

Together with timing, inertial and gravitational constraints are also incorporated into the imagined movement. Papaxanthis and colleagues (2002) examined the effect of movement direction and added mass to the duration of actual and imagined movements. Subjects executed or imagined arm movements in the sagittal and horizontal planes, in three different loading conditions: without added mass, with an added mass of 1 kg, and with an added mass of 1.5 kg. Whilst direction had no effect, the actual movements significantly increased in duration as a function of mass, as did those of the imagined movements. In light of these results, the authors suggested that "both inertial and gravitational constraints are accurately incorporated in the timing of the motor imagery process, which appears therefore to be functionally very close to the process of planning and performing the actual movement" (p. 447) (Papaxanthis et al., 2002).

Despite the fact that these studies, as well as numerous others, have shown similarities between these forms of movements, it is important to mention that some research did not find the same result for very short or long movement durations. Indeed, it was shown that movements whose duration was less than a few seconds were overestimated (Orliaguet & Coello, 1998), and movements whose duration was more than 30 seconds were underestimated (Grealy & Shearer, 2008; Hanyu & Itsukushima, 2000; Hanyu & Itsukushima, 1995). These discrepancies illustrate the difficulty for practitioners to interpret the possible discrepancy between imagined and actual times (Guillot et al., 2012).

Motor Imagery and Motor Expertise

The ability to form a mental image of a movement is thought to be dependent on individual motor expertise. This assumption has been supported by neuroimaging studies that compared brain activations in motor experts and novices (for review see also Debarnot, Sperduti, Di Rienzo, & Guillot, 2014). In a study on auditory motor imagery that involved experienced and novice musicians, by means of magnetoencephalography, Lotze and colleagues (2003) showed less brain activity in experts, although higher activation was found in regions devoted to motor functions.

Moving to the sport domain, it was shown that imagery abilities evolved with the evolution of motor performance, leading to different patterns of brain activation in experts and novices. For instance, in 2003, Ross and colleagues found that the brain's activation during MI of a golf swing correlated with the individual golf skill level (Ross, Tkach, Ruggieri, Lieber, & Lapresto, 2003). The pattern of cerebral activation in professional divers and novices was compared during MI of a diving task or a simple motor task by Wei and Luo (2010), who found significant differences between the two groups. Similar results were found in a study involving elite archers and novices (Chang, Lee et al., 2011). Overall, these data support the existence of distinct neural mechanisms during motor imagery in experts and novices.

Looking at behavioral data related to a mental chronometry paradigm, divergent patterns of results arise from MI literature. In an MI study on divers with different levels of expertise, Reed (2002) showed that the best springboard divers were the most accurate in imagining the dive with respect to divers at intermediate level and novices. Indeed, they found that the temporal difference between MI and its physical performance was lower in experts than in the other categories, suggesting that perfect technical knowledge gained by experts influenced MI results. Nevertheless, this result was not replicated by Guillot and colleagues (2004) in a study on MI performance in tennis players and gymnasts, in which they found that the durations of the imagined movements were higher than those of the executed movements irrespective of MI modality (visual or kinesthetic). In order to explain this result, they proposed that image accuracy would appear to be a more important factor than temporal characteristics of movement, leading to longer times dedicated to MI with respect to movement execution. Therefore, whether the expertise level alters/

facilitates the temporal equivalence between executed and imagined movement duration remains to be determined in future studies (Guillot et al., 2012). What seems that could be accepted, also by taking into consideration data on patients, is that if one cannot perform an action physically one cannot imagine it correctly, and the functional equivalence between the two movements might be lost (Olsson & Nyberg, 2010).

Calmels, Holmes, Lopez, and Naman (2006) did an in-depth evaluation of the isochrony between executed and imagined movements during the evaluation of a complex gymnastic vault considering the task in its entirety or disaggregating it into discrete temporal blocks. This procedure provided the opportunity to appraise the time course of mental processing. In a first session, elite gymnasts were asked to imagine the vault, which was considered to be composed of four stages, from their preferred perspective. During imagery, they were asked to tap their finger on their thigh at the beginning of each stage in order to monitor the stages' durations. In a second session, participants had to imagine the movement and then to execute it. Results showed that, although the time taken to imagine the entire vault was similar to the execution time, the temporal organization of the imagined and executed actions were different, and in some movement stages the MI duration was lower than the executed movement durations. The authors concluded that the results only partially support the functional equivalence between MI and movement execution. Therefore, especially in those motor acts that involve multiple components, further studies are needed to understand this point.

Motor Learning Through Action Observation and Motor Imagery

Action observation and motor imagery have been shown to activate neural circuits overlapping with those activated by movement execution. This similarity led neuroscientists to test, and subsequently show, their potential in evoking plastic mechanisms at a cortical level (which are necessary for motor learning to occur; Sanes and Donoghue, 2000), with considerable results in terms of motor learning. Indeed, despite the fact that physical practice is definitely crucial for the acquisition and the consolidation of new motor skills (Robertson, Pascual-Leone, & Miall, 2004), AO (Mattar & Gribble, 2005; Naish, Houston-Price, Bremner, & Holmes, 2014) and MI (Gentili & Papaxanthis, 2015; Gentili, Han, Schweighofer, & Papaxanthis, 2010; Pascual-Leone et al., 1995; Schuster et al., 2011) were successfully proposed as complementary methods for motor skill learning.

Motor Learning through Action Observation

The neural basis of motor learning is the possibility for the brain to develop plasticity in response to a changing environment. The occurrence of plastic phenomena in the brain, as well as the improvement of sensorimotor abilities, are considered evidence of motor learning. A number of studies have shown that these might occur after training via AO (action observation training - AOT). The first part described that passive observation of movement modulated cortical excitability in the onlookers' M1. However, only recent studies have shown that AOT can induce changes in M1 excitability that persist after the period of observation.

In a TMS study, Stefan and colleagues (2005) evaluated MEP amplitude and the probability of TMS-evoked movements to move in a certain direction. After observing a 30-min video showing thumb movements in a direction opposite to the baseline TMS-evoked direction (training target zone), "the probability of TMS-evoked movements to fall into the training target zone increased, the net acceleration of all TMS-evoked thumb movements was changed toward the direction of the observed movements, and the balance of M1 excitability was altered in favor of the agonist of the observed movements" (p. 9344) (Stefan et al., 2005). These modifications were substantially smaller but in agreement with those evoked after physical practice, and they thus suggest that AOT may induce specific long-lasting changes in motor representation. A similar evaluation methodology was also applied to elderly people, in which the effect of an AOT associated with motor training (MT) significantly enhanced the training effects compared with those induced by the administration of AOT and MT alone (Celnik et al., 2006). In the study of Zhang and colleagues (2011), MT+AOT improved the retention of the behavioral gain, i.e. increase of maximal velocity, when tested 30 minutes after the training. Authors concluded that AOT interacted with training-induced neuroplasticity and enhanced early consolidation of motor memories.

The temporal aspects of movements are one of the targets sensitive to changes induced by AOT. This point was specifically addressed by two studies of the same research group (Avanzino et al., 2015; Lagravinese, Bisio, Ruggeri, Bove, & Avanzino, 2017), which investigated whether AOT involving a sequence of finger opposition movements at a frequency (i.e., 3 Hz) higher than the spontaneous movement frequency (i.e., 2 Hz) might impact on M1 excitability and motor response. In the first TMS study (Avanzino et al., 2015), motor resonance during the observation of the 2 Hz-video and the 3 Hz-video was assessed before and after the exposition to AOT, during which participants observed a 10-minute video showing a 3 Hz-finger opposition movement sequence. Furthermore, their natural finger opposition rate was tested before and after AOT. Before AOT, M1 excitability increased more during the observation of the 2 Hz-video compared to when they observed faster movements (i.e., 3 Hz) in agreement with their spontaneous movement tempo (SMT) that was around 2 Hz. After AOT, SMT shifted towards 3 Hz and the motor resonance effect disappeared when looking at the 2 Hz video. This is an example showing how a brief period of AOT can modulate the response of the motor system. The second study (Lagravinese et al., 2017) tested the effects of multiple sessions of the same AOT over a week (one session every day). Results confirmed the performance gain, namely the shift of the SMT from 2 Hz to 3 Hz, and showed that AOT repeated over a week also led to a shift in the motor resonance; that is, MEP amplitude was significantly higher when looking at the 3 Hz video with respect to the 2 Hz video. Altogether, these results suggest that AOT can evoke changes to the observer's motor repertoire.

In this experiment, AOT was always followed by a subsequent motor test to evaluate changes to the SMT. One might propose that these tests might also have played an active role in evoking the changes observed in M1 excitability and SMT. The importance of providing a combined stimulation to evoke plasticity was stressed by a series of experiments during which Bisio *et al.* evaluated the effects of the administration of a paradigm that associated AO with a peripheral electrical stimulation (PNS) (Bisio, Avanzino, Gueugneau, et al., 2015; Bisio, Avanzino, Lagravinese, et al., 2015; Bisio, Avanzino, Biggio, Ruggeri, & Bove, 2017). In a first study, it was shown that AO-PNS protocol (15-min in duration) increased M1 excitability until 45 minutes after its administration, whilst this did not occur when AO and PNS were delivered alone (Bisio, Avanzino, Gueugneau, et al., 2015). Furthermore, this combined paradigm was proved to occlude the plastic increase of cortical excitability induced by motor learning (Bisio et al., 2017), similarly to what happened when protocols, known to evoke plasticity, interact with motor learning paradigms (Ziemann, Ilić, Pauli, Meintzschel, & Ruge, 2004). In light of these findings, the authors suggested that motor training and AO-PNS act on partially overlapping neuronal networks, which include M1, and that AO-PNS might be able to induce LTP-like plasticity in a similar way to overt movement execution. These results, when combined with the increased movement velocity gained by means of AO-PNS (Bisio, Avanzino, Lagravinese, et al., 2015), led the authors to conclude that when combined with a peripheral stimulation, AO is able to form a new motor memory.

In relation to the behavioral effect of AOT, the seminal paper by Mattar and Gribble (2005), in which they provide evidence that motor resonance promotes motor learning, must be cited. In this study, a group of participants observed a person learning to reach in a novel mechanical environment where a force field, imposed by a robotic arm, was applied to the participant's moving arm. When later they were tested moving in the same environment, they performed better than other subjects who observed similar movements but executed in a random force field that did not evoke learning; moreover, subjects who observed learning in a different environment performed worse.

Other evidence on the effects of AO on the following motor responses is provided by studies on motor priming and automatic imitation. Regarding motor priming, several studies have shown that the time to react to a stimulus (i.e., reaction time) was lower when the stimulus was in a position congruent to the position the subject has to assume, suggesting that AO promotes an improvement in motor performance (Brass et al., 2001; Press et al., 2007; Press, Bird, Walsh, & Heyes, 2008; Press et al., 2006). A kind of motor learning is the one observable during automatic imitation, an implicit mechanism during which the observer automatically changes their motor response to resemble the observed movement. Indeed, in a series of studies, it was shown that the features of the observed movement are automatically (and involuntarily) transferred to the following motor response, leading to a sort of implicit learning (Bisio et al., 2016; Bisio et al., 2012; Bisio et al., 2014; Kilner, Paulignan, & Blakemore, 2003).

Motor Learning through Motor Imagery

In their review, Olsson and Nyberg suggested that:

> "[t]he theoretical basis for motor imagery suggests that before execution of a voluntary movement, the brain has formed a motor representation that is believed to comprise the entire movement, including the plan as well as the intended result (Kandel, Schwartz, & Jessel, 2000). Moreover, since the motor representation supposedly precedes the execution then it could be detached from the execution and exist on its own (Jeannerod, 2006). Therefore, it can consciously be accessed during motor imagery and possibly the motor performance will be improved (Jeannerod, 1994; Jeannerod & Decety, 1995)."
>
> *(Olsson & Nyberg, 2010 p. 711)*

Based on that principle, a number of research studies applied MI paradigms, either by themselves or combined with physical practice, to test their potential to evoke cortical plasticity and improve motor performance (Driskell, Copper, & Moran, 1994; Feltz & Landers, 1983; Schuster et al., 2011). MI training is usually termed mental practice.

MI literature showing the beneficial effects of MI on motor performance dates back to the mid-1930s, when Sackett published two studies showing that subjects who mentally trained themselves to solve a maze performed better than others who did not mentally simulate maze resolution (Sackett, 1934, 1935). Shortly after, Perry evaluated the relative efficiency of actual practice and mental practice in different kinds of tasks ranging from simple voluntary movements and motor coordination to ideational activities, concluding that mental practice was effective in improving performance in a variety of tasks, but, when a movement was involved, actual practice was the most effective (Perry, 1939).

The first paper which summarized the results of 35 studies from 1934 to 1991 on the application of motor imagery to improve motor performance was published in 1994 by Driskell and colleagues and indicated that mental practice is an effective means for enhancing motor performance, although it is less effective than physical practice (Driskell et al., 1994). A number of studies have supported this conclusion. Particularly interesting are those presented by Gentili and colleagues (2006, 2010, 2015). In a series of studies, they tested the efficiency of mental practice compared to physical practice in improving motor performance; the improvement was evaluated by comparing the duration of overt (executed) and covert (imagined) movements during a motor learning paradigm. The task consisted in a reaching and pointing movement from a starting position to some final targets, whose order was previously memorized. In a first study (Gentili et al., 2006), after mental practice, participants observed a significant decrease in movement duration compared to the baseline condition. However, in agreement with Driskell's conclusion, motor performance improvement was greater after physical practice. Interestingly, they also observed a learning generalization, namely an enhancement of motor performance when it was executed in a different workspace. In a second study (Gentili et al., 2010), the authors evaluated the learning curve by comparing the trial-by-trial decrease in the duration of the executed and imagined movements. Although the learning rate was smaller during mental practice with respect to physical practice, movement duration significantly decreased in both groups compared with the baseline value, and this gain lasted until 24 hours after. This finding was replicated in a third study (Gentili & Papaxanthis, 2015), which added that the improvement in movement speed was higher in the dominant arm than in the non-dominant arm. All these findings have reinforced the idea that mental and physical practice share common neural mechanisms and activate the brain plastic phenomena that underlies motor learning.

One of the first neurophysiological studies providing direct evidence of plastic changes after mental practice was published by Pascual-Leone and colleagues (1995). They evaluated the modulation of MEP amplitude evoked by TMS during the acquisition of new fine motor skills. In particular, three groups of subjects – physical practice group, mental practice group, and control group - performed three different learning tasks over five consecutive days. The physical and mental practice groups had to learn a piano sequence and during the five days they trained physically or mentally according to the assigned group. The control group did not practice any sequence. Day-by-day motor performance was monitored by asking participants to play the piano sequence and testing the number of errors. Furthermore, the cortical maps of the muscles involved in this activity were acquired to evaluate changes in M1 cortical excitability. In the physical practice group, as well as in the mental practice group, the number of errors decreased day-by-day and the cortical area dedicated to controlling the muscle involved in playing piano significantly increased. These results were not observed in the control group, suggesting that mental practice, like physical practice, modulated the cortical motor representation of the trained muscles, evoking cortical plasticity.

More recently, the effectiveness of mental practice in evoking plastic changes in M1 excitability and motor performance improvements was assessed in a neurophysiological study by Bonassi et al. (2017), which combined MI with a peripheral nerve stimulation. Indeed, despite the fact that experimental evidence has suggested that the neural mechanisms activated during MI and movement execution are similar (similar feedforward models might be activated by the two kinds of movements), one crucial point that differentiates imagined and actual movements is the lack of peripheral sensory feedback during MI. In order to provide this sensory feedback, Bonassi and colleagues combined MI with concomitant peripheral electrical stimulation (ES) and tested MEP amplitudes and movement rate before and after this combined protocol (ESMI), MI alone and physical practice alone (PP). The task consisted in executing (PP) or imagining (MI and ESMI) finger-tapping movements at increasing rates. Results showed that, similarly to PP, ESMI increased movement rate and MEP amplitude, whilst no differences were observed after MI alone, thus suggesting the crucial role played by sensory afferences during mental practice in order to evoke plastic changes and motor learning.

Action Observation and Motor Imagery: Motor Enhancement in Sports

All the considerations presented in the previous parts of this paper have pointed out the role that action observation and motor imagery can play in motor learning. This part describes the most recent findings on the application of these techniques in sport science with a view to improving motor performance.

Application of Action Observation during Motor Learning in Sport

In the context of motor skill acquisition, demonstrations are a common instructional technique to convey information to the learner (Williams & Hodges, 2005), and the related learning process is called *observational learning* (Mattar & Gribble, 2005). Whereas effectiveness in learning simple motor skills has already been shown in previous parts of this paper, some studies have provided results on the successful applications of AO paradigms in learning complex motor skills such as those required during sport performance. In sport settings, model demonstrations are widely used by instructors as a teaching technique to facilitate acquisitions of new motor patterns. A meta-analysis of the effectiveness of observational learning techniques combined with physical practice has shown that it affords significant advantages over practice alone, and revealed a moderate effect in terms of improving movement dynamics, whilst a small effect was observed on movement outcome (Ashford, Bennett, & Davids, 2006).

There are several examples of the combination of observational learning and physical practice in sport settings.

Al-abood and colleagues (2001) compared the efficacy of visual demonstrations and verbal instructions on the acquisition of movement coordination during a dart-aiming task that was new to all participants. In order to evaluate the performance before and after training, movement outcomes, in term of scores reached during the throws, and kinematic parameters (coordination between upper and lower arm segments) were considered, and the results showed a significant improvement of all the parameters in the visual demonstration group with respect to the verbal instruction group, thus showing observational learning to be a valuable learning technique.

In 2002, Guadagnoli and colleagues examined the efficacy of video instructions with respect to verbal and self-guided instruction in improving golf performance in golfers (Guadagnoli, Holcomb, & Davis, 2002). The group that received the video instructions was trained by a professional teacher who used both verbal and video (video knowledge of the results) feedback on the performance, whilst the verbal group only received verbal feedback from the same teacher. Participants from the self-guided group practiced on their own. Before, the day after and two weeks after the four training sessions participants were tested, and asked to strike 15 golf balls. Distance and accuracy were considered as dependent variables and the results showed that in the second post-test the video group performed better than the others, suggesting that this combined technique might be a valuable tool to improve motor performance.

D'Innocenzo and colleagues (2016) went a step further by analyzing the effect of visual guidance for observational learning of the golf swing on a group of novices. During the observation of the model, visual guidance was put in place by superimposing transient colors to highlight the key features of the set up. Results were compared with those obtained when participants watched the same video without colors or a neutral video. The study showed that participants in the visual guidance group improved the swing execution and the improvement was maintained one week later, suggesting that, during observational learning, visual guidance might be crucial to accelerating motor skill acquisition.

Observational learning seems to be a promising coaching method also in weightlifting exercises as shown by the study of Sakadjian, Panchuk, & Pearce (2014), which compared the efficacy, in term of improvement in kinematic and kinetic measures during a power clean exercise, of a traditional coaching technique (during which participants received verbal feedback during practice), and action observation technique (during which subjects received similar verbal coaching and physical practice but also observed a video of a skilled model). This study showed that the coaching technique with AO resulted in significantly faster technique improvements and improvements in performance compared with traditional teaching methods.

The same was true for gymnastic exercises, as shown by Bouazizi et al.'s study (2014) comparing the efficacy of training based on the combination of AO and physical practice with physical practice alone. Indeed, measures of performance taken before and after training showed the effectiveness of observational learning techniques in improving motor performance.

All these studies, together with others (Hohmann, Obelöer, Schlapkohl, & Raab, 2016; Holding, Meir, & Zhou, 2017; Post, Aiken, Laughlin, & Fairbrother, 2016), converge on the efficacy of action observation as an additional technique to physical practice in order to promote faster learning. However, these studies have not directly tackled the information that learners perceive and acquire during observational learning. The next part will deal with this issue.

What Information from the Model Is Used by the Observer During Observational Learning in Sport?

A question raised by some authors concerns the specific information perceived and acquired during the learning process when observing a model on a video. Indeed, by identifying the nature of the information picked up by learners from the video demonstrations, one can enhance the content and the presentation of this information in the visual stimuli to promote skill acquisition.

One proposal is that observers focus mainly on the movement process (i.e., the spatiotemporal changes of body joints or extremities in relation to each other) (Scully & Newell, 1985), whilst another is that learners pay attention to the information that is helpful in achieving the movement goal (Wohlschläger et al., 2003). This issue becomes particularly important when what has to be learnt is a complex task as in the case of movement pertaining to sport actions.

The first hypothesis is based on the assumption that the perceived motion is minimized and used to constrain the reproduction of movement during observational learning (Scully & Newell, 1985). Indeed, according to this theory, a demonstration should be particularly effective when relative motion information of the movement is highlighted. This hypothesis was supported by the results of a study in which, in a series of experiments, participants practiced a ballet sequence following the presentation of a human model's video compared to a point-light display (PLD) (Johansson, 1973). PLD reduced information such as the shape and other aesthetic features of the stimuli, but highlighted the kinematic information. Results showed that participants who followed PLD performed better than those who viewed the human model. Nevertheless, this result was never replicated, and other groups only found that both kinds of stimuli led to improvements in motor performance when compared to learning without observing.

Horn et al.'s study (2002) assessed the efficacy in improving the outcome accuracy and the intra-limb coordination pattern during a kicking action in soccer obtained after the observation of a human model's video compared to a PLD. Following Scully and Newell's theory, they hypothesized that participants observing the minimalistic video would perform better (in terms of movement outcomes and coordination) than those viewing a video model. The hypothesis was not confirmed since the results showed that, in the two groups performing observational learning, there were gains in the global representation and temporal phasing of movement with respect to a control group, but no differences between them.

Point-light display was also used by Breslin and colleagues (2009) to evaluate the effect of information load, namely how much information concerning the model's body while moving is crucial to show participants in order to facilitate the learning process through observation. In their study, four groups of naïve subjects practiced a cricket bowling action. Before the intervention participants performed the target movement, their kinematics and performance outcome were noted. Then, they were assigned to four groups: one group listened to instructions on how to perform the action on audiotape, and the other three groups had a video demonstration showing the PLD generated on the movement of a semiprofessional bowler model. One group observed the full-body PLD, one group observed only the PLD of the right bowling arm and the last observed the motion of the wrists of both arms. Observation preceded movement execution. Participant's kinematics of the bowling arm became more similar to that of the model in the group observing the full-body movement and the bowling arm movement with respect to the other groups, suggesting that viewing end-effector constitutes crucial perceptual information in observational learning.

The same issue was tackled in a recent study by Ghorbani and Bund (2016), who tested which information is picked up by novice observers from a demonstration of a baseball-pitch as a to-be-learnt task. The study considered three demonstration groups (video of a human model, stick-figure, and PLD), who looked at the video before training, and a control group. Kinematic data relative to intra- and inter-limb coordination patterns and movement time were compared before and after training. The hypothesis according to which looking at the impoverished stimuli would allow focusing on motion details and thus improve motor performance did not find support, since no differences were found among demonstrations groups.

The conclusion of a review published in 2007 (Hodges, Williams, Hayes, & Breslin, 2007), which was aimed at understanding what is implicitly modeled by observers during observational learning, was that the scientific literature in sport neuroscience cannot give a conclusive answer, and this is still true at present.

Tips and Tricks

When planning training that makes use of AO techniques, some points need to be considered.

Among those, one might include the possibility for the observer to recognize the *biological origin* of the displayed movement. As already pointed out in the first part of this chapter, motor resonance mechanisms, namely the processes at the basis of the observational learning technique, can be evoked only if the observer is able to map the observed kinematics into own law of motion (Bisio et al., 2010; Bisio et al., 2014). This concept must not be confused with the possibility for learners to learn new motor patterns that are not in their own motor repertoire. Indeed, the law of motions pertains to all kinds of movement, irrespective of the experience a person has mastered with it. Namely, a novice to the sport of tennis automatically recognizes as biological the movement performed by Roger Federer even if they are not able to correctly handle a tennis racket. By contrast, in a virtual reality environment, virtual stimuli might not be recognized as biological even when performing very simple movements if their kinematics violates the biological law of motion. That has to be considered when researchers build artificial stimuli with the aim of using them during observation learning.

Another point that needs attention is the *context* in which the model's movement occurs. Indeed, a recent study showed that if the context is misleading with respect to what the subject is expecting, motor resonance mechanisms might not be triggered or be optimal to promote learning (Amoruso & Urgesi, 2016).

Then, a TMS study has shown the importance of the specificity of the effector and the observation perspective when creating the visual stimuli. Concerning the specificity of the effector, the first study providing evidence of the existence of an MNS in humans already showed that cortical excitability is maximal in the cortical region where the muscle involved in the observed movement is mapped (Fadiga et al., 1995). This result was confirmed by Maeda and colleagues (2002), who also found enhanced cortical excitability when observing a video in first- with respect to third-person perspective.

Furthermore, the instructions given to the subjects before the observation were shown to modulate the brain's activity during observation. This was the result of two studies (Decety et al., 1997; Suchan, Melde, Herzog, Hömberg, & Seitz, 2008) that, using PET, showed increased activity in areas associated with movement planning when the instruction given to participants was to observe and later imitate the gesture rather than recognize or judge its features.

Application of Motor Imagery during Motor Learning in Sport

Imagery used in practice routines is a well-established technique among sport experts such as professional athletes. Indeed, most elite athletes (70–90%) report they use MI for improving their performance (Hall, Rodgers, & Barr, 1990; Jones & Stuth, 1997). It must be noted that the use of MI as a training technique increases with the increase in the sport experience, and the use of mental practice appeared to be more effective for experienced trainees than for novices (Driskell et al., 1994). This point was formalized in two reviews (Debarnot et al., 2014; Olsson & Nyberg, 2010) which provided strong support for the existence of distinct neural mechanisms of motor expertise during MI as a function of the individual skill level, namely, borrowing the title of one of these studies "If you can't do it, you won't think it" (Olsson & Nyberg, 2010). Therefore, having motor experience with the task will increase the MI quality because it produces greater visual and kinesthetic awareness, and consequently, it improves the result of mental practice tasks. This information is particularly important when planning training based on mental practice in sport.

Several studies, ranging from individual to team sports, showed enhancement of sport performance with mental practice. Weinberg and colleagues (2003) investigated the relationship between the use and effectiveness of imagery in athletes from both individual and team sports. They concluded that for a closed sport (i.e., which takes place under fixed, unchanging environmental conditions), such as the high jump, it is much easier to know what to imagine since there is the possibility of preparing and imagining exactly what will take place. By contrast, during open sports (which are characterized by temporally or spatially changing environments) like soccer, athletes must be concerned with several factors that may impede the MI performance, and for this reason MI effectiveness might be reduced. Nevertheless, examples of MI application can be found in both sport types.

Concerning individual sports, since the early 1990s, evidence of the efficacy of MI has been provided for instance in strength performance, stretching and flexibility, athletics, gymnastics, tennis, and golf. In 1992, Yue and Cole first provided evidence that MI-related strength improvement may depend on changes in the central programming of the voluntary muscle contraction. Indeed, the group that practiced MI increased the maximal finger voluntary force with respect to the group who performed physical practice, and more than the control group (Yue & Cole, 1992). This result was subsequently confirmed in studies that considered single-joint movements, not specifically related to an ecological sport performance (Sidaway & Trzaska, 2005; Smith, Collins, & Holmes, 2003; Tenenbaum et al., 1995; Zijdewind, Toering, Bessem, Van der Laan, & Diercks, 2003), and also in a study testing whether combining MI with physical training might improve dynamic strength in sport exercises, namely bench press and sled leg press (Lebon, Collet, & Guillot, 2010).

A controversy exists on the efficacy of MI intervention on stretching and flexibility exercises. Vergeer and Roberts (2006) applied a four-week flexibility training program during which two groups of subjects experienced MI, whilst the third group was a control group who was not engaged in MI. Active and passive ranges of motion were assessed to evaluate the effectiveness of the intervention. A general improvement in flexibility was found in all groups, without differences among them, although the two groups who participated in MI interventions reported higher levels of comfort with respect to the control group. These results are at odds with those reported by Guillot and colleagues (2010), who compared flexibility scores in a group of synchronized swimmers before and after a five-week mental practice program that included stretching exercises in active and passive conditions. Significant increase in stretching performance was found in MI with respect to the control group.

The effectiveness of internal MI on high jumping performance was examined by Olsson, Jonsson, & Nyberg (2008), who tested whether jumping height, number of failed attempts, take-off angle, and bar clearance changed after a six-week training program during which two groups of active jumpers were trained with either the MI program or maintained their regular training. Results showed that bar clearance, a critical and very complex component of the high jump, significantly improved in MI groups with respect to the control group. Its complexity may be the reason why this component benefitted more than the others from this cognitive training technique.

An external focus during MI was adopted by Guillot and colleagues (2013) in a study assessing the efficacy of an MI training program associated with physical practice in improving accuracy and speed during an ecological serve test in tennis. During MI interventions, athletes were required to focus on ball trajectory and, in particular, to visualize the space above the net where the serve can be successfully hit. Results showed that MI in combination with physical practice improved tennis serve performance. Given Olsson *et al.*'s (2008) and Guillot *et al.*'s (2013) findings, it appears evident that a crucial factor that could impact on MI effectiveness is the MI perspective, a point that will be discussed in the following part.

A combination of internal and external MI was adopted by Brouziyne and Molinar (2005) in a study on golfers. This study examined how MI training combined with physical training affected the approach shot in beginner golfers. Three groups were recruited: one group received imagery combined with physical training, another only practiced physically, and the control group had no practice for five weeks. The imagery practice consisted of mentally representing a scene close to reality before each shot, moving the focus from the internal sensation to the external scene including the environment and the ball. The performance outcome was how close to the pin they were on a 50 m shot. The results showed that the group who received combined physical and imagery trainings improved significantly more than the group that only trained physically.

Although less frequent than in individual sports, some examples of the application of MI interventions in team sports are published in scientific literature. An example is a study by Blair and colleagues (1993), who administered to 22 participants (11 soccer player and 11 novices) an MI intervention which lasted a total of six weeks (two 15-minute sessions per week), and compared their performance in term of timing (time to complete the task) and accuracy (time penalties) to that of a control group who did not receive MI training. MI intervention consisted in both visual and kinesthetic MI with both and external and internal imagery perspectives. Results showed that the MI group improved more than the control group and that the improvement was observed in both experts and novices.

Tips and Tricks

In the previous part, successful examples of applying MI during training were described. Before planning to use mental practice during sport training, one should be familiar with some key aspects of MI.

Different kinds of MI were introduced. A first classification concerned MI modalities, namely visual and kinesthetic. It is conceivable that the degree to which MI modality impacts on mental practice effectiveness depends on the sport. Unfortunately, in sport domains there is a dearth of information on this issue. At present, two studies on dancers directly tackle this issue. Indeed, elite dancers can be considered as a special population of athletes who have trained extensively in both physical and mental domains, and may capitalize on the benefits of mental practice. Two studies assessed the content of dancer's images. One of them proposed a dance imagery questionnaire (S. Nordin & Cummin, 2006), and the other evaluated when dancers engage in MI practice (Nordin & Cumming, 2007). Unfortunately, they did not provide a final answer on which MI modality is the most effective in improving performance. In a first pilot study, Coker, Mclsaac, and Nilsen (2012) tested the effects of kinesthetic and visual imagery practice on two technical dance movements, and found that the benefits of the different modalities of MI are task-specific. In a second study, involving three groups of dancers, the same research group compared the effects of visual MI, kinesthetic MI, and a control condition involving a mental arithmetic task on plié and sauté, and failed to find any differences (Coker, McIsaac, & Nilsen, 2015). Therefore, whether MI modality affected MI effectiveness is still an open issue in dance, and also in other sports. Future studies need to focus on this aspect.

It was previously mentioned that within visual MI one might differentiate between first-person/internal and third-person/external perspectives. Hardy (1997) proposed that one perspective might be more effective for some tasks than for others (Hardy, 1997). In particular, an internal perspective may be superior for tasks that require positioning the body in relation to other external features. By contrast, an external perspective might exert a beneficial effect on tasks heavily dependent on form for their successful execution. This hypothesis was confirmed by two studies that examined the effects of training based on different visual MI perspectives on the performance of tasks where form was important, and tasks in which rehearsing the location in which a certain movement has to take place was crucial. Indeed, in Hardy and Callow's study (1999), the results of three experiments examining the effects of visual external and internal MI in karate and gymnastics (sports in which external and aesthetic components are important) offer strong support for the hypothesis that external visual imagery is superior to the internal one. Conversely, Callow *et al.*'s study (2013) on slalom performance (namely, a task that requires participants to move through a set course of gates) showed that, by training with internal visual MI, participants improved their accuracy more than by training with an external MI perspective. Another important feature of a motor task that needs to be considered when choosing between internal and external MI perspectives is whether the task involves open or closed skill movements. According to the hypothesis proposed by McLean and Richardson (1994), closed skill movements, which occur in a stable and predictable environment, would benefit more from the internal perspective, whilst open skill movements, in which environmental factors are constantly changing, would gain more from an external perspective. This theory was examined and confirmed by a recent study on tennis, a sport that requires both open skills during the serve, and closed skills during forehand and backhand (Dana & Gozalzadeh, 2017).

With regard to kinesthetic MI, one of the first things that needs to be considered is that MI ability depends on the sensory input. This is particularly evident in sports requiring the use of an implement, as in the case of tennis, table tennis, and golf. A behavioral study tested the role of the handled tool on the isochrony between MI and ME in tennis players (Bisio, Avanzino, Ruggeri, & Bove, 2014). When athletes imagined a forehand movement and held a tennis racket, the duration of imagined movements mirrored the duration of the real movement. Differently, isochrony was lost when they handled a tennis-like racket and an umbrella, suggesting that, although MI mainly relies on the activity of cortical motor regions, non-motor information—such as the use of a tool to practice movement—strongly affects MI. It is likely that daily practice with a tool causes the inclusion of the implement in motor plans, and consequently a mismatch between the afferent information and the information included in motor plans causes a decline in the MI performance. This hypothesis was supported by Wang *et al.*'s study (2014), which measured motor cortical excitability in badminton players during MI, and found an increase in MEP amplitude when athletes handled the badminton racket. They concluded that long-term training with a specific tool led to a functional reorganization in the motor related cortical network causing the inclusion of the tool in motor plans. Finally, long-lasting and daily experience with a tool was shown to modify the perception of the peripersonal space, namely the space of action, enlarging its boundaries in order to incorporate it (Biggio, Bisio, Avanzino, Ruggeri, & Bove, 2017). Therefore, one might conclude that the congruency between the information encoded in the motor repertoire and the afferent input, such as haptic information during hand-tool interaction, is crucial to evoking a correct motor image.

Matching the environmental context where mental practice takes place with that typical of the sport was shown to impact on MI quality. Guillot and colleagues (2005) compared autonomic nervous system responses (heart rate and skin conductance) in three conditions: (1) while experts in table tennis executed the sport gesture, (2) while they imagined it in a neutral laboratory context at a table, and (3) while they imagined it in an ecological context, namely in front of the table, wearing the typical clothes used during practice, and handling the racket. Results showed that both heart rate and skin conductance in the MI ecological condition significantly changed with respect to the neutral condition, and their values moved towards those obtained during the real movement execution, suggesting that the environmental context helps athletes to recreate during MI the physiological responses that characterize actual movement execution.

All these aspects are enumerated, together with others, in the PETTLEP model. The PETTLEP model is an evidence-based, seven-point checklist that includes physical, environmental, task, timing, learning, emotional, and perspective elements of imagery delivery. It highlights which areas need to be monitored in order to promote equivalence between MI and the corresponding physical task with the aim of enhancing the efficacy of MI practice. This model, which aims to provide a framework for the effective execution of MI interventions, was proposed by Holmes and Collins in 2001 (Holmes & Collins, 2001) and recently revised by Wakefield and Smith (2012). Here, a brief explanation of each component will be provided. For more detailed information on the features of the model, please refer to Holmes and Collins (2001) and Wakefield and Smith (2012).

The *physical* component "refers to the importance of making the imagery experience as physical as possible" (p. 3) (Wakefield & Smith, 2012), taking into account the posture adopted during the real execution of the task and also the implements used during the task. This enhances the vividness of the imagery. The *environment* component "relates to the place where the imagery is performed" and "should be as similar as possible to the performance environment" (p. 4) (Wakefield & Smith, 2012). The *task* component relates to the content of the imagery that should be appropriate to the skill level of the athletes. Indeed, as suggested at the beginning of part 4.2, having actual motor experience of the imagined movement is fundamental to produce high-quality images and to make the mental training successful. The *timing* component highlights the importance of the isochrony between imagined and real movements. The *learning* component suggests that "the content of the imagery should be adapted as the individual becomes more skilled" (p. 5) (Wakefield & Smith, 2012). The *emotions* component considers the fact that a competition is an emotion-laden experience, and thus, in order to recreate an image that is close to reality, one might add the emotional content typical of the competitive situation to the motor image. Finally, perspective refers to the importance of choosing the appropriate viewpoint during MI, as extensively discussed before.

Another idea that needs to be considered is the time of the day when mental practice is executed. Gueugneau *et al.* (2009) investigated whether a circadian fluctuation of the motor imagery process occurred by monitoring participants' imagined and actual movement duration of walking and writing movements every three hours from 8 am to 11 pm. Results showed that participants' ability to internally simulate their movements fluctuated significantly during the day, reaching isochrony between 2 pm and 8 pm, which is thought to be the best temporal range to execute MI intervention. These daily changes were not observed when the arm involved in MI was immobilized during the day suggesting that physical activity calibrates motor predictions on a daily basis (Gueugneau, Schweighofer, & Papaxanthis, 2015).

Psyching-up as a Technique to Empower Motor Performance in Sport

The importance of psychological skills training has been recognized for at least 30 years, and the number of athletes using psychological training strategies has increased. Psychological skills training techniques, known also as psyching-up techniques, are self-directed cognitive strategies used immediately prior or during movement execution that are designed to enhance physical performance, to increase enjoyment, or to achieve greater sport and physical activity self-satisfaction. Among these we will propose examples of the applications of self-talk, goal setting, and preparatory arousal to improve motor performance in sport.

Application of Self-Talk in Sport

Self-talk is a technique commonly used by sport psychologists during mental-skills training to regulate cognitions, emotion, behavior, and performance. Self-talk is a multidimensional construct that refers to self-verbalization and is used by athletes to direct sport-related thinking (James Hardy, 2006; Hardy, Oliver, & Tod, 2009).

The different dimensions of self-talk include (Hardy et al., 2009):

- *frequency*, namely how often the athletes use self-talk;
- *overtness* to other people, since self-talk might be either overt, potentially audible to others, or covert, inaudible to others. Although overt self-talk was initially preferred by researchers because it allows the monitoring of self-talk technique (Ming & Martin, 1996), feedback from participants has shown that it could be distracting (Masciana, Van Raalte, Brewer, Brandon, & Coughlin, 2001). For this reason, in many subsequent studies, participants have been advised to use covert self-talk (Harvey, Van Raalte, & Brewer, 2002);
- *valence*, namely the content of self-talk, which can range from positive to negative. Although a general agreement exists on the effects of positive self-talk in improving motor performance with respect to control, mixed results have been described when comparing positive and negative self-talk strategies and this may depend on athletes' interpretation of the content (Tod, Hardy, & Oliver, 2011);
- *motivation* that similarly to the valence refers to the content, but specifically to the fact that it could be motivating or demotivating;
- the *content*, why athletes make use of self-talk, from which derives the classification on instructional self-talk and motivational self-talk, in turn divided into several functions (Hardy, Gammage, & Hall, 2001). Instructional self-talk is designed to drive the attention focus on movement pattern, whilst motivation self-talk aims to build confidence (Zinsser, Bunker, & Williams, 2010), enhancing effort and creating a positive mood (Theodorakis, Weinberg, Natsis, Douma, & Kazakas, 2000). For this reason, Theodorakis *et al.* (2000) postulated the "matching hypothesis" proposing that "instructional self-talk would be better suited to skill, timing or precision-based tasks than motivational self-talk, whereas motivational self-talk would be optimal for strength or endurance-based movements" (p. 47) (Hardy et al., 2009).

Once self-talk has been defined and after having considered each dimension, the main question that needs to be tackled is the nature of the relationship between self-talk and performance, and if other factors beyond its dimensions moderate it by altering its direction, namely having a positive or a negative effect, and also the magnitude (Tod et al., 2011).

One of these was proposed in 1971 by Paivio in his dual coding theory that suggests that each person prefers encoding information either verbally or non-verbally, namely *verbal and non-verbal preference* (Paivio, 1971). One might hypothesize that athletes with strong preference for verbal processes would use self-talk more frequently than others.

Another conditioning factor might be the *belief in self-talk*. Since 1992 qualitative interviews reported that athletes believes that self-talk influences their competition performance (Gould, Eklund, & Jackson, 1992; Gould, Jackson, & Eklund, 1992). In a subsequent study on tennis players, athletes responded to a questionnaire about the effect of the influence of self-talk on their performance, and observations showed that believers won more points than non-believers (Van Raalte, Brewer, Rivera, & Petitpas, 1994).

Two recent review papers included athletes' *skill level* as a potential moderator (Hatzigeorgiadis, Zourbanos, Galanis, & Theodorakis, 2011; Tod et al., 2011) on the basis of previous research reporting differences in the use of self-talk between elite and non-elite athletes and between successful and unsuccessful athletes (Highlen & Bennett, 1983). To this purpose, it has been noted that novices tend to "talk" themselves through movement (Coker & Fischman, 2010) and make large use of instructional self-talk (Hardy et al., 2009). Although both review papers hypothesized that self-talk interventions might have a greater impact on novices than on expert athletes, Hatzigeorgiadis's meta-analysis concluded that the type of participant was a non-significant moderator, and that participants with different skill levels might benefit from self-talk (Hatzigeorgiadis et al., 2011).

Preference, belief in self-talk, and skill level are strictly related to individual characteristics. Other moderators consider situational factors that might influence the relationship between self-talk and performance. Among these we can mention task motor demand and difficulty, outcome performance, and the presence of significant others.

Concerning *motor demand*, the distinction can be made between tasks involving fine motor skills, requiring manual dexterity and accuracy, and tasks involving gross motor skills, requiring endurance and strength. Preliminary evidence by Hatzigeorgiadis (2006) suggests that self-talk helps athletes to focus their attention on the task. For this reason, in a subsequent study, the same author hypothesized that since tasks requiring precision need more attention than those requiring strength, self-talk would impact more on fine motor skills (Hatzigeorgiadis et al., 2011).

It was shown that self-talk was more often used for *moderately difficult tasks* than for tasks that are perceived as too hard (Fernyhough & Fradley, 2005). Progress within a game in terms of score (outcome performance) can have an effect on self-talk and its valence. Van Raalte and colleagues (2000) evaluated the antecedents of the use of positive and negative self-talk during a tennis match. Their findings showed that both point outcome and serving status influenced the likelihood of the use of self-talk. Conroy and Metzler (2004) added that participants used more positive self-talk while succeeding than while failing. The behavior and the language of significant people that are physically close to the athletes might affect the use and content of self-talk. For an athlete, a significant person might be a parent, a coach, as well as a team-mate or an opponent. Usually coaches promote the use of self-talk even if this promotion is unrelated to the frequency of athletes' self-talk, as suggested by Hardy and Hall (2006). A strict dependence on coaches' behavior and the use of positive and negative self-talk was reported by Zourbanos, Hatzigeorgiadis, & Theodorakis (2007), who showed that supportive coaches' behavior predicted athletes' positive self-talk, whilst negative behaviors such as distracting the athletes and acting inappropriately was associated with negative self-talk.

All the above-mentioned studies have provided successful examples of the application of the self-talk technique in sport. Many of these compared different kinds of self-talk and evaluated which was most successful in improving performance, also when compared to a control group. Most of them found that participants who engaged in self-talk were better than control participants, for example with regard to vertical jump height (Tod, Thatcher, Mcguigan, & Thatcher, 2009), knee extension strength (Theodorakis et al., 2000), and vertical jump performance and kinematics in male rugby union players (Edwards, Tod, & McGuigan, 2008). Again, self-talk has been found to improve soccer passing (Slimani et al., 2016) and badminton French short serve execution (Theodorakis et al., 2000); improved throw accuracy was described in water polo players after self-talk intervention (Hatzigeorgiadis, Theodorakis, & Zourbanos, 2004); self-talk was generally associated with increased muscular strength and power, whilst contrasting results were found in regard to *vis-à-vis* muscular endurance, as reported by a recent review paper (Tod, Edwards, McGuigan, & Lovell, 2015); and increased softball throwing accuracy was shown after self-talk intervention (Chang et al., 2014). All these studies are examples of successful applications of self-talk in sports and reviews on this matter conclude that self-talk has a great impact during training (Hatzigeorgiadis et al., 2011; Tod et al., 2011). For this reason, Hatzigeorgiadis *et al.* (2011) have suggested that coaches, educators, and athletes should be strongly advised to persist with their self-talk plans.

What is still missing is detailed information concerning the physiological effect of self-talk on autonomic nervous system responses and on the brain's activity in sport contexts. To the best of our knowledge, only one study associated self-talk intervention during skiing performance to the increase of heart rate, which marks the increase of the level of arousal (Rushall, Hall, Roux, Sasseville, & Rushall, 1988). Concerning brain activity, research performed on normal subjects and individuals with schizophrenia have shown the involvement of the Broca area (involved with the generation of self-talk) and of the lateral temporal and parietal cortices (involved in monitoring self-talk), including the Wernicke region, and have suggested that self-talk is not merely a psychological phenomenon but has specific physiological correlates (St Clair Gibson & Foster, 2007). Unfortunately, we are not aware of studies on the brain's activation during self-talk in sport and for this reason future research must deal with this issue.

Goal-Setting in Sport

A goal can be defined as the object or the aim of an action that can be internally driven or externally imposed. As suggested in a recent review by Swann and Rosenbaum "goal setting is one of the most widely applied and universally accepted strategies used to increase physical activity" (p. 1) (Swann & Rosenbaum, 2017). For this reason, establishing the right goal for the right person, at the right time might be crucial for the effectiveness of an intervention in sports.

Concerning the effect of goals setting on performance, Locke and Latham (2002) have affirmed that goals influence performance through four mechanisms:

- a goal has a directive function, meaning that participants direct their attention and effort to goal-relevant activities;
- a goal has an energizing function, namely the higher the goal, the higher the effort devoted to it;
- a goal influences persistence, and a hard goal prolongs the time devoted to reach it;
- a goal may affect arousal levels and the choice of the strategy, which in turn affects the action outcome.

Furthermore, in the same review, the authors considered a series of moderators of the goal-performance relationship: for instance, how committed participants are to the goal (goal commitment), how important the goal is for them (goal importance), and how they perceive progress in relation to the goal (feedback on performance).

Historically, goal setting techniques were designed to improve psychomotor performance (Locke & Bryan, 1966) and workers' productivity (Locke, Shaw, Saari, & Latham, 1981). In 1985, Locke and Latham provided the basis for the application of goal setting techniques to improve sport performance (Locke & Latham, 1985). Its effectiveness was afterwards confirmed by a meta-analysis (Kyllo & Landers, 1995), although more recent results challenged evidence on its efficacy with respect to a control group (Cobb, Stone, Anonsen, & Klein, 2000; McKay, King, Eakin, Seeley, & Glasgow, 2001).

Evidence supporting the use of goal setting in sport comes from Annesi's study, which proposed a goal-setting protocol on the exercise maintenance of new and returning exercisers, and showed that the measures of attendance and dropout were significantly better for the goal setting group than the control group (Annesi, 2002). Furthermore, a recent review on the effects of cognitive strategies on strength performance concluded that goal setting was reliably associated with increased strength performance, considering maximal strength, muscular endurance, and power for the evaluation (Tod et al., 2015).

Arousal and Sport

Arousal is a multidimensional construct defined as the cognitive and somatic reaction to an internal or an external stimulus. It is generally supposed that there is an optimal state of arousal for high performance. The optimal level of arousal is defined by the combination of cognitive and affective sensations (Hardy, Jones, & Gould, 1996), individual preferences (Hanin, 2000), and the requirements of the particular task or sport (Birrer & Morgan, 2010). All the strategies mentioned in this chapter (namely, action observation, motor imagery, self-talk, goal-setting) were proposed to regulate the arousal level, but results concerning the level of arousal and the outcome performance are contrasting. As suggested by Birrer and Morgan (2010), this might depend on two main factors that are strictly related to individual athletes' features, namely athletes' knowledge of their individual performance-facilitating state of arousal before and during the competition, and athletes' knowledge of their current level of arousal. Hanton and colleagues (2005) examined competition anxiety and performance-facilitating arousal states and proposed that athletes can interpret the intensity of anxiety-related symptoms or arousal as either facilitative or debilitative towards the performance.

Among the primary aims of sport scientists we can enlist understanding the relationship between arousal and performance, and identifying the best technique that athletes might use to regulate arousal in order to obtain the best performance (Gould & Udry, 1994). Several theories have been proposed to explain the regulation of arousal-performance relationship, namely the inverted-U-hypothesis (Gould & Krane, 1992), the catastrophe theory (Hardy, 1990), Hanin's optimal zone of functioning hypothesis (Hanin, 1980), multidimensional anxiety theory (Burton, 1990), and reversal theory (Kerr, 1985). Without going into detail, all these theories (Gould & Udry, 1994) imply that athletes become able to determine their optimal level of arousal, in agreement with Birrer and Morgan (2010) proposal.

Techniques to regulate arousal levels might be various, taking into account that sometimes athletes need to increase arousal level and other times to decrease it. Those techniques can be grouped into arousal energizing strategies and arousal reduction-stress management strategies (Gould & Udry, 1994). *Arousal energizing strategies* are necessary when athletes need to be charged-up to reach the optimal arousal level. An example might be the one reported by Perkins, Wilson, & Kerr (2001) on the effects of maximal strength performance in athletes, showing that significant increases in strength performance occurred in correspondence to high arousal levels. *Arousal reduction-stress management strategies* are applied when arousal level is considered too high and thus detrimental towards the performance. The most frequently used techniques include biofeedback, relaxation strategies, cognitive behavioral intervention, and mental preparations routine. We already described in detail mental preparation, with a particular focus on motor imagery training. In the next section, a brief explanation of the other techniques will be provided. Biofeedback interventions involve the use of instrumentation that provides individuals with information related to their physiological processes with the final aims of enhancing the performance by providing a route to self-regulation (for a review on its application in sport see Strack Linden, & Wilson, 2011). Among the kinds of biofeedback parameters, we can mention muscle activity, heart rate, skin conductance, and brain activity. Concerning the latter, a recent review provided examples of both successful and unsuccessful EEG-biofeedback trainings in various sports aimed at enhancing motor performance or regulating arousal level pre- and post-competition (Mirifar, Beckmann, & Ehrlenspiel, 2017). Relaxation strategies focus primarily on lowering physiological arousal and have the objective to prepare the subject to be skilled enough to be relaxed even in stressful situations. They are usually associated with the decrease of heart rate, oxygen consumption, respiration rate, and muscle activity (Gould & Udry, 1994). Cognitive behavioral interventions devote special attention on replacing negative self-statements and images with positive ones related to the desirable performance.

In conclusion, previous and current researches reveal that arousal regulation strategies can be used to influence athletes arousal level and thus to enhance the performance, although additional studies are needed to understand when, how, and with whom these methodologies will be most effective.

References

Abreu, A. M., Macaluso, E., Azevedo, R. T., Cesari, P., Urgesi, C., & Aglioti, S. M. (2012). Action anticipation beyond the action observation network: A functional magnetic resonance imaging study in expert basketball players. *European Journal of Neuroscience*, 35(10), 1646–1654. https://doi.org/10.1111/j.1460-9568.2012.08104.x

Aglioti, S. M., Cesari, P., Romani, M., & Urgesi, C. (2008). Action anticipation and motor resonance in elite basketball players. *Nature Neuroscience*, 11, 1109–1116. https://doi.org/10.1038/nn.2182

Al-abood, S. A., Davids, K., & Bennett, S. J. (2001). Specificity of task constraints and effects of visual demonstrations and verbal instructions in directing learners' search during skill acquisition. *Journal of Motor Behavior*, 33(3), 295–305. https://doi.org/10.1080/00222890109601915

Amoruso, L., & Urgesi, C. (2016). Contextual modulation of motor resonance during the observation of everyday actions. *NeuroImage*, 134, 74–84. https://doi.org/10.1016/j.neuroimage.2016.03.060

Annesi, J. J. (2002). Goal-setting protocol in adherence to exercise by italian adults. *Perceptual and Motor Skills*, 94(2), 453–458. https://doi.org/10.2466/pms.2002.94.2.453

Ashford, D., Bennett, S. J., & Davids, K. (2006). Observational modeling effects for movement dynamics and movement outcome measures across differing task constraints: A meta-analysis. *Journal of Motor Behavior*. https://doi.org/10.3200/JMBR.38.3.185-205

Avanzino, L., Lagravinese, G., Bisio, A., Perasso, L., Ruggeri, P., & Bove, M. (2015). Action observation: mirroring across our spontaneous movement tempo. *Scientific Reports*, 5(1), 10325. https://doi.org/10.1038/srep10325

Balser, N., Lorey, B., Pilgramm, S., Naumann, T., Kindermann, S., Stark, R., ... Munzert, J. (2014a). The influence of expertise on brain activation of the action observation network during anticipation of tennis and volleyball serves. *Frontiers in Human Neuroscience*, 8, 568. https://doi.org/10.3389/fnhum.2014.00568

Balser, N., Lorey, B., Pilgramm, S., Stark, R., Bischoff, M., Zentgraf, K., ... Munzert, J. (2014b). Prediction of human actions: Expertise and task-related effects on neural activation of the action observation network. *Human Brain Mapping*, 35(8), 4016–4034. https://doi.org/10.1002/hbm.22455

Biggio, M., Bisio, A., Avanzino, L., Ruggeri, P., & Bove, M. (2017). This racket is not mine: The influence of the tool-use on peripersonal space. *Neuropsychologia*, 103. https://doi.org/10.1016/j.neuropsychologia.2017.07.018

Binkofski, F., Amunts, K., Stephan, K. M., Posse, S., Schormann, T., Freund, H. J., ... Seitz, R. J. (2000). Broca's region subserves imagery of motion: A combined cytoarchitectonic and fMRI study. *Human Brain Mapping*, 11(4), 273–285. https://doi.org/10.1002/1097-0193(200012)11:4<273::AID-HBM40>3.0.CO;2-0

Birrer, D., & Morgan, G. (2010). Psychological skills training as a way to enhance an athlete's performance in high-intensity sports. *Scandinavian Journal of Medicine and Science in Sports*. https://doi.org/10.1111/j.1600-0838.2010.01188.x

Bishop, D. T., Wright, M. J., Jackson, R. C., & Abernathy, B. (2013). Neural bases for anticipation skill in soccer: An fMRI study. *J Sport Exerc Phychol*, 35(1), 98–109. https://doi.org/10.1126/science.1238409.

Bisio, A., Avanzino, L., Biggio, M., Ruggeri, P., & Bove, M. (2017). Motor training and the combination of action observation and peripheral nerve stimulation reciprocally interfere with the plastic changes induced in primary motor cortex excitability. *Neuroscience*, 348, 33–40. https://doi.org/10.1016/j.neuroscience.2017.02.018

Bisio, A., Avanzino, L., Gueugneau, N., Pozzo, T., Ruggeri, P., & Bove, M. (2015). Observing and perceiving: A combined approach to induce plasticity in human motor cortex. *Clinical Neurophysiology*, 126(6), 1212–1220. https://doi.org/10.1016/j.clinph.2014.08.024

Bisio, A., Avanzino, L., Lagravinese, G., Biggio, M., Ruggeri, P., & Bove, M. (2015). Spontaneous movement tempo can be influenced by combining action observation and somatosensory stimulation. *Frontiers in Behavioral Neuroscience*, 9(AUGUST). https://doi.org/10.3389/fnbeh.2015.00228

Bisio, A., Avanzino, L., Ruggeri, P., & Bove, M. (2014). The tool as the last piece of the athlete's gesture imagery puzzle. *Neuroscience*, 265. https://doi.org/10.1016/j.neuroscience.2014.01.050

Bisio, A., Casteran, M., Ballay, Y., Manckoundia, P., Mourey, F., & Pozzo, T. (2012). Motor resonance mechanisms are preserved in Alzheimer's disease patients. *Neuroscience*. https://doi.org/10.1016/j.neuroscience.2012.07.017

Bisio, A., Casteran, M., Ballay, Y., Manckoundia, P., Mourey, F., & Pozzo, T. (2016). Voluntary imitation in alzheimer's disease patients. *Frontiers in Aging Neuroscience*, 8(MAR). https://doi.org/10.3389/fnagi.2016.00048

Bisio, A., Sciutti, A., Nori, F., Metta, G., Fadiga, L., Sandini, G., & Pozzo, T. (2014). Motor Contagion during Human-Human and Human- Robot Interaction. *PLoS One*, 9(8), e106172. https://doi.org/10.1371/journal.pone.0106172

Bisio, A., Stucchi, N., Jacono, M., Fadiga, L., & Pozzo, T. (2010). Automatic versus voluntary motor imitation: Effect of visual context and stimulus velocity. *PLoS One, 5*(10). https://doi.org/10.1371/journal.pone.0013506

Blair, A., Hall, C., & Leyshon, G. (1993). Imagery effects on the performance of skilled and novice soccer players. *Journal of Sports Sciences, 11*(2), 95–101. https://doi.org/10.1080/02640419308729971

Blakemore, S. J., & Frith, C. (2005). The role of motor contagion in the prediction of action. In *Neuropsychologia* (Vol. 43, pp. 260–267). https://doi.org/10.1016/j.neuropsychologia.2004.11.012

Bonassi, G., Biggio, M., Bisio, A., Ruggeri, P., Bove, M., & Avanzino, L. (2017). Provision of somatosensory inputs during motor imagery enhances learning-induced plasticity in human motor cortex. *Scientific Reports, 7*(1). https://doi.org/10.1038/s41598-017-09597-0

Bonzano, L., Roccatagliata, L., Ruggeri, P., Papaxanthis, C., & Bove, M. (2016). Frontoparietal cortex and cerebellum contribution to the update of actual and mental motor performance during the day. *Scientific Reports, 6, 30126.* https://doi.org/10.1038/srep30126

Bouazizi, M., Azaiez, F., & Boudhba, D. (2014). Effects of learinng by video modelin on gymnastic performances among Tunisian students in the second year of secondary level. *Journal of Sports and Physical Education, 1*(5), 05–08.

Bove, M., Tacchino, A., Novellino, A., Trompetto, C., Abbruzzese, G., & Ghilardi, M. F. (2007). The effects of rate and sequence complexity on repetitive finger movements. *Brain Research, 1153*, 84–91. https://doi.org/10.1016/j.brainres.2007.03.063

Bove, M., Tacchino, A., Pelosin, E., Moisello, C., Abbruzzese, G., & Ghilardi, M. F. (2009). Spontaneous movement tempo is influenced by observation of rhythmical actions. *Brain Research Bulletin, 80*, 122–127. https://doi.org/10.1016/j.brainresbull.2009.04.008

Brass, M., Bekkering, H., & Prinz, W. (2001). Movement observation affects movement execution in a simple response task. *Acta Psychologica, 106*(1–2), 3–22. https://doi.org/10.1016/S0001-6918(00)00024-X

Breslin, G., Hodges, N. J., & Williams, A. M. (2009). Effect of information load and time on observational learning. *Research Quarterly for Exercise and Sport, 80*(3), 480–490. https://doi.org/10.1080/02701367.2009.10599586

Brouziyne, M., & Molinaro, C. (2005). Mental Imagery Combined with Physical Practice of Approach Shots for Golf Beginners. *Perceptual and Motor Skills, 101*(1), 203–211. https://doi.org/10.2466/pms.101.1.203-211

Buccino, G., Binkofski, F., Fink, G. R., Fadiga, L., Fogassi, L., Gallese, V., … Freund, H. J. (2001). Action observation activates premotor and parietal areas in a somatotopic manner: An fMRI study. *The European Journal of Neuroscience, 13*, 400–404. https://doi.org/ejn1385 [pii]

Burton, D. (1990). Multimodal stress management in sport: Current status and future direction. In J. Jones & L. Hardy (Eds.), *Stress and performance in sport* (pp. 171–201). Oxford: John Wiley.

Callow, N., & Hardy, L. (2004). The relationship between the use of kinaesthetic imagery and different visual imagery perspectives. *Journal of Sports Sciences, 22*(2), 167–177. https://doi.org/10.1080/02640410310001641449

Callow, N., Roberts, R., Hardy, L., Jiang, D., & Edwards, M. G. (2013). Performance improvements from imagery: Evidence that internal visual imagery is superior to external visual imagery for slalom performance. *Frontiers in Human Neuroscience, 7.* https://doi.org/10.3389/fnhum.2013.00697

Calmels, C., Holmes, P., Lopez, E., & Naman, V. (2006). Chronometric comparison of actual and imaged complex movement patterns. *Journal of Motor Behavior, 38*(5), 339–348. https://doi.org/10.3200/jmbr.38.5.339-348

Calvo-Merino, B., Glaser, D. E., Grèzes, J., Passingham, R. E., & Haggard, P. (2005). Action observation and acquired motor skills: An FMRI study with expert dancers. *Cerebral Cortex, 15*(8), 1243–1249. https://doi.org/10.1093/cercor/bhi007

Calvo-Merino, B., Grèzes, J., Glaser, D. E., Passingham, R. E., & Haggard, P. (2006). Seeing or doing? Influence of visual and motor familiarity in action observation. *Current Biology : CB, 16*, 1905–1910. https://doi.org/10.1016/j.cub.2006.10.065

Celnik, P., Stefan, K., Hummel, F., Duque, J., Classen, J., & Cohen, L. G. (2006). Encoding a motor memory in the older adult by action observation. *NeuroImage, 29*, 677–684. https://doi.org/10.1016/j.neuroimage.2005.07.039

Chang, Y. K., Ho, L. A., Lu, F. J. H., Ou, C. C., Song, T. F., & Gill, D. L. (2014). Self-talk and softball performance: The role of self-talk nature, motor task characteristics, and self-efficacy in novice softball players. *Psychology of Sport and Exercise, 15*(1), 139–145. https://doi.org/10.1016/j.psychsport.2013.10.004

Chang, Y., Lee, J. J., Seo, J. H., Song, H. J., Kim, Y. T., Lee, H. J., … Kim, J. G. (2011). Neural correlates of motor imagery for elite archers. *NMR in Biomedicine, 24*(4), 366–372. https://doi.org/10.1002/nbm.1600

Cobb, L. E., Stone, W. J., Anonsen, L. J., & Klein, D. A. (2000). The influence of goal setting on exercise adherence. *Journal of Health Education, 31*(5), 277–281. https://doi.org/10.1080/10556699.2000.10604703

Coker, C., & Fischman, M. (2010). Motor skill learning for effective coaching and performance. In *Applied sport psychology: Personal growth to peak performance* (pp. 21–41). Boston, MA: McGraw Hill.

Coker, E., McIsaac, T. L., & Nilsen, D. (2015). Motor imagery modality in expert dancers: An investigation of hip and pelvis kinematics in Demi-Plié and Sauté. *Journal of Dance Medicine & Science, 19*(2), 63–69. https://doi.org/10.12678/1089-313X.19.2.63

Coker, E., McIsaac, T., & Nilsen, D. (2012). Effects of kinesthet versus visual imagery practice on two technical dance movements. *Journal of Dance Medicine & Science, 16*(1), 36–39.

Conroy, D. E., & Metzler, J. N. (2004). Patterns of self-talk associated with different forms of competitive anxiety. *Journal of Sport & Exercise Psychology, 26*(1), 69–89. https://doi.org/10.1123/jsep.26.1.69

Craighero, L., Bello, A., Fadiga, L., & Rizzolatti, G. (2002). Hand action preparation influences the responses to hand pictures. *Neuropsychologia, 40*(5), 492–502.

Craighero, L., Jacono, M., & Mele, S. (2016). Resonating with the ghost of a hand: A TMS experiment. *Neuropsychologia, 84*, 181–192. https://doi.org/10.1016/j.neuropsychologia.2016.02.014

D'Innocenzo, G., Gonzalez, C. C., Williams, A. M., & Bishop, D. T. (2016). Looking to learn: The effects of visual guidance on observational learning of the golf swing. *PLoS One, 11*(5). https://doi.org/10.1371/journal.pone.0155442

Dana, A., & Gozalzadeh, E. (2017). Internal and external imagery effects on tennis skills among novices. *Perceptual and Motor Skills, 124*(5), 1022–1043. https://doi.org/10.1177/0031512517719611

Debarnot, U., Sperduti, M., Di Rienzo, F., & Guillot, A. (2014). Experts bodies, experts minds: How physical and mental training shape the brain. *Frontiers in Human Neuroscience, 8*. https://doi.org/10.3389/fnhum.2014.00280

Decety, J., Grèzes, J., Costes, N., Perani, D., Jeannerod, M., Procyk, E., … Fazio, F. (1997). Brain activity during observation of actions. Influence of action content and subject's strategy. *Brain, 120*(10), 1763–1777. https://doi.org/10.1093/brain/120.10.1763

Decety, J., Jeannerod, M., & Prablanc, C. (1989). The timing of mentally represented actions. *Behavioural Brain Research, 34*(1–2), 35–42. https://doi.org/10.1016/S0166-4328(89)80088-9

Decety, J., & Michel, F. (1989). Comparative analysis of actual and mental movement times in two graphic tasks. *Brain and Cognition, 11*(1), 87–97.

di Pellegrino, G., Fadiga, L., Fogassi, L., Gallese, V., & Rizzolatti, G. (1992). Understanding motor events: a neurophysiological study. *Experimental Brain Research, 91*(1), 176–180. https://doi.org/10.1007/BF00230027

Driskell, J. E., Copper, C., & Moran, A. (1994). Does mental practice enhance performance? *Journal of Applied Psychology, 79*(4), 481–492. https://doi.org/10.1037//0021-9010.79.4.481

Edwards, C., Tod, D., & McGuigan, M. (2008). Self-talk influences vertical jump performance and kinematics in male rugby union players. *Journal of Sports Sciences, 26*(13), 1459–1465. https://doi.org/10.1080/02640410802287071

Ehrsson, H. H., Geyer S., & Naito E. (2003). Imagery of voluntary movement of fingers, toes, and tongue activates corresponding body-part-specific motor representations. *Journal of Neurophysiology, 90*(5), 3304–3316. https://doi.org/10.1152/jn.01113.2002

Fadiga, L., Buccino, G., Craighero, L., Fogassi, L., Gallese, V., & Pavesi, G. (1998). Corticospinal excitability is specifically modulated by motor imagery: A magnetic stimulation study. *Neuropsychologia, 37*, 147–158. https://doi.org/10.1016/S0028-3932(98)00089-X

Fadiga, L., Craighero, L., Buccino, G., & Rizzolatti, G. (2002). Speech listening specifically modulates the excitability of tongue muscles: A TMS study. *European Journal of Neuroscience, 15*(2), 399–402. https://doi.org/10.1046/j.0953-816x.2001.01874.x

Fadiga, L., Fogassi, L., Pavesi, G., & Rizzolatti, G. (1995). Motor facilitation during action observation: A magnetic stimulation study. *Journal of Neurophysiology, 73*, 2608–2611.

Feltz, D. L., & Landers, D. M. (1983). The effects of mental practice on motor skill learning and performance: A meta-analysis. *Journal of Sports Psychology, 5*, 25–57.

Fernyhough, C., & Fradley, E. (2005). Private speech on an executive task: Relations with task difficulty and task performance. *Cognitive Development, 20*(1), 103–120. https://doi.org/10.1016/j.cogdev.2004.11.002

Gallese, V., Fadiga, L., Fogassi, L., & Rizzolatti, G. (1996). Action recognition in the premotor cortex. *Brain, 119*, 593–609.

Gallese, V., Fadiga, L., Fogassi, L., & Rizzolatti, G. (2002). Action representation and the inferior parietal lobule. *Common Mechanisms in Perception and Action Attention and Performance Vol XIX, 19*, 247–266.

Gallese, V., & Goldman, A. (1998). Mirror neurons and the simulation theory of mind-reading. *Trends in Cognitive Sciences*. https://doi.org/10.1016/S1364-6613(98)01262-5

Gallese, V., Keysers, C., & Rizzolatti, G. (2004). A unifying view of the basis of social cognition. *Trends in Cognitive Sciences*. https://doi.org/10.1016/j.tics.2004.07.002

Gangitano, M., Mottaghy, F. M., & Pascual-Leone, A. (2001). Phase-specific modulation of cortical motor output during movement observation. *Neuroreport*, *12*, 1489–1492. https://doi.org/10.1097/00001756-200105250-00038

Gao, Q., Duan, X., & Chen, H. (2011). Evaluation of effective connectivity of motor areas during motor imagery and execution using conditional Granger causality. *NeuroImage*, *54*(2), 1280–1288. https://doi.org/10.1016/j.neuroimage.2010.08.071

Gastaut, H. J., & Bert, J. (1954). EEG changes during cinematographic presentation. *EEG Clinical Neurophysiology*, *6*, 433–444. https://doi.org/10.1016/0013-4694(54)90058-9

Gavazzi, G., Bisio, A., & Pozzo, T. (2013). Time perception of visual motion is tuned by the motor representation of human actions. *Scientific Reports*, *3*, 1168. https://doi.org/10.1038/srep01168

Gentili, R., Han, C. E., Schweighofer, N., & Papaxanthis, C. (2010). Motor learning without doing: trial-by-trial improvement in motor performance during mental training. *Journal of Neurophysiology*, *104*, 774–783. https://doi.org/10.1152/jn.00257.2010

Gentili, R. J., & Papaxanthis, C. (2015). Laterality effects in motor learning by mental practice in right-handers. *Neuroscience*, *297*, 231–242. https://doi.org/10.1016/j.neuroscience.2015.02.055

Gentili, R., Papaxanthis, C., & Pozzo, T. (2006). Improvement and generalization of arm motor performance through motor imagery practice. *Neuroscience*, *137*(3), 761–772. https://doi.org/10.1016/j.neuroscience.2005.10.013

Gerardin, E., Sirigu, A., Lehéricy, S., Poline, J. B., Gaymard, B., Marsault, C., … Le Bihan, D. (2000). Partially overlapping neural networks for real and imagined hand movements. *Cerebral Cortex (New York, N.Y. : 1991)*, *10*(11), 1093–1104. https://doi.org/10.1093/cercor/10.11.1093

Ghorbani, S., & Bund, A. (2016). Observational learning of a new motor skill: The effect of different model demonstrations. *International Journal of Sports Science & Coaching*, *11*(4), 514–522.

Gould, D., Eklund, R. C., & Jackson, S. A. (1992). 1988 U.S. Olympic wrestling excellence: I. mental preparation, precompetitive cognition, and affect. *Sport Psychologist*, *6*(4), 358–382. https://doi.org/10.1123/tsp.6.4.358

Gould, D., Jackson, S. A, & Eklund, R. C. (1992). 1988 U.S. Olympic wrestling excellence: II. Thoughts and affect occurring during competition. *Sport Psychologist*, *6*(4), 383–402. Retrieved from http://search.ebscohost.com/login.aspx?direct=true&db=s3h&AN=20735381&site=ehost-live

Gould, D., & Krane, V. (1992). The arousal-athletic performance relationship: Current status and future directions. In T. Horn (Ed.), *Advances in Sport Psychology* (pp. 119–141). Champaign, IL: Human Kinetics.

Gould, D., & Udry, E. (1994). Psychological skills for enhancing performance: arousal regulation strategies. *Medicine and Science in Sports and Exercise*, *26*(4), 478–485. https://doi.org/10.1249/00005768-199404000-00013

Grealy, M. A., & Shearer, G. F. (2008). Timing processes in motor imagery. *European Journal of Cognitive Psychology*, *20*(5), 867–892. https://doi.org/10.1080/09541440701618782

Grèzes, J., & Decety, J. (2001). Functional anatomy of execution, mental simulation, observation, and verb generation of actions: A meta-analysis. *Human Brain Mapping*, *12*, 1–19. https://doi.org/10.1002/1097-0193(200101)12:1<1::AID-HBM10>3.0.CO;2-V

Guadagnoli, M., Holcomb, W., & Davis, M. (2002). The efficacy of video feedback for learning the golf swing. *Journal of Sports Sciences*, *20*(8), 615–622. https://doi.org/10.1080/026404102320183176

Gueugneau, N., Mauvieux, B., & Papaxanthis, C. (2009). Circadian modulation of mentally simulated motor actions: Implications for the potential use of motor imagery in rehabilitation. *Neurorehabilitation and Neural Repair*, *23*(3), 237–245. https://doi.org/10.1177/1545968308321775

Gueugneau, N., Schweighofer, N., & Papaxanthis, C. (2015). Daily update of motor predictions by physical activity. *Scientific Reports*, *5*. https://doi.org/10.1038/srep17933

Guillot, A., & Collet, C. (2005). Duration of mentally simulated movement: A review. *Journal of Motor Behavior*, *37*(1), 10–20. https://doi.org/10.3200/JMBR.37.1.10-20

Guillot, A., Collet, C., & Dittmar, A. (2004). Relationship between visual and kinesthetic imagery, field dependence-independence, and complex motors skills. *Journal of Psychophysiology*, *18*(4), 190–198. https://doi.org/10.1027/0269-8803.18.4.190

Guillot, A., Collet, C., & Dittmar, A. (2005). Influence of environmental context on motor imagery quality: An autonomic nervous system study. *Biology of Sport*, *22*(3), 215–226.

Guillot, A., Collet, C., Nguyen, V. A., Malouin, F., Richards, C., & Doyon, J. (2008). Functional neuroanatomical networks associated with expertise in motor imagery. *NeuroImage*, *41*(4), 1471–1483. https://doi.org/10.1016/j.neuroimage.2008.03.042

Guillot, A., Collet, C., Nguyen, V. A., Malouin, F., Richards, C., & Doyon, J. (2009). Brain activity during visual versus kinesthetic imagery: An fMRI study. *Human Brain Mapping*, *30*(7), 2157–2172. https://doi.org/10.1002/hbm.20658

Guillot, A., Desliens, S., Rouyer, C., & Rogowski, I. (2013). Motor imagery and tennis serve performance: The external focus efficacy. *Journal of Sports Science and Medicine*, *12*(2), 332–338. https://doi.org/10.1016/j.jshs.2014.12.008

Guillot, A., Di Rienzo, F., & Collet, C. (2014). The Neurofunctional Architecture of Motor Imagery. In *Advanced Brain Neuroimaging Topics in Health and Disease - Methods and Applications,* (Ms. Danije). InTech. https://doi.org/10.5772/58270

Guillot, A., Hoyek, N., Louis, M., & Collet, C. (2012). Understanding the timing of motor imagery: Recent findings and future directions. *International Review of Sport and Exercise Psychology*. https://doi.org/10.1080/1750984X.2011.623787

Guillot, A., Tolleron, C., & Collet, C. (2010). Does motor imagery enhance stretching and flexibility? *Journal of Sports Sciences*, *28*(3), 291–298. https://doi.org/10.1080/02640410903473828

Hall, C. R., Rodgers, W. M., & Barr, K. A. (1990). The use of imagery by athletes in selected sports. *The Sport Psychologist*, *4*(1), 1–10. https://doi.org/10.1123/tsp.4.1.1

Hanakawa, T., Immisch, I., Toma, K., Dimyan, M. A., Van Gelderen, P., & Hallett, M. (2003). Functional properties of brain areas associated with motor execution and imagery. *Journal of Neurophysiology*, *89*(2), 989–1002. https://doi.org/10.1152/jn.00132.2002

Hanin, Y. (1980). A study of anxiety in sports. In W. Straub (Ed.), *Sport psychology: An analysis of athlete behavior* (pp. 236–249). Ithaca, NY, Movement Publications.

Hanin, Y. (2000). *Emotions in sport*. Champaign, IL: Human Kinetics.

Hanton, S., Wadey, R., & Connaughton, D. (2005). Debilitative interpretations of competitive anxiety: A qualitative examination of elite performers. *European Journal of Sport Science*, *5*(3), 123–136. https://doi.org/10.1080/17461390500238499

Hanyu, K., & Itsukushima, Y. (1995). Cognitive distance of stairways distance, traversal time, and mental walking time estimations. *Environment and Behavior*, *27*(4), 579–591. https://doi.org/10.1177/0013916595274007

Hanyu, K., & Itsukushima, Y. (2000). Cognitive distance of stairways: A multi-stairway investigation. *Scandinavian Journal of Psychology*, *41*(1), 63–69. https://doi.org/10.1111/1467-9450.00172

Hardy, J. (2006). Speaking clearly: A critical review of the self-talk literature. *Psychology of Sport and Exercise*. https://doi.org/10.1016/j.psychsport.2005.04.002

Hardy, J., Gammage, K., & Hall, C. (2001). A descriptive study of athlete self-talk. *The Sport Psychologist*, *15*(3), 306–318. https://doi.org/10.1123/tsp.15.3.306

Hardy, J., & Hall, C. (2006). Exploring coaches' promotion of athlete self-talk. *Hellenic Journal of Psychology*, *3*, 134–149.

Hardy, J., Oliver, E., & Tod, D. (2009). A framework for the study and application of self-talk within sport. In S. Mellalieu & H. Sheldon (Eds.), *Advances in applied sport psychology a review* (pp. 37–74). New York, NY: Routledge.

Hardy, L. (1990). A catastrophe model of anxiety and performance. In *Stress and performance in sport* (pp. 81–106). Chichester, UK: Wiley.

Hardy, L. (1997). The coleman roberts griffith address: Three myths about applied consultancy work. *Journal of Applied Sport Psychology*, *9*(2), 277–294. https://doi.org/10.1080/10413209708406487

Hardy, L., & Callow, N. (1999). Efficacy of external and internal visual imagery perspectives for the enhancement of performance on tasks in which form is important. *Journal of Sport and Exercise Psychology*, *21*(2), 95–112. https://doi.org/10.1123/jsep.21.2.95

Hardy, L., Jones, G., & Gould, D. (1996). *Understanding psychological preparation for sport: Theory and practice of elite performers*. Chichester, UK: Wiley.

Harvey, D., Van Raalte, J., & Brewer, B. (2002). Relationship between self talk and golf performance. *International Sports Journal*, *6*, 84–91.

Hashimoto, R., & Rothwell, J. C. (1999). Dynamic changes in corticospinal excitability during motor imagery. *Experimental Brain Research*, *125*, 75–81. https://doi.org/10.1007/s002210050660

Hatzigeorgiadis, A. (2006). Instructional and motivational self-talk: An investigation on perceived self-talk functions. *Hellenic Journal of Psychology*, *3*(164–175).

Hatzigeorgiadis, A., Theodorakis, Y., & Zourbanos, N. (2004). Self-talk in the swimming pool: The effects of self-talk on thought content and performance on water-polo tasks. *Journal of Applied Sport Psychology*, *16*(2), 138–150. https://doi.org/10.1080/10413200490437886

Hatzigeorgiadis, A., Zourbanos, N., Galanis, E., & Theodorakis, Y. (2011). Self-talk and sports performance: A meta-analysis. *Perspectives on Psychological Science*, *6*(4), 348–356. https://doi.org/Doi 10.1177/1745691611413136

Hétu, S., Grégoire, M., Saimpont, A., Coll, M. P., Eugène, F., Michon, P. E., & Jackson, P. L. (2013). The neural network of motor imagery: An ALE meta-analysis. *Neuroscience and Biobehavioral Reviews*. https://doi.org/10.1016/j.neubiorev.2013.03.017

Heyes, C. (2011). Automatic imitation. *Psychological Bulletin*, *137*, 463–483. https://doi.org/10.1037/a0022288

Heyes, C., Bird, G., Johnson, H., & Haggard, P. (2005). Experience modulates automatic imitation. *Cognitive Brain Research*, *22*(2), 233–240. https://doi.org/10.1016/j.cogbrainres.2004.09.009

Hickok, G. (2009). Eight problems for the mirror neuron theory of action understanding in monkeys and humans. *Journal of Cognitive Neuroscience*, *21*(7), 1229–1243. https://doi.org/10.1162/jocn.2009.21189

Highlen, P., & Bennett, B. (1983). Elite divers and wrestlers: A comparison between open-and closed-skill athletes. *Journal of Sport Psychology*, 390–409. https://doi.org/10.1123/jsp.5.4.390

Hodges, N., Williams, A. M., Hayes, S., & Breslin, G. (2007). What is modelled during observational learning? *Journal of Sports Sciences*, *25*(5), 531–545. https://doi.org/10.1080/02640410600946860

Hohmann, T., Obelöer, H., Schlapkohl, N., & Raab, M. (2016). Does training with 3D videos improve decision-making in team invasion sports? *Journal of Sports Sciences*, *34*(8), 746–755. https://doi.org/10.1080/02640414.2015.1069380

Holding, R., Meir, R., & Zhou, S. (2017). Can previewing sport-specific video influence reactive-agility response time? *International Journal of Sports Physiology and Performance*, *12*(2), 224–229. https://doi.org/10.1123/ijspp.2015-0803

Holmes, P. S., & Collins, D. J. (2001). The PETTLEP approach to motor imagery: A functional equivalence model for sport psychologists. *Journal of Applied Sport Psychology*, *13*(1), 60–83. https://doi.org/10.1080/10413200109339004

Horn, R. R., Williams, A. M., & Scott, M. A. (2002). Learning from demonstrations: The role of visual search during observational learning from video and point-light models. *Journal of Sports Sciences*, *20*(3), 253–269. https://doi.org/10.1080/026404102317284808

Iacoboni, M. (2009). Imitation, empathy, and mirror neurons. *Annual Review of Psychology*, *60*, 653–670. https://doi.org/10.1146/annurev.psych.60.110707.163604

Iacoboni, M., Woods, R. P., Brass, M., Bekkering, H., Mazziotta, J. C., & Rizzolatti, G. (1999). Cortical mechanisms of human imitation. *Science*, *286*(5449), 2526–2528.

Jeannerod, M. (1994). The representing brain: Neural correlates of motor intention and imagery. *Behavioral and Brain Sciences*, *17*(2), 187. https://doi.org/10.1017/S0140525X00034026

Jeannerod, M. (2001). Neural simulation of action: A unifying mechanism for motor cognition. *NeuroImage*, *14*, S103–S109. https://doi.org/10.1006/nimg.2001.0832

Jeannerod, M. (2006). *Motor Cognition. Motor cognition: What actions tell the self.* https://doi.org/10.1093/acprof:oso/9780198569657.001.0001

Jeannerod, M., & Decety, J. (1995). Mental motor imagery: A window into the representational stages of action. *Current Opinion in Neurobiology*. https://doi.org/10.1016/0959-4388(95)80099-9

Johansson, G. (1973). Visual perception of biological motion and a model for its analysis. *Perception & Psychophysics*, *14*(2), 201–211. https://doi.org/10.3758/BF03212378

Jones, L., & Stuth, G. (1997). The uses of mental imagery in athletics: An overview. *Applied and Preventive Psychology*, *6*(2), 101–115. https://doi.org/10.1016/S0962-1849(05)80016-2

Kandel, E., Schwartz, J., & Jessel, T. (2000). *Principles of neural science 4th.* New York, NY: McGraw-Hill.

Kasai, T., Kawai, S., Kawanishi, M., & Yahagi, S. (1997). Evidence for facilitation of motor evoked potentials (MEPs) induced by motor imagery. *Brain Research*, *744*(1), 147–150. https://doi.org/10.1016/S0006-8993(96)01101-8

Kasess, C. H., Windischberger, C., Cunnington, R., Lanzenberger, R., Pezawas, L., & Moser, E. (2008). The suppressive influence of SMA on M1 in motor imagery revealed by fMRI and dynamic causal modeling. *NeuroImage*, *40*, 828–837. https://doi.org/10.1016/j.neuroimage.2007.11.040

Kerr, J. H. (1985). The experience of arousal: A new basis for studying arousal effects in sport. *Journal of Sports Sciences*, *3*(3), 169–179. https://doi.org/10.1080/02640418508729749

Kilner, J. M., Paulignan, Y., & Blakemore, S. J. (2003). An interference effect of observed biological movement on action. *Curr Biol*, *13*(6), 522–525.

Klatzky, R. L., Lederman, S. J., & Matula, D. E. (1991). Imagined haptic exploration in judgments of object properties. *Journal of Experimental Psychology: Learning, Memory, and Cognition*, *17*(2), 314–322. https://doi.org/10.1037/0278-7393.17.2.314

Kosslyn, S. M., Digirolamo, G. J., Thompson, W. L., & Alpert, N. M. (1998). Mental rotation of objects versus hands: Neural mechanisms revealed by positron emission tomography. *Psychophysiology*, *35*(2), 151–161. https://doi.org/10.1111/1469-8986.3520151

Kyllo, L. B., & Landers, D. M. (1995). Goal setting in sport and exercise - a research synthesis to resolve the controversy. *Journal of Sport & Exercise Psychology*, *17*(2), 117–137. https://doi.org/10.1123/jsep.17.2.117

Lagravinese, G., Bisio, A., Ruggeri, P., Bove, M., & Avanzino, L. (2017). Learning by observing: The effect of multiple sessions of action-observation training on the spontaneous movement tempo and motor resonance. *Neuropsychologia*, *96*, 89–95. https://doi.org/10.1016/j.neuropsychologia.2016.09.022

Landry, S. P., Pagé, S., Shiller, D. M., Lepage, J.-F., Théoret, H., & Champoux, F. (2014). Auditory imagery forces motor action. *Neuroreport*, (DECEMBER), 1–6. https://doi.org/10.1097/WNR.0000000000000307

Lebon, F., Collet, C., & Guillot, A. (2010). Benefits of motor imagery training on muscle strength. *Journal of Strength and Conditioning Research / National Strength & Conditioning Association*, 24(6), 1680–1687. https://doi.org/10.1519/JSC.0b013e3181d8e936

Leonardo, M., Fieldman, J., Sadato, N., Campbell, G., Ibanez, V., Cohen, L., … Hallett, M. (1995). A functional magnetic resonance imaging study of cortical regions associated with motor task execution and motor ideation in humans. *Human Brain Mapping*, 3, 83–92.

Li, S., Latash, M. L., & Zatsiorsky, V. M. (2004). Effects of motor imagery on finger force responses to transcranial magnetic stimulation. *Cognitive Brain Research*, 20(2), 273–280. https://doi.org/10.1016/j.cogbrainres.2004.03.003

Locke, E. A., & Bryan, J. F. (1966). Cognitive aspects of psychomotor performance: The effects of performance goals on level of performance. *Journal of Applied Psychology*, 50(4), 286–291. https://doi.org/10.1037/h0023550

Locke, E. A., & Latham, G. P. (1985). The Application of Goal Setting to Sports. *Journal of Sport Psychology*, 7(3), 205–222. https://doi.org/10.1123/jsp.7.3.205

Locke, E. A., & Latham, G. P. (2002). Building a practically useful theory of goal setting and task motivation: A 35-year odyssey. *American Psychologist*, 57(9), 705–717. https://doi.org/10.1037//0003-066X.57.9.705

Locke, E. A., Shaw, K. N., Saari, L. M., & Latham, G. P. (1981). Goal setting and task performance: 1969–1980. *Psychological Bulletin*, 90(1), 125–152. https://doi.org/10.1037/0033-2909.90.1.125

Lotze, M., & Halsband, U. (2006). Motor imagery. *Journal of Physiology Paris*, 99(4–6), 386–395. https://doi.org/10.1016/j.jphysparis.2006.03.012

Lotze, M., Montoya, P., Erb, M., Hülsmann, E., Flor, H., Klose, U., … Grodd, W. (1999). Activation of cortical and cerebellar motor areas during executed and imagined hand movements: An fMRI study. *Journal of Cognitive Neuroscience*, 11(5), 491–501. https://doi.org/10.1162/089892999563553

Lotze, M., Scheler, G., Tan, H. R. M., Braun, C., & Birbaumer, N. (2003). The musician's brain: Functional imaging of amateurs and professionals during performance and imagery. *NeuroImage*, 20(3), 1817–1829. https://doi.org/10.1016/j.neuroimage.2003.07.018

Maeda, F., Kleiner-Fisman, G., & Pascual-Leone, A. (2002). Motor facilitation while observing hand actions: Specificity of the effect and role of observer's orientation. *Journal of Neurophysiology*, 87, 1329–1335. https://doi.org/10.1152/jn.00773.2000

Malouin, F., Richards, C. L., Jackson, P. L., Dumas, F., & Doyon, J. (2003). Brain activations during motor imagery of locomotor-related tasks: A PET study. *Human Brain Mapping*, 19(1), 47–62. https://doi.org/10.1002/hbm.10103

Masciana, R., Van Raalte, J., Brewer, B., Brandon, M., & Coughlin, M. (2001). Effects of cognitive strategies on dart throwing performance. *International Sports Journal*, 5, 31–39.

Mattar, A. A. G., & Gribble, P. L. (2005). Motor learning by observing. *Neuron*, 46, 153–160. https://doi.org/10.1016/j.neuron.2005.02.009

McKay, H. G., King, D., Eakin, E. G., Seeley, J. R., & Glasgow, R. E. (2001). The diabetes network internet-based physical activity intervention: A randomized pilot study. *Diabetes Care*, 24(8), 1328–1334. https://doi.org/10.2337/diacare.24.8.1328

McLean, N., & Richardson, A. (1994). The role of imagery in perfecting already learned physical skills. In A. Sheikh & E. Korn (Eds.), *Imagery in sport and physical performance* (pp. 49–73). Amityville, NY: Baywood Publishing Company, Inc.

Miall, R. C., & Wolpert, D. M. (1996). Forward models for physiological motor control. *Neural Networks*. https://doi.org/10.1016/S0893-6080(96)00035-4

Ming, S., & Martin, G. L. (1996). Single-subject evaluation of a self-talk package for improving figure skating performance. *Sport Psychologist*, 10(3), 227–238. https://doi.org/10.1123/tsp.10.3.227

Mirifar, A., Beckmann, J., & Ehrlenspiel, F. (2017). Neurofeedback as supplementary training for optimizing athletes' performance: A systematic review with implications for future research. *Neuroscience and Biobehavioral Reviews*. https://doi.org/10.1016/j.neubiorev.2017.02.005

Mukamel, R., Ekstrom, A. D., & Kaplan, J. (2010). Report single-neuron responses in humans during execution and observation of actions. *Current Biology*, 20(8), 750–756. https://doi.org/10.1016/j.cub.2010.02.045

Munzert, J., Lorey, B., & Zentgraf, K. (2009). Cognitive motor processes: The role of motor imagery in the study of motor representations. *Brain Research Reviews*. https://doi.org/10.1016/j.brainresrev.2008.12.024

Naish, K. R., Houston-Price, C., Bremner, A. J., & Holmes, N. P. (2014). Effects of action observation on corticospinal excitability: Muscle specificity, direction, and timing of the mirror response. *Neuropsychologia*, 64, 331–348. https://doi.org/10.1016/j.neuropsychologia.2014.09.034

Nordin, S., & Cummin, J. (2006). Measuring the content of dancers' images: Development of the dance imagery questionnaire (DIQ). *Journal of Dance Medicine & Science*, 10, 85–98.

Nordin, S. M., & Cumming, J. (2007). Where, when, and how: A quantitative account of dance imagery. *Research Quarterly for Exercise and Sport*, 78(4), 390–395. https://doi.org/10.1080/02701367.2007.10599437

Olsson, C. J., Jonsson, B., & Nyberg, L. (2008). Internal imagery training in active high jumpers: Cognition and neurosciences. *Scandinavian Journal of Psychology*, 49(2), 133–140. https://doi.org/10.1111/j.1467-9450.2008.00625.x

Olsson, C. J., & Nyberg, L. (2010). Motor imagery: If you can't do it, you won't think it. *Scandinavian Journal of Medicine and Science in Sports*. https://doi.org/10.1111/j.1600-0838.2010.01101.x

Orliaguet, J. P., & Coello, Y. (1998). Differences between actual and imagined putting movements in golf: A chronometric analysis. *International Journal of Sport Psychology*, 29(2), 157–169.

Paivio, A. (1971). *Imagery and verbal processes*. New York, NY: Holt, Rinehart and Winston.

Papaxanthis, C., Schieppati, M., Gentili, R., & Pozzo, T. (2002). Imagined and actual arm movements have similar durations when performed under different conditions of direction and mass. *Experimental Brain Research*, 143(4), 447–452. https://doi.org/10.1007/s00221-002-1012-1

Parsons, L. M. (1987). Imagined spatial transformation of one's body. *Journal of Experimental Psychology General*, 116(2), 172–191. https://doi.org/10.1037/0096-3445.116.2.172

Pascual-Leone, A., Nguyet, D., Cohen, L. G., Brasil-Neto, J. P., Cammarota, A., & Hallett, M. (1995). Modulation of muscle responses evoked by transcranial magnetic stimulation during the acquisition of new fine motor skills. *Journal of Neurophysiology*, 74(3), 1037–1045. Retrieved from http://www.ncbi.nlm.nih.gov/pubmed/7500130

Perkins, D., Wilson, G. V, & Kerr, J. H. (2001). The effects of elevated arousal and mood on maximal strength performance in athletes. *Journal of Applied Sport Psychology*, 13(3), 239–259. Retrieved from http://articles.sirc.ca/search.cfm?id=S-791477%5Cnhttp://ezproxy.net.ucf.edu/login?url=http://search.ebscohost.com/login.aspx?direct=true&db=sph&AN=SPHS-791477&site=ehost-live%5Cnhttp://www.taylorandfrancis.com

Perry, H. M. (1939). The relative efficiency of actual and "imaginary" practice in five selected tasks. *Archives of Psychology*, 34, 5–75.

Piaget, J. (1952). Play, dreams and imitation in childhood. *Journal of Consulting Psychology*. https://doi.org/10.1037/h0052104

Porro, C. A., Francescato, M. P., Cettolo, V., Diamond, M. E., Baraldi, P., Zuiani, C., … di Prampero, P. E. (1996). Primary motor and sensory cortex activation during motor performance and motor imagery: A functional magnetic resonance imaging study. *The Journal of Neuroscience : The Official Journal of the Society for Neuroscience*, 16(23), 7688–7698. https://doi.org/8922425

Post, P. G., Aiken, C. A., Laughlin, D. D., & Fairbrother, J. T. (2016). Self-control over combined video feedback and modeling facilitates motor learning. *Human Movement Science*, 47, 49–59. https://doi.org/10.1016/j.humov.2016.01.014

Press, C., Bird, G., Walsh, E., & Heyes, C. (2008). Automatic imitation of intransitive actions. *Brain and Cognition*, 67(1), 44–50. https://doi.org/10.1016/j.bandc.2007.11.001

Press, C., Gillmeister, H., & Heyes, C. (2006). Bottom-up, not top-down, modulation of imitation by human and robotic models. *European Journal of Neuroscience*, 24(8), 2415–2419. https://doi.org/10.1111/j.1460-9568.2006.05115.x

Press, C., Gillmeister, H., & Heyes, C. (2007). Sensorimotor experience enhances automatic imitation of robotic action. *Proceedings of the Royal Society B: Biological Sciences*, 274(1625), 2509–2514. https://doi.org/10.1098/rspb.2007.0774

Raalte, J. L. Van, Brewer, B. W., Rivera, P. M., & Petitpas, A. J. (1994). The relationship between observable self-talk and competitive junior Tennis players' match performances. *Journal of Sport & Exercise Psychology*, 16, 400–415. https://doi.org/10.1123/jsep.16.4.400

Reed, C. L. (2002). Chronometric comparisons of imagery to action: Visualizing versus physically performing springboard dives. *Memory & Cognition*, 30(8), 1169–1178. https://doi.org/10.3758/BF03213400

Richardson, A. (1967). Mental practice: A review and discussion. Part I. *Research Quarterly. American Association for Health, Physical Education and Recreation*, 38(1), 95–107. https://doi.org/10.1080/10671188.1967.10614808

Di Rienzo, F., Collet, C., Hoyek, N., & Guillot, A. (2014). Impact of neurologic deficits on motor imagery: A systematic review of clinical evaluations. *Neuropsychology Review*. https://doi.org/10.1007/s11065-014-9257-6

Rizzolatti, G., & Craighero, L. (2004). The mirror-neuron system. *Annu Rev Neurosci*, 27, 169–192. https://doi.org/10.1146/annurev.neuro.27.070203.144230

Rizzolatti, G., Fadiga, L., Fogassi, L., & Gallese, V. (1999). Resonance behaviors and mirror neurons. *Arch Ital Biol*, 137(2–3), 85–100.

Rizzolatti, G., Fadiga, L., Gallese, V., & Fogassi, L. (1996). Premotor cortex and the recognition of motor actions. *Brain Res Cogn Brain Res*, 3(2), 131–141.

Rizzolatti, G., Fogassi, L., & Gallese, V. (2001). Neurophysiological mechanisms underlying the understanding and imitation of action. *Nature Reviews. Neuroscience, 2*(9), 661–670. https://doi.org/10.1038/35090060

Rizzolatti, G., Fogassi, L., & Gallese, V. (2002). Motor and cognitive functions of the ventral premotor cortex. *Current Opinion in Neurobiology.* https://doi.org/10.1016/S0959-4388(02)00308-2

Robertson, E. M., Pascual-Leone, A., & Miall, R. C. (2004). Opinion: Current concepts in procedural consolidation. *Nature Reviews Neuroscience, 5*(7), 576–582. https://doi.org/10.1038/nrn1426

Romani, M., Cesari, P., Urgesi, C., Facchini, S., & Aglioti, S. M. (2005). Motor facilitation of the human cortico-spinal system during observation of bio-mechanically impossible movements. *NeuroImage, 26.* https://doi.org/10.1016/j.neuroimage.2005.02.027

Ross, J. S., Tkach, J., Ruggieri, P. M., Lieber, M., & Lapresto, E. (2003). The mind's eye: Functional MR imaging evaluation of golf motor imagery. *AJNR. American Journal of Neuroradiology, 24*(6), 1036–1044. Retrieved from http://www.ncbi.nlm.nih.gov/pubmed/12812924

Rossini, P. M. (1999). Corticospinal excitability modulation to hand muscles during movement imagery. *Cerebral Cortex, 9*(2), 161–167. https://doi.org/10.1093/cercor/9.2.161

Roth, M., Decety, J., Raybaudi, M., Massarelli, R., Delon-Martin, C., Segebarth, C., ... Jeannerod, M. (1996). Possible involvement of primary motor cortex in mentally simulated movement: A functional magnetic resonance imaging study. *Neuroreport.* https://doi.org/10.1097/00001756-199605170-00012

Ruffino, C., Papaxanthis, C., & Lebon, F. (2017). Neural plasticity during motor learning with motor imagery practice: Review and perspectives. *Neuroscience, 341,* 61–78. https://doi.org/10.1016/j.neuroscience.2016.11.023

Rushall, B. S., Hall, M., Roux, L., Sasseville, J., & Rushall, A. C. (1988). Effects of three types of thought content instructions on skiing performance. *Sport Psychologist, 2*(4), 283–297. https://doi.org/10.1123/tsp.2.4.283

Sackett, R. S. (1934). The relationship between amount of symbolic rehearsal and retention of a maze habit. *Journal of General Psychology, 10,* 376–395.

Sackett, R. S. (1935). The relationship between amount of symbolic rehearsal and retention of a maze habit. *Journal of General Psychology, 13*(1), 113–130. https://doi.org/10.1080/00221309.1935.9917869

Sakadjian, A., Panchuk, D., & Pearce, A. J. (2014). Kinematic and kinetic improvements associated with action observation facilitated learning of the power clean in Australian footballers. *Journal of Strength and Conditioning Research, 28*(6), 1613–1625. https://doi.org/10.1519/JSC.0000000000000290

Sanes, J. N., & Donoghue, J. P. (2000). Plasticity and primary motor cortex. *Annual Review of Neuroscience, 23,* 393–415. https://doi.org/10.1146/annurev.neuro.23.1.393

Saygin, A. P., Wilson, S. M., Hagler, D. J., Bates, E., & Sereno, M. I. (2004). Point-light biological motion perception activates human premotor cortex. *The Journal of Neuroscience : The Official Journal of the Society for Neuroscience, 24*(27), 6181–6188. https://doi.org/10.1523/JNEUROSCI.0504-04.2004

Schuster, C., Hilfiker, R., Amft, O., Scheidhauer, A., Andrews, B., Butler, J., ... Ettlin, T. (2011). Best practice for motor imagery: A systematic literature review on motor imagery training elements in five different disciplines. *BMC Medicine, 9*(1), 75. https://doi.org/10.1186/1741-7015-9-75

Sciutti, A., Bisio, A., Nori, F., Metta, G., Fadiga, L., Pozzo, T., & Sandini, G. (2012). Measuring Human-Robot Interaction Through Motor Resonance. *International Journal of Social Robotics, 4*(3). https://doi.org/10.1007/s12369-012-0143-1

Scully, D., & Newell, K. (1985). The acquisition of motor skills: Towards a visual epception perspective. *Journal of Human Movement Studies, 12,* 169–187.

Sidaway, B., & Trzaska, A. R. (2005). Can mental practice increase ankle dorsiflexor torque? *Physical Therapy, 85*(10), 1053–1060.

Singer, T. (2006). The neuronal basis and ontogeny of empathy and mind reading: Review of literature and implications for future research. *Neuroscience and Biobehavioral Reviews.* https://doi.org/10.1016/j.neubiorev.2006.06.011

Slimani, M., Bragazzi, N. L., Tod, D., Dellal, A., Hue, O., Cheour, F., ... Chamari, K. (2016). Do cognitive training strategies improve motor and positive psychological skills development in soccer players? Insights from a systematic review. *Journal of Sports Sciences.* https://doi.org/10.1080/02640414.2016.1254809

Smith, D., Collins, D., & Holmes, P. (2003). Impact and mechanism of mental practice effects on strength. *International Journal of Sport and Exercise Psychology, 1*(3), 293–306. https://doi.org/10.1080/1612197X.2003.9671720

St Clair Gibson, A., & Foster, C. (2007). The role of self-talk in the awareness of physiological state and physical performance. *Sports Medicine.* https://doi.org/10.2165/00007256-200737120-00003

Stecklow, M. V., Infantosi, A. F. C., & Cagy, M. (2010). EEG changes during sequences of visual and kinesthetic motor imagery. *Arquivos de Neuro-Psiquiatria, 68*(4), 556–561. https://doi.org/10.1590/S0004-282X2010000400015

Stefan, K., Cohen, L. G., Duque, J., Mazzocchio, R., Celnik, P., Sawaki, L., ... Classen, J. (2005). Formation of a motor memory by action observation. *The Journal of Neuroscience : The Official Journal of the Society for Neuroscience, 25*, 9339–9346. https://doi.org/10.1523/JNEUROSCI.2282-05.2005

Stinear, C., & Byblow, W. (2004). Modulation of corticospinal excitability and intracortical inhibition during motor imagery is task-dependent. *Experimental Brain Research, 157*(3). https://doi.org/10.1007/s00221-004-1851-z

Stinear, C. M., & Byblow, W. D. (2003). Motor imagery of phasic thumb abduction temporally and spatially modulates corticospinal excitability. *Clinical Neurophysiology, 114*(5), 909–914. https://doi.org/10.1016/S1388-2457(02)00373-5

Stinear, C. M., Byblow, W. D., Steyvers, M., Levin, O., & Swinnen, S. P. (2006). Kinesthetic, but not visual, motor imagery modulates corticomotor excitability. *Experimental Brain Research, 168*, 157–164. https://doi.org/10.1007/s00221-005-0078-y

Stinear, C. M., Fleming, M. K., & Byblow, W. D. (2006). Lateralization of unimanual and bimanual motor imagery. *Brain Research, 1095*(1), 139–147. https://doi.org/10.1016/j.brainres.2006.04.008

Strack, B., Linden, M., & Wilson, V. (Eds.). (2011). History of biofeedback in sport. In *Biofeedback and neurofeedback applications in sportpsychology* (pp. 21–45). Wheat Ridge, CO: Association for Applied Psychophysiology and Biofeedback.

Suchan, B., Melde, C., Herzog, H., Hömberg, V., & Seitz, R. J. (2008). Activation differences in observation of hand movements for imitation or velocity judgement. *Behavioural Brain Research, 188*(1), 78–83. https://doi.org/10.1016/j.bbr.2007.10.021

Swann, C., & Rosenbaum, S. (2017). Do we need to reconsider best practice in goal setting for physical activity promotion? *British Journal of Sports Medicine*, bjsports-2017-098186. https://doi.org/10.1136/bjsports-2017-098186

Tenenbaum, G., Bar-Eli, M., Hoffman, J. R., Jablonovski, R., Sade, S., & Shitrit, D. (1995). The effect of cognitive and somatic psyching-up techniques on isokinetic leg strength performance. *Journal of Strength and Conditioning Research, 9*(1), 3–7. https://doi.org/10.1519/00124278-199502000-00001

Theodorakis, Y., Weinberg, R., Natsis, P., Douma, I., & Kazakas, P. (2000). The effects of motivational versus instructional self-talk on improving motor performance. *Sport Psychologist (Champaign, IL), 14*(3), 253–271. https://doi.org/10.1123/tsp.14.3.253

Tod, D., Edwards, C., McGuigan, M., & Lovell, G. (2015). A systematic review of the effect of cognitive strategies on strength performance. *Sports Medicine.* https://doi.org/10.1007/s40279-015-0356-1

Tod, D., Hardy, J., & Oliver, E. (2011). Effects of self-talk: A systematic review. *Journal of Sport and Exercise Psychology, 33*(5), 666–687. https://doi.org/10.1123/jsep.33.5.666

Tod, D. A., Thatcher, R., Mcguigan, M., & Thatcher, J. (2009). Effects of instructional and motivational self-talk on the vertical jump. *Journal of Strength and Conditioning Research, 23*(1), 196–202. https://doi.org/10.1519/JSC.0b013e3181889203

Tomasello, M., Kruger, A. C., & Ratner, H. H. (1993). Cultural learning. *Behavioral and Brain Sciences, 16*(3), 495. https://doi.org/10.1017/S0140525X0003123X

Tremblay, F., Tremblay, L. E., & Colcer, D. E. (2001). Modulation of corticospinal excitability during imagined knee movements. *Journal of Rehabilitation Medicine, 33*(5), 230–234. https://doi.org/10.1080/165019701750419635

Van Raalte, J. L., Cornelius, A. E., Hatten, S. J., & Brewer, B. W. (2000). The antecedents and consequences of self-talk in competitive tennis. *Journal of Sport & Exercise Psychology.* https://doi.org/10.1123/jsep.22.4.345

Vergeer, I., & Roberts, J. (2006). Movement and stretching imagery during flexibility training. *Journal of Sports Sciences, 24*(2), 197–208. https://doi.org/10.1080/02640410500131811

Wakefield, C., & Smith, D. (2012). Perfecting practice: Applying the PETTLEP model of motor imagery. *Journal of Sport Psychology in Action, 3*(1), 1–11. https://doi.org/10.1080/21520704.2011.639853

Wang, Z., Wang, S., Shi, F. Y., Guan, Y., Wu, Y., Zhang, L. L., ... Zhang, J. (2014). The effect of motor imagery with specific implement in expert badminton player. *Neuroscience, 275*, 102–112. https://doi.org/10.1016/j.neuroscience.2014.06.004

Wei, G., & Luo, J. (2010). Sport expert's motor imagery: Functional imaging of professional motor skills and simple motor skills. *Brain Research, 1341*, 52–62. https://doi.org/10.1016/j.brainres.2009.08.014

Weinberg, R., Butt, J., Knight, B., Burke, K. L., & Jackson, A. (2003). The relationship between the use and effectiveness of imagery: An exploratory investigation. *Journal of Applied Sport Psychology, 15*(1), 26–40. https://doi.org/10.1080/10413200305398

Williams, A. M., & Hodges, N. J. (2005). Practice, instruction and skill acquisition in soccer: Challenging tradition. *Journal of Sports Sciences, 23*(6), 637–650. https://doi.org/10.1080/02640410400021328

Wohlschläger, A., Gattis, M., & Bekkering, H. (2003). Action generation and action perception in imitation: An instance of the ideomotor principle. *Philosophical Transactions of the Royal Society of London. Series B, Biological Sciences, 358*, 501–515. https://doi.org/10.1098/rstb.2002.1257

Wright, M. J., Bishop, D. T., Jackson, R. C., & Abernethy, B. (2010). Functional MRI reveals expert-novice differences during sport-related anticipation. *Neuroreport, 21*(2), 94–98. https://doi.org/10.1097/WNR.0b013e328333dff2

Wright, M. J., Bishop, D. T., Jackson, R. C., & Abernethy, B. (2011). Cortical fMRI activation to opponents' body kinematics in sport-related anticipation: Expert-novice differences with normal and point-light video. *Neuroscience Letters, 500*(3), 216–221. https://doi.org/10.1016/j.neulet.2011.06.045

Yahagi, S., & Kasai, T. (1998). Facilitation of motor evoked potentials (MEPs) in first dorsal interosseous (FDI) muscle is dependent on different motor images. *Electroencephalography and Clinical Neurophysiology - Electromyography and Motor Control, 109*(5), 409–417. https://doi.org/10.1016/S0924-980X(98)00041-1

Yahagi, S., & Kasai, T. (1999). Motor evoked potentials induced by motor imagery reveal a functional asymmetry of cortical motor control in left- and right-handed human subjects. *Neuroscience Letters, 276*(3), 185–188. https://doi.org/10.1016/S0304-3940(99)00823-X

Yue, G., & Cole, K. J. (1992). Strength increases from the motor program: Comparison of training with maximal voluntary and imagined muscle contractions. *Journal of Neurophysiology, 67*(5), 1114–1123. https://doi.org/10.1152/jn.1992.67.5.1114

Zhang, X., de Beukelaar, T. T., Possel, J., Olaerts, M., Swinnen, S. P., Woolley, D. G., & Wenderoth, N. (2011). Movement observation improves early consolidation of motor memory. *The Journal of Neuroscience : The Official Journal of the Society for Neuroscience, 31*, 11515–11520. https://doi.org/10.1523/JNEUROSCI.6759-10.2011

Ziemann, U., Ilić, T. V, Pauli, C., Meintzschel, F., & Ruge, D. (2004). Learning modifies subsequent induction of long-term potentiation-like and long-term depression-like plasticity in human motor cortex. *The Journal of Neuroscience : The Official Journal of the Society for Neuroscience, 24*, 1666–1672. https://doi.org/10.1523/JNEUROSCI.5016-03.2004

Zijdewind, I., Toering, S. T., Bessem, B., Van der Laan, O., & Diercks, R. L. (2003). Effects of imagery motor training on torque production of ankle plantar flexor muscles. *Muscle and Nerve, 28*(2), 168–173. https://doi.org/10.1002/mus.10406

Zinsser, N., Bunker, L., & Williams, J. (2010). Cognitive techniques for building confidence and enhancing performance. In *Applied sport psychology: Personal growth to peak performance* (pp. 305–335). Boston, MA: Mc Graw Hill.

Zourbanos, N., Hatzigeorgiadis, A., & Theodorakis, Y. (2007). A preliminary investigation of the relationship between athletes' self-talk and coaches' behaviour and statements. *International Journal of Sports Science & Coaching, 2*(1), 57–66. https://doi.org/10.1260/174795407780367195

Neurofeedback Research in Sport

A Critical Review of the Field

Andrew M. Cooke, Eduardo Bellomo, Germano Gallicchio, and Christopher Ring

Neurofeedback, otherwise known as "brain-training", is in vogue. The famous Australian golfer, Jason Day (world number one at the time of writing this chapter), reportedly uses neurofeedback to allow him to "get in the zone", claiming that his "mental game has improved 110% since working with the [neurofeedback] system" (Australian Associated Press, 2013). Having recorded top-four finishes in all four of golf's major championships during the past five years, including winning the 2015 PGA Championship and accruing estimated earnings in excess of $33 million (All time money list, 2016), it is hard to argue against his training methods. Day is not the only one; consider the Italian soccer team, who reportedly used state-of-the-art brain training to help mastermind their penalty kick victory over France in the final of the 2006 World Cup (Wilson, Peper, & Moss, 2006). Similarly, consider the Canadian short-track speed skating team, who used neurofeedback to help them achieve five medals, including two golds, at the 2010 Vancouver Winter Olympic Games (Beauchamp, Harvey, & Beauchamp, 2012). From these success stories, one could create a compelling argument for the use of neurofeedback training as a tool to help ensure the optimal performance of athletes, especially under pressure-laden conditions, where optimal performance matters the most. However, despite an increasing "in vogue" status supported by high-profile successes, neurofeedback is far from being a mainstream intervention in elite sport. This chapter will review the available evidence and consider some of the reasons why neurofeedback training remains only a minor player in applied sport science. We especially focus on exploring some key methodological shortcomings and interpretational caveats that pervade much of the extant neurofeedback research. In doing so, this chapter will provide a concise introduction to neurofeedback training, and a critical and balanced view of the current state of knowledge regarding neurofeedback and sport performance. We also offer some guidelines for future research, which we hope will stimulate more high-quality neurofeedback experiments to further interrogate and unearth its putative performance-enhancing qualities in the years and decades to come.

What Is Neurofeedback?

Neurofeedback, sometimes termed "brain training", is biofeedback for the brain. In essence, it involves recording and displaying an individual's brain activity (e.g., in the form of graphs on a computer screen), in real-time, while encouraging the individual to develop strategies to control their brain activity levels. Two questions often posed when neurofeedback is described in this way are: (a) how can someone learn to take control of their brain activity and (b) why might this be useful? The answer to the latter question is straightforward. Indeed, it is well established that our movements are controlled by our brain, and distinct patterns of brain activity characterise optimal and suboptimal movement outcomes. For instance, in the clinical domain research has established distinct patterns of brain activity that are associated with suboptimal movement control in people with Parkinson's Disease, compared to healthy age-matched populations (e.g., Defebvre et al., 1994; Magnani, Cursi, Leocani, Volonte, & Comi, 2002). Similarly, in sport, there are differences in brain activity between highly skilled experts and less skilled novices (e.g., Cooke et al., 2014) as well as between successful and unsuccessful performances within an expert population (e.g., Babiloni et al., 2008). Thus, there is a rationale for encouraging sportsmen and sportswomen to consistently produce patterns of brain activity that we know to be associated with optimal movements, while avoiding those that characterise suboptimal movements. Doing so could reduce the likelihood of movement errors, a putative benefit not to be dismissed!

The answer to the first question, how can someone learn to control their brain activity, derives from some of the origins of behavioural science, namely, Skinner's work on operant conditioning (e.g., Skinner, 1963). In brief, he provided compelling evidence in a series of studies to show that organisms can learn to regulate their behaviour around positive and negative feedback (i.e., learn to augment behaviours that are accompanied by positive feedback and suppress those that are accompanied by negative feedback) (for review see Iversen, 1992). Neurofeedback training applies these operant conditioning principles. First, by displaying brain activity in real-time, neurofeedback affords individuals the opportunity to practice strategies to alter their brain activity levels. Importantly, this practice can be supplemented by positive and negative feedback to help individuals recognise what the desired pattern of brain activity looks and feels like. For example, if the optimal brain activity involves suppressing a particular brainwave frequency (e.g., alpha waves) by 25% compared to a resting baseline, the computer receiving the brain activity data can be set to provide positive feedback, such as the silencing of a high-pitch tone, or the smooth playing of a video on the screen, whenever alpha waves are reducing towards and below the 25% threshold. Meanwhile, negative feedback, such as the intensification of a tone, or the distortion of on-screen images, would occur if alpha waves increase above the desired level. In this way, participants are able to learn how to self-regulate their brain activity levels, specifically recognizing how to produce a desired state, while reducing the likelihood of sub-optimal cortical activation patterns.

Having introduced the concept of neurofeedback training, the next section provides a brief overview of how a neurofeedback intervention can be implemented. The main body of the chapter will then critique available evidence to assess the efficacy of neurofeedback training in sport, and allow the reader to form their own opinion about whether a neurofeedback intervention in their sport/with their athletes would be worthwhile.

Neurofeedback: Getting Started

By their very nature, neurofeedback interventions require the possession of some equipment capable of recording brain activity. Neurofeedback can be based on brain measures including functional magnetic resonance imaging (fMRI), near-infrared spectroscopy (NIRS), magnetoencephalography (MEG), and electroencephalography (EEG) (e.g., Thibault, Lifshitz, & Raz, 2016). However, EEG is currently the recording method of choice among neurofeedback researchers and practitioners in sport for two principal reasons. First, it is possible to deliver EEG-based neurofeedback in ecologically valid settings such as while golfers practice putting on the putting green (e.g., Arns, Kleinnijenhuis, Fallahpour, & Breteler, 2008). The same cannot be said for fMRI and MEG, which both require participants to remain largely motionless inside specialised laboratories and scanners. Second, EEG is comparatively low cost. Wireless EEG systems start from a few hundred dollars, while the other imaging systems costs upward of $50,000, with costs as high as $2 million for a high-specification fMRI scanner (all prices 2016). Such costs are prohibitive to all but the very wealthiest professional sports organizations. Accordingly, EEG-based neurofeedback will be the focus for the remainder of this chapter.

Neurofeedback equipment and protocol. The basic requirements of an EEG neurofeedback setup are: (a) an EEG amplifier and recording electrodes; (b) a computer with screen and speakers to display the acquired signals in visual and/or auditory form; and (c) software to allow the user to customise which elements of the EEG signal are fed back. Each of these components are illustrated in Figure 13.1.

It should be noted that there are a wide range of systems on the market. Some key features to help distinguish between higher and lower specification models are electrode type (active are better than passive), sample rate (higher sample rates allow more rapid and detailed feedback of the signal, >200 Hz required to permit the recording of the full gamma frequency range), and the resolution of the analog to digital convertor (higher the better, the latest systems provide 24 bit resolution). The specifications of the computer may also have some bearing on the effectiveness of the neurofeedback training. The minimum specifications are laid out by the manufacturers of the various EEG systems. Most systems will operate on any computer. In general, the more processing speed (typically > 2GHz), and the greater the RAM memory (typically > 1GB), the better. A dedicated graphics card can also be helpful in facilitating smooth and detailed visual feedback.[1]

Once a neurofeedback system is in place, the procedure to instrument participants for a neurofeedback training session ranges from a few minutes to around half an hour depending on the number of electrodes being attached. Figure 13.1A illustrates a participant instrumented for a neurofeedback training session in our laboratory. The key preparatory stages associated with neurofeedback instrumentation are summarised in Figure 13.2.

As shown in Figure 13.2, the final step prior to the commencement of neurofeedback training involves setting the thresholds to provide positive and negative feedback. It should be noted that

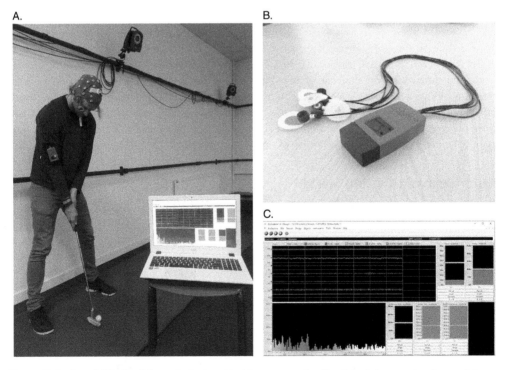

Figure 13.1 Panel (A): Participant instrumented for a neurofeedback training session in our laboratory. Panel (B): Example neurofeedback amplifier with recording electrodes. Panel (C): Screenshot of example neurofeedback software, with thresholds displayed as horizontal lines on each of the five bar charts.

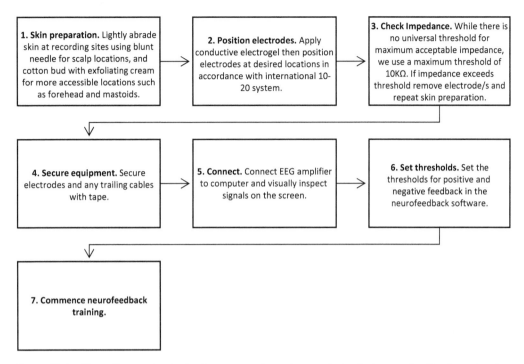

1. **Skin preparation.** Lightly abrade skin at recording sites using blunt needle for scalp locations, and cotton bud with exfoliating cream for more accessible locations such as forehead and mastoids.

2. **Position electrodes.** Apply conductive electrogel then position electrodes at desired locations in accordance with international 10-20 system.

3. **Check Impedance.** While there is no universal threshold for maximum acceptable impedance, we use a maximum threshold of 10KΩ. If impedance exceeds threshold remove electrode/s and repeat skin preparation.

4. **Secure equipment.** Secure electrodes and any trailing cables with tape.

5. **Connect.** Connect EEG amplifier to computer and visually inspect signals on the screen.

6. **Set thresholds.** Set the thresholds for positive and negative feedback in the neurofeedback software.

7. **Commence neurofeedback training.**

Figure 13.2   Flow diagram to depict key preparatory stages of a typical neurofeedback protocol.

this step is not strictly necessary since simply displaying real-time brain activity on the screen is sufficient to allow participants to practice strategies to modify their activation levels. However, the addition of thresholds to provide feedback will likely expedite learning through the principals of operant conditioning. When adopted, this step is of critical importance in determining the outcome of the neurofeedback intervention. The key issue of what to feedback (i.e., what thresholds to set) is discussed at length in the form of a critical review of the extant sport neurofeedback literature in the following sections.

Neurofeedback in Sport: What to Feedback and Does It Work? A Critical Review

There are two approaches that can be used to establish a rationale for what portion of brain activity to train and why this training ought to be beneficial for individual athletes, termed herein the *prescription approach* and the *data-driven approach*. The prescription approach is underscored by neuroscientific literature on the functional significance of individual measures of the EEG signal (e.g., spectral power in a specific frequency band). The basic premise is that a practitioner consults their knowledge of EEG functional significance and uses this to prescribe a particular kind of training that is theorised to be beneficial, based on the individual requirements of the athlete. For instance, activity in the 8–12 Hz frequency-band of the EEG spectrum (commonly termed "alpha power") is thought to have an inverse relation with cortical activity (e.g., Pfurtscheller, 1992). Thus, if an athlete reported struggling to perform under high-pressure conditions due to being unable to produce the required levels of relaxation, a practitioner may *prescribe* a neurofeedback training intervention to increase alpha power on the premise that increased alpha power is associated with reduced cortical activity (e.g., Beauchamp et al., 2012). Of course, a key caution with this approach is that our understanding of the functional significance of EEG activity is somewhat limited, and rapidly evolving. For example, while increased alpha power has been interpreted to reflect cortical areas at rest in the past (e.g., Pfurtscheller, 1992), more recent literature argues a more active role of increased alpha in functionally suppressing activity in task-irrelevant brain regions (e.g., Klimesch, 2012). Accordingly, it is crucial for practitioners to remain up to date with the latest scientific literature to inform any neurofeedback prescriptions they offer.

In contrast to the prescription approach, the data-driven approach to neurofeedback involves observing patterns of EEG activity associated with expert and/or successful performances, and training athletes to recognise and replicate these patterns at all times. This approach could see considerable variation in the neurofeedback training provided across different athletes. For instance, the data-driven approach would recommend different EEG scalp locations, frequencies, and thresholds depending on the sport, to reflect known inter-sport differences in the optimal patterns of cortical activity (for review see Cooke, 2013). This differs from the prescription approach, which often prescribes the same intervention, regardless of sport, to all athletes reporting similar symptoms (e.g., increase alpha power as a universal prescription to enhance relaxation/inhibition). Both approaches have merits and there are some pockets of encouraging evidence (but not unequivocal evidence), to suggest that both can be effective in the sport domain. We elaborate on the key evidence below.

Neurofeedback in Sport: Prescription Approach

To date, the prescription approach to neurofeedback has been mainly concerned with increasing relaxation and attentional control (e.g., alpha power training or sensorimotor rhythm training), or increasing creativity (e.g., alpha to theta ratio training). The studies we review below to evaluate these prescription-based protocols are also summarised alongside a wider complement of prescription neurofeedback studies in sport in Table 13.1.

Alpha power training. Spectral power in the alpha frequency band (around 8–12 Hz) has an inverse relation with cortical activity, whereby relatively low levels of alpha power are associated with cortical activation, and relatively high levels of alpha power are associated with inactivity and/or active inhibition (Klimesch, Sauseng, & Hanslmayr, 2007; Pfurtscheller, 1992). To this end, it has been reasoned that neurofeedback training to increase baseline alpha power should facilitate relaxation (e.g., Nowlis & Kamiya, 1970) and selective attention by inhibiting irrelevant cortical activity and thereby maximizing the amount of resources available for deployment to task relevant processes (e.g., Klimesch et al., 2007). To examine this notion, Dekker, Van den Berg, Denissen, Sitskoorn, and Van Boxtel (2014) trained six elite gymnasts to increase their baseline alpha power, while a control group of six elite gymnasts received equivalent training in the beta band (i.e., training of a randomly changing 4 Hz bandwidth somewhere between 16–36 Hz), which was not hypothesised to influence relaxation or attention. The purpose of this group was to control for the possibility that any benefits of the neurofeedback intervention could have been driven by placebo effects associated with exposure to neurofeedback equipment and attention from experimenters. Alpha power was operationalised as ±2 Hz from each individual's alpha peak, as identified at a baseline session (see Klimesch, Pfurtscheller, Mohl, & Schimke, 1990). Participants attended ten training sessions, each consisting of 24 minutes of auditory neurofeedback based on power at C3 and C4 electrodes, referenced to left and right earlobes, respectively. Specifically, participants sat in a comfortable chair and listened to their favourite songs, with the sound quality determined by their alpha power (or beta power for members of the control group). Relative alpha power (i.e., power in the 8–12 Hz band divided by sum of total power in 4–35 Hz band) over the most recent four second window (updated every 125 ms), was computed and compared with the level achieved in the previous four second window. When the current alpha power exceeded that produced in the previous time window, an increase in the richness and fullness of the music (proportional to the extent to which alpha exceeded the previous level) occurred. In contrast, the music became

Table 13.1 Summary of prescription neurofeedback studies in sport

Paper	Sport	Participants receiving neurofeedback intervention	What was fed back?	Was neurofeedback associated with changes in cortical activity at post-test?	Was neurofeedback associated with changes in performance at post-test?	Main limitation(s)
Beauchamp et al. (2012)	Speed skating	20 expert (development squad or national team) speed skaters	Increase alpha power and decrease beta power at Cz.	Not assessed	Not assessed, although it was noted that team ranking improved during the period when the intervention was active.	No post-test assessments. No control groups. Neurofeedback intervention coincided with numerous other biofeedback, psychological skills, and technical training interventions so unable to make any specific conclusions about neurofeedback training.
Dekker et al. (2014)	Gymnastics	12 expert gymnasts / trampolinists from national performance centre	Increase baseline alpha power at C3 and C4.	No	Not assessed	No pre-test or post-test measures of performance.
Kavussanu et al. (1998)	Basketball	12 recreational basketball players	Practice at increasing and decreasing 0.5 Hz – 32 Hz power over right and left temporal cortex.	Not assessed, but data during training sessions indicated that EEG changes did manifest when neurofeedback signal was present.	Yes – partial. Sub-group analyses comparing biggest and smallest responders to the neurofeedback training (in terms of changes in EEG activity during training sessions) showed improved performance in the biggest responders.	Neurofeedback intervention coincided with heart rate and muscle activity biofeedback so unable to make any specific conclusions about neurofeedback training.
Raymond et al. (2005)	Sport Dance	Six college-level dancers	Theta power to exceed alpha power at Pz.	Not assessed	Yes	Lack of pre-test and post-test EEG assessment prevents improved performance from being unequivocally linked to neurofeedback intervention.

(Continued)

Paper	Sport	Participants receiving neurofeedback intervention	What was fed back?	Was neurofeedback associated with changes in cortical activity at post-test?	Was neurofeedback associated with changes in performance at post-test?	Main limitation(s)
Ros et al. (2009)	Ophthalmic surgery	10 trainee ophthalmic surgeons	Increase SMR at Cz.	Not assessed	Yes	Lack of pre-test and post-test EEG assessment prevents performance from being unequivocally linked to neurofeedback intervention.
Rostami et al. (2012)	Rifle shooting	12 expert marksmen	Increase SMR power at C3 and theta power to exceed alpha power at Pz.	Not assessed	Yes	Lack of pre-test and post-test EEG assessment prevents performance from being unequivocally linked to neurofeedback intervention.
Shaw et al. (2012)	Gymnastics	11 college gymnasts	Increase SMR and decrease theta power at Cz.	No	Yes	Lack of EEG changes imply that improvements in performance not attributable to neurofeedback training. Neurofeedback intervention coincided with heart rate variability biofeedback.
Sherlin et al. (2013)	Baseball	Five professional baseball players from development squad of a Major League Baseball team	Combination of increase and decrease low and high frequency power over combination of frontal, central and parietal electrode locations.	Yes	Not assessed	No test of the effects of neurofeedback training on performance.
Sherlin et al. (2015)	Golf	16 top division collegiate golfers	Details not provided – unclear whether this study followed prescription or data-driven approach	Not assessed	Yes	No information about the neurofeedback protocol used. No pre- or post-test EEG data.

thinner and more distant during epochs when alpha power decreased (see van Boxtel et al., 2012). Participants received no instructions other than to sit back and relax.

Analyses comparing EEG alpha power in pre- and post-intervention tests revealed no significant changes in alpha power. However, in spite of the null effects of the intervention on cortical activity, the alpha power group reported feeling in better "physical shape" and achieving greater "mental balance" than members of the control group as the training progressed. The study thus offers some indication that alpha power training could have some benefits, yet it is clearly subject to a number of shortcomings. First and foremost, the lack of change in cortical activity from pre- to post-intervention test questions the effectiveness of the neurofeedback protocol in training participants to self-regulate their levels of alpha power. However, this could be an artefact of low statistical power since the mean alpha levels did increase marginally in the experimental group, and this identical protocol has previously proved successful at significantly increasing alpha power in a larger sample of non-athletes (i.e., van Boxtel et al., 2012). Notwithstanding, the reliance on self-report rather than objective performance data or measures of relaxation limits any conclusions concerning the effectiveness of this form of prescribed alpha-power training on sporting performance or calmness under pressure. It is recommended that future studies incorporate an objective performance assessment and measures of psychological stress both before and after the neurofeedback intervention in order for any outcome effects to be more readily assessed.

Sensorimotor rhythm training. While the functional significance of the sensorimotor rhythm (SMR; power in the 12–15 Hz range, strongest in sensorimotor cortex) is not as well established as alpha power, there is reasonable evidence linking enhanced SMR power with increased attention and reduced motor interference during perceptual processing (e.g., Gruzelier, Egner, & Vernon, 2006; Kober et al., 2015). Accordingly, Shaw, Zaichkowsky, and Wilson (2012) prescribed a neurofeedback intervention to increase SMR power, with the overarching aim of improving balance beam performance in a sample of eleven college gymnasts. The gymnasts underwent ten training sessions to increase SMR (13–15 Hz) power at the Cz electrode (with reference electrode on right ear lobe and ground electrode on the left ear lobe) to exceed 2.5µV. In addition to increasing SMR power, they were simultaneously trained to ensure theta (4–7 Hz) power was below 10µV (12.5µV for three participants for whom 10µV was too difficult). In brief, high-levels of eyes-open theta power have been associated with inattention and fatigue, and characterise attention-deficit-hyperactivity-disorder (Gruzelier, 2009). Accordingly, it was reasoned that decreased theta power alongside increased SMR power would provide the best means of training the gymnasts to reduce sensorimotor interference and increase their attention, and recognise how to call upon these states during their balance beam routine. Each training session was 15 minutes in duration, with the first five sessions utilizing visual neurofeedback (i.e., participants viewed visual displays of the SMR and theta signals on a screen) while the final five sessions combined visual neurofeedback with an auditory tone to indicate when the desired thresholds had been met. The addition of the tone in the final sessions afforded participants the opportunity to look away from the computer screen, thereby reducing the risk of participants becoming reliant on the visual displays when self-regulating cortical power.

Similar to Dekker et al. (2014), results revealed no change in EEG activity from pre- to post-intervention tests. However, results indicated pre-test to post-test improvements in performance ratings for artistry and execution elements of the balance beam routine. Moreover, there was a significant deterioration in performance in the month following the neurofeedback intervention withdrawal. This implies that the intervention was indeed beneficial for the period over which it was carried out, but the performance benefits were not sustained once the training ceased.

The beneficial performance effects during this intervention are certainly encouraging, and represents a strength when compared to the previously described Dekker et al. (2014) experiment, which did not assess objective performance. However, the lack of pre-test to post-test changes in EEG activity remains a concern and could imply that the improvement in performance that was achieved by the gymnasts was not directly attributable to the neurofeedback that they received. This study was also subject to three additional limitations which should be considered. First, all participants also undertook a heart rate variability biofeedback training program in parallel with the neurofeedback intervention. Accordingly, the extent to which the performance findings are attributable to the neurofeedback versus the heart rate variability training are unknown. Second, the use of a 2.5μV fixed threshold for SMR power for all participants could have limited the effectiveness of the protocol by not taking into account individual differences in baseline SMR power. For instance, training to increase SMR power above 2.5μV would be considerably easier for a participant with an SMR power baseline close to this threshold compared to someone whose baseline is further away. To address this issue, thresholds could have been based on a percentage change from an individual's baseline rather than a fixed value for all (e.g., Ring, Cooke, Kavussanu, McIntyre, & Masters, 2015). Finally, the drop in performance that was observed after the training ended could suggest that any benefits were driven by a placebo effect associated with the presence of the biofeedback equipment and experimenter. A sham-feedback control group akin to the random beta-training group used by Dekker et al. (2014) could have been included in the study design to test this possibility.

A study of SMR neurofeedback that did contain a control group was conducted by Rostami, Sadeghi, Karami, Abadi, and Salamati (2012). They trained 12 elite marksmen to increase SMR power while concurrently inhibiting high-beta (20–30 Hz) power. Participants in the neurofeedback group attended fifteen training sessions in which they had to increase SMR power (13–15 Hz) over C3 (referenced to C4, with ground electrode on the right ear lobe) while avoiding a concurrent increase in high-beta power (20–30 Hz). The latter feature of the intervention was presumably designed to help ensure that the increase SMR power training did not spill over to higher frequency bands. Each thirty minute training session was preceded a two-minute baseline recording. Participants were rewarded on a visual display each time they increased SMR power above baseline level for 500ms, in the absence of a concurrent increase in beta power. If participants received rewards for more than 90% of any training session, then the SMR threshold level was increased above baseline level for subsequent sessions to facilitate progression.

Encouragingly, results revealed that neurofeedback training was associated with improvements in shooting accuracy from pre- to post-intervention shooting tests, while the performance of the control group, who received no neurofeedback training, was unchanged. This finding adds to the results of Shaw et al. (2012) to offer further promising evidence of the effectiveness of increase SMR neurofeedback interventions in sport. However, there are once again a series of limitations, which lessen the impact of these results. First, no pre-test and post-test measures of EEG are reported, so the hypothesised effects of the training on cortical activity at post-test (i.e., increased SMR power) cannot be confirmed. Second, like the Shaw et al. (2012) study, it is unfortunate that these participants also simultaneously completed a separate neurofeedback intervention targeting alpha and theta power. Accordingly, while the main focus of the manuscript concerned SMR power, it is impossible to say with certainty that the SMR intervention was responsible for the beneficial performance effects. Finally, while the presence of a non-neurofeedback control group is better than no control group at all, it would have been desirable to include a sham-neurofeedback control group who received comparable exposure to neurofeedback equipment and experimenters in order to evaluate and take account of potential placebo effects.

Given these limitations of existing prescription-based SMR power studies in sport, it is worth reviewing a final SMR neurofeedback study conducted outside of sport. Specifically, Ros and colleagues (2009) subjected 10 trainee ophthalmic surgeons to eight neurofeedback training sessions, each 30-minutes in duration, aimed at increasing SMR power at Cz (referenced to linked ears). Participants were rewarded, indicated by the movement of a spaceship on a video game, when they increased SMR by 80% from their baseline, in the absence of concurrent increases in theta (4–7 Hz) and high-beta (22–30 Hz) power. Members of the experimental group were compared to both a non-neurofeedback control group ($N = 8$) and a separate neurofeedback group who received alpha and theta neurofeedback training ($N = 10$). Results indicated a benefit of SMR training on performance, with completion time of a simulated cataract operation improving from pre- to post-intervention among members of the SMR training group only. In addition to faster completions, the SMR group also demonstrated a pre- to post-intervention test improvement in technique, as indexed by a 4.1% improvement on a technique rating scale completed by two experienced consultant ophthalmic surgeon observers. Performance among members of the control group and the alternative neurofeedback group was unchanged.

Although outside of sport, this study is of interest since the sensorimotor precision demands combined with the dire consequences of errors faced by surgeons may represent similar pressures and demands to those experienced in elite sport. The inclusion of both non-neurofeedback and alternative neurofeedback control groups are a strength of this study. That selective performance benefits emerged in the increase SMR neurofeedback group provides good evidence that the beneficial effects of neurofeedback are genuine and not due to placebo. However, this study is still limited by a lack of EEG measurement at pre-test and post-test sessions. Like the study of Rostami et al. (2012), this design limitation prevents the observed beneficial effects of neurofeedback training on performance from being directly associated with neurofeedback-induced changes in cortical activation.

In sum, there is encouraging evidence to suggest that training to increase SMR power can be prescribed to help increase perceptual processing and inhibit sensorimotor interference in precision sports. However, more research needs to be done, addressing some of the limitations cited above, before the effectiveness of such protocols can be unequivocally confirmed.

Alpha-theta training. The origins of alpha-theta training stem from evidence that innovative ideas (e.g., high creativity) often occur during the transition period between wakefulness and sleep (Gruzelier, 2009). Training to encourage theta power to exceed alpha power while the eyes are closed is designed to replicate the brain state that occurs during the wakefulness-sleep transition (i.e., hypnogogia). Raymond, Sajid, Parkinson, and Gruzelier (2005) conducted an alpha-theta neurofeedback intervention in a sample of six college level sport-dancers, compared to two matched groups of eight dancers who received either heart rate variability biofeedback training, or no training (i.e., control group). The neurofeedback intervention consisted of 10 sessions, each of 20-minutes duration, divided into one-minute blocks interspersed with brief breaks to help ensure that no participant actually fell asleep. Training was delivered based on activity at the Pz electrode, referenced to the ear lobes. In this study, alpha power was operationalised as ±1.5 Hz from the peak in the 8–12 Hz range, while the frequency 4 Hz below the individual alpha peak was used as the median point of a 3 Hz theta band. Since alpha-theta training requires participants to close their eyes, the feedback was auditory, with a "babbling brook" played when alpha was higher than theta, and "crashing waves" played when theta was higher than alpha. As the latter represented the desired state, participants were asked to visualise themselves dancing whenever they heard the crashing waves sound.

Results showed that overall dance performance, as rated by qualified judges, improved from pre-intervention to post-intervention tests to a greater extent among members of the neurofeedback group compared to members of the control group. However, the heart rate variability biofeedback group also improved to a greater extent than the controls, raising the possibility that the improvements recorded in both biofeedback groups were placebo effects driven by the additional exposure to equipment and experimenters that these groups experienced. To counter this argument, it is worth noting that scores on the subscales of the dance assessment measure (which are combined to formulate the overall score), revealed that neurofeedback training was associated with an improvement in dancer timing that was absent in both control and heart rate variability groups. This provides evidence of specific benefits on an aspect of coordination (i.e., timing) within movement tasks that may be attributed to alpha-theta neurofeedback training. However, caution should be expressed once again due to the lack of pre- and post-test EEG assessment, a common limitation in the prescription neurofeedback field.

Further caution about the widespread effectiveness of alpha-theta neurofeedback training is advised in light of the lack of benefits of alpha-theta neurofeedback in the previously reported study of neurofeedback in trainee ophthalmic surgeons (i.e., Ros et al., 2009). Indeed, Ros et al. (2009) showed benefits of SMR neurofeedback, but alpha-theta neurofeedback failed to promote performance benefits over and above those recorded by non-neurofeedback controls. Given the differences in functional significance of SMR (e.g., argued to reduce sensorimotor interference) and alpha-theta (e.g., concerned with the enhancement of creativity), it is not surprising that the SMR training was more effective for the surgery task, which likely affords little opportunity to deviate from the standard operating procedure and exhibit creative flair. These data add further weight to the viewpoint that prescription neurofeedback training should be carefully designed and specifically tailored to the sport and athlete in question. There is likely no single intervention that can be prescribed to deliver universal effectiveness. However, increasing SMR power does seem a useful means of promoting perceptual focus and fine motor control in accuracy tasks, while alpha-theta training may be the prescription of choice for athletes wishing to enhance their movement timing and creativity.

Neurofeedback in Sport: Data-Driven Approach

Compared to prescription neurofeedback studies, data-driven neurofeedback studies tend to benefit from higher ecological validity. Specifically, the training can occur in ecologically valid environments (e.g., while standing and holding a golf putter), and during real sport tasks (e.g., while striking putts). In contrast, prescription-based neurofeedback studies typically take place in a quiet and comfortable setting (e.g., comfortable chair in front a computer screen) that is removed from the sporting arena. A summary table of data-driven neurofeedback studies in sport is provided at the end of this section (Table 13.2), while a written critique of some of the most influential studies is provided next.

The seminal study of data-driven neurofeedback in sport was conducted by Landers and colleagues in 1991. They investigated the effects of neurofeedback in 16 experienced but sub-elite archers. The choice of EEG variable, electrode locations, and thresholds for the neurofeedback intervention were drawn from earlier research noting that elite marksmen and archers displayed a relatively lower activation of the left- compared to the right-hemisphere of the brain, during target aiming (e.g., Hatfield, Landers, & Ray, 1984; Salazar et al., 1990). Informed by these "expert-model" data, Landers et al. (1991) reasoned that training pre-elite archers to decrease left-hemisphere activity during aiming should enhance performance. Accordingly, two recording electrodes were attached (one over left temporal cortex and one over right temporal cortex), along with a reference electrode (right mastoid) and ground electrode (right earlobe). Participants attended a single-neurofeedback training session where they initially faced a computer screen displaying two moving horizontal bars to reflect EEG slow potentials (the relative shifts in voltage in baseline EEG) at each recording electrode. Eight participants assigned to a "correct" neurofeedback group were asked to move the bottom bar on the screen to the right. This occurred when they produced a negative voltage shift of their slow potential recorded at the left-hemisphere electrode. Initially they were required to produce a -16μV shift, upon which the words "good trial" would appear on the screen. With each good trial, the negativity threshold was updated by -2μV, until a criterion reduction of -40μV was achieved. Once this was achieved, the whole procedure was repeated with participants now adopting their shooting stance while controlling the moving bars. In all, the neurofeedback training lasted between 45 and 75 minutes depending on how quickly each participant reached the criterion level. Eight participants assigned to an "incorrect" neurofeedback group underwent an identical protocol except they were instructed to move the top bar

Table 13.2 Summary of data-driven neurofeedback studies in sport

Paper	Sport	Participants receiving neurofeedback intervention	What was fed back?	Was neurofeedback associated with changes in cortical activity at post-test?	Was neurofeedback associated with changes in performance at post-test?	Main limitation(s)
Arns et al. (2008)	Golf putting	Six experienced golfers (M handicap = 12.3)	Reduction of a combination of theta, alpha, sensory motor rhythm and/or beta power in the final moments preceding putts at FPz	Not assessed, but data during training sessions indicated that EEG changes did manifest when neurofeedback signal was present.	Not assessed, although performance was better during neurofeedback training sessions compared to training sessions without neurofeedback being present.	No post-test so unable to assess whether participants learned to alter EEG and whether this associated with improved performance.
Berka et al. (2010)	Rifle shooting	37 novices with no previous experience	Increase pre-shot alpha power at Fz and Cz.	Yes – partial. Increases in 9–10 Hz power (i.e., a small portion of the 8–12 Hz band that was trained).	Yes	Respiration-based biofeedback occurred simultaneously with neurofeedback so unclear which had strongest influence on performance.
Cheng et al. (2015a)	Golf putting	Eight expert golfers (M handicap = 0)	Increase pre-putt SMR power at Cz.	Yes	Yes	Relatively small sample
Kao et al. (2014)	Golf putting	Three expert golfers (M handicap = 0)	Reduce pre-putt theta power at Fz.	No	Yes	Small sample. Lack of EEG changes imply that improvements in performance not attributable to neurofeedback training.
Landers et al. (1991)	Archery	Eight pre-elite archers	Increase negative amplitude of slow-potential recorded over left temporal cortex.	No	Yes	Lack of EEG changes imply that improvements in performance not attributable to neurofeedback training.
Ring et al. (2015)	Golf putting	12 experienced golfers (M handicap = 23)	Reduce pre-putt theta and high-alpha power at Fz.	Yes	No	Neurofeedback and sham control group both improved performance to a similar extent from pre- to post-test. Any benefits of EEG neurofeedback training might be due to placebo effect.
Sherlin et al. (2015).	Golf	16 top division collegiate golfers	Details not provided – unclear whether this study followed prescription or data-driven approach	Not assessed	Yes	No information about the neurofeedback protocol used. No pre- or post-test EEG data.

on the screen, which reflected voltage shifts in the slow potential recorded at the right-hemisphere electrode. Like some of the previously described prescription-based neurofeedback studies, the purpose of this sham control group was to examine the possibility of placebo effects.

Within-group comparisons revealed that the "correct" neurofeedback group improved their accuracy from pre- to post-intervention archery tests, while accuracy among members of the "incorrect" neurofeedback group got worse. This finding represents the first data-driven example of neurofeedback training being used to enhance performance in sport. However, EEG assessment revealed no between-group differences in left-hemisphere EEG activity during the post-test. This indicates that the neurofeedback training protocol did not cause members of the left-hemisphere neurofeedback group to suppress left-hemisphere function. Consequently, the improvement in performance that was achieved by this group may not be directly attributable to the neurofeedback that they received.

A similar finding was recently reported by Kao, Huang, and Hung (2014). They trained three expert golfers to reduce frontal-midline theta power (4–8 Hz) below the mean level recorded during ten successful putts in a pre-intervention test. The rationale for choosing frontal-midline theta training was based on data from 20 skilled golfers, showing that lower frontal-midline theta power in the three-seconds preceding backswing distinguished best from worst putts (i.e., Kao, Huang, & Hung, 2013). Results indicated improvements in putting accuracy in the post-intervention tests, but these were not accompanied by the hypothesised reductions in frontal-midline theta power. Taken together, these studies both offer promising evidence of benefits of data-driven neurofeedback on performance, but the impact of both findings is limited by the lack of accompanying EEG changes after completion of training.

Building on these experiments, a study from our lab (i.e., Ring et al., 2015) was able to demonstrate the effectiveness of data-driven neurofeedback training at modifying post-intervention EEG power. We applied the data-driven approach to a sample of recreational golfers. The choice of EEG variable, electrode locations, and thresholds for this neurofeedback intervention were informed by research demonstrating a reduction in frontal-midline theta power (4–7 Hz) and high-alpha power (10–12 Hz) in the final two seconds preceding golf putts, which was greater in experts compared to novices, and for holed compared to missed putts (e.g., Cooke et al., 2014; Kao et al., 2013). Using these "expert-model" and "successful performance" data, we trained a sample of 12 recreational golfers to reduce their frontal mid-line theta and high-alpha power (i.e., Fz electrode, with reference and ground electrodes at right and left mastoids, respectively) before initiating putts, while a control group of twelve recreational golfers received false neurofeedback. Our neurofeedback training intervention consisted of three separate one-hour sessions where participants heard an auditory tone, which varied in pitch, based on their real-time theta and high-alpha power. The tone was set to silence when they produced a reduction in power, relative to their own individual baseline, exceeding 18.2%, 36.4%, and 54.6% for theta, and 26.8%, 53.6%, and 80.4% for high-alpha, in the first, second, and third training sessions, respectively. Crucially, by adopting an auditory form of neurofeedback, we were able to provide this training while participants practiced their putting. Participants addressed the ball on an artificial putting green, and attempted to silence the tone while in their putting stance. When the tone was successfully turned off (i.e., when the desired theta and high-alpha power reduction had been achieved), participants were cued to putt. In this way, our intervention was designed not only to train participants to produce the desired state, but also to couple this state with the initiation of the golf putting movement. This simultaneous presentation of real-time neurofeedback during task-performance represents a useful advancement on the protocols adopted by Landers et al. (1991) and Kao et al. (2014). Members of the control group underwent an identical protocol, except the tone that they heard was not contingent on their brain activity and, thus, they received no systematic brain training. Accordingly, our sham neurofeedback group was designed to control for any possible placebo effects, but with less risk of impairing performance than the "incorrect" feedback control group used in Landers and colleagues (1991) design.

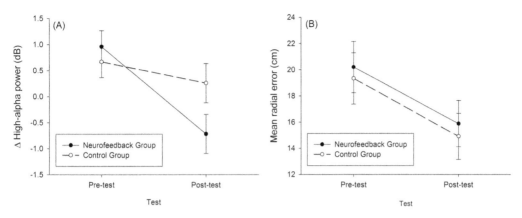

Figure 13.3 Panel (A): Mean high-alpha power (relative to baseline) at Fz during three seconds prior to movement displayed group by test interaction. Panel (B): Mean radial error (i.e., average distance from hole) of 2.4 m putts displayed main effect for test but no group by test interaction. Error bars depict standard error of the means. Data presented in full by Ring et al. (2015) http://dx.doi.org/10.1016/j.psychsport.2014.08.005

Results demonstrated a positive effect of the neurofeedback training on pre-movement EEG activity at a post-intervention test. Specifically, there was a group by test interaction effect characterised by a pre-intervention to post-intervention reduction in frontal-midline pre-movement theta and high-alpha power in members of the neurofeedback group only (Figure 13.3A). This study provides some of the first evidence that neurofeedback training can be delivered in a sport-training environment to teach athletes to self-regulate their brain activity. However, this positive EEG finding was somewhat offset by performance data revealing that both "correct" and "sham" neurofeedback groups displayed similar improvements in putting accuracy from the pre- to the post-intervention putting tests (Figure 13.3B). In accord with the studies described earlier, this result further indicates that any improvements in performance may not be directly attributable to the neurofeedback training received.

While all of these studies support the potential of data-driven neurofeedback in either shaping brain activity *or* improving performance, they fall short of providing unequivocal evidence of its efficacy. One study that does point towards data-driven neurofeedback training producing selective changes in both brain activity *and* performance was conducted by Cheng and colleagues (2015a). Their neurofeedback training focused on SMR power (12–15 Hz) at the central-midline. This was informed by their observation in a prior study that expert dart players displayed higher SMR power than novices in the two seconds preceding dart release (Cheng et al., 2015b). It was argued that augmented SMR power reflected a reduced cognitive interference with sensorimotor information processing, which could be a feature of autonomous and skilled performance.

Cheng and colleagues (2015a) adopted a similar training intervention as utilised by Ring et al. (2015). Eight pre-elite golfers assigned to a neurofeedback group attended four to six hours of neurofeedback training during which an acoustic tone was sounded when they increased their SMR power above their mean level of SMR power during successful putts recorded in the pre-intervention test. The sounding of the tone served as a cue to putt. Eight pre-elite golfers assigned to a control group underwent the same protocol except the feedback they received was false (i.e., random tone). Results revealed a significant group by test interaction for performance, with only the correct neurofeedback group improving their putting accuracy from the pre-intervention to the post-intervention putting accuracy test. Results also revealed that the correct neurofeedback group produced a greater pre-intervention to post-intervention test increase in

SMR power compared to the control group in the time window spanning 1.5 seconds to one second before the initiation of putts.

These findings provide arguably the most compelling support to date for the efficacy of neurofeedback as an intervention to enhance sporting performance. Importantly, Cheng et al.'s (2015a) data-driven approach yielded selective changes in both cortical activity and performance in an experimental group, and not in a sham control group, thereby ruling out the possibility of placebo effects. A slight peculiarity of this study is that the data used to inform the neurofeedback intervention were extracted from darts players rather than golfers. Normally, one would advise caution at applying the data-driven approach outside of the sport in which the original expert-model/ successful performance data were generated due to well-established variability in the optimal EEG profiles across different sports (e.g., Cooke, 2013). However, on this occasion the outcome was successful. It is interesting to note that in both prescription and data-driven neurofeedback approaches, interventions focused on the SMR band have yielded the most encouraging results. This could reflect increased SMR power being a part of the EEG spectrum that does generalise as a feature of optimal performance across multiple fine-motor accuracy tasks. On this basis, increased SMR neurofeedback appears an especially promising tool for practitioners and coaches operating in precision and accuracy based-sports. Indeed, given the results of Cheng et al. (2015b), there is already foundation for a data-driven neurofeedback study investigating the effectiveness of this intervention in the sport of darts.

Finally, a slight variant on the data-driven approach adopted by the four studies reviewed above was described by Arns and colleagues (2008). Rather than adopting an "expert-model", they adopted a "successful performance" model that was truly individualised for each participant. Specifically, they conducted individual comparisons of cortical activity associated with the best (i.e., holed) and worst (i.e., missed) putts during a baseline session. This resulted in customised neurofeedback for each participant, involving the reduction of a combination of theta (4–8 Hz), alpha (8–12 Hz), sensory motor rhythm (13–15 Hz), and/or beta (15–30 Hz) power in the final moments preceding putts. This individualisation differs from the "successful performance" model adopted by Ring et al. (2015), since in that study the successful performance profile was extracted from group mean data distinguishing holed and missed putts in a previous study (i.e., Cooke et al., 2014), and, thus, did not account for potential individual differences from one performer to the next.

Having established individualised feedback profiles for each of their six participants, Arns et al. (2008) adopted a crossover design with all participants completing 12 blocks of putts, with concurrent auditory neurofeedback training (i.e., putt when the tone turns off) being provided in the even- but not the odd-numbered blocks. Results revealed that participants holed more putts during the blocks in which they received neurofeedback compared to those in which they did not. These encouraging results further endorse an individualised approach to neurofeedback training, suggesting that practitioners may take an athlete-specific rather than a sport-specific approach when customizing neurofeedback thresholds. These recommendations further underscore the caution that should be applied when generalizing data across sports or applying a prescription-based neurofeedback solution.

While the results of Arns et al. (2008) provide useful insights into the individualisation that may be required to optimise the effectiveness of future neurofeedback training, there are also some limitations of their design. First, the lack of a control group could render this study susceptible to placebo effects whereby improved performances were elicited by the presence of the neurofeedback system and auditory tone, rather than by changes in cortical activity per se. Moreover, the lack of a post-test retention session in this study as compared to all of the others described in this section prevent any firm conclusions about the extent to which participants learned to control the tone. It is noteworthy, and somewhat disappointing, that performance deteriorated every time the neurofeedback signal was removed and participants putted without hearing the tone.

In sum, the increased SMR neurofeedback protocol adopted by Cheng et al. (2015a) offers clear promise as a tool to enhance the putting performance of golfers, and the throwing accuracy of darts players. While generalising this intervention to other sports without expert model data to confirm that increased SMR power is a feature of optimal performance would be a risk, it could be one that pays dividends for tasks that share the precision and accuracy features of darts and putting. For tasks where no prior optimal-performance data are available, the adoption of the individualised approach to neurofeedback exemplified by Arns et al. (2008) would seem a good option. This simply requires a pre-test session/s to identify individualised features of optimal performance. The subsequent intervention and thresholds would then be designed to reward the production of optimal performance EEG features.

Methodological Recommendations for Future Neurofeedback Interventions

It should be clear by now that while there are pockets of suggestive evidence to endorse neurofeedback training in sport, most studies to date are affected by one or more potentially serious methodological flaws. The presence of these flaws considerably limits the extent to which the proposed benefits of neurofeedback can be attributed unequivocally to neurofeedback interventions. We recommend that future studies adopt more rigorous experimental designs to address some of the previous shortcomings. A comprehensive set of neurofeedback protocol recommendations have been laid by some recent reviews (e.g., Gruzelier, 2014; Rogala et al., 2016). In addition to the points tabled in those reviews, we highlight some considerations especially pertinent to the field of sport neurofeedback research in the sections below. By following these principles, future researchers can play an important role in adding further clarity to the sport neurofeedback field.

1   Sport neurofeedback research should ensure the amount of learned self-regulation is assessed. The main tenet of neurofeedback training is that participants can learn to self-regulate a selective feature of their brain activity. While most previous studies quantified the change in behaviour (e.g., any performance improvement) consequent to neurofeedback training, it is surprising to note that very few studies (e.g., Cheng et al., 2015a; Ring et al., 2015) have reported the changes in the targeted brain activity consequent to neurofeedback training. Future research testing the presence of differences in the targeted brain activity from pre-training to post-training should provide evidence to confirm that participants indeed learned to emit the desired brain activity.

2   The relation between learned self-regulation and behavioural changes should be assessed at the individual level to help establish the causal process through which changes in performance are accounted for by changes in brain activity. Not all participants learn to self-regulate the targeted brain activity to the same extent: some may learn better than others (e.g., Kavussanu, Crews, & Gill, 1998). Accordingly, the participants who show the largest change in the targeted brain activity should also show the largest behavioural (performance) change. With this in mind, mediation analyses could be used to formally test the link between the change in learned self-regulation and change in performance (cf. Kavussanu et al., 1998). Further, it is possible to investigate whether this link is moderated by factors such as experience and training history.

3   A suitable control group should always be included in the design. It is assumed that, when present, the performance benefits of neurofeedback training are due to the alteration of the targeted brain activity. However, to support this causal relation a series of alternative interpretations need to be ruled out. Performance improvement could be attributed to the following: the passing of the time; expectancy (placebo) effect; increased self-efficacy; and increased effort (motivation). These alternative interpretations can be excluded by control groups that receive no training; some form of training other than neurofeedback (e.g., discovery learning); sham neurofeedback

training (e.g., standard non-contingent neurofeedback to control for the amount of feedback and yoked non-contingent neurofeedback to also control for the success rate); contingent but irrelevant neurofeedback training (e.g., non-neural feedback that is not linked with performance); and contingent and relevant neurofeedback training but inversely related to performance (e.g., decrease activity when increased activity is expected to aid performance). The inclusion of all these control groups is clearly unfeasible in a single investigation. However, a series of studies could address all these points and exclude them one by one. In doing so, it would be important for said study/studies to randomly allocate participants to groups, ideally with some form of blinding (single or double).

4   There are a number of important design choices that researchers must consider when developing their neurofeedback training protocols. For instance, the training schedule (e.g., the number of sessions, the duration of each session, the inter-session interval) will likely influence the effectiveness of the neurofeedback intervention (Rogala et al., 2016). Decisions about the volume of training will need to weigh up the pros (e.g., faster learning) and cons (e.g., tiredness, demotivation) of the components that make up the training schedule. The modality of the feedback signal (e.g., auditory, visual) will depend on whether the neurofeedback training is to be provided in a realistic performance environment (e.g., while the athlete is preparing to move) or in a context removed from the real performance situation (e.g., sitting in front of a computer screen). While it may be better to have multimodal feedback, at least at the start of training, visual feedback cannot be used in realistic performance environments requiring visual aiming. Although instantaneous feedback that is provided in real time to the athlete might seem optimal, it should be borne in mind that delayed (terminal) feedback that is provided after completing the movement may be more appropriate in some motor learning situations (e.g., Schmidt, Lange, & Young, 1990). Similarly, the frequency of the feedback needs to be considered because if it is provided every time, learners may become over-reliant on the feedback (see Arns et al., 2008), which could hamper performance when the feedback is no longer available (e.g., Winstein & Schmidt, 1990). Therefore, it is recommended that the feedback frequency be reduced across the course of training.[2]

5   In closing, it should also be noted that studies to date have typically included relatively few participants, and, therefore, the chance of finding genuine effects is hampered by inadequate statistical power. Future research with larger and/or more specialist samples (e.g., homogenous sample of elite performers within a single-sport) could address this issue.

Future Research Directions

In addition to adhering to the methodological considerations outlined above, there are a number of theoretical avenues and considerations that future neurofeedback studies would do well to pursue. For instance, it is possible that the low rate of learned self-regulation reported by previous sport neurofeedback experiments could be linked to the well-known inverse problem in EEG recording. Namely, participants could successfully learn to alter the targeted signal recorded from scalp electrodes in different ways, potentially even by altering non-neural activity. To highlight the plausibility of such reasoning, we offer an interpretation of the effects of alpha-theta neurofeedback training, which does not involve changes in neural activity. These studies typically train participants to increase theta power relative to alpha power at electrodes placed on the parieto-occipital region in an attempt to replicate the well-known changes in brain activity associated with what happens to theta and alpha power when we fall asleep (e.g., Gruzelier, 2009). However, this change could also be explained through a peripheral non-neural mechanism involving changes to muscle tone. Namely, muscle activity contaminates higher frequencies more than lower frequencies (e.g., alpha more than theta), and, therefore, a reduction in muscle activity, such as head and facial muscles in neck, jaw, and forehead, could result in reduced power likely to affect alpha frequency more than theta frequency. Thus, reduced muscle tone could explain both the modified alpha-theta power ratio and the increased hypnogogic state. While we do not necessarily say that this is the case, we point out that this explanation could confound the relationship between cortical activity and neurofeedback outcomes. A number of strategies could be employed in future studies to help minimise this confounding. First, researchers could control for non-neural activity by measuring it. For example, muscle activity, ocular activity, ventilation, and other non-neural physiological activity can be recorded and used to constrain the feedback so that these indices do not unduly influence the neurofeedback protocol (e.g., Ring et al., 2015). Second, researchers could move away from using signals recorded directly on the scalp as the feedback to using signals based on estimates of the sources (i.e., neural generators) of the signals recorded on the scalp. For example, studies could explore the efficacy of low resolution electromagnetic tomography (LORETA) neurofeedback in teaching participants to self-regulate their brain activity (Congedo, Lubar, & Joffe, 2004). Such studies would afford more confident assertions that any training-induced changes in the recorded EEG are attributed to modified neural activity. They would also afford researchers exciting opportunities to more precisely target specific brain regions (e.g., motor areas) within their training protocols.

Second, researchers could explore the utility of new neurofeedback training protocols based on the latest findings in the field of sport neuroscience. For example, protocols could be developed to focus on signals other than power recorded in a single channel on the scalp. A rationale for such training can be drawn from recent research reporting that experts display less alpha connectivity between the left temporal and the frontal regions of the cortex than novices (e.g., Gallicchio, Cooke, & Ring, 2016). Cross-regional alpha connectivity has been computed as a form of consistency of cross-channel phase lag over trials (e.g., magnitude-squared coherence, inter-site phase clustering). These indices must be computed as the average of multiple trials and therefore cannot be fed back easily on a trial-by-trial basis. However, by computing these indices as the consistency across time instead of trials (e.g., Cohen, 2014) future researchers could explore the efficacy of connectivity neurofeedback training in sport performance.

Similarly, in response to recent evidence highlighting increases in the regional gating of cortical alpha power as a feature of motor learning and control (e.g., Gallicchio, Cooke, & Ring, 2017), future neurofeedback protocols could be designed to encourage optimal gating of alpha for a given sport. Specifically, Gallicchio et al. (2017) found that task-irrelevant brain regions show higher alpha power than task-relevant brain regions during preparation for golf putts, with this effect intensifying with practice. In line with the inhibitory function attributed to cortical alpha (Klimesch et al., 2007), activity in regions with higher alpha power is inhibited more than the activity in regions showing lower alpha power. Consequently, the results were interpreted to reflect resources being "gated" away from task-irrelevant regions (e.g., temporal regions) and towards task-relevant regions (e.g., central-frontal regions) during preparation for putts (see also Jensen & Mazaheri, 2010). Future multi-channel EEG neurofeedback studies could focus on the ratio of alpha power at central compared to peripheral scalp locations to maximise alpha gating in self-paced aiming sports.

In addition, future neurofeedback protocols could train participants to produce patterns of cortical activity within individualised zones of optimal functioning, rather than single-thresholds based on the successful performance approach adopted by previous data-driven neurofeedback studies (e.g., Arns et al., 2008; Cheng et al., 2015a). For instance, recent work by Bertollo and colleagues (e.g., Bertollo et al., 2016) has argued that optimal performance can occur within two separate zones. Specifically, it can manifest as highly fluent, efficient, and automatic processing, which may be associated with low-levels of cortical activity, or it can manifest through highly effortful and controlled processing, which may be associated with high-levels of cortical activity (e.g., Bertollo et al., 2016). Accordingly, future neurofeedback protocols may be specifically tailored for upcoming events depending on the expected zone most likely to support success (e.g., outdoor events in unpredictable/highly adverse weather conditions may demand more effortful processing to support success, compared to events in "perfect" conditions, which may be more likely to benefit from automaticity).

Finally, it is noted that neurofeedback training provides researchers with an exciting opportunity to manipulate selective features of brain activity and then observe its direct consequences on thoughts, feelings, and actions. For example, a wealth of studies have revealed that expert athletes show relatively lower activation in the left temporal region of the cortex compared to novices, in preparation for movement execution (for review see Cooke, 2013; Hatfield, Haufler, Hung, & Spalding, 2004). Based on the view that the left temporal region hosts language areas (e.g., Wexler, 1980), this effect has been interpreted as experts relying on less verbal declarative processing than novices (e.g., Zhu, Poolton, Wilson, Maxwell, & Masters, 2011). However, this interpretation is based on reverse inference. In other words, left temporal activity has been linked to numerous cognitive processes, including memory and audition, as well as verbal declarative language (e.g., LaBar & Phelps, 1998; Zatorre & Belin, 2001). Accordingly, neurofeedback training can be used as an experimental manipulation to test causal relationships between patterns of brain activation (e.g., reduced activity in the left temporal region), psychological state (e.g., cognition, emotion, motivation), and performance (e.g., more precise movements). For instance, researchers could test this causal process by teaching participants to down-regulate activity of the left temporal region and observe changes in the verbal descriptive activity (e.g., amount of self-talk). Thus, neurofeedback can be used by researchers as an intervention to test cause-and-effect relationships and elucidate a clearer picture of the functional significance of various aspects of the EEG signal recorded at different locations.

Conclusion

This chapter set out to provide a brief introduction to neurofeedback training followed by a comprehensive and critical review of the extant sport neurofeedback literature. The outcome of the literature review points to some encouraging evidence for neurofeedback as a tool that may enhance sporting performance in some circumstances, but the jury is most definitely still out. We hope that by consistently highlighting some key limitations within the extant research field, researchers will be better equipped to conduct more rigorous tests of the putative benefits of neurofeedback training in the future. We hope that our recommendations for future research based on some of the latest sport neuroscience findings will also stimulate more high-quality neurofeedback experiments in due course. While the current research base falls short of providing indisputable evidence to support the use of neurofeedback training in sport, this does not deter our enthusiasm for the potential of neurofeedback to yield clear and consistent benefits in the future. Sport neurofeedback, and sport neuroscience in general, are young and dynamic research fields. With constant advancements in brain imaging technology alongside evolutions in our understanding of the functional meaning of brain signals related to sport performance, the years and decades to come promise to be exciting and fruitful times for sport psychophysiology researchers, coaches, and athletes alike.

Notes

1 For more specific and comprehensive guidance on neurofeedback equipment and operating systems, please consult manufacturer guidelines.
2 We recognise that our recommendations pertaining to most issues raised in this paragraph (e.g., frequency and duration of training) fall short of providing firm direction as to the optimal solutions.

This is quite simply because the current evidence base is insufficiently developed to allow strong recommendations to be made. It is a challenge for future researchers to uncover optimal frequencies, durations, and tapering schedules for neurofeedback training in sport.

References

All time money leaders. (2016, July 12). Retrieved from: http://espn.go.com/golf/moneylist/_/tour/alltime

Arns. M., Kleinnijenhuis, M., Fallahpour, K., & Breteler, R. (2008). Golf performance enhancement and real-life neurofeedback training using personalized event-locked EEG profiles. *Journal of Neurotherapy, 11*, 11–18.

Australian Associated Press. (2013, March 6). Jason Day's brain training boosts his golf form. *The Australian*. Retrieved from www.theaustralian.com.au/

Babiloni, C., Del Percio, C., Iacoboni, M., Infarinato, F., Lizio, R., Marzano, N., … Eusebi, F. (2008). Golf putt outcomes are predicted by sensorimotor cerebral EEG rhythms. *Journal of Physiology, 586*, 131–139.

Beauchamp, M. K., Harvey, R. H., & Beauchamp, P. H. (2012). An integrated biofeedback and psychological skills training program for Canada's Olympic short-track speedskating team. *Journal of Clinical Sport Psychology, 6*, 67–84.

Berka, C., Behneman, A., Kintz, N., Johnson, R., & Raphael, G. (2010). Accelerating training using interactive neuro-educational technologies: Applications to archery, golf and rifle marksmanship. *The International Journal of Sport and Society, 1*(4), 87–104.

Bertollo, M., di Fronso, S., Filho, E., Conforto, S., Schmid, M., Bortoli, L., … Robazza, C. (2016). Proficient brain for optimal performance: The MAP model perspective. *PeerJ, 4:e2082.* http://dx.doi.org/10.7717/peerj.2082

Cheng, M., Huang, C., Chang, Y., Koester, D., Schack, T., & Hung, T. (2015a). Sensorimotor rhythm neurofeedback enhances golf putting performance. *Journal of Sport & Exercise Psychology, 37*, 626–636.

Cheng, M., Hung, C., Huang, C., Chang, Y., Lo, L., Shem, C., & Hung, T. (2015b). Expert-novice differences in SMR activity during dart throwing. *Biological Psychology, 110*, 212–218.

Cohen, M. X. (2014). *Analyzing neural time series data: Theory and practice.* Cambridge, MA: MIT Press.

Congedo, M., Lubar, J. F., & Joffe, D. (2004). Low resolution electromagnetic tomography neurofeedback. *Transactions on Neural Systems and Rehabilitation Engineering, 12*, 387–397.

Cooke, A. (2013). Readying the head and steadying the heart: A review of cortical and cardiac studies of preparation for action in sport. *International Review of Sport & Exercise Psychology, 6*, 122–138.

Cooke, A., Kavussanu, M., Gallicchio, G., Willoughby, A., McIntyre, D., & Ring, C. (2014). Preparation for action: Psychophysiological activity preceding a motor skill as a function of expertise, performance outcome, and psychological pressure. *Psychophysiology, 51*, 374–384.

Defebvre, L., Bourriez, J., Dujardin, K., Derambure, P., Destee, A., & Guieu, J. (1994). Spatiotemporal study of Bereitschaftspotential and event-related desynchronization during voluntary movement in Parkinson's Disease. *Brain Topography, 6*, 237–244.

Dekker, M. K. J., Van den Berg, B. R., Denissen, A. J. M., Sitskoorn, M. M., & Van Boxtel, G. J. M. (2014). Feasibility of eyes open alpha power training for mental enhancement in elite gymnasts. *Journal of Sports Sciences, 32*, 1550–1560.

Gallicchio, G., Cooke, A., & Ring, C. (2016). Lower left temporal-frontal connectivity characterizes expert and accurate performance: High-alpha T7-Fz connectivity as a marker of conscious processing during movement. *Sport, Exercise & Performance Psychology, 5*, 14–24.

Gallicchio, G., Cooke, A., & Ring, C. (2017). Practice makes efficient: Cortical alpha oscillations are associated with improved golf putting performance. *Sport, Exercise and Performance Psychology, 6*, 89–102.

Gruzelier, J. H. (2009). A theory of alpha/theta neurofeedback, creative performance enhancement, long distance functional connectivity and psychological integration. *Cognitive Processing, 10*, 101–109.

Gruzelier, J. H. (2014). EEG-neurofeedback for optimising performance III: A review of methodological and theoretical considerations. *Neuroscience and Biobehavioral Reviews, 44*, 159–182.

Gruzelier, J. H., Egner, T., & Vernon, D. (2006). Validating the efficacy of neurofeedback for optimising performance. *Progress in Brain Research, 159*, 421–431.

Hatfield, B.D., Haufler, A.J., Hung, T., & Spalding, T.W. (2004). Electroencephalographic studies of skilled psychomotor performance. *Journal of Clinical Neurophysiology, 21*, 144–156.

Hatfield, B. D., Landers, D. M., & Ray, W. J. (1984). Cognitive processes during self-paced motor performance: An electroencephalographic profile of skilled marksmen. *Journal of Sport Psychology, 6*, 42–59.

Iversen, I. H. (1992). Skinner's early research from reflexology to operant conditioning. *American Psychologist, 47*, 1318–1328.

Jensen, O., & Mazaheri, A. (2010). Shaping functional architecture by oscillatory alpha activity: Gating by inhibition. *Frontiers in Human Neuroscience, 4,* http://dx.doi.org/10.3389/fnhum.2010.00186

Kao, S., Huang, C., & Hung, T. (2013). Frontal midline theta is a specific indicator of optimal attentional engagement during skilled putting performance. *Journal of Sport & Exercise Psychology, 35,* 470–478.

Kao, S., Huang, C., & Hung, T. (2014). Neurofeedback training reduces frontal midline theta and improves putting performance in expert golfers. *Journal of Applied Sport Psychology, 26,* 271–286.

Kavussanu, M., Crews, D.J., & Gill, D.L. (1998). The effects of single versus multiple measures of biofeedback on basketball free throw shooting performance. *International Journal of Sport Psychology, 29,* 132–144.

Klimesch, W. (2012). Alpha-band oscillations, attention, and controlled access to stored information. *Trends in Cognitive Sciences, 16,* 606–617.

Klimesch, W., Pfurtscheller, G., Mohl, W., & Schimke, H. (1990). Event-related desynchronization, ERD-mapping and hemispheric differences for words and numbers. *International Journal of Psychophysiology, 8,* 297–308.

Klimesch, W., Sauseng, P., & Hanslmayr, S. (2007). EEG alpha oscillations: The inhibition-timing hypothesis. *Brain Research Reviews, 53,* 63–88.

Kober, S. E., Witte, M., Stangl, M., Valjamae, A., Neuper, C., & Wood, G. (2015). Shutting down sensorimotor interference unblocks the networks for stimulus processing: An SMR neurofeedback training study. *Clinical Neurophysiology, 126,* 82–95.

LaBar, K. S., & Phelps, E. A. (1998). Arousal-mediated memory consolidation: Roles of the medial temporal lobe in humans. *Psychological Science, 9,* 490–493.

Landers, D. M., Petruzzello, S. J., Salazar, W., Crews, D. J., Kubitz, K. A., Gannon, T. L., & Han, M. (1991). The influence of electrocortical biofeedback on performance in pre-elite archers. *Medicine and Science in Sports and Exercise, 23,* 123–129.

Magnani, G., Cursi, M., Leocani, L., Volonte, M. A., & Comi, G. (2002). Acute effects of L-dopa on event-related desynchronisation in Parkinson's disease. *Neurological Sciences, 23,* 91–97.

Nowlis, D. P., & Kamiya, J. (1970). Control of electroencephalographic alpha rhythms through auditory feedback and the associated mental activity. *Psychophysiology, 6,* 476–484.

Pfurtscheller, G. (1992). Event-related synchronization (ERS): An electrophysiological correlate of cortical areas at rest. *Electroencephalography and Clinical Neurophysiology, 83,* 62–69.

Raymond, J., Sajid, I., Parkinson, L. A., & Gruzelier, J. H. (2005). Biofeedback and dance performance: A preliminary investigation. *Applied Psychophysiology and Biofeedback, 30,* 65–73.

Ring, C., Cooke, A., Kavussanu, M., McIntyre, D. B., & Masters, R. S. W. (2015). Investigating the efficacy of neurofeedback training for expediting expertise and excellence in sport. *Psychology of Sport & Exercise, 16,* 118–127.

Rogala, J., Jurewicz, K., Paluch, K., Kublik, E., Cetnarski, R., & Wrobel, A. (2016). The do's and don'ts of neurofeedback training: A review of the controlled studies using healthy adults. *Frontiers in Human Neuroscience, 10,* 301.

Ros, T., Moseley, M. J., Bloom, P. A., Benjamin, L., Parkinson, L. A., & Gruzelier, J. H. (2009). Optimising microsurgical skills with EEG neurofeedback. *BMC Neuroscience, 10,* 87.

Rostami, R., Sadeghi, H., Karami, K. A., Abadi, M. A., & Salamati, P. (2012). The effects of neurofeedback on the improvement of rifle shooters' performance. *Journal of Neurotherapy, 16,* 264–269.

Salazar, W., Landers, D. M., Petruzzello, S. J., Han, M. W., Crews, D. J., & Kubitz, K. A. (1990). Hemispheric asymmetry, cardiac response, and performance in elite archers. *Research Quarterly for Exercise and Sport, 61,* 351–359.

Schmidt, R. A., Lange, C., & Young, D. E. (1990). Optimizing summary knowledge of results for skill learning. *Human Movement Science, 9,* 325–348.

Shaw, L., Zaichkowsky, L., & Wilson, V. (2012). Setting the balance: Using biofeedback and neurofeedback with gymnasts. *Journal of Clinical Sport Psychology, 6,* 47–66.

Sherlin, L. H., Ford, N. C. L., Baker, A. R., & Troesch, J. (2015). Observational report of the effects of performance brain training in collegiate golfers. *Biofeedback, 43,* 64–72.

Sherlin, L. H., Larson, N. C., & Sherlin, R. M. (2013). Developing a performance brain training approach for baseball: A process analysis with descriptive data. *Applied Psychophysiology & Biofeedback, 38,* 29–44.

Skinner, B. F. (1963). Operant Behavior. *American Psychologist, 18,* 503–515.

Thibault, R. T., Lifshitz, M., & Raz, M. (2016). The self-regulating brain and neurofeedback: Experimental science and clinical promise. *Cortex, 74,* 247–261.

Van Boxtel, G. J. M., Denissen, A. J. M., Jager, M., Vernon, D., Dekker, M. K. J., Mihajlovic, V., & Sitskoorn, M. M. (2012). A novel self-guided approach to alpha activity training. *International Journal of Psychophysiology, 83,* 282–294.

Wexler, B. E. (1980). Cerebral laterality and psychiatry: A review of the literature. *American Journal of Psychiatry, 137,* 279–291.

Wilson, V. E., Peper, E., & Moss, D. (2006). "The mind room" in Italian soccer training: The use of bio-feedback and neurofeedback for optimum performance. *Biofeedback, 34*, 79–81.

Winstein, C. J., & Schmidt, R. A. (1990). Reduced frequency of knowledge of results enhances motor skill learning. *Journal of Experimental Psychology: Learning, Memory and Cognition, 16*, 677–691.

Zatorre, R. J., & Belin, P. (2001). Spectral and temporal processing in human auditory cortex. *Cerebral Cortex, 11*, 946–953.

Zhu, F.F., Poolton, J.M., Wilson, M.R., Maxwell, J.P., & Masters, R.S.W. (2011). Neural coactivation as a yardstick of implicit motor learning and the propensity for conscious control of movement. *Biological Psychology, 87*, 66–73.

14

Neurofeedback in Sport
Theory, Methods, Research, and Efficacy

Tsung-Min Hung and Ming-Yang Cheng

Introduction

Reaching superior performance is the goal of every athlete. Neurofeedback training (NFT) is a way to maintain an adaptive level of concentration for optimal performance by way of regulating cortical brain activity. This chapter covers relevant information regarding the application of NFT in enhancing sports performance. The aims of this chapter are three-fold. First, to provide both the theoretical and methodological basis of NFT in sport performance. Secondly, to evaluate the quality of studies regarding this line of research, with a particular focus on methodological critiques regarding how to evaluate the effects of NFT on sports performance. Finally, we conclude with several directions for future studies.

Fundamentals of NFT

The mind and action are interconnected. NFT offers insight into how the mind works. Since Kamiya (1968) first showed that humans can self-regulate cortical activity in the alpha frequency band by instrumental/operant conditioning, NFT has been applied in various domains such as neurological, cognitive, and motoric performance, which has shed light on its potential benefits. The basic assumption of EEG NFT is: change the EEG, change the behavior (Vernon, 2005). Therefore, the goal of EEG NFT is to maintain EEG within an optimal zone that has been associated with a desirable behavior by the audio or visual feedback in real time. The participant is expected to enter and maintain the specific optimal zone without the assistance of an NFT device after the learning process.

There are five elements that are considered the pillars of NFT (Enriquez-geppert, Huster, & Herrmann, 2017). The first is that the variables of NFT are based on psychophysiological measurements, such as high temporal resolution electroencephalography (EEG) and magnetoencephalography (MEG), which are the ideal options for real-time NFT. Apart from these, high spatial resolution functional magnetic resonance imaging (fMRI) and near-infrared spectroscopy (NIRS) are increasingly developed. Given the nature of sport performance, a measurement based on real-time that can be applied in the real field is the ideal candidate for NFT. Hence, EEG NFT is highly suitable in sport domain, compared to other psychophysiological measurements (Thompson, Steffert, Ros, Leach, & Gruzelier, 2008).

The second is online data-preprocessing. Once the EEG recording is set up, connecting the NFT device to the computer is the next step. A computer is required to extract the specific EEG activity to manipulate, and also to send real-time audio or visual feedback back to participants. In general, the main function of the NFT program is comparing the recorded EEG activity and the threshold set before the training. During the stage of EEG recording, a preliminary purification of the cortical signal by removing the identified eye and muscle artifacts is the main task. The eye artifacts in particular can easily affect amplitude, which is transferred from the EEG, and falsely lead to regulation of eye movement instead of cortical activity.

The third is feature-extraction, which means to pull out the meaningful EEG signals for manipulation. Generally, feature-extraction can be a specific EEG frequency band that is considered related to a certain cognitive performance. The choice of incorrect extraction has been reported and linked to performance reduction in NFT (Zich et al., 2015).

The fourth is the generation of a feedback signal. This refers to a sensory stimulus that represents the status of the extracted feature. Meanwhile, the sensory stimulus also serves as a bridge to help the participant learn how to regulate EEG. This signal can be in audio, visual, or other modalities, and can have more than one modality simultaneously. Nevertheless, the goal of these feedback elements is to connect the targeted characteristic or feature of brain activity to a specific threshold.

Last but not the least are the characteristics of the participant. Under an EEG NFT, participants are actively engaged in training and continuously try to modulate their EEG to the threshold. Hence, to keep up motivation (Kleih & Kübler, 2013) and positive mood state (Subramaniam & Vinogradov, 2013) during training has been reported to be relevant to the prediction of individual learning success in NFT. This topic has been emphasized by recent studies in NFT, especially regarding the classification of responder and non-responder (Weber, Köberl, Frank, & Doppelmayr, 2011). Hence, the trainer should instruct participants in the protocol of NFT to make the training clearer and more transparent. It is important to note that this step is easily underestimated yet extremely crucial, because the trust of the participants regarding the NFT leads to a successful training. The trainer must therefore carry out the explanation carefully; otherwise, in a worst case, an irreversible placebo effect is created in the control group.

NFT has been applied to enhance cognitive functioning or to normalize deviating brain activity in patients. For example, Alpha NFT has been linked to performance enhancement on cognitive tasks. Alpha frequency amplitude is reported to be inversely related to the numbers of activated neuronal populations (Jensen & Mazaheri, 2010), suggesting inhibited neural cortical activity during the presence of alpha power. Lower alpha desynchronization in the range of about 6–10 Hz is obtained in response to a variety of non-task and non-stimulus specific factors, which may be best subsumed under the term 'attention'. It is topographically widespread over the entire scalp and probably reflects general task demands and attentional processes (Klimesch, 1999). Upper alpha desynchronization in the range of about 10–12 Hz is topographically restricted and develops during the processing (Klimesch, 1999), and is related to inhibition of unnecessary cortical regions in successful task performance (Cooper, Croft, Dominey, Burgess, & Gruzelier, 2003; Jensen & Mazaheri, 2010). Augmented alpha NFT has been shown to improve the performance of mental rotation enhancement (Hanslmayr, Sauseng, Doppelmayr, Schabus, & Klimesch, 2005), Matrix Rotation task (Riecansky & Katina, 2010), and working memory (Reis et al., 2016).

In a study employing exogenous theta oscillations by the transcranial alternating current stimulation (tACS) to a mid-frontal scalp region during an executive functioning task, tACS led to enhanced behavioral performance compared to alpha band tACS. This result suggests frontal midline theta power as causally contributing to executive functioning (Van Driel, Sligte, Linders, Elport, & Cohen, 2015). In the field of NFT, previous studies have shown that augmented frontal midline theta power is associated with cognitive processing enhancement (Mitchell, McNaughton, Flanagan, & Kirk, 2008), and reduced frontal midline theta power in response to demanding tasks seems to be associated with reduced task performance in healthy participants (Donkers et al., 2011) as well as in patients (Schmiedt, Brand, Hildebrandt, & Basar-Eroglu, 2005).

Sensorimotor rhythm (SMR) NFT contributes to reduction in the severity of ADHD symptoms and poor performance in various attention-demanding tasks. SMR has been reported to be most prominent in the central scalp regions of the sensorimotor cortex (Blankertz et al., 2010; Pfurtscheller & Neuper, 1997; Sterman, 1996). Higher SMR power is associated with the mental state of relaxed alertness (Kober, Witte, Ninaus, Neuper, & Wood, 2013), attention, short-term memory, and memory consolidation (Doppelmayr & Weber, 2011; Egner & Gruzelier, 2004; Gruzelier, Egner, & Vernon, 2006; Hoedlmoser et al., 2008; Tinius & Tinius, 2000; Vernon, 2005; Vernon et al., 2003). Augmented SMR training has been shown to improve attentional processing as well as reduce inattentive behavior in neurotypical participants and participants with ADHD (Arns, de Ridder, Strehl, Breteler, & Coenen, 2009; Egner & Gruzelier, 2004; Kropotov et al., 2005; Lubar & Shouse, 1976; Mann, Sterman, & Kaiser, 1996; Tansey, 1984; Tansey & Bruner, 1983; Vernon et al., 2003). Moreover, augmented SMR training has been shown to enhance performance in spatial rotation tasks, suggesting a more efficient attentional processing regulatory control of the somatosensory and sensorimotor pathways (Doppelmayr & Weber, 2011).

NFT Studies in Sport Performance Enhancement

Theta

The origin of frontal midline theta activity has been related to the anterior cingulate cortex (ACC), which is believed to deal with cognitive and behavioral control (Asada, Fukuda, Tsunoda, Yamaguchi, & Tonoike, 1999). As an indicator of attentional processes, previous studies have shown that the enhanced theta activity in the medial prefrontal cortex after response error is related to volitional attentional control (Dayan & Cohen, 2011). In the context of visuomotor and sensorimotor performances, higher frontal midline theta power has also been associated with expert performance in comparison to novices (Baumeister, Reinecke, Liesen, & Weiss, 2008; Doppelmayr, Finkenzeller, & Sauseng, 2008). Higher theta power prior to movement execution may indicate that skilled athletes perform the task with an effective top-down initiated focused attention in meeting the demands of information processing and attentional control (Baumeister et al., 2013). However, within intraindividual comparison studies, better performance was preceded by lower (Kao, Huang, & Hung, 2013) and more stable (Chuang, Huang, & Hung, 2013) frontal midline theta power, compared with that of poor performance in skilled athletes. These findings suggest that a more stable and lower sustained attention allocation resulted in better performance compared to the over investment of attention reflected by higher theta power at the frontal region.

The limited studies on NFT using frontal midline theta have shown promising results. Kao, Huang, and Hung (2014) demonstrated that a single session of NFT targeted at reducing frontal midline theta power facilitated golf putting performance in three highly skilled golfers. This evidence suggested that sustained attention was stabilized through the theta NFT and led to improved putting performance. However, related studies that employed combined EEG frequency components including theta have shown inconsistent results. Raymond, Sajid, Parkinson, and Gruzelier (2005) demonstrated that 10 sessions of increasing Theta and inhibiting Alpha (frequencies based on IAF bands) at Pz improved dancing performance in an experimental group compared to a control group. However, a recent study failed to show a positive effect on dancing performance after 10 sessions of increasing Theta (5–8 Hz) and inhibiting Alpha (8–11 Hz) at Pz (Gruzelier, Thompson, Redding, Brandt, & Steffert, 2014). As the number of studies is limited, it is difficult to conclude whether theta NFT or its variant is effective in improving motor performance. Future studies should look for a more convergent protocol to examine this issue.

Alpha

Alpha power is commonly defined as the frequency band within 8–12 Hz, which has been related to cortical inhibition and relaxation (Klimesch, 1996). Recent studies have suggested that alpha power could be further classified into lower alpha power (8–10 Hz), a general state of attention, and higher alpha power (10–12 Hz), which reflects task-specific attention allocation.

In the context of sport performance, higher alpha power at the left temporal cortex has been linked to reduced interference from verbal-analytical processes during the preparation period in successful sport performance. For example, rifle marksmen exhibited significantly greater alpha power at T3 during a preparation period when compared to novices in rifle shooting performance (Haufler, Spalding, Santa Maria, & Hatfield, 2000). The similar trend of left temporal alpha has also been demonstrated in another study. These results may indicate how a verbal-analytical suppression process is critical to the preparation period in target shooting sports, suggesting that a higher order of motor planning underpins superior shooting performance. On the other hand, parietal alpha power has also been studied in sport performance. Previous studies have reported that expert golfers performing better at putting performance compared to novices demonstrated a significantly higher parietal alpha power at the parietal sites, indicating that superior putting performance was preceded by economical processing of the sensorimotor information (Baumeister et al., 2008).

Research findings in alpha NFT were inconsistent. A NFT study targeted at increasing alpha power in the left hemisphere showed improved archery performance, in comparison to the control group (Landers et al., 1991). However, gymnasts reported small improvements in sleep quality, mental shape, and physical shape but not for stress, arousal, and perceived training experiences after a ten-session NFT targeted at increasing Alpha band at C3 and C4 sites (Dekker, Van den Berg, Denissen, Sitskoorn, & Van Boxtel, 2014). Similarly, studies that employed combined EEG frequency components including alpha also showed inconsistent results. For example, Rostami, Sadeghi, Karami, Abadi, and Salamati (2012) reported that 15 sessions of NFT targeted at increasing Alpha (8–12 Hz) and Theta (4–8 Hz) while inhibiting high Beta (20–30 Hz) at Pz improved rifle shooting performance, compared to the non-trained control group. While Raymond et al. (2005) reported an improvement in dancing performance after inhibiting Alpha and increasing Theta at Pz based on individual alpha frequency (IAF), Gruzelier, Thompson, et al. (2014) failed to observe improvements in dancing performance after NFT targeted at inhibiting Alpha (8–11 Hz) and increasing Theta (5–8 Hz) at Pz site. Furthermore, golfers failed to enhance putting performance after receiving a protocol of inhibiting high Alpha (10–12 Hz) and Theta (4–8 Hz) activity at the Fz site in comparison to a control group (Ring, Cooke, Kavussanu, McIntyre, & Masters, 2015). The discrepancy within these studies could be attributed to methodological heterogeneity. Moreover, the rationale for choosing the NFT target was not empirically tested in some of these studies, which also contributed to the inconsistent findings.

SMR

SMR is thought to generate from the somatosensory relay nuclei of the thalamus, known as ventrobasal nuclei (Sterman, 1996, 2000). Therefore, SMR is most observable in the central regions, especially the sensorimotor cortex (Blankertz et al., 2010; Pfurtscheller & Neuper, 1997; Sterman, 1996). The reduced transmission of thalamus and the sensorimotor cortex results in an attenuated or inhibited processing of sensorimotor information (Sterman, 2000), which is reflected by increased SMR.

Higher SMR power has been linked with better motor performance, suggesting that a more silent and efficient process at the sensorimotor cortex is beneficial to motor performance. Previous reports have shown that increased SMR activity inhibits the somatosensory information flow to the motor cortex with subsequent improvements in memory and attentional performance (Kober et al., 2015). These results suggest that superior performance was related to reduced cortical activation (Del Percio et al., 2011), especially in the movement-related cortical area (Di Russo, Pitzalis, Aprile, & Spinelli, 2005). These findings infer that higher SMR activity in improved cognitive performance is related to reduced motor-related processing while maintaining alertness in the nucleus activity between thalamus and sensorimotor cortex.

In the context of sport performance, Cheng, et al. (2015) compared the SMR power between expert dart-throwers and the novices in a dart-throwing task and demonstrated that the expert dart-throwers exhibited significantly higher SMR power in the preparation period than that of the novices. This result suggests that skilled performance is a result of less interference in the information processing during preparation. Similarly, Cheng et al. (2017) investigated personal best and worst pistol shooting performances and found that the best performances were preceded by higher SMR power compared to the worst performances, suggesting an improved processing efficiency in superior performance. These findings and interpretations are consistent with the psychomotor efficiency hypothesis proposed by Hatfield and Hillman (2001).

As for SMR NFT in sports, Cheng et al. (2015) reported significant improvement in putting performance after eight sessions of augmented SMR NFT compared to a control group, suggesting a higher psychomotor efficiency prior to putting movement execution as a result of NFT. Moreover, the ability of maintaining higher SMR power before putting was also observed in the NFT group compared to the control group. Given the negative correlation between SMR power and the sensorimotor cortex, higher SMR power has been suggested as an index of higher level of psychomotor efficiency, which might lead to a more automatic movement execution in sports performance (Cheng et al., 2017). This view has been supported by previous studies in the context of cognitive control, which suggest that the voluntary control of increased SMR NFT is linked with facilitated cognitive processing, in which interference is reduced and perceptual and memory functions maintained (Egner & Gruzelier, 2001; Gruzelier, Inoue, Smart, Steed, & Steffert, 2010; Ros et al., 2009).

Similarly, a mixed biofeedback protocol including increasing SMR (13–15 Hz) and inhibiting Theta (4–7 Hz) at Cz and T3 sites, together with heart rate variability (HRV) biofeedback in an uncontrolled gymnastics study also showed a positive effect on balance (Shaw, Zaichkowsky, & Wilson, 2012). However, no changes in HRV, sensorimotor rhythm, and theta power were observed. On the contrary, Paul et al. (Paul, Ganesan, Sandhu, & Simon, 2012) reported no significant improvement on archery performance after twelve sessions of increasing SMR NFT while inhibiting high Beta (22–26 Hz) and Theta (4–7 Hz) at the Cz site in four weeks in the experimental group compared to control group. Notably, the archers reported a significant increment on SMR/theta ratio after NFT. Similar training protocol of increasing SMR (12–15 Hz) and inhibiting Beta (22–37 Hz) and Theta (4–8 Hz) at C3 and C4 sites also exhibited positive effects on reducing anxiety in swimmers compared to a control group (Faridnia, Shojaei, & Rahimi, 2012). In a sample of athletes from mixed sports, 20 sessions of increasing SMR (12–15 Hz) concomitant with inhibiting Theta (4–7 Hz) and high Beta (21–35 Hz) at C3 and C4 led to significant improvements in the levels of autotelic engagement and mental arithmetic performance compared to a control group (Mikicin, 2015). The NFT study targeted at SMR power was effective in increasing SMR activity, which is a precedent in improved motor performance. However, the mixed target results including SMR were less consistent. Given the limited number of studies in this area, more replications with more consistent methodological considerations are required to further clarify the effectiveness of SMR and its related approach in improving motor performance.

Moreover, caution should be exercised when applying SMR NFT on novices because the characteristic cortical activity in superior motor performers contrasts with the pattern in novices, which has been characterized by heavy reliance on working memory (Beilock, Carr, MacMahon, & Starkes, 2002) as well as monitoring of somatosensory information (Loze, Collins, & Holmes, 2001; Schröter & Leuthold, 2009) when executing motor skills. As motor learning proceeds, suppression of SMR power is progressively increased (Quandt & Marshall, 2014).

Methodological Issues

Similar to all other scientific endeavors, research on NFT in sport should follow the same levels of scientific rigidity. To some extent, applying NFT is similar to training in sport; that is, to reasonably record the baseline and observe the change from the baseline as training proceeds. Moreover, to apply NFT more efficiently, finding the right number of repetitions and duration is also quite important. In the following paragraphs, practical yet important issues such as measurements and validations are raised to provide a more complete picture of NFT in sport performance.

Before the NFT: The Selection of Training Target

The rationale of selecting specific training targets should be empirically examined. For example, training targets derived from sport performance-based studies is recommended. Although previous studies have shown the positive effects on sport performance after NFT, several studies failed to report the beneficial effects of NFT. One possible explanation for the lack of significant training effects from NFT is the selection of NFT targets with a relatively weak evidence for a connection of the selected NFT target to sport performance. For instance, Gruzelier, Thompson, et al. (2014) adopted a ten-session training with the protocol of inhibiting alpha while increasing theta at Pz in dancers' performance. The rationale for selecting this protocol was based on the beneficial effect of NFT for creativity (Green & Green, 1977). However, no other evidence for an association between lower alpha concomitant increased theta and better dancing performance has been provided. Similarly, although one study reported an improvement in rifle shooting after 15 training sessions of increasing SMR while inhibiting beta at C3 and C4, the rationale for using this training target was missing in the report (Rostami et al., 2012). Therefore, the selection of training targets is recommended to be based on evidence originated from the previous expert-novice comparison (Cheng et al., 2015; Doppelmayr et al., 2008; Haufler et al., 2000) or an intraindividual-based performance comparison design (Cheng et al., 2017; Chuang et al., 2013; Kao et al., 2013). With this solid foundation for NFT target selection, the effects of NFT can be systematically investigated.

Before the NFT: Setup the Threshold

To achieve optimal training effects, a personalized training threshold should be established (Arns, Kleinnijenhuis, Fallahpour, & Breteler, 2008; Cheng et al., 2015). Given individual differences as well as a possible nonlinear manner in the relationship between levels of EEG power and specific motor performance, the threshold should be individually determined. An empirical approach to determine personalized thresholds would be to derive the EEG power by averaging the specific EEG frequency band from trials with the successful performance of specific athletes. For example, in an eight-session NFT study, Cheng et al. (2015) extracted the successful trials (trials which putt in the hole) in the pre-test from each participant and calculated a mean EEG power as the training threshold for each golfer. Furthermore, to define a proper adjustment for the following training, they also computed the standard deviation from the mean of each participant. The personalized standard deviation was used as an adjustment when they changed the training difficulty.

During Training: Evaluate Trainability within Sessions

EEG state can fluctuate on a daily basis. Therefore, focusing on the change between each session may be a more practical approach to identifying the learning progress from neurofeedback training and the ability to control their EEG (Dempster & Vernon, 2009). For instance, Cheng et al. (2015) focused on the successful training ratio, which was defined as the amount of time that the participant successfully entered the designated threshold in a 30-second period (the time of each training trial). A higher ratio indicated better control of EEG. An increased ratio throughout the training in a single session may have indicated that the athlete achieved better control of target EEG during the training. This result could be attributed to the consistent strategy used by participants in the whole training session. On the other hand, no significant changes should have been expected in the control group, in which they received sham feedback instead of authentic feedback from themselves.

Baseline Increment

Investigating baseline changes is another way to show enhanced controllability on NFT in participants. Previous studies have evaluated the threshold variation within day-to-day sessions and suggested that increased threshold could serve as a marker for improvement of controllability due to neurofeedback training (Doppelmayr & Weber, 2011). For example, using the regression line slope as an indicator of NFT performance (Escolano, Olivan, Lopez-Del-Hoyo, Garcia-Campayo, & Minguez, 2012; Witte, Kober, Ninaus, Neuper, & Wood, 2013; Zoefel, Huster, & Herrmann, 2011), Zoefel et al. (2011) found only high alpha (IAF to IAF+2 Hz) training exhibited a visible change in baseline EEG; no changes were observed in low alpha and low beta when compared to its baselines. The training threshold based on the mean from previous sessions has also been applied as an adaptive threshold of EEG band power (Reichert, Kober, Neuper, & Wood, 2015). For example, Cheng et al. (2015) compared the baseline threshold among sessions and found that training threshold was significantly elevated after the first and second training sessions. That is, the high level of the training threshold was maintained throughout the following six sessions, suggesting that participants learned to control SMR power after the first and second training sessions and maintained the ability in remaining training sessions.

Frequency Band Specificity

Adjacent frequency bands can be altered by NFT as well (Nan et al., 2012). The first evaluation regarding the NFT is to verify whether only the trained band is altered after NFT while the other frequency bands stay unchanged. Frequency band specificity can be evaluated within daily training sessions or compared between the pre-test and the post-test.

However, as the complex processing of the cortex, the evidence of frequency band specificity is inconclusive in the performance of cognitive tasks (Gruzelier, 2014b). For example, concomitant change of beta power during training has been reported after augmented SMR NFT (Ghoshuni, Firoozabadi, Khalilzadeh, Reza, & Golpayegani, 2012; Schabus et al., 2014). Furthermore, Ros et al. (2013) found that down-regulating alpha power was accompanied by concurrent changes in the theta and beta bands. Similar findings of non-specificity has also been reported by a study examining the trainability of frontal midline theta which demonstrated concomitant changes at theta, alpha, and beta bands after eight sessions of NFT on both a training group and pseudo-training group (Enriquez-Geppert et al., 2014). However, Cheng et al. (2015) were able to demonstrate the frequency band specificity of NFT by showing the lack of significant change on flanking frequency bands (theta, alpha, low beta, and high beta) after eight sessions of augmented SMR NFT in a golf putting task. The discrepancy regarding frequency band specificity among these studies could be attributed to differences in the type of learning, attention, motivation, effort, reinforcement monitoring, etc., which may invoke several bands during training. Hence, future research should record and report the EEG based on a wider spectrum recording, which can further our understanding of the effects caused by the NFT on adjacent frequency bands.

Topographical Specificity

Topographical specificity refers to whether a concurrent change of cortical activity in areas other than the training site is observed after NFT. Generally, the comparison of cortical activity between the training site and surrounding cortical regions has been used as a measurement of topographical specificity. Evaluating topographical specificity is crucial because it is a way to see whether behavioral changes are tightly connected to the changes generated solely from the training site. However, whether cortical activation altered by NFT is spatially specific at the training site remains in question. Based on research thus far, a spread or a concurrent change in the neighboring regions has been reported. For example, Cheng et al. (2015) found a concurrent change in Pz after eight sessions of augmented SMR training at Cz for putting performance, suggesting the NFT training targeting to reduce activation of sensorimotor cortex has spillover to affect the parietal region. Given the claim that SMR originates in the centro-parietal region (Grosse-Wentrup, Schölkopf, & Hill, 2011), whether the observed SMR changed in Pz after Cz NFT should be considered as an evidence for non-topographical specificity remains a debatable issue. However, the spillover effect was more clearly demonstrated in a NFT study in cognitive tasks, which reported that a marginally increased alpha power was found at the P3, O1, F7, and T3 after a down regulation of theta NFT based on the abnormally high theta power at F4, C3, P3, F7, F8, and T6 (Becerra et al., 2012). As suggested by previous studies, the concurrent changes in areas other than the training site after NFT remains one of the factors that should be anticipated before training starts. It is recommended that future NFT studies examine cortical activity at not only the training site, but also at adjacent sites and other more remote regions of the brain so that the cortical mechanism underlying NFT may be further understood.

Responder vs. Non-Responder

The non-responder refers to those participants who do not show expected change via NFT. Previous NFT and Brain–Computer Interface (BCI) studies have reported that non-responders comprise 15–30% of the participants (Allison & Neuper, 2009; Enriquez-Geppert et al., 2014; Zoefel et al., 2011). The non-responders could be due to individualized susceptibility to NFT; however, little explanation for being a non-responder has been provided at present.

Evidence has shown that the difference between responder and non-responder can be assessed by resting-state EEG activity. For example, SMR power in the left lateral central electrodes, e.g. C5, C3, CP5, and CP3 in the eyes-open condition, best predicted performance under augmented SMR training (Reichert et al., 2015). This evidence is in line with a SMR BCI study by Blankertz et al. (2010), which reported that participants exhibited better control over SMR power when they showed a higher SMR power within the left central region in the eyes open condition before training started. Hence, the topological distribution of SMR power in the left central region between responders and non-responders in the eyes open condition may serve as a preliminary measurement for screening non-responders in subsequent training.

Other Issues for NFT in Sport Performance

The number of optimal training sessions is still under debate. However, based on previous studies, at least eight sessions are recommended. The positive effects of NFT have been reported in dance performance (Raymond, Sajid, et al., 2005), archery (Paul et al., 2012), swimming (Faridnia et al., 2012), gymnastics (Dekker et al., 2014; Shaw et al., 2012), rifle shooting (Rostami et al., 2012), and golf putting (Cheng et al., 2015). This is in line with previous studies that reported performance enhancement in attention and working memory (Vernon et al., 2003), microsurgery skills (Ros et al., 2009), perceptual integration and recognition memory (Keizer, Verment, & Hommel,

2010; Keizer, Verschoor, Verment, & Hommel, 2010; Salari, Büchel, & Rose, 2014), and cognitive creativity (Gruzelier, Foks, Steffert, Chen, & Ros, 2014) after eight sessions of NFT. Hence, we can preliminarily conclude that eight training sessions might be the minimum for generating an expected effect. In the elderly, a positive outcome was obtained within 30 and 31 to 35 (Angelakis et al., 2007; Becerra et al., 2012), but not with four sessions (Lecomte & Juhel, 2011). These studies suggest that elderly participants may require more NFT sessions for an observable effect. Therefore, eight sessions of NFT are tentatively suggested as the minimum required protocol for young healthy participants, while more sessions might be needed for older participants.

A remaining question is how long each training session should last. The ideal duration of a single training session remains unknown. A short training session may be less likely to see changes in performance and cortical activity. However, a long training session may make exhaust participants. Furthermore, the ability to sustain attention may be reduced because of tiredness generated by NFT. Gruzelier (2014a) reported that after 15-minutes of SMR ratio NFT whereby a positive effect on calmness ratings was observed, a rise in tiredness was also observed. Although several reports have shown positive effects from training for duration of 20 to 30 minutes (Cheng et al., 2015; Ghaziri et al., 2013; Raymond, Sajid, et al., 2005; Rostami et al., 2012), the possible concentration and motivation costs resulting from an extended training session should be considered when designing training protocols.

The interval between training sessions must also be addressed. Current evidence is inconclusive. However, an interval between one or two days might be the ideal option. Vernon et al. (2009) suggested that interval of training sessions extended over a period of days are more effective than finishing the trainings within a single day. Furthermore, Ros et al. (2009) found that trainee microsurgeons exhibited better surgical skills in the second half of an eight-session training course for SMR ratio training, which varied from 8.5 days compared to the first half training, 4.8 days. This argument should be considered for future studies, as some have failed to show the positive effects of a series of NFT training sessions within a day (Albert, Simmons, & Walker, 1974; Nan et al., 2015).

Direction for Future Studies

Research in NFT and sport is still in its infancy and the number of high quality studies is still very limited. Therefore, more studies are needed to accumulate more knowledge regarding this noninvasive approach for self-regulating cortical activity. Given the methodological heterogeneity among previous studies, future studies should consider adopting a more standardized approach to systematically examine the relationship between different EEG frequency bands and motor performance. Furthermore, a relationship between a specific EEG frequency band and motor performance should be established before moving into a NFT study employing that specific frequency band as the training target. This logic has been followed by the left temporal alpha, frontal midline theta, and SMR, for which a relationship between the specific EEG frequency band and motor performance was observed in an expert-novice comparison design (Cheng et al., 2015; Doppelmayr et al., 2008; Haufler et al., 2000) and an intraindividual good-poor performance comparison design (Cheng et al., 2017; Chuang et al., 2013; Kao et al., 2013).

Studies conducted by single-session NFT can not only examine evidence of learning, but also the cognitive and affective outcomes generated in an extremely limited time. Although limited training sessions are not feasible for the discussion of long-term changes in behavioral and cognitive performance, single-session NFT provides a possibility for practical application in the sports domain. Previous studies have shed light on potential improvement with single-session NFT, which enhanced pre-elite archers' performance with augmented SCPs NFT at T3 (Landers et al., 1991) and also improved golf putting performance with down regulating theta at Fz (Kao et al., 2014).

Future studies should aim to evaluate the retention effect of NFT. The evidence of this issue has been argued, however, no study has been able to provide a conclusive suggestion as yet. How long training effects last is not only a scientific question, but also a critical factor determining the acceptance of NFT as well as the method of using NFT on sports performers. For example, athletes might use this information for scheduling their NFT session alongside their training and competition schedules so that the NFT effects may be maximized with efficient time allocation. Again, retention effect should be investigated at the level of performance and cortical activities. This issue should be combined with the aforementioned suggestions to investigate the effects of NFT in terms of the number of sessions and the interval of each session.

There is a knowledge gap regarding the relationship between NFT and motor imagery. Establishing a connection between motor imagery and the targeted EEG activity is important. A concrete motor imagery can basically link with the targeted EEG activity. However, trainers should help athletes to figure out whether there might be another crucial motor imagery which can establish a stronger connection with the targeted EEG. For example, Cheng et al. (2015) carried out NFT on 16 pre-elite golfers and found only three main motor imageries selected by the golfers that were related to better putting performance: A clearer trajectory between the ball to the hole, smoother shoulder rotation, and clearer visual imagery of the golf ball. They put forth that participants who successfully adjusted EEG to the designated threshold saw improved putting performance. However, little evidence has been provided regarding the detailed usage of motor imagery and its effect on NFT.

Methods on how to increase training difficulty should be specified. There are several ways to increase training difficulty. First, the trainer can ask athletes to increase their successful training ratio on a single session, e.g. increase the ratio from 50% to 75%. Secondly, training duration can be lengthened. For example, if the trainers ask athletes to maintain 50% of the successful training ratio, then the goal would be to achieve this ratio for an extended duration, e.g. from 30 seconds to 40 seconds. Likewise, the trainer can also ask athletes to achieve the target ratio with more sessions in a daily training. Finally, the threshold level can be heightened. This might be the most intuitive way to increase training difficulty. However, this should be considered as the last step because a tiny rise in threshold could build up a disproportionate training difficulty. This could cause some frustration for participants and result in loss of confidence and motivation for training. Furthermore, athletes might start to doubt whether the motor imagery they use links with the target EEG activity.

The rationale for adopting the individualized frequency band for NFT is to avoid the delineation of spectral bands which could be varied between individuals and with age (Klimesch, 1999). Previous studies have adopted the individualized frequency band in NFT in sport (Raymond, Sajid, et al., 2005; Raymond, Varney, Parkinson, & Gruzelier, 2005).

Future research investigating performance in real-world competitions after lab NFT is also encouraged. The ecological or external validity of NFT has yet to be examined. The conditions in the real world, obviously, cannot be compared directly to conditions in the laboratory (Walsh, 2014). Hence, future studies should consider applying NFT to a field to validate the effects of NFT, especially performance measurements and the training itself.

The trainer-participant interface should be further elaborated in future studies. This topic is getting more important because the relationship between the trainer and the participant plays a critical role in terms of the effectiveness of training. As previous studies have suggested, when trainers come across to participants, social interaction is generated that might lead to placebo responses established by beliefs and expectations (Benedetti, Carlino, & Pollo, 2011).

Besides the effects of NFT on behavior outcomes, self-report ratings regarding NFT should be encouraged. The relative factors in sport performance are dependent on the type of movement. However, some common psychological construct, such as attention, mood, motivation, and control are highly valuable for understanding the learning process, especially when it comes to long-term NFT. These additional reports may clarify the variability and relation to performance (Gruzelier, 2014b).

Conclusion

This chapter aims to provide a methodological review for the effects of EEG NFT on sport performance. The discussion of methodological issues and the suggestions for future studies are the highlight of this chapter.

The accumulated reports conclude a positive effect from EEG NFT. However, several issues are yet to be resolved. First, the most important issue by far is the selection of an appropriate training target with strong evidence for its connection to motor performance. Second is how to verify training effects in terms of frequency specificity and topographical specificity is important for understanding mechanisms underlying the training. Third, the screening criteria before application of EEG NFT are an important issue due to a certain ratio of non-responders found in previous studies. Finally, how to design a reasonable and effective training protocol is a highlight for future studies, especially consideration of the optimal number of trainings and training session duration. In regard to ecological validity, hosting training in the field instead of in a lab would significantly boost the value of applying EEG NFT in sport performance enhancement.

EEG NFT is a way to link the mind and behavior, which provides a means of exploring a more efficient way to enhance or sustain superior motor performance. Based on the studies we have summarized in this chapter, an advanced EEG NFT study is recommended that integrates supplied measurements to systematically verify whether the change of target EEG is interconnected to projected behavior. Considering the complex nature of sport performance, establishing a specific EEG NFT protocol for specific sports is highly recommended.

References

Albert, I. B., Simmons, J., & Walker, J. (1974). Massed and spaced practice in alpha enhancement. *Perceptual and Motor Skills*, *39*(3), 1039–1042. https://doi.org/10.2466/pms.1974.39.3.1039

Allison, B., & Neuper, C. (2009). Could anyone use a BCI? In *Brain Computer Interfaces* (p. 409). https://doi.org/10.1007/978-1-84996-272-8

Angelakis, E., Stathopoulou, S., Frymiare, J. L., Green, D. L., Lubar, J. F., & Kounios, J. (2007). EEG neurofeedback: A brief overview and an example of peak alpha frequency training for cognitive enhancement in the elderly. *The Clinical Neuropsychologist*, *21*(1), 110–129. https://doi.org/10.1080/13854040600744839

Arns, M., de Ridder, S., Strehl, U., Breteler, M., & Coenen, A. (2009). Efficacy of neurofeedback treatment in ADHD: The effects on inattention, impulsivity and hyperactivity: A meta-analysis. *Clinical EEG and Neuroscience*, *40*(3), 180–189. https://doi.org/10.1177/155005940904000311

Arns, M., Kleinnijenhuis, M., Fallahpour, K., & Breteler, R. (2008). Golf performance enhancement and real-life neurofeedback training using personalized event-locked EEG profiles. *Journal of Neurotherapy*, *11*(4), 11–18. https://doi.org/10.1080/10874200802149656

Asada, H., Fukuda, Y., Tsunoda, S., Yamaguchi, M., & Tonoike, M. (1999). Frontal midline theta rhythms reflect alternative activation of prefrontal cortex and anterior cingulate cortex in humans. *Neuroscience Letters*, *274*(1), 29–32. https://doi.org/10.1016/S0304-3940(99)00679-5

Baumeister, J., Reinecke, K., Liesen, H., & Weiss, M. (2008). Cortical activity of skilled performance in a complex sports related motor task. *European Journal of Applied Physiology*, *104*(4), 625–631. https://doi.org/10.1007/s00421-008-0811-x

Baumeister, J., Von Detten, S., Van Niekerk, S. M., Schubert, M., Ageberg, E., & Louw, Q. A. (2013). Brain activity in predictive sensorimotor control for landings: An EEG pilot study. *International Journal of Sports Medicine*, *34*(12), 1106–1111. https://doi.org/10.1055/s-0033-1341437

Becerra, J., Fernández, T., Roca-Stappung, M., Díaz-Comas, L., Galán, L., Bosch, J., … Harmony, T. (2012). Neurofeedback in healthy elderly human subjects with electroencephalographic risk for cognitive disorder. *Journal of Alzheimer's Disease : JAD*, *28*(2), 357–367. https://doi.org/10.3233/JAD-2011-111055

Beilock, S. L., Carr, T. H., MacMahon, C., & Starkes, J. L. (2002). When paying attention becomes counterproductive: Impact of divided versus skill-focused attention on novice and experienced performance of sensorimotor skills. *Journal of Experimental Psychology: Applied*, *8*(1), 6–16. https://doi.org/10.1037/1076-898X.8.1.6

Benedetti, F., Carlino, E., & Pollo, A. (2011). Hidden administration of drugs. *Clinical Pharmacology & Therapeutics*, *90*(5), 651–661. https://doi.org/10.1038/clpt.2011.206

Blankertz, B., Sannelli, C., Halder, S., Hammer, E. M., Kübler, A., Müller, K. R., ... Dickhaus, T. (2010). Neurophysiological predictor of SMR-based BCI performance. *NeuroImage*, *51*(4), 1303–1309. https://doi.org/10.1016/j.neuroimage.2010.03.022

Cheng, M. Y., Huang, C. J., Chang, Y. K., Koester, D., Schack, T., & Hung, T. M. (2015). Sensorimotor rhythm neurofeedback enhances golf putting performance. *Journal of Sport and Exercise Psychology*, *37*(6), 626–636. https://doi.org/10.1123/jsep.2015-0166

Cheng, M. Y., Hung, C. L., Huang, C. J., Chang, Y. K., Lo, L. C., Shen, C., & Hung, T. M. (2015). Expert-novice differences in SMR activity during dart throwing. *Biological Psychology*, *110*, 212–218. https://doi.org/10.1016/j.biopsycho.2015.08.003

Cheng, M. Y., Wang, K. P., Hung, C. L., Tu, Y. L., Huang, C. J., Dirk, K., ... Hung, T. M. (2017). Higher power of sensorimotor rhythm is associated with better performance in skilled air-pistol shooters. *Psychology of Sport and Exercise*, *32*. https://doi.org/https://doi.org/10.1016/j.psychsport.2017.05.007

Chuang, L. Y., Huang, C. J., & Hung, T. M. (2013). The differences in frontal midline theta power between successful and unsuccessful basketball free throws of elite basketball players. *International Journal of Psychophysiology*, *90*(3), 321–328. https://doi.org/10.1016/j.ijpsycho.2013.10.002

Cooper, N. R., Croft, R. J., Dominey, S. J. J., Burgess, A. P., & Gruzelier, J. H. (2003). Paradox lost? Exploring the role of alpha oscillations during externally vs. internally directed attention and the implications for idling and inhibition hypotheses. *International Journal of Psychophysiology*, *47*(1), 65–74. https://doi.org/10.1016/S0167-8760(02)00107-1

Dayan, E., & Cohen, L. G. (2011). Neuroplasticity subserving motor skill learning. *Neuron*, *72*(3), 443–454. https://doi.org/10.1016/j.neuron.2011.10.008

Dekker, M. K. J., Van den Berg, B. R., Denissen, A. J. M., Sitskoorn, M. M., & Van Boxtel, G. J. M. (2014). Feasibility of eyes open alpha power training for mental enhancement in elite gymnasts. *Journal of Sports Sciences*, *32*(16), 1550–1560. https://doi.org/10.1080/02640414.2014.906044

Del Percio, C., Iacoboni, M., Lizio, R., Marzano, N., Infarinato, F., Vecchio, F., ... Babiloni, C. (2011). Functional coupling of parietal alpha rhythms is enhanced in athletes before visuomotor performance: A coherence electroencephalographic study. *Neuroscience*, *175*, 198–211. https://doi.org/10.1016/j.neuroscience.2010.11.031

Dempster, T., & Vernon, D. J. (2009). Identifying indices of learning for alpha neurofeedback training. *Applied Psychophysiology Biofeedback*, *34*(4), 309–318. https://doi.org/10.1007/s10484-009-9112-3

Di Russo, F., Pitzalis, S., Aprile, T., & Spinelli, D. (2005). Effect of practice on brain activity: An investigation in top-level rifle shooters. *Medicine and Science in Sports and Exercise*, *37*(9), 1586–1593. https://doi.org/10.1249/01.mss.0000177458.71676.0d

Donkers, F. C. L., Schwikert, S. R., Evans, A. M., Cleary, K. M., Perkins, D. O., & Belger, A. (2011). Impaired neural synchrony in the theta frequency range in adolescents at familial risk for schizophrenia. *Frontiers in Psychiatry*, *2*, 51. https://doi.org/10.3389/fpsyt.2011.00051

Doppelmayr, M., Finkenzeller, T., & Sauseng, P. (2008). Frontal midline theta in the pre-shot phase of rifle shooting: Differences between experts and novices. *Neuropsychologia*, *46*(5), 1463–1467. https://doi.org/10.1016/j.neuropsychologia.2007.12.026

Doppelmayr, M., & Weber, E. (2011). Effects of SMR and theta/beta neurofeedback on reaction times, spatial abilities, and creativity. *Journal of Neurotherapy*, *15*(2), 115–129. https://doi.org/10.1080/10874208.2011.570689

Egner, T., & Gruzelier, J. H. (2001). Learned self-regulation of EEG frequency components affects attention and event-related brain potentials in humans. *Neuroreport*, *12*(18), 4155–4159. https://doi.org/10.1097/00001756-200112210-00058

Egner, T., & Gruzelier, J. H. (2004). EEG biofeedback of low beta band components: Frequency-specific effects on variables of attention and event-related brain potentials. *Clinical Neurophysiology*, *115*(1), 131–139. https://doi.org/10.1016/S1388-2457(03)00353-5

Enriquez-geppert, S., Huster, R. J., & Herrmann, C. S. (2017). EEG-Neurofeedback as a tool to modulate cognition and behavior : A review tutorial. *Frontiers in Human Neuroscience*, *11*(February), 1–19. https://doi.org/10.3389/fnhum.2017.00051

Enriquez-Geppert, S., Huster, R. J., Scharfenort, R., Mokom, Z. N., Zimmermann, J., & Herrmann, C. S. (2014). Modulation of frontal-midline theta by neurofeedback. *Biological Psychology*, *95*(1), 59–69. https://doi.org/10.1016/j.biopsycho.2013.02.019

Escolano, C., Olivan, B., Lopez-Del-Hoyo, Y., Garcia-Campayo, J., & Minguez, J. (2012). Double-blind single-session neurofeedback training in upper-alpha for cognitive enhancement of healthy subjects.

In *Proceedings of the Annual International Conference of the IEEE Engineering in Medicine and Biology Society, EMBS* (pp. 4643–4647). https://doi.org/10.1109/EMBC.2012.6347002

Faridnia, M., Shojaei, M., & Rahimi, A. (2012). The effect of neurofeedback training on the anxiety of elite female swimmers. *Annals of Biological Research, 3*(2), 1020–1028. Retrieved from http://scholarsresearch library.com/ABR-vol3-iss2/ABR-2012-3-2-1020-1028.pdf

Ghaziri, J., Tucholka, A., Larue, V., Blanchette-Sylvestre, M., Reyburn, G., Gilbert, G., … Beauregard, M. (2013). Neurofeedback training induces changes in white and gray matter. *Clinical EEG and Neuroscience, 44*(4), 265–272. https://doi.org/10.1177/1550059413476031

Ghoshuni, M., Firoozabadi, M., Khalilzadeh, M. A., Reza, M., & Golpayegani, H. (2012). The effect of sensorimotor rhythm enhancing neurofeedback on power of adjacent frequency bands. *Biomedical Engineering: Applications, Basis and Communications, 24*(4), 307–312. https://doi.org/10.1142/S1016237212500238

Green, E., & Green, A. (1977). Beyond biofeedback. *Beyond Biofeedback*. New York: Delacorte Press. Retrieved from http://ovidsp.ovid.com/ovidweb.cgi?T=JS&PAGE=reference&D=psyc2&NEWS=N&AN=1979-00452-000

Grosse-Wentrup, M., Schölkopf, B., & Hill, J. (2011). Causal influence of gamma oscillations on the sensorimotor rhythm. *NeuroImage, 56*(2), 837–842. https://doi.org/10.1016/j.neuroimage.2010.04.265

Gruzelier, J. H. (2014a). Differential effects on mood of 12–15 (SMR) and 15–18 (beta1) Hz neurofeedback. *International Journal of Psychophysiology, 93*(1), 112–115. https://doi.org/10.1016/j.ijpsycho.2012.11.007

Gruzelier, J. H. (2014b). EEG-neurofeedback for optimising performance. III: A review of methodological and theoretical considerations. *Neuroscience and Biobehavioral Reviews, 44*, 159–182. https://doi.org/10.1016/j.neubiorev.2014.03.015

Gruzelier, J. H., Egner, T., & Vernon, D. J. (2006). Chapter 27 validating the efficacy of neurofeedback for optimising performance. *Progress in Brain Research, 159*, 421–431. https://doi.org/10.1016/S0079-6123(06)59027-2

Gruzelier, J. H., Foks, M., Steffert, T., Chen, M. J. L., & Ros, T. (2014). Beneficial outcome from EEG-neurofeedback on creative music performance, attention and well-being in school children. *Biological Psychology, 95*(1), 86–95. https://doi.org/10.1016/j.biopsycho.2013.04.005

Gruzelier, J. H., Inoue, A., Smart, R., Steed, A., & Steffert, T. (2010). Acting performance and flow state enhanced with sensory-motor rhythm neurofeedback comparing ecologically valid immersive VR and training screen scenarios. *Neuroscience Letters, 480*(2), 112–116. https://doi.org/10.1016/j.neulet.2010.06.019

Gruzelier, J. H., Thompson, T., Redding, E., Brandt, R., & Steffert, T. (2014). Application of alpha/theta neurofeedback and heart rate variability training to young contemporary dancers: State anxiety and creativity. *International Journal of Psychophysiology, 93*(1), 105–111. https://doi.org/10.1016/j.ijpsycho.2013.05.004

Hanslmayr, S., Sauseng, P., Doppelmayr, M., Schabus, M., & Klimesch, W. (2005). Increasing individual upper alpha power by neurofeedback improves cognitive performance in human subjects. *Applied Psychophysiology Biofeedback, 30*(1), 1–10. https://doi.org/10.1007/s10484-005-2169-8

Hatfield, B. D., & Hillman, C. H. (2001). The psychophysiology of sport. *Handbook of Sport Psychology*, 362–386. Retrieved from http://kch.illinois.edu/research/labs/neurocognitive-kinesiology/files/Articles/Hatfield_2001_ThePsychophysiologyOfSport.pdf

Haufler, A. J., Spalding, T. W., Santa Maria, D. L., & Hatfield, B. D. (2000). Neuro-cognitive activity during a self-paced visuospatial task: Comparative EEG profiles in marksmen and novice shooters. *Biological Psychology, 53*(2–3), 131–160. https://doi.org/10.1016/S0301-0511(00)00047-8

Hoedlmoser, K., Pecerstorfer, T., Gruber, G., Anderer, P., Doppelmayr, M., Klimesch, W., & Schabus, M. (2008). Instrumental conditioning of human sensorimotor rhythm (12–15 Hz) and its impact on sleep as well as declarative learning. *Sleep, 31*(10), 1401–1408. https://doi.org/10.5665/sleep/31.10.1401

Jensen, O., & Mazaheri, A. (2010). Shaping functional architecture by oscillatory alpha activity: Gating by inhibition. *Frontiers in Human Neuroscience, 4*. https://doi.org/10.3389/fnhum.2010.00186

Kamiya, J. (1968). Conscious control of brain waves. *Psychology Today, 1*, 57–60.

Kao, S. C., Huang, C. J., & Hung, T. M. (2013). Frontal midline theta is a specific indicator of optimal attentional engagement during skilled putting performance. *Journal of Sport & Exercise Psychology, 35*(5), 470–478.

Kao, S. C., Huang, C. J., & Hung, T. M. (2014). Neurofeedback training reduces frontal midline theta and improves putting performance in expert golfers. *Journal of Applied Sport Psychology, 26*(3), 271–286. https://doi.org/10.1080/10413200.2013.855682

Keizer, A. W., Verment, R. S., & Hommel, B. (2010). Enhancing cognitive control through neurofeedback: A role of gamma-band activity in managing episodic retrieval. *NeuroImage, 49*(4), 3404–3413. https://doi.org/10.1016/j.neuroimage.2009.11.023

Keizer, A. W., Verschoor, M., Verment, R. S., & Hommel, B. (2010). The effect of gamma enhancing neurofeedback on the control of feature bindings and intelligence measures. *International Journal of Psychophysiology*, *75*(1), 25–32. https://doi.org/10.1016/j.ijpsycho.2009.10.011

Kleih, S. C., & Kübler, A. (2013). Empathy, motivation, and P300 BCI performance. *Frontiers in Human Neuroscience*, *7*. https://doi.org/10.3389/fnhum.2013.00642

Klimesch, W. (1996). Memory processes brain oscilliations and EEG synchronization memory processes, brain oscillations and EEG synchronization. *International Journal of Psychophysiology*, *43*(1–2), 61–100.

Klimesch, W. (1999). EEG alpha and theta oscillations reflect cognitive and memory performance: A review and analysis. *Brain Research Reviews*, *29*(2–3), 169–195. https://doi.org/10.1016/S0165-0173(98)00056-3

Kober, S. E., Witte, M., Ninaus, M., Neuper, C., & Wood, G. (2013). Learning to modulate one's own brain activity: The effect of spontaneous mental strategies. *Frontiers in Human Neuroscience*, *7*(October), 1–12. https://doi.org/10.3389/fnhum.2013.00695

Kober, S. E., Witte, M., Stangl, M., Väljamäe, A., Neuper, C., & Wood, G. (2015). Shutting down sensorimotor interference unblocks the networks for stimulus processing: An SMR neurofeedback training study. *Clinical Neurophysiology*, *126*(1), 82–95. https://doi.org/10.1016/j.clinph.2014.03.031

Kropotov, J. D., Grin-Yatsenko, V. A., Ponomarev, V. A., Chutko, L. S., Yakovenko, E. A., & Nikishena, I. S. (2005). ERPs correlates of EEG relative beta training in ADHD children. *International Journal of Psychophysiology*, *55*(1), 23–34. https://doi.org/10.1016/j.ijpsycho.2004.05.011

Landers, D. M., Petruzzello, S. J., Salazar, W., Crews, D. J., Kubitz, K. A., Gannon, T. L., & Han, M. (1991). The influence of electrocortical biofeedback on performance in pre-elite archers. *Medicine & Science in Sports & Exercise*, *23*(1), 123–129. https://doi.org/10.1249/00005768-199101000-00018

Lecomte, G., & Juhel, J. (2011). The effects of neurofeedback training on memory performance in elderly subjects. *Psychology*, *2*(8), 846–852. https://doi.org/10.4236/psych.2011.28129

Loze, G. M., Collins, D., & Holmes, P. S. (2001). Pre-shot EEG alpha-power reactivity during expert air-pistol shooting: A comparison of best and worst shots. *Journal of Sports Sciences*, *19*(9), 727–733. https://doi.org/10.1080/02640410152475856

Lubar, J. F., & Shouse, M. N. (1976). EEG and behavioral changes in a hyperkinetic child concurrent with training of the sensorimotor rhythm (SMR) – A preliminary report. *Biofeedback and Self-Regulation*, *1*(3), 293–306. https://doi.org/10.1007/BF01001170

Mann, C. A., Sterman, M. B., & Kaiser, D. A. (1996). Suppression of EEG rhythmic frequencies during somatomotor and visuo-motor behavior. *International Journal of Psychophysiology*, *23*(1–2), 1–7. https://doi.org/10.1016/0167-8760(96)00036-0

Mikicin, M. (2015). The autotelic involvement of attention induced by EEG neurofeedback training improves the performance of an athlete's mind. *Biomedical Human Kinetics*, *7*(1), 58–65. https://doi.org/10.1515/bhk-2015-0010

Mitchell, D. J., McNaughton, N., Flanagan, D., & Kirk, I. J. (2008). Frontal-midline theta from the perspective of hippocampal "theta." *Progress in Neurobiology*. https://doi.org/10.1016/j.pneurobio.2008.09.005

Nan, W., Qu, X., Yang, L., Wan, F., Hu, Y., Mou, P., ... Rosa, A. (2015). Beta/theta neurofeedback training effects in physical balance of healthy people. In *World Congress on Medical Physics and Biomedical Engineering, June 7–12, 2015, Toronto, Canada* (pp. 1213–1216). Springer. https://doi.org/10.1007/978-3-319-19387-8_294

Nan, W., Rodrigues, J. P., Ma, J., Qu, X., Wan, F., Mak, P. U. P. I., ... Rosa, A. (2012). Individual alpha neurofeedback training effect on short term memory. *International Journal of Psychophysiology*, *86*(1), 83–87. https://doi.org/10.1016/j.ijpsycho.2012.07.182

Paul, M., Ganesan, S., Sandhu, J. S., & Simon, J. V. (2012). Effect of sensory motor rhythm neurofeedback on psycho-physiological, electro-encephalographic measures and performance of archery players. *Ibnosina Journal of Medicine and Biomedical Sciences*, *4*(2), 32–39. Retrieved from http://journals.sfu.ca/ijmbs/index.php/ijmbs/article/view/221

Pfurtscheller, G., & Neuper, C. (1997). Motor imagery activates primary sensorimotor area in humans. *Neuroscience Letters*, *239*(2–3), 65–68. https://doi.org/10.1016/S0304-3940(97)00889-6

Quandt, L. C., & Marshall, P. J. (2014). The effect of action experience on sensorimotor EEG rhythms during action observation. *Neuropsychologia*, *56*(1), 401–408. https://doi.org/10.1016/j.neuropsychologia.2014.02.015

Raymond, J., Sajid, I., Parkinson, L. A., & Gruzelier, J. H. (2005). Biofeedback and dance performance: A preliminary investigation. *Applied Psychophysiology Biofeedback*, *30*(1), 65–73. https://doi.org/10.1007/s10484-005-2175-x

Raymond, J., Varney, C., Parkinson, L., & Gruzelier, J. H. (2005). The effects of alpha/theta neurofeedback on personality and mood. *Cognitive Brain Research*, *23*(2–3), 287–292. https://doi.org/10.1016/j.cogbrainres.2004.10.023

Reichert, J. L., Kober, S. E., Neuper, C., & Wood, G. (2015). Resting-state sensorimotor rhythm (SMR) power predicts the ability to up-regulate SMR in an EEG-instrumental conditioning paradigm. *Clinical Neurophysiology, 126*(11), 2068–2077. https://doi.org/10.1016/j.clinph.2014.09.032

Reis, J., Portugal, A. M., Fernandes, L., Afonso, N., Pereira, M., Sousa, N., & Dias, N. S. (2016). An alpha and theta intensive and short neurofeedback protocol for healthy aging working-memory training. *Frontiers in Aging Neuroscience, 8*, 157. https://doi.org/10.3389/fnagi.2016.00157

Riecansky, I., & Katina, S. (2010). Induced EEG alpha oscillations are related to mental rotation ability: The evidence for neural efficiency and serial processing. *Neuroscience Letters, 482*(2), 133–136. https://doi.org/10.1016/j.neulet.2010.07.017

Ring, C., Cooke, A., Kavussanu, M., McIntyre, D., & Masters, R. (2015). Investigating the efficacy of neurofeedback training for expediting expertise and excellence in sport. *Psychology of Sport and Exercise, 16*(P1), 118–127. https://doi.org/10.1016/j.psychsport.2014.08.005

Ros, T., Moseley, M. J., Bloom, P. A., Benjamin, L., Parkinson, L. A., & Gruzelier, J. H. (2009). Optimizing microsurgical skills with EEG neurofeedback. *BMC Neuroscience, 10*(1), 87. https://doi.org/10.1186/1471-2202-10-87

Ros, T., Théberge, J., Frewen, P. A., Kluetsch, R., Densmore, M., Calhoun, V. D., & Lanius, R. A. (2013). Mind over chatter: Plastic up-regulation of the fMRI salience network directly after EEG neurofeedback. *Neuroimage, 65*, 324–335.

Rostami, R., Sadeghi, H., Karami, K. A., Abadi, M. N., & Salamati, P. (2012). The effects of neurofeedback on the improvement of rifle shooters' performance. *Journal of Neurotherapy, 16*(4), 264–269. https://doi.org/10.1080/10874208.2012.730388

Salari, N., Büchel, C., & Rose, M. (2014). Neurofeedback training of gamma band oscillations improves perceptual processing. *Experimental Brain Research, 232*(10), 3353–3361. https://doi.org/10.1007/s00221-014-4023-9

Schabus, M., Heib, D. P. J., Lechinger, J., Griessenberger, H., Klimesch, W., Pawlizki, A., … Hoedlmoser, K. (2014). Enhancing sleep quality and memory in insomnia using instrumental sensorimotor rhythm conditioning. *Biological Psychology, 95*(1), 126–134. https://doi.org/10.1016/j.biopsycho.2013.02.020

Schmiedt, C., Brand, A., Hildebrandt, H., & Basar-Eroglu, C. (2005). Event-related theta oscillations during working memory tasks in patients with schizophrenia and healthy controls. *Brain Research. Cognitive Brain Research, 25*(3), 936–947. https://doi.org/10.1016/j.cogbrainres.2005.09.015

Schröter, H., & Leuthold, H. (2009). Motor programming of rapid finger sequences: Inferences from movement-related brain potentials. *Psychophysiology, 46*(2), 388–401. https://doi.org/10.1111/j.1469-8986.2008.00772.x

Shaw, L., Zaichkowsky, L., & Wilson, V. (2012). Setting the balance: Using biofeedback and neurofeedback with gymnasts. *Journal of Clinical Sport Psychology, 6*(1), 47–66. https://doi.org/10.1123/jcsp.6.1.47

Sterman, M. B. (1996). Physiological origins and functional correlates of EEG rhythmic activities: Implications for self-regulation. *Biofeedback and Self-Regulation, 21*(1), 3–33. https://doi.org/10.1007/BF02214147

Sterman, M. B. (2000). Basic concepts and clinical findings in the treatment of seizure disorders with EEG operant conditioning. *Clinical EEG (Electroencephalography)*. https://doi.org/10.1177/155005940003100111

Subramaniam, K., & Vinogradov, S. (2013). Improving the neural mechanisms of cognition through the pursuit of happiness. *Frontiers in Human Neuroscience, 7*(August), 452. https://doi.org/10.3389/fnhum.2013.00452

Tansey, M. A. (1984). EEG sensorimotor rhythm biofeedback training: Some effects on the neurologic precursors of learning disabilities. *International Journal of Psychophysiology, 1*(2), 163–177. https://doi.org/10.1016/0167-8760(84)90036-9

Tansey, M. A., & Bruner, R. L. (1983). EMG and EEG biofeedback training in the treatment of a 10-year-old hyperactive boy with a developmental reading disorder. *Biofeedback and Self-Regulation, 8*(1), 25–37. https://doi.org/10.1007/BF01000534

Thompson, T., Steffert, T., Ros, T., Leach, J., & Gruzelier, J. H. (2008). EEG applications for sport and performance. *Methods, 45*(4), 279–288. https://doi.org/10.1016/j.ymeth.2008.07.006

Tinius, T. P., & Tinius, K. A. (2000). Changes after EEG biofeedback and cognitive retraining in adults with mild traumatic brain injury and attention deficit hyperactivity disorder. *Journal of Neurotherapy, 4*(2), 27–44. https://doi.org/10.1300/J184v04n02_05

Van Driel, J., Sligte, I. G., Linders, J., Elport, D., & Cohen, M. X. (2015). Frequency band-specific electrical brain stimulation modulates cognitive control processes. *PLoS ONE, 10*(9). https://doi.org/10.1371/journal.pone.0138984

Vernon, D. J. (2005). Can neurofeedback training enhance performance? An evaluation of the evidence with implications for future research. *Applied Psychophysiology Biofeedback, 30*(4), 347–364. https://doi.org/10.1007/s10484-005-8421-4

Vernon, D. J., Dempster, T., Bazanova, O., Rutterford, N., Pasqualini, M., & Andersen, S. (2009). Alpha neurofeedback training for performance enhancement: Reviewing the methodology. *Journal of Neurotherapy*, *13*(4), 214–227. https://doi.org/10.1080/10874200903334397

Vernon, D. J., Egner, T., Cooper, N., Compton, T., Neilands, C., Sheri, A., & Gruzelier, J. H. (2003). The effect of training distinct neurofeedback protocols on aspects of cognitive performance. *International Journal of Psychophysiology*, *47*(1), 75–85. https://doi.org/10.1016/S0167-8760(02)00091-0

Walsh, V. (2014). Is sport the brain's biggest challenge? *Current Biology*, *24*(18), R859–R860. https://doi.org/10.1016/j.cub.2014.08.003

Weber, E., Köberl, A., Frank, S., & Doppelmayr, M. (2011). Predicting successful learning of SMR neurofeedback in healthy participants: Methodological considerations. *Applied Psychophysiology Biofeedback*, *36*(1), 37–45. https://doi.org/10.1007/s10484-010-9142-x

Witte, M., Kober, S. E., Ninaus, M., Neuper, C., & Wood, G. (2013). Control beliefs can predict the ability to up-regulate sensorimotor rhythm during neurofeedback training. *Frontiers in Human Neuroscience*, *7*. https://doi.org/10.3389/fnhum.2013.00478

Zich, C., Debener, S., Kranczioch, C., Bleichner, M. G., Gutberlet, I., & De Vos, M. (2015). Real-time EEG feedback during simultaneous EEG-fMRI identifies the cortical signature of motor imagery. *NeuroImage*, *114*, 438–447. https://doi.org/10.1016/j.neuroimage.2015.04.020

Zoefel, B., Huster, R. J., & Herrmann, C. S. (2011). Neurofeedback training of the upper alpha frequency band in EEG improves cognitive performance. *NeuroImage*, *54*(2), 1427–1431. https://doi.org/10.1016/j.neuroimage.2010.08.078

15

We Think, Therefore We Are

A Social Neuroscience Perspective on Team Dynamics, Hyper-Brains, and Collective Minds

Edson Filho and Gershon Tenenbaum

Descartes' "I think, therefore I am" observation symbolizes the birth of modern Western philosophy and highlights the functional role of the human mind. In this chapter, we extend Descartes' observation from "I" to "we" processes in team dynamics research. The notion of "collective mind" is an integral part of many team processes described in the Sport, Exercise, and Performance Psychology literature. In fact, scholars have been interested in evolving models to capture the abstract notion of team processes, such as cohesion, team mental models, and collective efficacy (Filho & Tenenbaum, 2015). Most of these models have been psychometric in nature; that is, concerned with identifying the reflective or formative indicators of team processes. Furthermore, research on team dynamics has also focused on the development of statistically reliable models linking team processes within a nomological network consisting of inputs, throughputs, and outputs (Carron, Hausenblas, & Eys, 2005; Filho, Tenenbaum, & Yang, 2015b). Most recently, the growth of social neuroscience has ushered new approaches to the study of team dynamics, particularly those focused on capturing the reflective and formative indicators of team processes through peripheral and central psychophysiological methods. The purpose of this chapter is to introduce the theories and methodologies that lay the foundation for the study of hyper-brains and collective minds in interactive motor tasks at large, and the sports domain in particular. We advanced applied implications stemming from the research conducted thus far, and conclude by discussing future research avenues on this realm.

Theoretical Background

Philosophers have discussed the notion of "mind" for centuries, at least since Aristotle. However, to this day, no clear answer has emerged on the mechanisms governing the mind and its impingent faculty of consciousness. What we know thus far is that the information processing capacity of different species is linked to their ability to establish complex social concepts and groups (*the social brain hypothesis*; see Dunbar, 1998). Some animal beings have a brain (physical entity) but do not seem to have a conscious mind. This so-called *mind/brain problem* is central to the study of group dynamics across disciplines (Coulter & Sharrock, 2007). Instinct may govern group behavior in some species that do not possess a mind, whereas a *collective consciousness* (see Durkheim, 2014) might explain, at least in part, complex group interactions in humans, including team dynamics in sport and exercise settings. Working teams can only perform complex tasks and synchronized actions in space and time (coordination) if its members can "read" each other's minds.

Theory of Mind

Briefly stated, Theory of Mind (TOM) is concerned with our minds ability to "read other minds" (Vogeley et al., 2001). In other words, "How do I know what you are thinking and how do you know what I am thinking" is a fundamental question that TOM tries to address. Without knowing each other's mental states, goal-oriented (intentional) and highly coordinated group behavior is unlikely to take place in the natural world. As TOM is a meta-theory (i.e., "a theory of theories"), two sub-theories have proposed answers to its fundamental question, namely *theory-theory* and *simulation theory*.

Theory-theory proposes that human beings have an innate, endowed capability to understand each other's mental states (Goldman, 2012). Evidence for this theory abounds from both the human and natural sciences. In the human sciences realm, the classic works by Piaget and Vygotsky support the idea that the human brain will naturally develop in complexity and, eventually, can abstract what others are thinking. Chomsky's (1965) theory of language also touches on the idea that human beings have an endowed capacity for acquiring language, and that the ability to communicate complex knowledge rests in part on the ability to read each other's mental states. In the natural sciences realm, the discovery of the putative mirror neuron system and the mentalizing network supports the notion that human beings can read each other minds (Clark & Dumas, 2015). Specifically, the discovery of the putative mirror neurons suggests that the brain is naturally structured for "neuronal firing" when observing others doing things we do. It is for this reason, at least in part, that we can experience vicarious neural activity, and thus empathize and understand how others think and feel (Rizzolatti & Craighero, 2004). The mentalizing network allows for complex cognitive processing, including attributing mental states to one another and meta-cognitive thinking (e.g., reflection) about the self and others (Clark & Dumas, 2015). Together, these two systems provide the neural substrate to allow mind reading to take place in the natural world.

Simulation theory, as the name suggests, rests on the notion that we can simulate each other's mental states based on our own mental representations (Leudar, Costall, & Francis, 2004). As such, some individuals, due to their previous experiences and genetic make-up, are better at reading people's minds. If we take the aphorism that the human mind is like a computer, it is clear that some computational models are better than others because of their hardware, software, or a combination of both. Support from simulation theory abounds from research with autism (Goldman, 2012). Autistic individuals can have difficulty recognizing when to empathize with others because they often struggle with perspective-taking abilities. Apart from clinical studies, research on empathy seems to suggest that our ability to read each other's minds can be enhanced through myriad routes, including perception and communication training (Sevdalis & Raab, 2014).

We take on an interpretive pluralist approach insofar that the synthesis of both theory-theory and simulation theory, rather than each sub-theory individually, is most likely to bear fruits to scholars and practitioners interested in team dynamics (see Wilkinson & Ball, 2012). Since the era of Socrates and Plato, millennia have gone by and the nature-nurture debates lives on, likely because both nature and nurture contribute to the body-mind functioning and our ability to read minds. What is more central to our discussion is that working teams depend on our minds' ability to show shared and complementary mental models that can be captured through scientific methods.

Methodological Considerations

Criticism of the idea of "collective mind" stems from the lack of evidence that such a phenomenon exists and can deal with the vast amount of information being exchanged by a group of individuals engaged in an interdependent task (see Silva, Garganta, Araújo, Davids, & Aguiar, 2013). To circumvent this criticism, and move evidence-practice forward (Figure 15.1), we suggest that scholars adopt a stepwise methodological approach by (1) using multi-person monitoring to reliably quantify and capture activity among a group of people engaged in interdependent tasks, (2) advancing interactive research paradigms addressing both cooperative and competitive motor tasks, and (3) using multi-modal assessment of central and peripheral outcome variables, while controlling for behavioral and contextual co-variates.

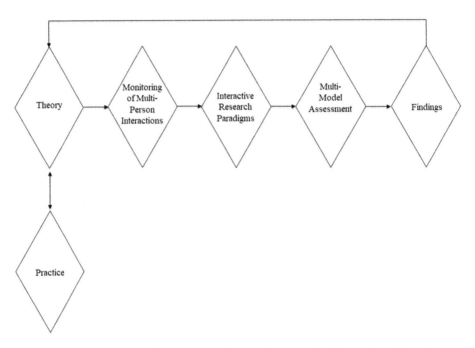

Figure 15.1 Stepwise schematic heuristics to advance theory and evidence-based practice in team dynamics, hyper-brains, and collective minds.

Step 1: Reliable Monitoring of Multi-Person Interactions

To reliably measure team processes through psychophysiological monitoring, it is important to (1) ensure that the data acquisition apparatus from different individuals is time-locked, and (2) conduct baseline assessments to quantify the state of homeostasis (equilibrium) of the different individuals.

First, there is consensus that the reliable synchronization of multiple devices is paramount whether one adopts a *time-based* or *event-based* research design (see Blascovich, Vanman, Mendes, & Dickerson, 2011). In time-based studies, the unit of analysis is a time-window that can be defined *a priori* as based on theory and previous research, or *a posteriori* via inductive bottom-up analysis. In an event-based design, the unit of analysis is defined around a triggered event (e.g., "t_0"), which in turn allows one to assess what happened before or after a given event. Timing is crucial across research designs because without a time dimension (either empirical or theoretical) it is impossible to establish "what leads to what" (i.e., input-output relations) in a given nomological network (Hawking, 1989; Popper, 2005). The same point-in-time or the same unit of analysis must be contrasted across multiple individuals. As Montague et al. (2002) averred, data collection must be "started at the same time and allowed to run in parallel" (p. 1160).

It follows that push-button and software generated triggers are common ways to synchronize in time multiple data recordings from different individuals. In fact, Babiloni and Astolfi (2014, p.78) have noted that the best method to synchronize two systems is by using an "external trigger that reaches all of the acquisition machines" at the same time (see also Lindenberger, Li, Gruber, & Müller, 2009). For instance, when studying cooperative juggling, we have synchronized two EEG systems through the use as a push-button trigger (Figure 15.2, left panel). Noteworthy, if two data acquisition systems of different makes are used to collect data, one must be cautious of inter-equipment variability, which interferes with the reliability of the data acquisition. For instance, two different EEG systems might not have the same number of channels (e.g., 23 channels versus 32 channels) or be able to collect data at the same sample frequency (e.g., 256 Hz versus 521 Hz). As such, adjustments before, during and after data collection must be executed to ensure that "apples are being compared to apples and oranges to oranges." Finally, an alternative method to ensure the reliable monitoring from multi-person interactions is to use the same single device to collect data from two or more individuals. For instance, some biofeedback systems allow the user to input data from two or more people at the same time (Figure 15.2, right panel).

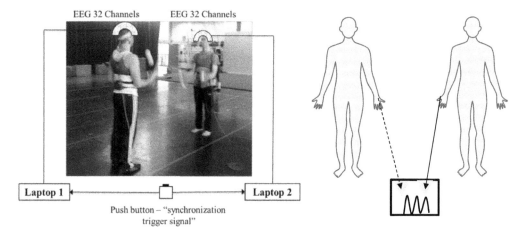

Figure 15.2 Example of the juggling paradigm wherein two jugglers have their psychophysiological responses monitored at the same time. A push-button trigger is used to synchronize the systems in time (left panel). Schematic representation of a same device synchronization wherein two individuals have their physiological responses (e.g., galvanic skin response) inputted into the same data acquisition hardware (right panel).

Second, baseline assessments are required to test whether changes beyond chance level occurred due to the experimental condition (e.g., experimental manipulation check). Furthermore, in multi-person studies, baselines are used to standardize and compare the responses across individuals. Specifically, different individuals show different bio-psycho-social responses to a given stimuli akin to the notion of *individual response stereotype* (Stern, Ray, & Quigley, 2001). Moreover, according to the *law of initial values* (see Wilder, 1967), changes in psychophysiological functioning depend on the pre-stimulus levels, with higher changes expected if the pre-stimulus levels are low than if the pre-stimulus levels are high. Importantly, there is no set-in-stone guideline for how long a baseline assessment should last. Rather, the assessment should be long enough to capture a stable pre-stimulus signal within normal ranges (to ensure the equipment is working properly) that allows for subsequent data filtering and analysis (Tenenbaum & Filho, 2018). For instance, if during data collection heart rate values are above realistic normal ranges (> 220 bpm), the researcher must check whether the hardware (e.g., equipment and sensors) is properly connected, and/or the software is working correctly.

Step 2: Advancing Interactive Research Paradigms

Since the discovery of the mirror neurons in the 1980s (for a review see Rizzolatti & Craighero, 2004), and the emergence of social neuroscience in the 1990s (see Cacioppo & Berntson, 1992), there has been scant research on the monitoring of psychophysiological responses with healthy individuals in general, and during interactive motor tasks in particular (Filho, Bertollo, Robazza, & Comani, 2015a). The bulk of the research has been centered on clinical populations (Schilbach et al., 2013). Another portion of the research has targeted healthy individuals, however primarily through observational paradigms (Di Paolo & De Jaegher, 2012; Konvalinka & Roepstorff, 2012). In observational paradigms, social stimuli are presented and individuals' psychophysiological responses to that stimuli are recorded. That is, an individual engages in action, while another remains disengaged as a mere observer. The input is thus unidirectional rather than reciprocal and multi-factorial (Figure 15.3).

Given that Sport, Exercise, and Performance Psychology researchers primarily study healthy populations engaged in action (Filho & Tenenbaum, 2015), it is paramount to advance research based on interactive paradigms and coupled with multi-modal psychophysiological measurements targeting both central and peripheral physiological mechanisms (Figure 15.4). First, central and peripheral functional connections in the body differ when people are actively engaged in social interaction, compared to when people are only mere observers of social exchanges (see Di Paolo & De Jaegher, 2012; Konvalinka & Roepstorff, 2012). Importantly, not all interactions are made equal. Virtual interactions through the internet and virtual reality exchanges have been found to differ from in-person social exchanges (Dumas, Lachat, Martinerie, Nadel, & George, 2011). Second, highly interactive tasks require continuous involvement of various individuals, and thereby social loafing is less likely to occur (Filho et al., 2015a).

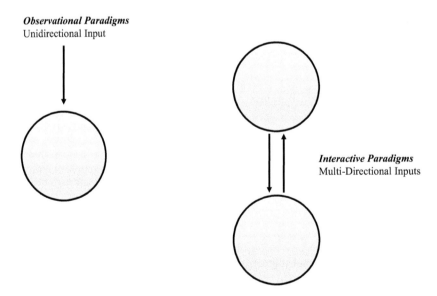

Figure 15.3 Observational paradigms allow for unidirectional inputs. Interactive paradigms are characterized by multi-directional inputs between the interacting subjects.

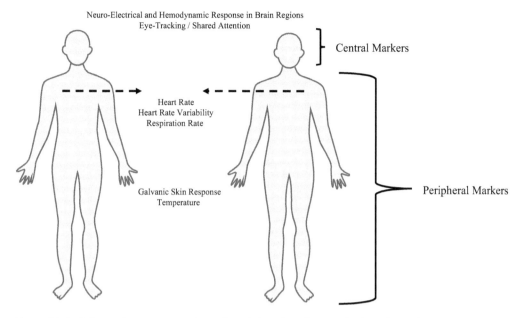

Neuro-Electrical and Hemodynamic Response in Brain Regions
Eye-Tracking / Shared Attention

Central Markers

Heart Rate
Heart Rate Variability
Respiration Rate

Galvanic Skin Response
Temperature

Peripheral Markers

Figure 15.4 Schematic representation of peripheral and central physiological markers used to study abstract psychological concepts.

Degree and Type of Interactivity

If we abide by the logic of measurement development (for a review see Tenenbaum & Filho, 2015), the degree of interactivity for a given task can be conceptualized within a continuum ranging from *Highly Passive* to *Highly Interactive*. Diachronic tasks ("I play and then you play"; turn-taking approaches) are distinct from interactive tasks ("We continuously play together"; concurrent acting approaches). Furthermore, we can scale the type of task within a continuum ranging from *Highly Cooperative* to *Highly Competitive*. Individuals join and remain in groups to cooperate and outcompete one another and other groups (Carron et al., 2005). That is, cooperation and competition can be among individuals in a group (You and Me in cooperation; You versus Me in intra-group competition), or among groups at large (We and Them; We versus Them). It follows that a 2x2 matrix can be used to inform multi-person research according to its *degree* and *type* of interactivity (Figure 15.5). Of note, certain research paradigms may be more or less suitable to certain measurement tools. For instance, hyper-scanning studies using fMRI are not as mobile as multi-person monitoring using heart rate monitors. Where possible, to allow for triangulation of information, multi-modal assessment of central and peripheral markers is advisable. For instance, in any given study or applied intervention, it is advisable to collect and triangulate data on different peripheral and central physiological markers, such as galvanic skin response, heart rate, and brain waves in different frequency (alpha, beta, theta) bands (Figure 15.5). Triangulation of information helps to bring about new insights as well as rule out alternative explanations for a given phenomenon or performance situation. To this matter, collecting subjective report data is also imperative to the study of abstract (latent variables) psychological concepts at the group-level of analysis, such as cohesion, team mental models, and collective efficacy (Tenenbaum & Filho, 2018).

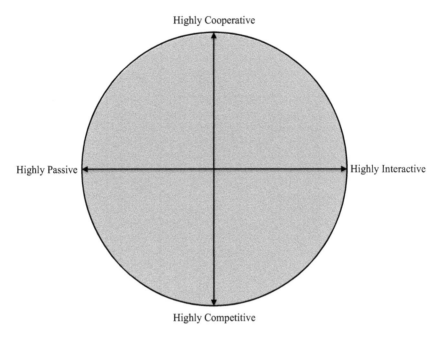

Figure 15.5 Matrix of degree (highly passive versus highly interactive) and type (highly cooperative versus highly competitive) of research paradigm.

Step 3: Multi-Modal Assessment of Psychophysiological Markers

As we have discussed throughout, social neuroscience is concerned with finding the neural mechanisms underpinning abstract social constructs (e.g., leadership, cohesion, team mental models) and explaining complex group behavior. To advance understanding of abstract team processes that populate our individual and collective minds, it is important to map peripheral and central psychophysiological responses. There are various markers of peripheral psychophysiological responses, with electrocardiogram (EKG), electrodermal activity, electromyography (EMG), and respiration response being among the most commonly used in the Sport, Exercise and Performance Psychology domain (Tenenbaum & Filho, 2018). Guidelines on how to collect data using these measures are beyond the scope of this chapter and have been detailed elsewhere (Blascovich et al., 2011; Stern et al., 2001). Again, when using these measurement tools in multi-person studies, it is critical to ensure the systems are synchronized and that individuals' variations are accounted for (see Step 1, Figure 15.1).

Joint attention and hyper-brain studies have been considered as measurement approaches of central markers of team processes across domains (Babiloni & Astolfi, 2014; Montague et al., 2002). If people involved in group work are gazing at the same location, it is inferred that they are paying attention to the same cues, and this information can be correlated to measures of performance to derive meaning. In hyper-scanning studies, scholars are primarily interested in functional hyper-connectivity measures, including estimates of coherence, partial directed coherence, phase locking value, circular correlation coefficient, and Kraskov's Mutual Information. In a nutshell, the idea behind studies targeting hyper-brains, joint attention, or synchronization of psychophysiological markers is to partial out the variance evolving from the social interaction from other sources of variability including the individuals', teams', tasks', and contextual characteristics (Filho et al., 2015a).

Individuals' characteristics, such as age, gender, personality, body composition, health status, hormonal status (e.g., women in menopause), and skill-level (e.g., experts versus novices) have been shown to influence team processes (Blascovich et al., 2011). The characteristics of the team (e.g., size, period of existence, and stage of development) are also related to variability in team processes (Carron et al., 2005). In addition, task characteristics, beyond the degree and type of interaction, are thought to influence the coupling of individuals' peripheral and central psychophysiological markers (Filho et al., 2015a). For instance, altering the difficulty of the task (e.g., slow vs fast paced interactions) has been shown to influence hyper-brains connectivity in interactive motor tasks (Filho et al., 2016). As well, contextual manipulations (e.g., priming effects, social evaluation threat) have been shown to influence psychophysiological responses in groups (see Blascovich et al., 2011). Overall, individuals are performing interdependent tasks within teams that are bounded to contexts. Therefore, *individual x team x task x context* iterative effects must be considered in advancing psychophysiological research and practice on working teams (Figure 15.6).

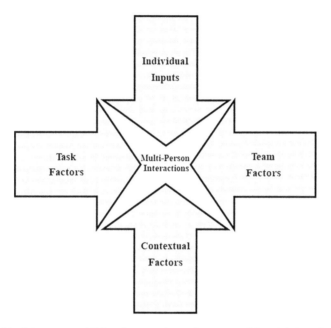

Figure 15.6   Individual (e.g., age, skill-level), team (e.g., size, tenure/historicity), task (e.g., complexity, degrees of freedom), and contextual factors (e.g., high x low-pressure environment) inter-act and should be taken into account in multi-person studies and interventions.

Applied Remarks

Evidence-based practice guidelines for practitioners interested in enhancing team functioning can be derived from recent research on the peripheral and central mechanisms that underpin successful social interactions in myriad tasks, including game and card playing, music playing, and coop-erative juggling. In particular, research has highlighted the role of coupled psychophysiological responses in leadership and supported the idea that team processes are intertwined in a reciprocal linkage (see Bandura, 1997) insofar that they are both cause and effect, and changes in one process influences another and vice-versa.

Leadership

Across domains of human interest, research on leadership has been mostly shaped by the leader-follower dichotomy (Filho & Rettig, 2016). In a nutshell, scholars are interested in examining what makes some individuals leaders and others followers, as well as the mechanisms that allow for successful leaders and followers' well-being, satisfaction, and optimal performance. Of note, hyper-brain studies on the leader-follower dichotomy have yielded some insights on the science of leadership in interactive tasks. For instance, a seminal hyper-scanning study on card playing revealed that leaders show a higher global cortical activation than followers (Babiloni et al., 2007). It might be that being a leader, in the sense of *initiating action*, requires greater cognitive resources than being a follower.

Previous research on guitar duets (Sänger, Müller, & Lindenberger, 2012; 2013) and spontaneous imitation of hand movements among dyadic groups (Dumas, Martinerie, Soussignan, & Nadel, 2012; Dumas, Nadel, Soussignan, Martinerie, & Garnero, 2010) has also revealed that asymmetries in between-brain interactions can differentiate leaders from followers in motor tasks. That is, the space-time patterns of brain activation (i.e., different parts of the brain of leaders and followers are activated at different times during social interaction) for leaders and followers engaged in motor tasks, such as guitar duet playing and imitative gestural interactions, tend to differ. In the same vein, recent research on cooperative dyadic juggling has suggested that spatial-temporal hyper-brain dynamics might indeed illuminate the leader-follower dichotomy (Filho et al., 2015a; Filho et al., 2016). Individuals with greater skills are more likely to lead by initiating and engaging in adaptive behaviors because they are not as cognitively invested in the interactive task, compared to their less-skilled teammates (Filho et al., 2016; see Figure 15.7). High-skilled individuals have more advanced mental representations and thus can operate in a more "automatic pilot" mode, akin to the *neural-efficiency hypothesis* (see Bertollo et al., 2016; Grabner, Neubauer, & Stern, 2006), compared to their less-skilled teammates.

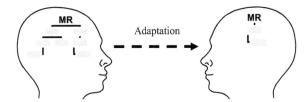

Figure 15.7   More skilled and experienced individuals (left panel) possess more developed Mental Representations (MR) and thus can lead and adapt to less skilled individuals (right panel) in interactive situations (based on Filho et al., 2016; 2017).

The Reciprocal Linkage among Cohesion, Team Mental Models, and Collective Efficacy

Empirical research has confirmed the assertion that team processes are connected in a systemic fashion (Filho et al., 2015b). Specifically, the Integrated Framework of Team Dynamics (IFTD) suggests that cohesion, team mental models, and collective efficacy differ from one another, yet co-vary and influence, through either direct or indirect means, team outcomes (Figure 15.8).

In terms of cohesion, which represents the strength of a group of individuals' social and tasks bonds (see Carron et al., 2005), research on hyper-brains in diachronic game-theory tasks has consistently shown that cooperating individuals (i.e., high attraction to the group task) show a higher interpersonal brain synchronization, in comparison to when defecting one another (Fallani et al., 2010). Physical touching in social interactions has also been shown to increase synchronization of peripheral responses, namely electrodermal and cardiovascular activity (Chatel-Goldman, Congedo, Jutten, & Schwartz, 2014). Moreover, neuroimaging research has revealed that love partners show a shared and complementary coding of emotion distributed in their brain networks that is unique to their relationship, and likely coupled with their non-verbal communication

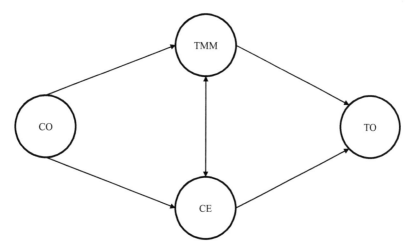

Figure 15.8 Integrated Framework of Team Dynamics (IFTD) in sports (Adapted from Filho, Tenenbaum, & Yang, 2015b). Cohesion (CO) is exogenous to Team Mental Models (TMM) and Collective Efficacy (CE), which in turn are correlated and influence Team Outcomes (TO).

exchanges (Anders, Heinzle, Weiskopf, Ethofer, & Haynes, 2011). As such, to increase cohesion, practitioners must work towards increasing psychophysiological synchronization among individuals. As well, practitioners can infer cohesiveness from the degrees of psychophysiological synchronization among a group of people.

Team Mental Models (TMM), which represents a team's shared and complementary mental representations, is thought to form the basis for team coordination (see Filho & Tenenbaum, 2012). Research in music has highlighted the synchronization of cardiovascular responses among members of a choir engaged in concurrent singing, thus suggesting that group coordination is partially dependent on shared psychophysiological synchronization (Müller & Lindenberger, 2011). Hyper-scanning research on dyadic guitar playing has also corroborated the notion that shared inter-brain links underpin team coordination (Lindenberger et al., 2009; Sänger et al., 2012). Specifically, periods of coordinated guitar playing were preceded by inter-brain synchronization in the delta and theta frequency ranges. Also noteworthy, Astolfi and colleagues (2012) collected simultaneous EEG recordings of dyadic teams of airplane pilots during a simulated flight mission and observed a network of shared functional connections between the brains of the two pilots during the take-off and landing, which are the crucial phases of a flight.

Furthermore, hyper-brain research with cooperative jugglers has revealed that shared and complementary peripheral (heart and breathing rate patterns) and inter-brains synchronization (i.e., alpha and theta inter-brain coherence) are related to team coordination (Filho et al., 2016; Filho, Pierini, Robazza, Tenenbaum, & Bertollo, 2017). Additionally, shared understanding hinges on simultaneous in-phase coordination of cerebral activity across communicators (Stolk et al., 2014). As such, practitioners must consider implementing multi-person bio-neurofeedback sessions. If teammates learn to co-regulate their shared and complementary psychophysiological responses, they are more likely to be "at the right place at the right time doing the right thing." Moreover, teaching groups of people communication skills may change how their brains link during verbal exchanges.

Collective efficacy is another important team process that represents teammates' trust in the team as a whole (see Feltz, Short, & Sullivan, 2008). It has been demonstrated that interpersonal synchronization influences the individual's abilities to trust somebody else (Krueger et al., 2007). Specifically, in a classic hyper-brain scanning study on the neural correlates of trust, Krueger and colleagues (2007) showed that different types of trust, namely conditional and unconditional, selectively activated different parts of the brain. Altogether, there is mounting evidence that different team processes are linked to different electrical and hemodynamic spatiotemporal dynamics within and between brains.

Concluding Remarks

In this chapter, we provided an interpretative analysis of how the idea of "mind" at the individual level of analysis and "collective minds" at the group level of analysis is central to the study of teams. We highlighted the main tenets of Theory of Mind insofar that "reading other minds" seems to be both an endowed ability and a developed skill that allows one to empathize with and simulate what goes on inside other people's heads. We advanced a stepwise methodological heuristic to inform research on this matter in Sport, Exercise, and Performance Psychology. From our vantage point, the reliable multi-modal monitoring of interactive tasks can advance understanding of the peripheral and central markers underpinning important team processes, including leadership and the reciprocal linkage among cohesion, team mental models, coordination, and collective efficacy. If we understand the reflective and formative psychophysiological markers of these constructs that populate the notion of "collective mind," multi-person evidence-based bio-neurofeedback protocols can be advanced in the near future.

Finally, we concede that research in this area is in its infancy, particularly inquiries using interactive research paradigms. Expanding research on current paradigms on card tasks/playing (Babiloni et al., 2007), rhythm and music (Sänger et al., 2013), aviation (Astolfi et al., 2012), and spontaneous hand gesture imitation in vivo and online (Dumas et al., 2011) are warranted. The level of interactivity of each one of these paradigms varies greatly (Figure 15.2), and thus should be considered accordingly by researchers and practitioners with different needs and interests. Within the Sport, Exercise, and Performance Psychology domain, *the juggling paradigm* is a promising method forward (for a review see Filho et al., 2015). Like research on self-paced sports which has advanced our understanding of the athletes' brain, dyadic juggling may advance research in hyper-brains in terms of both learning and performance, and with respect to individual-team-task-context factors. Residual issues in the hyper-scanning research across domains include studies using dynamic causal modelling to assess causality in hyper-brain networks, especially in studies tapping into the leader-follower dichotomy. Methodologically, it is important to advance studies beyond dyadic interactions, particularly in hyper-scanning. Manipulating individuals, teams, tasks, and contextual characteristics may shed light on the issue of residual synchronization in multi-person studies. Specifically, is the observed synchronization in psychophysiological responses between two or more people attributed to the people themselves, the team as a whole, the task at hand, or the context? This question must be further studied to advance the science of hyper-brains and collective minds, and its corollary of meta-cognitive concepts, including the notion of "mind reading" and the idea of *collective consciousness*.

References

Anders, S., Heinzle, J., Weiskopf, N., Ethofer, T., & Haynes, J. D. (2011). Flow of affective information between communicating brains. *Neuroimage, 54*, 439–446. doi: 10.1016/j.neuroimage.2010.07.004

Astolfi, L., Toppi J., Borghini G., Vecchiato G., He, E. J., Roy A., ... Babiloni, F. (2012). Cortical activity and functional hyperconnectivity by simultaneous EEG recordings from interacting couples of professional pilots. *Paper presented at the IEEE Engineering in Medicine and Biology Society Annual Conference* (pp. 4752–4755). doi: 10.1109/EMBC.2012.6347029.

Babiloni, F., & Astolfi, L. (2014). Social neuroscience and hyperscanning techniques: Past, present and future. *Neuroscience & Biobehavioral Reviews, 44*, 76–93. doi: 10.1016/j.neubiorev.2012.07.006

Babiloni, F., Cincotti, F., Mattia, D., Fallani, F. D. V., Tocci, A., Bianchi, L., … Astolfi, L. (2007, August). High resolution EEG hyperscanning during a card game. In *Engineering in Medicine and Biology Society, 2007. EMBS 2007. 29th Annual International Conference of the IEEE* (pp. 4957–4960). IEEE.

Bandura, A. (1997). *Self-efficacy: The exercise of control.* New York, NY: W. H. Freeman.

Bertollo, M., di Fronso, S., Filho, E., Conforto, S., Schmid, M., Bortoli, L., … Robazza, C. (2016). Proficient brain for optimal performance: The MAP model perspective. *PeerJ.* 1–26. doi: 10.7717/peerj.2082

Blascovich, J., Vanman, E., Mendes, W. B., & Dickerson, S. (2011). *Social psychophysiology for social and personality psychology.* Thousand Oaks, CA: Sage Publications.

Cacioppo, J. T., & Berntson, G. G. (1992). Social psychological contributions to the decade of the brain: Doctrine of multilevel analysis. *American Psychologist, 47,* 1019–1028.

Carron, A. V., Hausenblas, H. A., & Eys, M. A. (2005). *Group dynamics in sport* (3rd ed.). Morgantown, WV: Fitness Information Technology.

Chatel-Goldman, J., Congedo, M., Jutten, C., & Schwartz, J. L. (2014). Touch increases autonomic coupling between romantic partners. *Frontiers in Behavioral Neuroscience, 8.* doi: 10.3389/fnbeh.2014.00095

Chomsky, N. (1965). *Aspects of the theory of syntax.* Cambridge, MA: MIT Press.

Clark, I., & Dumas, G. (2015). Toward a neural basis for peer-interaction: What makes peer-learning tick? *Frontier in Psychology,* 1–12. doi: 10.3389/fpsyg.2015.00028

Coulter, J., & Sharrock, W. W. (2007). *Brain, mind, and human behavior in contemporary cognitive science: Critical assessments of the philosophy of psychology.* Lewiston, NY: Edwin Mellen Press.

Di Paolo, E., & De Jaegher, H. (2012). The interactive brain hypothesis. *Frontiers in Human Neuroscience, 6.* doi: 10.3389/fnhum.2012.00163

Dumas, G., Lachat, F., Martinerie, J., Nadel, J., & George, N. (2011). From social behaviour to brain synchronization: Review and perspectives in hyperscanning. *IRBM, 32,* 48–53. doi: 10.1016/j.irbm.2011.01.002

Dumas, G., Martinerie, J., Soussignan, R., & Nadel, J. (2012). Does the brain know who is at the origin of what in an imitative interaction? *Frontiers in Human Neuroscience, 6,* 1–11. doi: 10.3389/fnhum.2012.00128

Dumas, G., Nadel, J., Soussignan, R., Martinerie, J., & Garnero, L. (2010). Inter-brain synchronization during social interaction. *PLoS ONE, 5*(8). E121166. doi: 10.1371/journal.pone.0012166

Dunbar, R. I. (1998). The social brain hypothesis. *Brain, 9,* 178–190.

Durkheim, E. (2014). *The division of labor in society.* New York, NY: Free Press.

Fallani, F. D. V., Nicosia, V., Sinatra, R., Astolfi, L., Cincotti, F., Mattia, D., … Babiloni, F. (2010). Defecting or not defecting: How to "read" human behavior during cooperative games by EEG measurements. *PloS One, 5,* e14187. doi: 10.1371/journal.pone.0014187

Feltz, D. L., Short, S. E., & Sullivan, P. J. (2008). *Self-efficacy in sport.* Champaign, IL: Human Kinetics.

Filho, E., & Tenenbaum, G. (2012). Team mental models in sports: An overview. In R. Schinke (Ed.), *Athletic insight's writings in sport psychology.* Hauppauge, NY: Nova Science Publishers, Inc.

Filho, E., & Tenenbaum, G. (2015). Sports psychology. *Oxford bibliographies.* Oxford, UK: Oxford University Press.

Filho, E., Bertollo, M., Robazza, C., & Comani, S. (2015a). The juggling paradigm: A novel social neuroscience approach to identify neuropsychophysiological markers of team mental models. *Frontiers in Psychology,* 1–6. doi: 10.3389/fpsyg.2015.00799

Filho, E., Tenenbaum, G., & Yang, Y. (2015b). Cohesion, team mental models, and collective efficacy: Towards an integrated framework of team dynamics in sport. *Journal of Sports Sciences, 33,* 641–653. doi: 10.1080/02640414.2014.957714

Filho, E., & Rettig, J. (2016). Intergroup conflict management strategies from a Nobel Peace Laureate: The case of Jose Ramos-Horta. *Basic and Applied Social Psychology, 38,* 351–361. doi: 10.1080/01973533.2016.1221348

Filho, E., Bertollo, M., Tamburro, G., Schinaia, L., Chatel-Goldman, J., di Fronso, S., … Comani, S. (2016). Hyperbrain features of team mental models within a juggling paradigm: A proof of concept. *PeerJ,* 1–38. doi: 10.7717/peerj.2457

Filho, E., Pierini, D., Robazza, C., Tenenbaum, G., & Bertollo, M. (2017). Shared mental models and intra-team psychophysiological patterns: A test of the juggling paradigm. *Journal of Sports Sciences, 35,* 112–123. doi: 10.1080/02640414.2016.1158413

Goldman, A. I. (2012). Theory of mind. In E. Margolis, R. Samuels, & S. Stich. (Eds.). *Oxford handbook of philosophy and cognitive science.* Oxford, UK: Oxford University Press.

Grabner, R. H., Neubauer, A. C., & Stern, E. (2006). Superior performance and neural efficiency: The impact of intelligence and expertise. *Brain Research Bulletin, 69,* 422–439. doi: 10.1016/j.brainresbull.2006.02.009

Hawking, S. (1989). *A brief history of time: From big bang to black holes.* London, UK: Bantam Books.

Konvalinka, I., & Roepstorff, A. (2012). The two-brain approach: How can mutually interacting brains teach us something about social interaction? *Frontiers in Human Neuroscience, 6.* doi: 10.3389/fnhum.2012.00215

Krueger, F., McCabe, K., Moll, J., Kriegeskorte, N., Zahn, R., Strenziok, M., ... Grafman, J. (2007). Neural correlates of trust. *Proceedings of the National Academy of Sciences, 104*, 20084–20089. doi: 10.1073/pnas.0710103104

Leudar, I., Costall, A., & Francis, D. (2004). Theory of mind: A critical assessment. *Theory Psychology, 14*, 571–578. doi: 10.1177/0959354304046173

Lindenberger, U., Li, S. C., Gruber, W., & Müller, V. (2009). Brains swinging in concert: Cortical phase synchronization while playing guitar. *BMC Neuroscience, 10*, 1–12. doi: 10.1186/1471-2202-10-22

Montague, P. R., Berns, G. S., Cohen, J. D., McClure, S. M., Pagnoni, G., Dhamala, M., ... Fisher, R. E. (2002). Hyperscanning: Simultaneous fMRI during linked social interactions. *NeuroImage, 16*, 1159–1164. doi: 10.1006/nimg.2002.1150

Müller, V., & Lindenberger, U. (2011). Cardiac and respiratory patterns synchronize between persons during choir singing. *PloS ONE, 6*, e24893. doi: 10.1371/journal.pone.0024893

Popper, K. (2005). *The logic of scientific discovery.* New York, NY: Routledge.

Rizzolatti, G., & Craighero, L. (2004). The mirror-neuron system. *Annual Reviews of Neuroscience, 27*, 169–192. doi: 10.1146/annurev.neuro.27.070203.144230

Sänger, J., Müller, V., & Lindenberger, U. (2012). Intra- and interbrain synchronization and network properties when playing guitar in duets. *Frontiers in Human Neuroscience, 6*, 1–19. doi: 10.3389/fnhum.2012.00312

Sänger, J., Müller, V., & Lindenberger, U. (2013). Directionality in hyperbrain networks discriminates between leaders and followers in guitar duets. *Frontiers in Human Neuroscience, 7*, 1–14. doi: 10.3389/fnhum.2013.00234

Schilbach, L., Timmermans, B., Reddy, V., Costall, A., Bente, G., Schlicht, T., & Vogeley, K. (2013). A second-person neuroscience in interaction. *Behavioral and Brain Sciences, 36*, 441–462. doi: 10.1017/S0140525X12002452

Sevdalis, V., & Raab, M. (2014). Empathy in sports, exercise, and the performing arts. *Psychology of Sport and Exercise, 15*, 173–179. doi:10.1016/j.psychsport.2013.10.013

Silva, P., Garganta, J., Araújo, D., Davids, K., & Aguiar, P. (2013). Shared knowledge or shared affordances? Insights from an ecological dynamics approach to team coordination in sports. *Sports Medicine, 43*, 765–772. doi: 10.1007/s40279-013-0070-9

Stern, R. M., Ray, W. J., & Quigley, K. S. (2001). *Psychophysiological recording.* Oxford, UK: Oxford University Press.

Stolk, A., Noordzij, M. L., Verhagen, L., Volman, I., Schoffelen, J. M., Oostenveld, R., ... Toni, I. (2014). Cerebral coherence between communicators marks the emergence of meaning. *Proceedings of the National Academy of Sciences, 111*, 18183–18188. doi: 10.1073/pnas.1414886111

Tenenbaum, G., & Filho, E. (2015). Measurement considerations in performance psychology. In. M. Raab, B. Lobinger, S. Hoffmann, A. Pizzera, & S. Laborde (Eds.), *Performance psychology: Perception, action, cognition, and emotion* (pp. 31–44). Philadelphia, PA: Elsevier.

Tenenbaum, G., & Filho, E. (2018). Psychosocial measurement issues in sports and exercise settings. *Oxford research encyclopedia of psychology.* Oxford, UK: Oxford University Press.

Vogeley, K., Bussfeld, P., Newen, A., Herrmann, S., Happé, F., Falkai, P., ... Zilles, K. (2001). Mind reading: Neural mechanisms of theory of mind and self-perspective. *Neuroimage, 14*, 170–181. doi: 10.1006/nimg.2001.0789

Wilder, J. (1967). *Stimulus and response: The law of initial value.* Bristol, UK: Wright.

Wilkinson, M. R. & Ball, L. J. (2012). Why studies of autism spectrum disorders have failed to resolve the theory theory versus simulation theory debate. *Review of Philosophy and Psychology, 3*, 263–291. doi:10.1007/s13164-012-0097-0

Section III

Clinical Sport Neuroscience and Psychophysiology

16

Neuroanatomy and Cellular Mechanisms of Sports-Related Concussion and Traumatic Brain Injury

Kenneth Perrine, Suzanne Zuckerman, and Philip E. Stieg

Introduction

Concussion and mild traumatic brain injury (TBI) have become increasingly publicized over the last decade both in the scientific literature and the lay media. The incidence of concussions is estimated to be 1.4 million reported cases per year, with ~200,000 cases of physical activity or sports-related concussions per year [1, 2]. However, these figures are likely to be underestimates from under-reporting, and the CDC estimates that there are between 1.6 million and 3.8 million treated and untreated concussions related to sport each year. The suicides of several prominent NFL football players with dementia or depression received international publicity, and histopathological studies of the brains of a number of these players [3–5] led to a resurgence of research on a type of tauopathy termed "chronic traumatic encephalopathy" formerly known as dementia pugilistica from older literature on boxers [6]. In conjunction with reports of deaths of young athletes from "second impact syndrome" and blast-related injuries sustained by soldiers in the Middle East conflicts these studies led to a near-hysteria in the media culminating in television specials and widely read popular books [7]. However, the neuropathology and neuroanatomy of concussion have been lacking in these popular press outlets, yet our knowledge of the mechanisms of concussion, especially in relation to sports-related injuries, has made steady progress in the scientific literature. The current chapter will present summaries of the most recent research on the neuropathology and neuroanatomy of concussion, starting from the macroscopic levels of damage as seen in severe TBI to the cellular mechanisms that are affected in both concussion and TBI. The relationship of the neuroanatomical substrate of concussion to actual cognitive and behavioral functioning will also be presented.

Definitions

The definition of <u>concussion</u> has evolved considerably over the decades. A consensus statement from a panel of experts at the fifth international conference on concussion in sport held in Berlin [8] generated the following definition of a Sports Related Concussion (SRC):

> … a traumatic brain injury induced by biomechanical forces. Several common features that may be utilised in clinically defining the nature of a concussive head injury include:
> SRC may be caused either by a direct blow to the head, face, neck or elsewhere on the body with an impulsive force transmitted to the head.

1 SRC typically results in the rapid onset of short-lived impairment of neurological function that resolves spontaneously. However, in some cases, signs and symptoms evolve over a number of minutes to hours.

2 SRC may result in neuropathological changes, but the acute clinical signs and symptoms largely reflect a functional disturbance rather than a structural injury and, as such, no abnormality is seen on standard structural neuroimaging studies.

3 SRC results in a range of clinical signs and symptoms that may or may not involve loss of consciousness. Resolution of the clinical and cognitive features typically follows a sequential course. However, in some cases symptoms may be prolonged.

The clinical signs and symptoms cannot be explained by drug, alcohol, or medication use, other injuries (such as cervical injuries, peripheral vestibular dysfunction, etc.) or other co-morbidities (e.g., psychological factors or coexisting medical conditions).

The transient derangement of neurological functioning often results from a sudden deceleration phenomenon of the brain's movement within the cranium from an abrupt cessation of movement as in a motor vehicle accident or collisions between players in athletic competition. Similar impairment can occur from a direct blow to the head from a foreign object (assaults, some sports injuries) or from abrupt changes in ambient pressure as in the blast injuries sustained in military action. Regardless of the mechanism, most concussions share a constellation of symptoms. These include physical signs and symptoms, cognitive impairment, emotional changes and sleep disturbances. Physical signs and symptoms consist of any of the following: headache, "pressure in the head", nausea or vomiting, neck pain, balance problems, fatigue, double vision, dizziness or vertigo, feeling "slowed down", sensitivity to light (photophobia), sensitivity to sound (phonophobia) or looking dazed. Cognitive impairment consists of any of the following: mentally "foggy", poor concentration, poor memory, repeating questions, slowed responses or being confused about events. Emotional changes consist of any of the following: irritability, sadness, being more emotional than usual or feeling anxious. Sleep disturbances consist of any of the following: drowsiness, insomnia, sleeping more than usual or sleeping less than usual (Table 16.1).

Loss of consciousness (LOC) is not necessarily present in concussion, and if present is usually brief compared to a more serious injury. There also may be a period of retrograde amnesia in which events prior to the injury are not recalled, or post-traumatic amnesia in which new

Table 16.1 Typical symptoms of a concussion

Physical	Cognitive	Emotional	Sleep
Headache	Mentally "foggy"	Irritability	Drowsiness
"Pressure in head"	Poor concentration	Sadness	Insomnia
Nausea/vomiting	Confused about recent events	More emotional than usual	Sleeping more than usual
Neck pain	Poor memory	Nervous/Anxious	Sleeping less than usual
Balance problems	Repeats questions		
Dizziness/vertigo	Slowed responses		
Double vision			
Fatigue			
Feels "slowed down"			
Sensitivity to light			
Sensitivity to noise			
Looks dazed			

memories are not formed and the first recollection after the injury is well after resumption of any loss of consciousness. Patients frequently confuse loss of consciousness with post-traumatic amnesia; even though witnesses may report only a few seconds or a minute of LOC, the patient will unwittingly insist they were unconscious until they woke up in the emergency room (Figure 16.1).

Concussions represent the mildest degree of traumatic brain injury (TBI), which, for the purposes of this chapter, will exclude injuries resulting in positive neuroimaging. Some definitions of concussion suggest using "mild" to represent LOC of less than 1 hour or post-traumatic amnesia of less than 30 minutes [9]. The most recent version of the International Classification of Diseases [10] uses the term "concussion" when there is no LOC or LOC for less than 30 minutes, and "traumatic brain injury" when there is LOC with different codes assigned for the duration of LOC. Athletes, especially those in professional or collegiate level sports with high incidences of bodily contact, often report having a "ding", their "bell rung", or "seeing stars" for a brief period of time (seconds) after a head injury, but these phenomena are very transient and the athletes can "shake off" the feeling and return to play with absolutely no subsequent symptoms. It is unclear if these represent the mildest degree of concussion. In general, most concussions remit with no residual symptoms after 10 days, whereas TBI symptoms can persist for years or indefinitely [11] (Figure 16.2).

Some patients report persisting symptoms after the expected recovery phase that are labeled as <u>Post Concussion Syndrome</u> (PCS), which was originally used to describe the initial period of time following a concussion. Most symptoms of PCS include: headache, dizziness, and irritability commonly presented with psychological symptoms such as depression, anxiety, and stress [12, 13]. The combination of symptoms associated with PCS, are influenced not only by biology and psychology, but also by societal pressures, making this presentation bio–psycho–social.

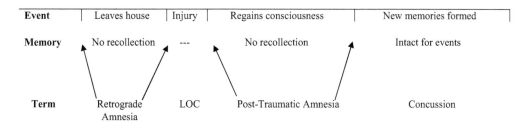

Figure 16.1   Timeline of Retrograde Amnesia, LOC, Post-Traumatic Amnesia.

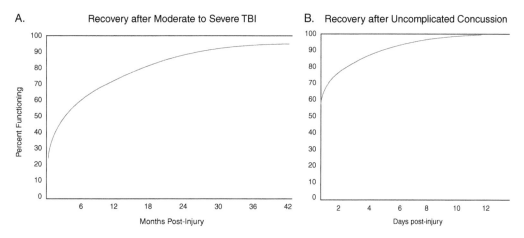

Figure 16.2   Recovery patterns after TBI and concussion.

Mechanisms of Damage in TBI

TBI can occur from several different but often overlapping mechanisms. There can be direct impact to the head from an external object such as another player's helmet, assaults, the head striking the ground in a fall, or penetration of the head with projectiles. These types of injury can result in skull fractures. However, impact to another part of the body can be transmitted to the head and brain, such as landing on the back or buttocks in a fall. Other than an object striking the head directly, there is frequently an acceleration/deceleration phenomenon in which the head is moving at a particular velocity and is abruptly stopped (e.g., in a motor vehicle accident) but the brain continues to move forward within the skull vault. The brain, which is not held rigidly in place within the cranium, can move forward/backward or other directions several times before coming to rest. This movement can result in "coup-contrecoup" injuries in which the brain impacts the skull anteriorly and then bounces back to strike the occiput posteriorly. However, the brain and head are rarely moving in a completely straight direction, and rather than exerting linear forces, the injury can induce rotational forces in which the brain rotates somewhat upon the brainstem or the brainstem itself rotating to some degree (Figure 16.3).

Patients who are in civil litigation with personal injury lawsuits, seeking compensation from worker's compensation or disability, or those with psychiatric problems such as somatization may report "concussions" from unlikely events such as banging their head on a shelf or cabinet upon standing, striking the headboard of their bed from sitting back too quickly, or having non-credible impacts from objects such as a few cereal boxes falling on their head. Unfortunately, these latter patients can make up the majority of cases presenting to emergency rooms or concussion clinics due in part to the publicity that has been produced in the media over the last decade. For example, the authors see patients in a concussion clinic or receive calls from a concussion hotline, and there was a dramatic increase in calls and visits after the film "Concussion" regarding chronic traumatic encephalopathy [14] was released in December, 2016.

The mechanisms responsible for classic concussion without positive neuroimaging will be discussed initially, and the neuroanatomy of complicated concussions in which there is some degree of parenchymal damage and of more moderate to severe TBI will also be briefly reviewed.

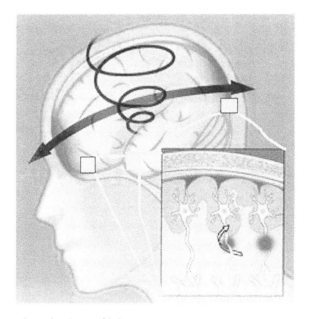

Figure 16.3 Forces and mechanisms of injury.

Mechanisms of Concussion in Sport

Out of 11 sports, the NCAA determined American football, men's ice hockey, and women's soccer to have the greatest number of reported sports related concussions [15]. Over four years, the NCAA analyzed 1,670 concussions reported across differing sports. Men's wrestling, men's ice hockey, and women's ice hockey emerged as the sports with the highest overall concussion rates [15]. Men's football, women's volleyball, women's gymnastics, men's and women's ice hockey, men's and women's basketball, and men's and women's lacrosse all had a greater number of concussions occur during practice rather than during a game. Sports such as cheerleading, cycling, roller and inline skating, ice-skating, kickboxing, and mixed martial arts can result in concussion or TBI, however, there is little research that has been done on these activities [16, 17].

The following mechanisms of injury, broken down by sport, can lead to concussion:

Boxing

An integral goal of competition is to attack the head and face of the opponent, which can result in concussion or TBI [18]. Punches thrown from the shoulder (i.e. roundhouse or hook) do not only accrue more force, but may also land on an angle and produce rotational force. A straight punch such as a forward jab will gather less force and will not generate rotation [6]. A common mechanism of injury is player contact with opponent followed by player contact with surface.

Wrestling

The most common mechanism of injury is player contact during takedown [15, 19].

Football

The most common mechanisms of injury include player contact while blocking and player contact while tackling [15]. Other mechanisms of injury include hitting helmet to helmet, head to shoulder, or head to ground. Blows can also be transmitted from the body to the head [8]. If hit in the helmet, the temporal areas are most commonly struck [20]. In high school football, running plays are a primary mechanism of injury [19].

Women's Gymnastics

The most common mechanism of injury is surface contact during the floor routine [15].

Women's Volleyball

The most common mechanisms of injury are player contact with the surface or player contact while digging or making a defensive play [15, 21]. Defensive specialists and outside hitters can be the most at risk for concussion on the collegiate level whereas middle blockers and setters can be the most at risk on the high school level.

Women's Field Hockey

The most common mechanisms of injury are player contact while handling the ball, player contact while running, and stick contact during general play [15]. The mechanisms of colliding with another player can result in blows to the side of the head while the player is looking at the ball or looking in a different direction at time of impact [22]. Midfielders and attacking forwards are positions with high risk of receiving a concussion, which may be due to them needing to run at high speeds and colliding with defenders that can be larger in size [22].

Ice Hockey

The most common mechanism of injury for men is player contact during checking while the most common mechanisms for women are player contact during general play and contact with the boards [15, 20]. In addition, female ice hockey players have more contact with the ice than male players and male players have a higher risk of taking an elbow to the head or shoulder. If hit in the helmet the temporal areas are most commonly struck.

Baseball/Softball

The most common mechanism of injury for softball is ball contact while fielding [15]. Regarding baseball, collision between players is most common in the minor leagues as a mechanism of concussion while contact with a batted ball is the most common mechanism in the major leagues. A large number of concussions occur at home plate, in the infield, and in the outfield [23]. Most of the incidents that result in concussion at home plate involve the catcher. The catcher has the highest risk of receiving a concussion because of his or her fielding position, the number of pitches they catch, and batting. They are the players exposed to the most situations for injury.

Basketball

The most common mechanism of injury for men is player contact while defending. The most common mechanism of injury for women is player contact during general play [15]. Contact with the ground or surrounding equipment can also be a mechanism of concussion. Being hit by another player's elbow is also of high risk for this sport, especially during rebounding or defensive play [24].

Soccer

A key aspect of the game is the use of the head for controlling and advancing the ball. The most common mechanism of injury for both men and women athletes is player contact while heading the ball. If hit in the head the temporal areas are most commonly struck [20]. Head injury can result from an elbow to the head, arm/hand to the head, or a head to the head [25]. In addition, involvement of the goalkeeper can increase the probability of head injury.

Lacrosse

The most common mechanism of injury for men is player contact during general play. The most common mechanisms of injury for women are player contact while defending and stick contact while defending [15]. Male lacrosse players can be most at risk for head injury in the moments of offensive play before collision during which the players may not have possession of the ball but will be attempting to pick up a loose ball or handling a ball [26]. Head injury can also result from compound mechanisms, such as contact with an opponent's stick followed by contact with a ball, another player, or the surface [27].

Rugby

The common mechanisms of injury are head-high tackle, head contact with the surface, head contact with the opponent's body, head contact with the opponent's lower limb, and head to head contact [28]. All positions are susceptible to concussion and have approximately between a 0.3% and an 11.4% chance of injury [29].

Neck Musculature

Anatomy, such as muscle mass, changes depending on gender and can affect the frequency and recovery time of TBI and concussions. This difference is now recognized in analyses of soccer ball heading with athletes. Having symmetrical strength in neck flexors and extensors can reduce head acceleration during heading and may reduce the risk of repetitive low-impact injuries [30]. Female athletes have decreased flexor and extensor strength, smaller head mass, shorter head-neck segment length, and decreased neck girth when compared with the musculature of male athletes. Musculoskeletal strength in the neck increases as neck girth and head-neck segment mass increases [31]. In soccer, women are approximately 2.4 times more likely to experience a concussion when they have the same time of exposure to the sport as men [32]. This higher rate of injury could be in part due to these differences in muscle strength and density. Without having strong neck musculature, there is more acceleration of the head during impacts in sport, which generates more velocity onto the brain inside the skull.

Developmental Attributes

Children and teenagers are in a vital period when the brain is continuing to strengthen connections between neurons, the body is going through puberty, and further developing bone and muscle. This period of development can also place a child at greater risk than adults for head injury resulting in concussion or moderate to severe TBI [33]. Children have larger heads as compared to their bodies than adults, the cranial bones are thinner, neck and shoulder muscles are underdeveloped, the subarachnoid space is larger, and the myelination of axons is incomplete. Thinner cranial bones may not be able to endure severe impacts. Underdeveloped neck and shoulder muscles cannot counteract against acceleration and lower the force at which the skull makes contact with another object or person. Having a larger subarachnoid space provides room for the brain to move within the skull and cause further injury to the brain tissue. Unprotected axons are more prone to shearing and tearing during head injury as opposed to when myelinated [18, 34].

Children, teenagers, and young adults have a higher risk of diffuse brain swelling secondary to TBI. "Second impact syndrome" refers to a second concussion sustained shortly after a previous concussion [35, 36]. This phenomenon was originally characterized as sudden death following a recent previous concussion due to rapid cerebral swelling [37]. Diffuse cerebral swelling is now considered a common complication of TBI that is most often seen in children and young adults and is not a direct result of a prior concussion [38]. After the release of the original research proposed by Cantu (1998), the 17 cases of athletes whose cause of death had been determined to be second impact syndrome were re-evaluated. The true cause of death for those individuals was subdural hematoma [39].

Head injury can result from increased exposure to a multitude of varying mechanisms varying drastically across sports. The characteristics of the hit itself such as whether the force was linear or rotational, if the player was in motion during the hit, or if the player was exposed to multiple contacts will determine the severity of the injury. Depending upon the severity, the player can develop a concussion with exclusively cellular disturbances or a traumatic brain injury with both cellular changes and positive neuroimaging findings.

Cellular Changes

Within the first minute post-impact, the environment and chemistry of neurons and glial cells change drastically [40]. Glutamate and other neurotransmitters are released into the extracellular fluid. The increased neurotransmitters with positive charges bind to receptors on the post-synaptic membrane (compared to the outside, the internal environment of the neuron is negative, running approximately between -60 and -70 mV, which is an attractive voltage to ions with positive charges in the external environment) leading to depolarization of the cellular membrane (increased positive voltage) on the post-synaptic neuron. Depolarization opens ionic channels resulting in derangements of the cell membrane potential, including an influx of calcium and sodium. The calcium levels can remain elevated for up to four days post-injury, while sodium normalizes within a few minutes. Calcium can enter a cell by means of ligand-gated and voltage-gated ion channels. Ligand-activated ion channels require a neurotransmitter to open or close while voltage-gated ion channels open when the cell membrane becomes positively charged. Normally, neurotransmitters are removed from the synapse quickly and efficiently by means of specialized enzymes or neighboring cells, however, these mechanisms have difficulty keeping up with the amount of positively charged ions flowing into the extracellular fluid and are simultaneously affected by the process of neuroinflammation. During the prolonged state of activation, neurofilament side-arms, an integral part of a neuron's cytoskeleton, can collapse due to phosphorylation by the influx of calcium ions.

While glutamate, sodium, and calcium are gathering in the synapses, potassium is pushed out of the intracellular space by the stretching and shearing of axonal processes. The sodium-potassium pump controlling ionic transport increases to normalize the ionic gradient, which requires more energy production with adenosine triphosphate (ATP). The mitochondria attempt to buffer increased calcium. Glucose uptake rises, followed by reduction of ATP levels. The release of glutamate produces over-activation of N-methyl-D-aspartate (NMDA) receptors and an influx of calcium into the mitochondria with further hyperglycolysis. Hyperglycolysis is followed by hypoglycolysis as the cell attempts to stabilize glucose metabolism from a state of competing glucose supply vs. demand. The increasing ATP production leads to more oxygen converting into water and the formation of superoxides. The resulting byproducts of oxygen ions, free radicals, and peroxides otherwise known as reactive oxygen species create oxidative stress, damage to proteins, DNA and lipids, and can potentially trigger generalized cell death (apoptosis) [41]. Caspases are cysteine proteases that, when activated, cleave enzymes and proteins involved in maintaining cell structure, signal transduction, transcription and DNA repair thus creating apoptosis [42]. Synaptophysin, a protein involved in the movement of synaptic vesicles in the synaptic cleft, increases depending of the severity of the injury disrupting synaptic vesicles for up to a month post-injury.

During this period of cellular insult, microglia and astrocytes are drawn to the area where there is a loss of afferents and efferents, which is known as acute neuroinflammation. If there is a disruption of the blood brain barrier upon injury, which is typically associated with moderate to severe TBI and not concussion, then leukocytes infiltrate the area in addition to glial cells [43]. The astrocytes mediate the movement of fluids between the intracellular and extracellular space, uptake glutamate, eliminate free radicals, buffer K+, and reduce excitotoxicity [44]. During acute neuroinflammation, astrocytes take part in building and maintaining the antioxidant defense of the brain. The antioxidants produced by these glial cells prevent damage to the reticular activating system. The microglia invade the damaged area and release microparticles that are small membrane-bound bodies that contain cytoplasm, cholesterol, phospholipids, and receptors [45]. Microglia microparticles induce neuroinflammation and activation of glial cells. The combined activation of astrocytes and microglia protect neurons from the influx of glutamate in the environment and promote healing. If the damage is severe and the activation of glial cells continues, neuroinflammation could then become chronic with glial cells becoming pushed beyond their limits and then promoting neurotoxicity rather than healing.

Extracellular Changes

The cellular changes outlined above generally occur within minutes to hours post-injury. However, the secondary effect on extracellular mechanisms can be longer lasting. Cerebral blood flow to the brain decreases, reaches a plateau between one to two minutes post-impact, and remains until symptoms begin to diminish after four to 10 days [46]. The cerebral metabolic rate of glucose consumption initially rises, peaking at about six minutes post-injury, and returns to baseline after approximately 20 minutes. Glucose metabolism begins dropping after 12 hours and remains below normal for up to 10 days post-impact. The hypometabolism in the thalamus, brainstem, and cerebellum correlates with the level of consciousness when PET imaging is obtained in human TBI patients, suggesting that concussions may have a shorter course of glucose hypometabolism than moderate and severe TBI [47].

Lactate follows the same pattern as glucose consumption with initial increases over 20 minutes followed by reduction in days post-injury. Changes in metabolism occur almost immediately after a concussion. Most of the research on these changes utilizes animal models permitting invasive studies of cellular and extracellular mechanisms that would not be possible in humans. However, there has been some research in concussed athletes utilizing Magnetic Resonance Spectroscopy (MRS) that shows decreased N-acetylaspartylglutamic acid (NAA) in the first few days post-injury [48]. NAA is one of the most prominent metabolites in human cerebral tissue that is detected on MRS, which is synthesized during conditions of high-energy or energy surplus. Such an environment is created when ATP and acetyl-CoA are in high concentration [49, 50].

Hormonal Changes

The pituitary gland produces and distributes a multitude of hormones into the blood stream such as growth hormone, thyroid-stimulating hormone, follicle-stimulating hormone, luteinizing hormone, alpha melanocyte-stimulating hormone, prolactin, adrenocorticotropic hormone, vasopressin, and oxytocin, which are all regulated through the hypothalamus. After a head injury, this communication can become disrupted and could result in long-term dysfunction of the pituitary gland. The length of dysfunction could be as broad as three months to 23 years post injury [18]. Changes in pituitary hormone levels correlate with cognitive dysfunction following TBI, however hormone disturbances are not permanent and can be treated with hormone replacement therapy [51]. There can also be damage to the thyroid that is proportional to the degree of injury and neurologic impairment, which can cause decreased levels of triiodothyronine and thyroxine and increased levels of thyrotropin [52].

Diffuse Axonal Injury

Damage to the white matter of the brain resulting from acceleration/deceleration (AD) forces in TBI was attributed to sheer strains by Holbourn [53, 54] who used a gelatin model to emulate human head trauma. Diffuse degeneration of white matter with development of retraction balls representing severed axons with extrusion of axoplasm, but without damage to the cortex, was later described by Strich [54–56]. Ommaya and Gennarelli [57–59] began examining the neuropathology of TBI based on the mechanical insult, which they termed as either static (slowly applied forces) or dynamic (rapid, with forces less than 200 ms). They found that a dynamic insult was far more common in most head injuries, with strong rapid forces resulting in cerebral contusions, primary brain lesions, and skull fractures as well as concussion. They hypothesized that cerebral concussion was a graded set of syndromes after head injury in which "the severity of disturbance in level and content of consciousness is caused by mechanically induced strains affecting the brain in a centripetal sequence of disruptive effects on function and structure" that begins superficially in mild cases and extends inwards in more severe levels to the deep diencephalic-mesencephalic structures. They also noted the presence of retrograde and post-traumatic amnesia corresponding to the severity of injury. Of note, the concussions produced by the rotation model had "g" forces from 348 to 1,025, all of which resulted in concomitant subdural and subarachnoid hemorrhages, while those that applied linear impact of comparable g forces did not produce concussion and more sporadic and focal hemorrhages. These animal models showed that rotation determined severity.

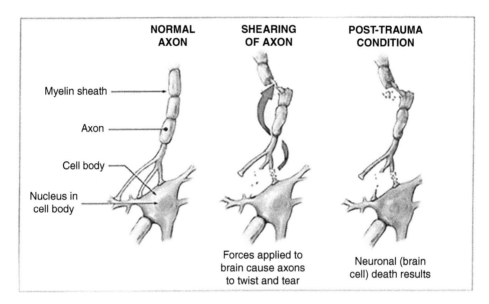

Figure 16.4 DAI.

However, the direction of impact also related to severity as well: sagittal (front-back) impacts resulted in the best recovery, lateral (side-side) injuries produced coma or severe disability, with oblique injuries falling in between (Figure 16.4).

The term "diffuse axonal injury" (DAI) was applied to this pathology by Adams et al. and Gennarelli et al. in the early 1980s [58]. Models using percussion and acceleration forces in animals produced significant strides in understanding the resultant effect on white matter. Gennarelli [58] confirmed that the angle of rotational forces exerted on the brain could account for coma in primates. He and his colleagues (1996) proposed four stages of damage approximating the degree of axonal stretch and strain, with effects of amount, location and severity of axonal damage. However, all of the primates who sustained Stage 1 (mildest) axonal injury had pathology primarily of brief ionic fluxes at the nodes of Ranvier. Stage 2 injury had cytoskeletal damage that was reversible over time. Gaetz later proposed that the depth of the lesion visible on MRI was associated with the duration of LOC resulting from deep grey matter and brainstem lesions [60, 61]. He also noted that cortical function drives the reticular activating system, which could account for some of the derangement of consciousness after TBI. He also stressed that traumatic brain injuries produce cellular and intercellular neurochemical, immunoreactive and inflammatory changes that may be the primary cause of neurophysiologic dysfunction from trauma.

Giza and Hovda [40, 62] have explored this "cascade" of biochemical changes in great detail, adding much to what we know of the process of damage induced by concussion. Especially with regards to the role of glutamate and the ensuing energy crisis, which are mitigated by the intervention of glial cells. The authors expanded upon the biochemical outcomes of cytoskeletal damage, axonal dysfunction, altered neurotransmission, inflammation, and even cell death (Figures 16.5 and 16.6).

Gaetz [54] concluded that the term DAI is a misnomer, given that the axonal damage is not *diffuse*. Instead, he suggested that the term Traumatic Axonal Injury (TAI) is a more accurate description of the white matter injuries resulting from TBI. However, despite the fact that very few head injuries and especially concussions do not produce diffuse axonal changes, the term DAI has persisted in the literature.

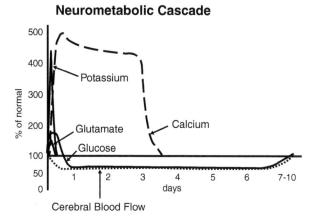

Figure 16.5 **Neurometabolic Cascade**. Reprinted from The New Neurometabilic Cascade of concussion, by Giza and Hovda. Retrieved from Neurosurgery Copyright 2014.

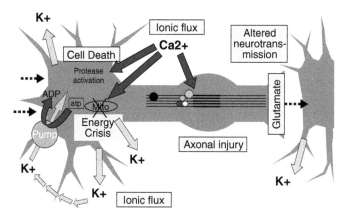

Figure 16.6 **Neurometabolic Cascade of mTBI**. Reprinted from The New Neurometabilic Cascade of concussion, by Giza and Hovda. Retrieved from Neurosurgery Copyright 2014.

Chronic Traumatic Encephalopathy

Chronic traumatic encephalopathy (CTE) was originally diagnosed as "dementia pugilistica" in boxers in the late 1920s who presented with motor symptoms such as unsteady gait and poor equilibrium that is similar to motor dysfunction in individuals who have damage to the pyramidal tracts, extrapyramidal system, or cerebellum [63]. These boxers, who were once called "punch drunk" by the popular media, began to deteriorate in motor, cognitive, and behavioral functioning later in life. This pattern of deterioration has recently been reported in some athletes from various other sports such as soccer and American football, especially in those with major depressive disorder.

The neuropathology of CTE was originally described in boxers as having neurofibrillary tangles, with a locus in the medial temporal lobe and brainstem tegmentum; neuronal loss in the substantia nigra; scarring of the cerebellar tonsils; and cavum septi pellucidi [64]. In 2005 and 2006, Omalu and colleagues released two case studies, including detailed autopsies of CTE in two professional American football players [3, 4]. The first report described an athlete who presented with diffuse amyloid plaques, neutrophil threads (NT), and NFTs in the neocortex. In contrast, the second report described an athlete who presented with NTs and NFTs, but no diffuse amyloid plaques. Player two had cavum septi pellucidi while player one did not. Neither had gross atrophy of the brain. Both players had long careers with the NFL and had few concussions on record. The pathology of CTE within sports and between sports is difficult to correlate. Some players were exposed to several concussions spread out over time and some to multiple repetitive concussions. In addition, these players are also susceptible to diseases like Parkinson's and Alzheimer's that are similar tauopathies. McKee [5, 65–67] extended Omalu's findings to a large cohort of retired NFL players whose brains were donated by their families due to dementia or severe depression. She defined CTE as a pathologically distinct tauopathy characterized by irregular formation of p-tau focused around blood vessels that can be visually and microscopically analyzed.

One of the hallmarks of CTE and other neurodegenerative diseases (e.g., Alzheimer's disease, Parkinson's disease, and frontotemporal dementias) is the dysfunction or misfolding of proteins. A prevalent dysfunction is the hyperphosphorylation of tau protein, which appears in CTE and various other diseases known as tauopathies. The tau protein has a major role in the formation and structural integrity of microtubules, which are important for the structure of axons and transport of materials between the cell body and the synapses [68]. The phosphorylation of tau can trigger the formation of neuronal filaments that accumulate within the neuron and can lead to cell death. Hyperphosphorylation of tau (p-tau) can cause it to group together in an insoluble form commonly referred to as neurofibrillary tangles (NFT). Tau protein can be expressed in the human brain in six different forms. The distinct pathology of tau and the relationship between its hyperphosphorylation and neurodegenerative disease is still currently unknown.

The biological pathology of CTE could be separated into four stages based on distribution and density of p-tau deposition. Stage I CTE was identified as exhibiting peripheral p-tau NFTs in the depths of the sulci and perivascular areas. The brains in stage I are typically of normal weight, meaning the brains have not begun to atrophy significantly, even though they start to show areas of neutrophil neurites and astrocytic tangles. In stage II, NFTs develop on the gyri in close proximity from the epicenters of p-tau in the depths of the sulci. Similar to stage I, brains in stage II CTE are also described as normal in weight. In stage III, the presentation includes overall cerebral atrophy, septal abnormalities, dilation of the ventricles, and deformation of the walls of the third ventricle. Stage III brains begin to atrophy and exhibit depigmentation in structures such as the locus coeruleus and the substantia nigra. In addition, there can be thinning of structures like the corpus callosum, which is a bundle of white matter fibers that connects the right and left hemispheres. Stage IV brains present with further atrophy in the medial temporal lobe, hypothalamus, thalamus, and mammillary bodies. These brains are markedly underweight. Stage IV CTE brains showed p-tau formations throughout the cortical and subcortical grey and white matter, accompanied with neuronal loss and gliosis (activation of the glial cells).

Until further research is completed, concussion, mild TBI and sub-concussive blows cannot be thought of as a progression or a predictor of CTE. There are several prospective research studies that are currently underway, including the LEGEND research study, or, Longitudinal Examination to Gather Evidence of Neurodegenerative Disease, which is prospectively examining living athletes and is open for enrollment [69]. Once the longitudinal prospective studies are completed, they will help identify CTE and help differentiate it from other dementias.

Sub-Concussive Brain Injury

Sub-concussive blows are defined as head impacts that do not result in clinically observable deficits or are subjectively symptomatic. However, there are recent findings that suggest repetitive low-impact head trauma can have an effect on brain functioning that is observable up to 24 hours post incident [70]. In 2000, 17,549 players in High School, Division I, II, and III College football reported just over 1,000 injuries within three football seasons [71]. The most common symptoms the football players reported were headache, dizziness, and confusion. Twenty-eight percent of injuries accompanied by a headache cleared in less than 24 hours. The mechanisms of sub-concussive blows are different from the mechanisms that can lead to concussion. Sub-concussive head injury does not result in retrograde amnesia (losing memory from before the injury), loss of consciousness immediately after impact, or post-traumatic amnesia (not encoding events for a period of time after the injury). Athletes typically describe sub-concussions as "getting their bell rung", "seeing stars" or "ringing in the ears". Also unlike concussions, these blows to the head are succinct and appear to resolve rapidly.

Balance and trunk control are abilities provided by the vestibular system, which consists of the peripheral vestibular apparatus, the ocular system, postural muscles, the brainstem, cerebellum, and the cortex [72]. The peripheral vestibular system is located in the inner ear and consists of the bony labyrinth and the membranous labyrinth. The bony labyrinth consists of the cochlea, the vestibule, and the semicircular canals which all work in tandem with the membranous labyrinth. The cochlea translates vibrations in the air into neural signals by the use of specialized hair cells that are interpreted as sound by the cortex. The vestibule contains the saccule and the utricle, which detect the orientation of the head in space and linear acceleration [73, 74]. The otolithic organs are composed of sensory hair cells, otoconia, and a layer of gelatin. These organs are positioned at a 90-degree angle with one horizontal and one vertical. The hair cells sit inside the gelatin layer, which is topped with the otoconia. The otoconia are like tiny rocks. When the head moves, these rocks are pushed naturally by gravity. When the otoconia move, they bend the gelatin layer and the hair cells sitting inside. If the hair cells bend in a certain direction, they depolarize and send signals down the vestibular nerve. A condition called benign paroxysmal positional vertigo can result from head trauma that displaces the otoconia in the utricle. This can cause brief spells of vertigo and is most common in traumatic brain injury [75].

The semicircular canals house the semicircular ducts, which detect rotation of the head [76]. Information obtained from the sensory stimuli captured in the peripheral vestibular system is sent to the vestibular ganglion, a bundle of bipolar cells that sense afferent impulses from the hair cells and send efferent impulses up the vestibulocochlear nerve. The vestibular ganglion produces the vestibular nerve, which combines with the cochlear nerve to create the vestibulocochlear nerve [77]. This nerve travels with the facial nerve that passes through the mastoid process, a bone protrusion behind the ear. The vestibular nerve continues to travel in tandem with the cochlear nerve through the petrous temporal bone to the posterior fossa and enters the brainstem at the mid-pons junction [72]. The vestibular nerve separates from the cochlear nerve and projects afferent fibers toward the vestibular nuclear complex in the pons. The vestibular nuclear complex consists of four main nuclei that process vestibular input. The inferior vestibular nucleus receives information from the utricle and saccule, also called the otolithic organs, that was transported by the vestibular nerve and sends those neural signals to the other three nuclei in addition to the cerebellum, which is the monitor of vestibular sensation and performance [77].

The vestibular system also integrates visual and proprioceptive information that helps the cortex maintain gaze and posture stability. Disruption of this system could explain some of the balance and other vestibular symptoms that patients describe with concussion. Problems with maintaining eye movements can cause dizziness with head movement, blurred vision, and nausea. Both the vestibular system and the oculomotor system work in tandem so that these problems do not occur. The oculomotor system is responsible for the generation of six different eye movements: saccades (rapid eye movements that bring new images onto the fovea), smooth pursuits (track slow-moving objects), vergence (directs both foveae on the same object), vestibulo–ocular reflex (keeps images steady on the fovea), optokinetic nystagmus (track large moving objects), and gaze holding (stabilizes images). These eye movements are generated by specialized nuclei of the premotor oculomotor brainstem. These oculomotor circuits are primarily separate both in physical location within the brainstem or pontine tegmentum and function. The pathways of all types of eye movement go through the medial longitudinal fasciculus (MLF) [73, 78]. White matter projections extend from the semicircular canal and the otolithic organs to the MLF. Afferents and efferents of the anterior portion of the semicircular canals make contact with the oculomotor complex and the oculomotor nucleus to control eye muscles on both eyes. The afferents and efferents of the posterior semicircular canal also innervate muscles on both eyes; however, the circuitry travels through the trochlear nucleus and the oculomotor complex. The otolithic organs have afferent projections in the vestibular nerve. The vestibulo-ocular reflex (VOR) originates from the semicircular canals to stabilize images on the fovea during rapid head movement [75]. Head trauma may disrupt the connection between the otolithic organs and the ocular muscles mediated by the VOR, which may lead to movement-related dizziness. The vestibular spinal reflex (VSR) transports information from the otolithic organs about spinal and leg musculature for balance strategies, which helps the body maintain an upright posture during movement [75]. The vestibulocollic reflex (VCR) controls the neck muscles and promotes the stabilization of the head during movement by integrating information from the otolithic organs.

Repetitive sub-concussive head injuries may lead to decreased density of white matter bundles as suggested by diffusion tensor imaging (DTI) studies [79, 80]. While some neuropsychological studies of sub-concussive blows have not shown a clear and prominent connection between number or severity of impact and cognitive impairment, others have discovered neurological sequele following brief repetitive sub-concussive head injury that can last up to 24 hours after the event [70, 81]. However, there still stands growing consideration for sub-concussive injuries and their short-term effects on behavior and cognition, which is beginning to incorporate long-term effects such as chronic traumatic encephalopathy. The inclusion of sub-concussive head injuries in the morbidity of CTE would explain why some individuals diagnosed with CTE did not have multiple recorded concussions [4]. Sub-concussive blows are subtler in appearance than concussion and may go unnoticed for longer periods of time while still contributing to the potential risk for the development of CTE later in life. Sub-concussive head impacts can occur from hits to any part of the head or body and can include rotational forces, which contribute to the shearing and tearing of axons. Damage to axons can then trigger the activation of glial cells and, just as with many biological processes, the more exposure to injury and the need for the body's injury response system can result in perturbations on a cellular level. However, the exact mechanisms and evidence for a role of either concussive or sub-concussive blows in CTE is still unknown and is not recognized as definitive by the International Conference on Concussion in Sport [8].

Pathological Damage in More Severe TBI

There are a number of macroscopic pathological processes than can occur after a moderate to severe TBI that are usually seen on routine neuroimaging such as CT scans or MRI. These can include contusions resulting from the brain striking the skull, or several different types of hemorrhage. Most of these processes result in more serious TBI and by many criteria are not regarded as concussions [82]. However, these pathological changes warrant review.

Epidural Hematoma

One of the most serious consequences of TBI is an epidural hematoma. This type of bleeding occurs from a rupture of an artery running along the dura (the outermost and relatively thick covering of the brain within the skull), most commonly the middle meningeal artery from a fracture of the temporal bone. Because the vessel is under arterial pressure, the blood pumps from the rupture at a rapid rate, causing a large amount of bleeding and a dramatic rise in intracranial pressure that can cause herniation of the brain or a skull fracture with venous bleeding into the epidural space. Those caused by venous oozing often exhibit a lucid period. However, most patients with epidural hematomas die in the field before they arrive at an Emergency Department where, if they survived, undergo emergency neurosurgery to evacuate the clots and control the bleeding.

Subdural Hematoma

Subdural hematomas occur as a result of bleeding veins or arteries between the dura and the second covering of the brain, the underlying arachnoid mater. The arachnoid is a thinner, filmy covering of the brain. Thin bridging veins drain from much of the convexity into the venous sinuses through the arachnoid mater. These veins can be stretched and are vulnerable to rupture after trauma. Subdural hematomas ooze blood under lower venous pressure or under the high pressure of arteries. Consequently, subdural hematomas can develop slowly over time (hours to even days), which is why one of the major precautions after a concussion is to be observant of any deterioration (worsening headaches, deteriorating mental status, etc.) with periodic checks of the patient in the initial hours after a head injury. Usually, a CT scan in the Emergency Department can detect subdural hematomas, although sometimes they can develop more slowly and not be detectable until after an ED visit. The treatment for SDH depends on the size and severity. Acute large SDH are often evacuated with an open craniotomy when the blood clots are more viscous, whereas subacute SDH can often be drained through a burr hole after having liquefied. Smaller SDH are gradually absorbed, and are simply monitored over time with serial CT scans. Because of the location of the veins typically involved in SDH, they usually occur along the convexity of the brain, within the interhemispheric fissure, or between the occipital lobe and cerebellum.

Other Hemorrhages

Several other types of arterial hemorrhages can occur after TBI. *Subarachnoid hemorrhages* arise from smaller arterioles bleeding between the arachnoid and the pia, the third and innermost of the meningeal layers of tissue surrounding the brain. Blood from these hemorrhages frequently disperse throughout a region of the subarachnoid space rather than remaining restricted to the site of the rupture, and can cause abnormalities not associated with a given location. *Intracerebral hemorrhages* bleed into the actual brain substance rather than remaining in the coverings of the brain, and can cause significant damage to brain function depending on the location of the hemorrhage and the surrounding brain substance. *Intraventricular hemorrhages* can occur with subarachnoid or intraparenchymal hemorrhages in which the bleeding enters the ventricles deep within the brain. Significant intraventricular hemorrhages can result in hydrocephalus caused by the pressure of blocked cerebrospinal fluid expanding the size of the ventricles and causing acute raised intracranial pressure.

Raised Intracranial Pressure and Herniations

Any of these hemorrhages or associated edema can produce some degree of movement of the brain from its usual location. *Midline shift* is a movement of one side of the brain towards the other across the midline. *Mass effect* is the pressure exerted on the brain, including the ventricles and sulci, from the increased brain pressure. *Herniations* are protrusions of brain parenchyma across or through structures into other brain regions; these include *falcine herniation* in which one mesial portion of the brain herniates beneath the falx to the other side, *uncal herniation* in which the anterior mesial and inferior bulge of the temporal lobe herniates through the tentorial incisura to exert pressure on the brainstem; and tonsillar herniation in which the cerebellar tonsils herniate through the foramen magnum to exert pressure on the brainstem.

Kenneth Perrine et al.

Macroscopic Damage from Contusions

In addition to damage induced by larger vessel hemorrhages, contusions can occur where the brain impacts the skull. These are bruises that arise from bleeding of capillary beds or venules, and are restricted to the area where the brain strikes the skull. These contusions are usually visible on CT scans.

Frontal and Occipital Poles

The frontal pole is the most anterior portion of the brain positioned immediately behind the anterior frontal bone. Because the brain is often moving forward at the time of an injury, this type of contusion is very common. Damage to the occipital pole is often a result of coup contrecoup forces.

Gyrus Rectus and Orbital Frontal Gyri

The orbital frontal region of the brain is the undermost surface of the brain posterior to the orbits. The basilar skull in this region is rather rough, and contusions can develop from the brain abrading against the skull. Also common are contusions of the gyrus rectus, the most mesial of the ventral frontal lobes almost to midline, where the olfactory bulb and tract receives olfactory cells from the nasal region and proceeds posteriorly. This area is situated on top of the cribriform plate, which has rather sharp ridges on the surface of the ethmoid bone, and the crista galli, which is a medial ridge projecting superiorly from the cribriform plate. However, the angle and thickness at which CT scans are performed frequently do not allow visualization of contusions from the cribriform plate or crista galli, which are far better visualized on MRI. These types of contusions frequently cause anosmia, short term memory problems and personality changes.

Mesial Frontal Region

The two hemispheres of the brain at and near the midline and anterior to the corpus callosum can sustain contusions from energy transmitted posteriorly or laterally to the falx, the part of the dura in the midline separating the two hemispheres. The anterior and mesial aspects of the frontal gyri and cingulate gyrus are in this region. Contusions in this area can cause personality and behavioral changes.

Temporal Pole

The temporal pole is the most anterior tip of the temporal lobe, situated immediately posterior to and abutting the sphenoid wing. Because of its far anterior location and proximity to bone, it is prone to developing contusions from the brain moving forward and abruptly stopping. Contusions in this area, if extreme, can cause problems with proper name retrieval and memory.

Encephalomalacia

Encephalomalacia is softening of the brain parenchyma. It occurs after the injury causes intracerebral hemorrhages or surface contusions. The brain has specialized cells called macrophages that "clean up" debris or unnatural substances in the brain substance. Once this process is completed, the part of the brain that sustained the damage and that was disposed of loses the glial support structures and softens, along with neuronal and axonal death. Encephalomalacia is a (late-occurring) consequence of parenchymal lesions that is evident on CT or MRI months after injury.

Neuroimaging

Neuroimaging is especially important if a more complicated concussion is suspected. More serious concussions that would indicate neuroimaging include neck pain or tenderness, double vision, weakness or tingling/burning in arms or legs, severe or increasing headaches, seizures or convulsions, loss of consciousness, deteriorating conscious state, vomiting, or increasingly restless, agitated or combative behavior (SCAT-5).

Skull X-Ray

Skull roentgenography visualizes calcium and is especially sensitive for imaging bone and, in particular, skull fractures. This imaging technique is also sometimes sensitive to midline shifts because as humans age there are some structures in the brain, such as the falx cerebri and the choroid plexus, which calcify. The falx cerebri is part of the dura mater that extends into the depths of the longitudinal fissure that separates both halves of the brain at midline and appears clearly on a skull X-ray, which are both characteristics used to identify midline shift. However, CT scans can show skull fractures quite well, so there is usually no reason to expose a patient to more radiation with skull X-rays.

Computed Tomography

Computerized tomography (CT) is a sensitive and reliable imaging program for assessing bone fractures, hemorrhage, contusions, and spinal trauma. It is the initial imaging technique of choice given its wide availability and rapid acquisition allowing for emergent intervention if necessary [9, 83]. CT is also used to assess herniation, hydrocephalus, edema, swelling, midline shift, and any other gross deformations of the brain or pathological changes between the brain and the skull [84]. CT can reveal hyperdensities indicative of contusions as well as adjacent vasogenic edema. An advantage of CT is the early detection of secondary effects of TBI such as herniations and cerebral edema. Mass effect or raised intracranial pressure evident on CT can cause subfalcine, transtentorial, or tonsillar herniation which can result in significant impairment and which are potentially reversible if detected early. This imaging technique, however, is not sensitive to subtle intra-parenchymal changes such as bleeding within the brain that can cause grey and white matter damage [85]. CT scans are typically the first line of medical care for patients admitted for head trauma because it is easily accessible, there are no contraindications for administration, and they can identify common gross symptomology of severe head injury. The main downside to the use of CT scans is the exposure to radiation, especially if multiple CT scans have been performed before in children.

Magnetic Resonance Imaging

Magnetic Resonance Imaging (MRI) is a primary imaging technique for the detection and characterization of more subtle effects of TBI, in which cerebral atrophy is commonly a consistent outcome [86–88]. Some studies maintain that the severity of chronic acute or subacute cerebral atrophy in combination with cognitive-behavioral sequele is predictive of prolonged cerebral atrophy after recovery from TBI [87, 89] MRI is more sensitive than CT to soft tissue injuries such as edema, hyperaemia from autoregulatory dysfunction, and cytotoxic edema. Brain swelling is especially problematic in pediatric head trauma [90]. MRI also allows a number of different sequences, each of which has advantages in identifying different types of pathology. Diffusion weighted imaging (DWI) is sensitive to both edema and stroke. Susceptibility weighted imaging (SWI) is an MRI technique that is particularly sensitive to the presence of blood products, beyond the capabilities of CT scans. Gradient echo (GRE) sequences is another type of MRI technique that is not as powerful or clear as an SWI, however, it is sensitive to iron deposition and the byproducts of blood, which can be positive indicators of hemorrhage [91]. Functional MRI can be used in later investigations to examine network connectivity, both in task paradigms and in the resting state, which reveals impact on default node networks [92–99].

Diffusion Tensor Imaging

Diffusion Tensor Imaging (DTI) is a new but primarily research-oriented MRI technique that can show disruptions of white matter tracts within the brain. These axonal processes connect neuronal regions to cortical areas (association tracts), or between cortex and subcortical structures (projection tracts), or between the two hemispheres (commissural bundles such as the corpus callosum and anterior/posterior commissures). DTI utilizes the unique characteristics of water molecules within axonal processes. At rest, water molecules in the brain show Brownian motion (random movements with no distinct pattern). However, given that water molecules are bound within a confined, unidirectional space within axons, the motion is more uniform and directed within a tensor that can be detected with special software and hardware in modern MRI models. Several measures can then be computed to depict the movement of the water molecules within the tracts. Fractional anisotropy (FA) assesses the uniformity of the direction of water molecule flow, ranging from 0 (random movement) to 1 (anisotropic movement in one direction). Mean diffusivity (MD) is a measure of the rate of diffusion or ellipsoid "size" of the water molecules in all directions within a voxel. Other measurements can be derived, including apparent diffusion coefficients (ADC maps), and directional axial diffusivity (AD) and radial diffusivity (RD). These quantified measures can be applied to a whole brain histogram, voxel-based analysis within specific tracts, region of interest (ROI) analyses examining brain regions identified a priori (e.g., corpus callosum, cingulum bundle), and tractography in which a "seed" is placed within a known fiber bundle and only axons comprising that bundle will be displayed and analyzed [100, 101].

DTI has been studied intensively as a biomarker for concussion and more severe TBI. Asken et al. [100] reviewed DTI findings from adult civilian, military, and sports-related concussion in a systematic critical review. Eighty-six eligible articles meeting inclusion criteria were included. They found significant contradictions between the eligible articles, with "widespread but inconsistent differences in white matter diffusion metrics" in analyses utilizing the typical measures employed in DTI studies. A number of confounding variables were identified, including control group variability, methods of statistical analyses, description or quantification of regions of interest, and the presence or absence of functional disturbances. They also noted that DTI studies of non-injury variables such as socioeconomic status and the presence of psychiatric disorders such as Attention Deficit Hyperactivity Disorder or Major Depressive Disorder significantly affected and confounded the findings in brain injured samples. Asken et al. and others [101, 102] conclude that DTI is not yet an accepted technique for identifying specificity in clinical samples of post-concussion syndrome.

Integrating the Concepts

Now that the neuroanatomical basis of concussion and TBI have been explained in detail, the key concepts can be used to gain an even deeper understanding when putting them in the context of an injured athlete. For example, let's use the following scenario of an athlete who becomes injured during a play in order to take a closer look at how concussions can present, and be evaluated and managed:

A 21-year-old male varsity lacrosse player, Mark, catches the eye of his opponent, who gains possession of the ball and is about to pass it. Mark tries to intercept the opponent making the pass and collides with him. Mark's head hits the opponent's shoulder and snaps back and to the side.

Mark's head hits the ground, his left temple smacking against the turf. Mark lays on the ground for several minutes with apparent brief loss of consciousness before being escorted off the field by an athletic trainer.

The athletic trainer can see that Mark is unsteady on his feet when walking to the sidelines and he appears to be in a daze. The athletic trainer pulls him out of the game and has him sit on the sidelines. The trainer should administer a Sport Concussion Assessment Tool fifth edition (SCAT-5) to assess the signs and symptoms of concussion. The SCAT-5 includes a list of observable signs of concussion, orientation/memory questions, the Glasgow Coma Scale, a concussion symptom checklist, a cervical spine assessment, history of risk factors, a neurological screening, and a balance examination [103, 104]. The King-Devick test is also frequently used to assess visual scanning [105]. Over the next hour, his eyes appear more focused and he seems to have come around. The athletic trainer asks Mark if he remembers being hit in the head on the field. He does not remember attempting an interception, being knocked down by an opponent's shoulder, hitting the ground, or walking off the field. This difficulty would be described as a combination of retrograde amnesia, a brief loss of consciousness, and post-traumatic amnesia. Mark continues to complain of dizziness and headache. His headache worsens and nausea and vomiting develops, which alarms the athletic trainer who suspects a possible subdural hematoma and calls an ambulance to transfer Mark to the hospital. In the emergency department, both a CT scan of the brain and the cervical spine are within normal limits. Mark is discharged from the hospital and goes home. He has difficulty sleeping later that night.

The next morning, he has continuing symptoms of dizziness and headache as well as sensitivity to light and sound, anxiety, feeling in a fog, difficulty with memory and concentration, mild balance problems, and tinnitus. Mark's primary care physician refers him to a neurologist where he has a neurological examination that is normal. Mark is given an MRI of the brain which is also normal. The neuroradiologist rightfully deferred performing DTI due to lack of enrollment in a research study given that DTI should currently be used only for research. The neurologist recommends a consultation with a neuropsychologist at a concussion clinic. Mark is administered a testing battery similar to the NFL/NHL assessment by a neuropsychologist. The results indicate mild attention and concentration problems along with mild balance problems on the Balance Error Scoring System (BESS) [106]. The neuropsychologist recommends a day or two of rest, but not complete isolation, with gradual return to work or school. The athletic trainer gives him a schedule of a gradual exercise regimen following CDC guidelines.

During a follow-up phone conversation with the neuropsychologist five days later, Mark happily reports that his symptoms slowly improved and now he is symptom free and back at school full-time, but worried about returning to sports. The neuropsychologist re-evaluates Mark and his results are within normal limits, indicating that he can resume vigorous exercise and non-contact practice. He is then referred to a sports-medicine doctor for final clearance to return to play.

This typical scenario highlights a number of neuroanatomical deficits in concussion. The normal CT and MRI scans are classic in showing the absence of this macroscopic damage to the brain. Mark's head was subjected to two different mechanical forces during his collision. The first is a rotational force, which causes the head to snap back at an angle and the brain to twist on top of the brainstem within the cranium. The rotational recoil was produced when Mark's head made contact with the player's shoulder while they were both moving at top speed. The head is abruptly stopped by the opponent's shoulder and rotates; however, the brain continues to move forward until it pushes up against the anterior skull. Following the rapid deceleration, the head is then accelerated backward in the opposite direction, which pushes the brain against the posterior skull, possibly causing a coup contrecoup injury. However, the lack of positive neuroimaging rules out this brain injury. The second force is a translational force, which does not produce as much damage within the brain as a rotational force. The translational force occurred when Mark's head hit the ground.

When Mark's head hit the ground, he landed on his left temple. A significant portion of the peripheral vestibular system structures lies within the temporal bone. The impact could stimulate and even over-stimulate these structures. Overstimulation of the cochlea, the organ responsible for interpreting sound, can cause tinnitus ("ringing in the ears"). In this situation, a large amount of force applied to the temporal region could cause a shifting of the otoconia within the otolithic organs. The metabolic cascade characteristic of concussions or microstructural changes could slow signal processing [107]. Slowed signal processing could affect the quality of the vestibulo-ocular reflex and the oculomotor system. Information from the peripheral vestibular system must be passed along to the eye muscles and organized by the cortex in order to stabilize images on the fovea. If visual images are unstable, dizziness and difficulty maintaining posture while moving could result. Proprioception uses optic flow (peripheral sensory stimuli that the cortex interprets as motion) in combination with limb position orientation to stabilize the body during simple standing and movement [108, 109]. Disruption of proprioception could cause imbalance.

Mark's symptoms of brief retrograde amnesia, loss of consciousness, post-traumatic amnesia, and cognitive symptoms are explanatory by the initial phase of the biochemical cascade with an acute spike in potassium and an influx of calcium into the cell bodies and axons. The signs and symptoms Mark experiences on post-injury day one are very consistent with hyperglycolysis and diminished cerebral blood flow (see Figure 16.4). The resolution of symptoms in less than a week are consistent with the return of calcium to normal and the return of cerebral blood flow and glucose to normal levels. If a post-mortem autopsy were performed, histopathology of the brain would not show any DAI, because his injury was a mild uncomplicated concussion.

Conclusion

Millions of head injuries sustained during participation in sports go unreported every year, with the majority of these injuries being sub-concussive blows, concussions, and mild TBI. *Sub-concussive blows* usually resolve completely within seconds and thus easily go unnoticed by other athletes, the athletic trainer and the coach. Many athletes refer to these as "dings" or "having their bell rung". *Concussion* results in a range of clinical signs and symptoms that may or may not involve loss of consciousness, which is usually brief. Common symptoms of concussion include physical signs and symptoms, cognitive impairment, emotional changes and sleep disturbances. Concussion and mild TBI can be caused by a variety of different mechanisms or a combination of mechanisms such as head to head, head to shoulder, head to elbow, head to ground and head to equipment, all of which can cause abrupt acceleration and sudden deceleration of the brain, or to an indirect hit to the body that transfers to the head (i.e. falling on the back from height that transmits forces to the head). *Moderate to severe TBI* often occurs from a direct impact to the head (i.e. a projectile, assaults, falls, etc.), more intense acceleration/deceleration forces (i.e. motor ve-hicle accidents), and stronger rotational forces. There are likely to be differences in these forces in various sports-related concussions.

An important factor of whether an injury will result in temporary deficits in neurological functions or LOC depends upon the type of force. Translational forces are much weaker than rotational forces. In cases of moderate to severe TBI, there are often strong rotational forces, lon-ger loss of consciousness, more prolonged *retrograde amnesia*, and longer *post-traumatic amnesia*. The former amnesia involves loss of memories from before the injury and can be reported for seconds, minutes, hours, or even days prior to injury. The latter amnesia involves loss of memory for a pe-riod of time following the injury, despite being awake and often alert. Many patients will confuse post-traumatic amnesia for being unconscious.

Gender and development can be protective factors in head injury. Physical differences be-tween men and women such as increased neck musculature and symmetrical strength in extensors and flexors can help stabilize the head in men. Children and teenagers do not have complete myelination until adulthood, which makes them more vulnerable to serious complications of concussion. *Cerebral edema* or *hemorrhages* can cause increased intracranial pressure, mass effect, midline shift, and herniation in more severe TBI. Concussion usually affects brain metabolism that does not result in macroscopic injury to the brain. If a concussion were to escalate to the point of some damage being visible on a CT or MRI scan, it is usually referred to as a *complicated* concussion. Head injury in both concussion and TBI results in cellular and extra-cellular changes in neurotransmitters and ionic balances resulting in metabolic abnormalities. Recovery from concussion generally takes seven to 10 days as the metabolic cascade resolves. More prolonged symptoms are much less common, and if extending to more than six weeks post-injury may be attributable to complex extraneous factors rather than neurophysiological damage.

The possible long-term consequences of repeated head injury resulting in CTE have been on the minds of parents, coaches, medical providers, news reporters and researchers. However, the support for a clinical correlate to this neuropathological process is being heavily debated in the scientific literature and has not yet been examined with prospective well-designed epidemiological studies. The number of athletes who develop CTE is only a fraction of the total number of athletes exposed to concussion or sub-concussive blows.

Concussions significantly affect biopsychosocial functioning. In sports-related injuries it is important for coaches, athletic trainers, nurses, and physicians to understand the underlying mechanisms of concussion to improve the awareness and management of brain related injuries. Armed with this knowledge, more informed decisions can be made for return to practice, return to play, return to school, and return to work.

References

1. [CDC], C.f.D.C.a.P. 2010.
2. Analytics, C., *EndNote X7*. 2017.
3. Omalu, B.I., et al., Chronic Traumatic Encephalopathy in a National Football League Player. *Neurosurgery*, 2005. **57**(1): pp. 128–134.
4. Omalu, B.I., et al., Chronic Traumatic Encephalopathy in a National Football League Player: Part II. *Neurosurgery*, 2006. **59**(5): pp. 1086–1092; discussion 1092–1093.
5. McKee, A.C., et al., Chronic Traumatic Encephalopathy in Athletes: Progressive Tauopathy Following Repetitive Head Injury. *Journal of Neuropathology and Experimental Neurology*, 2009. **68**(7): pp. 709–735.
6. Jordan, B.D., Neurologic Aspects of Boxing. *Archives of Neurology*, 1987. **44**(4): pp. 453–459.
7. Fainaru-Wada, M. and S. Fainaru, *League of Denial: The NFL, Concussions, and the Battle for Truth*. 2013, New York: Crown Archetype.
8. McCrory, P., et al., Consensus Statement on Concussion in Sport—The 5th International Conference on Concussion in Sport Held in Berlin, October 2016. *British Journal of Sports Medicine*, 2017. **51**(11): pp. 838–847.
9. McCrea, H.J., et al., Concussion in Sports. *Sports Health*, 2013. **5**(2): pp. 160–164.
10. World Health Organization, *ICD-10: International Statistical Classification of Diseases and Related Health Problems/World Health Organization*. 2004, Geneva: World Health Organization.
11. McCrory, P., et al., Consensus Statement on Concussion in Sport: The 3rd International Conference on Concussion in Sport Held in Zurich, November 2008. *Journal of Athletic Training*, 2009. **44**(4): pp. 434–448.
12. McCrea, M., et al., Official Position of the Military TBI Task Force on the Role of Neuropsychology and Rehabilitation Psychology in the Evaluation, Management, and Research of Military Veterans with Traumatic Brain Injury. *The Clinical Neuropsychologist*, 2008. **22**(1): pp. 10–26.
13. Ferguson, R.J., et al., Postconcussion Syndrome Following Sports-Related Head Injury: Expectation as Etiology. *Neuropsychology*, 1999. **13**(4): pp. 582–589.
14. Landesman, P., *Concussion*. 2015, Sony Pictures. 123 minutes.
15. Zuckerman, S.L., et al., Epidemiology of Sports-Related Concussion in NCAA Athletes from 2009–2010 to 2013–2014: Incidence, Recurrence, and Mechanisms. *The American Journal of Sports Medicine*, 2015. **43**(11): pp. 2654–2662.
16. Hutchison, M.G., et al., Head Trauma in Mixed Martial Arts. *The American Journal of Sports Medicine*, 2014. **42**(6): pp. 1352–1358.

17. Ling, H., J. Hardy, and H. Zetterberg, Neurological Consequences of Traumatic Brain Injuries in Sports. *Molecular and Cellular Neuroscience*, 2015. **66**(Part B): pp. 114–122.

18. National Research Council and Committee on Sports-Related Concussions in Youth, *Sports-Related Concussions in Youth: Improving the Science, Changing the Culture.* 2014, Washington, D.C.: National Academies Press.

19. Marar, M., et al., Epidemiology of Concussions Among United States High School Athletes in 20 Sports. *The American Journal of Sports Medicine*, 2012. **40**(4): pp. 747–755.

20. Delaney, J.S., A. Al-Kashmiri, and J.A. Correa, Mechanisms of Injury for Concussions in University Football, Ice Hockey, and Soccer. *Clinical Journal of Sport Medicine*, 2014. **24**(3): pp. 233–237.

21. Reeser, J.C., et al., A Comparison of Women's Collegiate and Girls' High School Volleyball Injury Data Collected Prospectively Over a 4-Year Period. *Sports Health*, 2015. **7**(6): pp. 504–510.

22. Rossiter, M. and M. Challis, Concussion in Field Hockey: A Retrospective Analysis into the Incidence Rates, Mechanisms, Symptoms and Recovery of Concussive Injuries Sustained by Elite Field Hockey Players. *BMJ Open Sport — Exercise Medicine*, 2017. **3**(1): p. e000260.

23. Green, G.A., et al., Mild Traumatic Brain Injury in Major and Minor League Baseball Players. *The American Journal of Sports Medicine*, 2015. **43**(5): pp. 1118–1126.

24. Zuckerman, S.L., et al., Mechanisms of Injury as a Diagnostic Predictor of Sport-Related Concussion Severity in Football, Basketball, and Soccer: Results from a Regional Concussion Registry. *Neurosurgery*, 2016. **63**(CN_suppl_1): pp. 102–112.

25. Andersen, T.E., et al., Mechanisms of Head Injuries in Elite Football. *British Journal of Sports Medicine*. 2004. **38**(6): pp. 690–696.

26. Lincoln, A.E., et al., Video Incident Analysis of Concussions in Boys' High School Lacrosse. *The American Journal of Sports Medicine*, 2013. **41**(4): pp. 756–761.

27. Barber Foss, K.D., et al., Epidemiology of Injuries in Men's Lacrosse: Injury Prevention Implications for Competition Level, Type of Play, and Player Position. *The Physician and Sports Medicine*, 2017. **45**(3): pp. 224–233.

28. Hinton-Bayre, A.D., G. Geffen, and P. Friis, Presentation and Mechanisms of Concussion in Professional Rugby League Football. *Journal of Science and Medicine in Sport*, 2004. **7**(3): pp. 400–404.

29. Kirkwood, G., et al., Concussion in Youth Rugby Union and Rugby League: A Systematic Review. *British Journal of Sports Medicine*, 2015. **49**(8): pp. 506–510.

30. Dezman, Z.D.W., E.H. Ledet, and H.A. Kerr, Neck Strength Imbalance Correlates with Increased Head Acceleration in Soccer Heading. *Sports Health*, 2013. **5**(4): pp. 320–326.

31. Bretzin, A.C., et al., Sex Differences in Anthropometrics and Heading Kinematics among Division I Soccer Athletes: A Pilot Study. *Sports Health*, 2017. **9**(2): pp. 168–173.

32. Fuller, C., A. Junge, and J. Dvorak, A Six Year Prospective Study of the Incidence and Causes of Head and Neck Injuries in International Football. *British Journal of Sports Medicine*, 2005. **39**(Suppl 1): pp. i3–i9.

33. Lovell, M.R. and V. Fazio, Concussion Management in the Child and Adolescent Athlete. *Current Sports Medicine Reports*, 2008. **7**(1): pp. 12–15.

34. Gómez, J.E. and A.C. Hergenroeder, New Guidelines for Management of Concussion in Sport: Special Concern for Youth. *Journal of Adolescent Health*, 2013. **53**(3): pp. 311–313.

35. Karlin, A.M., Concussion in the Pediatric and Adolescent Population: "Different Population, Different Concerns". *PM&R*, 2011. **3**(10, Supplement 2): pp. S369–S379.

36. Meehan, W.P., A.M. Taylor, and M. Proctor, The Pediatric Athlete: Younger Athletes with Sport-Related Concussion. *Clinics in Sports Medicine*, 2011. **30**(1): pp. 133–x.

37. Cantu, R.C., Second-Impact Syndrome. *Clinics in Sports Medicine*, 1998. **17**(1): pp. 37–44.

38. McCrory, P., Does Second Impact Syndrome Exist? *Clinical Journal of Sport Medicine: Official Journal of the Canadian Academy of Sport Medicine*, 2001. **11**(3): pp. 144–149.

39. Thomas, M., et al., Epidemiology of Sudden Death in Young, Competitive Athletes Due to Blunt Trauma. *Pediatrics*, 2011. **128**(1): pp. e1–e8.

40. Giza, C.C. and D.A. Hovda, The New Neurometabolic Cascade of Concussion. *Neurosurgery*, 2014. **75**(Suppl 4): pp. S24–S33.

41. Clapham, D.E., Calcium Signaling. *Cell*, 2007. **131**(6): pp. 1047–1058.

42. Knoblach, S.M., et al., Multiple Caspases are Activated after Traumatic Brain Injury: Evidence for Involvement in Functional Outcome. *Journal of Neurotrauma*, 2002. **19**(10): pp. 1155–1170.

43. Streit, W.J., R.E. Mrak, and W.S.T. Griffin, Microglia and Neuroinflammation: A Pathological Perspective. *Journal of Neuroinflammation*, 2004. **1**: p. 14.

44. Pekny, M. and M. Nilsson, Astrocyte Activation and Reactive Gliosis. *Glia*, 2005. **50**(4): pp. 427–434.

45. Kumar, A., et al., Microglial-Derived Microparticles Mediate Neuroinflammation after Traumatic Brain Injury. *Journal of Neuroinflammation*, 2017. **14**(1): p. 47.

46. Meier, T.B., et al., Recovery of Cerebral Blood Flow Following Sports-Related Concussion. *JAMA Neurology*, 2015. **72**(5): pp. 530–538.

47. Hattori, N., et al., Correlation of Regional Metabolic Rates of Glucose with Glasgow Coma Scale after Traumatic Brain Injury. *Journal of Nuclear Medicine*, 2003. **44**(11): pp. 1709–1716.

48. Henry, L.C., et al., Neurometabolic Changes in the Acute Phase after Sports Concussions Correlate with Symptom Severity. *Journal of Neurotrauma*, 2009. **27**(1): pp. 65–76.

49. Stefano Signoretti, et al., Biochemical and Neurochemical Sequelae Following Mild Traumatic Brain Injury: Summary of Experimental Data and Clinical Implications. *Neurosurgical Focus*, 2010. **29**(5): p. E1.

50. Vagnozzi, R., et al., Assessment of Metabolic Brain Damage and Recovery Following Mild Traumatic Brain Injury: A Multicentre, Proton Magnetic Resonance Spectroscopic Study in Concussed Patients. *Brain*, 2010. **133**(11): pp. 3232–3242.

51. Zetterberg, H., D.H. Smith, and K. Blennow, Biomarkers of Mild Traumatic Brain Injury in Cerebrospinal Fluid and Blood. *Nature Reviews. Neurology*, 2013. **9**(4): pp. 201–210.

52. Woolf, P.D., et al., Thyroid Test Abnormalities in Traumatic Brain Injury: Correlation with Neurologic Impairment and Sympathetic Nervous System Activation. *The American Journal of Medicine*, 1988. **84**(2): pp. 201–208.

53. Holbourn, A.H.S., Mechanics of Head Injuries. *The Lancet*, 1943. **242**(6267): pp. 438–441.

54. Gaetz, M., The Neurophysiology of Brain Injury. *Clinical Neurophysiology*, 2004. **115**(1): pp. 4–18.

55. Strich, S.J., Diffuse Degeneration of the Cerebral White Matter in Severe Dementia Following Head Injury. *Journal of Neurology, Neurosurgery, and Psychiatry*, 1956. **19**(3): pp. 163–185.

56. Strich, S., Shearing of Nerve Fibres as a Cause of Brain Damage Due to Head Injury: A Pathological Study of Twenty Cases. *The Lancet*, 1961. **278**(7200): pp. 443–448.

57. Ommaya, A.K. and T.A. Gennarelli, Cerebral Concussion and Traumatic Unconsciousness Correlation of Experimental and Clinical Observations on Blunt Head Injuries. *Brain*, 1974. **97**(4): pp. 633–654.

58. Gennarelli, T.A., et al., Diffuse Axonal Injury and Traumatic Coma in the Primate. *Annals of Neurology*, 1982. **12**(6): pp. 564–574.

59. Gennarelli, T.A., L.E. Thibault, and D.I. Graham, *Diffuse Axonal Injury: An Important Form of Traumatic Brain Damage. The Neuroscientist*, 1998. **4**(3): pp. 202–215.

60. Levin, H.S., et al., Serial MRI and Neurobehavioural Findings after Mild to Moderate Closed Head Injury. *Journal of Neurology, Neurosurgery and Psychiatry*, 1992. **55**(4): pp. 255–262.

61. Wilson, J.T., et al., Early and Late Magnetic Resonance Imaging and Neuropsychological Outcome after Head Injury. *Journal of Neurology, Neurosurgery and Psychiatry*, 1988. **51**(3): pp. 391–396.

62. Giza, C.C. and D.A. Hovda, The Neurometabolic Cascade of Concussion. *Journal of Athletic Training*, 2001. **36**(3): pp. 228–235.

63. Perrine, K., et al., The Current Status of Research on Chronic Traumatic Encephalopathy. *World Neurosurgery*, 2017. **102**(Supplement C): pp. 533–544.

64. Corsellis, J.A.N., C.J. Bruton, and D. Freeman-Browne, The Aftermath of Boxing. *Psychological Medicine*, 2009. **3**(3): pp. 270–303.

65. Armstrong, R.A., et al., A Quantitative Study of Tau Pathology in 11 Cases of Chronic Traumatic Encephalopathy. *Neuropathology and Applied Neurobiology*, 2017. **43**(2): pp. 154–166.

66. Cherry, J.D., et al., Microglial Neuroinflammation Contributes to Tau Accumulation in Chronic Traumatic Encephalopathy. *Acta Neuropathologica Communications*, 2016. **4**(1): pp. 112.

67. McKee, A.C., et al., The Neuropathology of Sport. *Acta Neuropathol*, 2014. **127**.

68. Wolfe, M.S., The Role of Tau in Neurodegenerative Diseases and Its Potential as a Therapeutic Target. *Scientifica*, 2012. **2012**: p. 796024.

69. Trials, C. *LEGEND*. Available from: https://clinicaltrials.gov/ct2/show/NCT02798185?cond=chronic+traumatic+encephalopathy&rank=3.

70. Hwang, S., et al., Vestibular Dysfunction after Subconcussive Head Impact. *Journal of Neurotrauma*, 2016. **34**(1): pp. 8–15.

71. Guskiewicz, K.M., et al., Epidemiology of Concussion in Collegiate and High School Football Players. *The American Journal of Sports Medicine*, 2000. **28**(5): pp. 643–650.

72. Khan, S. and R. Chang, Anatomy of the Vestibular System: A Review. *NeuroRehabilitation*, 2013. **32**(3): pp. 437–443.

73. Frohman, T.C., et al., Pearls & Oy-sters: The Medial Longitudinal Fasciculus in Ocular Motor Physiology. *Neurology*, 2008. **70**(17): pp. e57–e67.

74. Barrett, V.J.M., M.H. Tan, and J.S. Elston, Recurrent Third Nerve Palsy as the Presenting Feature of Neurofibromatosis 2. *Journal of Neuro-Ophthalmology*, 2012. **32**(4): pp. 329–331.

75. Wallace, B. and J. Lifshitz, Traumatic Brain Injury and Vestibulo-Ocular Function: Current Challenges and Future Prospects. *Eye and Brain*, 2016. **8**: pp. 153–164.

76. Lee, S., O. Abdel Razek, and B. Dorfman, *Vestibular System Anatomy.* Retrieved from: Emedicine. medscape.com/article/883956-overview aw2aab6c10. Accessed August, 2011. **30**: p. 2012.

77. Hain, T. and J. Helminski, *Anatomy and Physiology of the Normal Vestibular System in Vestibular Rehabilitation.* 2007, Philadelphia, PA: FA Davis Co.

78. Rüb, U., et al., Functional Neuroanatomy of the Human Premotor Oculomotor Brainstem Nuclei: Insights from Postmortem and Advanced in Vivo Imaging Studies. *Experimental Brain Research*, 2008. **187**(2): pp. 167–180.

79. Bahrami, N., et al., Subconcussive Head Impact Exposure and White Matter Tract Changes Over a Single Season of Youth Football. *Radiology*, 2016. **281**(3): pp. 919–926.

80. Mayinger, M.C., et al., White Matter Alterations in College Football Players: A Longitudinal Diffusion Tensor Imaging Study. *Brain Imaging and Behavior*, 2018. **12**(1): pp. 44–53.

81. Belanger, H.G., R.D. Vanderploeg, and T. McAllister, Subconcussive Blows to the Head: A Formative Review of Short-Term Clinical Outcomes. *The Journal of Head Trauma Rehabilitation*, 2016. **31**(3): pp. 159–166.

82. Gennarelli, T.A. and D.I. Graham, Neuropathology of the Head Injuries. *Seminars in Clinical Neuropsychiatry*, 1998. **3**(3): pp. 160–175.

83. Currie, S., et al., Imaging Assessment of Traumatic Brain Injury. *Postgraduate Medical Journal*, 2016. **92**(1083): pp. 41–50.

84. Rincon, S., R. Gupta, and T. Ptak, Chapter 22-Imaging of Head Trauma, in *Handbook of Clinical Neurology*, J.C. Masdeu and R.G. González, Editors. 2016, New York: Elsevier. pp. 447–477.

85. Mutch, C.A., J.F. Talbott, and A. Gean, Imaging Evaluation of Acute Traumatic Brain Injury. *Neurosurgery Clinics of North America*, 2016. **27**(4): pp. 409–439.

86. Strain, E.C., Drug Use and Sport—A Commentary on: Injury, Pain and Prescription Opioid Use among Former National Football League Football Players by Cottler et al. *Drug and Alcohol Dependence*, 2011. **116**(1): pp. 8–10.

87. Haugen, K.K., T. Nepusz, and A. Petróczi, The Multi-Player Performance-Enhancing Drug Game. *PLOS ONE*, 2013. **8**(5): p. e63306.

88. Gregory, A.J.M. and R.W. Fitch, Sports Medicine: Performance-Enhancing Drugs. *Pediatric Clinics of North America*, 2007. **54**(4): pp. 797–806.

89. Ilyuk, R.D., et al., Hostility and Anger in Patients Dependent on Different Psychoactive Drugs. *Activitas Nervosa Superior*, 2012. **54**(3/4): pp. 125–134.

90. Bennett Colomer, C., et al., Delayed Intracranial Hypertension and Cerebral Edema in Severe Pediatric Head Injury: Risk Factor Analysis. *Pediatric Neurosurgery*, 2012. **48**(4): pp. 205–209.

91. Bigler, E.D., Systems Biology, Neuroimaging, Neuropsychology, Neuroconnectivity and Traumatic Brain Injury. *Frontiers in Systems Neuroscience*, 2016. **10**(55): pp. 1–23.

92. van den Heuvel, M.P. and H.E. Hulshoff Pol, Exploring the Brain Network: A Review on Resting-State fMRI Functional Connectivity. *European Neuropsychopharmacology*, 2010. **20**(8): pp. 519–534.

93. Leech, R. and D.J. Sharp, The Role of the Posterior Cingulate Cortex in Cognition and Disease. *Brain*, 2014. **137**(1): pp. 12–32.

94. Sharp, D.J., et al., Default Mode Network Functional and Structural Connectivity after Traumatic Brain Injury. *Brain*, 2011. **134**(8): pp. 2233–2247.

95. Bonnelle, V., et al., Default Mode Network Connectivity Predicts Sustained Attention Deficits after Traumatic Brain Injury. *The Journal of Neuroscience*, 2011. **31**(38): pp. 13442–13451.

96. Bonnelle, V., et al., Salience Network Integrity Predicts Default Mode Network Function after Traumatic Brain Injury. *Proceedings of the National Academy of Sciences*, 2012. **109**(12): pp. 4690–4695.

97. Hillary, F.G., et al., Changes in Resting Connectivity During Recovery from Severe Traumatic Brain Injury. *International Journal of Psychophysiology*, 2011. **82**(1): pp. 115–123.

98. Cauda, F., et al., Disrupted Intrinsic Functional Connectivity in the Vegetative State. *Journal of Neurology, Neurosurgery and Psychiatry*, 2009. **80**(4): pp. 429–431.

99. Soddu, A., et al., Identifying the Default-Mode Component in Spatial IC Analyses of Patients with Disorders of Consciousness. *Human Brain Mapping*, 2012. **33**(4): pp. 778–796.

100. Asken, B.M., et al., Diffusion Tensor Imaging (DTI) Findings in Adult Civilian, Military, and Sport-Related Mild Traumatic Brain Injury (mTBI): A Systematic Critical Review. *Brain Imaging and Behavior*, 2017. **12**(2): pp. 585–612.

101. Niogi, S.N. and P. Mukherjee, Diffusion Tensor Imaging of Mild Traumatic Brain Injury. *The Journal of Head Trauma Rehabilitation*, 2010. **25**(4): pp. 241–255.

102. Assaf, Y. and O. Pasternak, Diffusion Tensor Imaging (DTI)-Based White Matter Mapping in Brain Research: A Review. *Journal of Molecular Neuroscience*, 2008. **34**(1): pp. 51–61.

103. Jennett, B. and M. Bond, Assessment of Outcome after Severe Brain Damage: A Practical Scale. *The Lancet*, 1975. **305**(7905): pp. 480–484.

104. Echemendia, R.J., et al., The Sport Concussion Assessment Tool 5th Edition (SCAT5). *British Journal of Sports Medicine*, 2017. **51**: pp. 843–850.
105. Galetta, K.M., et al., The King-Devick Test as a Determinant of Head Trauma and Concussion in Boxers and MMA Fighters. *Neurology*, 2011. **76**(17): pp. 1456–1462.
106. Iverson, G.L. and M.S. Koehle, Normative Data for the Balance Error Scoring System in Adults. *Rehabilitation Research and Practice*, 2013. **2013**: pp. 846418.
107. Fife, T.D. and D. Kalra, Persistent Vertigo and Dizziness after Mild Traumatic Brain Injury. *Annals of the New York Academy of Sciences*, 2015. **1343**(1): pp. 97–105.
108. Horiuchi, K., M. Ishihara, and K. Imanaka, The Essential Role of Optical Flow in the Peripheral Visual Field for Stable Quiet Standing: Evidence from the Use of a Head-Mounted Display. *PLOS ONE*, 2017. **12**(10): p. e0184552.
109. Dietz, V., Proprioception and Locomotor Disorders. *Nature Reviews Neuroscience*, 2002. **3**: p. 781.

The Neuropsychology of Concussion

Richard O. Temple

Introduction

Sport-related concussions have gained enormous attention over the past decade by scientists, medical professionals, and the athletic community at large (coaches, athletes, parents, school administrators, professional sports executives, etc.). Despite the increased visibility of this health epidemic, however, concussions, whether from sport or other injury mechanisms, are largely an "invisible injury," at least to all but the most sophisticated of neuroimaging techniques. Thus, concussions are largely defined by their functional impact, including clinical signs and symptoms, rather than any visually evident neuropathology. As such, clinical assessment methods with demonstrated sensitivity, specificity, reliability, and validity are needed to provide a clear picture of a concussion syndrome. Given the spectrum of physical, cognitive, and emotional symptoms characteristic of concussion, medical professionals with expertise in those areas of assessment and treatment are needed to provide that perspective. In this chapter, the role of the clinical neuropsychologist will be discussed in the accurate assessment and effective treatment of sport-related concussion. Although the focus of this chapter is clinical neuropsychology, it is acknowledged that a neuropsychologist alone cannot fully conceptualize or treat a given case. A multidisciplinary team is needed. Thus, the role of the neuropsychologist on such a team will be articulated.

Neuropsychology and the Clinical Neuropsychologist

Clinical neuropsychology can be defined as:

> a specialty in professional psychology that applies principles of assessment and intervention based upon the scientific study of human behavior as it relates to normal and abnormal functioning of the central nervous system. The specialty is dedicated to enhancing the understanding of brain–behavior relationships and the application of such knowledge to human problems.
>
> *(American Psychological Association)*

The National Academy Of Neuropsychology (NAN) defines a clinical neuropsychologist as:

> a professional within the field of psychology with special expertise in the applied science of brain–behavior relationships. Clinical neuropsychologists use this knowledge in the assessment, diagnosis, treatment, and/or rehabilitation of patients across the lifespan with neurological, medical, neurodevelopmental and psychiatric conditions, as well as other cognitive and learning disorders. The clinical neuropsychologist uses psychological, neurological, cognitive, behavioral, and physiological principles, techniques and tests to evaluate patients'

neurocognitive, behavioral, and emotional strengths and weaknesses and their relationship to normal and abnormal central nervous system functioning. The clinical neuropsychologist uses this information and information provided by other medical/healthcare providers to identify and diagnose neurobehavioral disorders, and plan and implement intervention strategies. The specialty of clinical neuropsychology is recognized by the American Psychological Association and the Canadian Psychological Association. Clinical neuropsychologists are independent practitioners (healthcare providers) of clinical neuropsychology and psychology.

(NAN Position Paper, 2001)

From these definitions, one can discern the role of the neuropsychologist in both assessment and intervention of neurologically based conditions. Specific expertise in brain-behavior relationships is emphasized. Further, the multi-disciplinary nature of neuropsychology is emphasized, which is necessary for the proper addressing of any complex neurological condition.

Neurocognitive Sequelae of Concussion

Concussions result from some external force acting on the head, resulting in linear and rotational forces (see Chapter 16). Thus, cognitive deficits seen following concussion are often diffuse and heterogeneous. Given the architecture of the brain and cranial vault, as well as a tendency for contact on the front of the head, the frontal lobes are very often involved. Common cognitive deficits following concussion are most often found in the areas of attention, processing speed, executive functioning, and memory. However, given the diffuse nature of a closed head injury, other deficits can result as well. Therefore, assessment of other cognitive domains (e.g., language, visuospatial skills, sensorimotor functioning) is critical to obtain a comprehensive clinical picture of the individual post-concussion. Karr, Areshenkoff, and Garcia-Barrera (2014) presented data from a meta-analytic review of cognitive consequences of concussion, showing "staggering variability" in effect sizes across studies. These results speak further to the heterogeneity of concussion sequelae, and the importance of individualized assessment of the individual with concussion to discern his/her unique pattern of functioning.

Numerous studies have been published on the time course of recovery from concussion, and predictors of prolonged recovery. McCrea et al. (2012) conducted a large study of concussion recovery (570 concussed athletes and 166 controls). They found that 10% of athletes experienced a protracted symptom recovery (i.e., greater than seven days) that was associated with longer recovery on neurocognitive testing. At 45–90 days post-injury, the prolonged group reported elevated symptoms, without accompanying deficits on neurocognitive or balance testing. Prichep et al. (2013) performed EEG tests on 65 male athletes with concussion, within 24 hours of their concussion, and at post-concussion days eight and 45. Players were classified as having a "mild" or "moderate" concussion by their symptom report. The moderate group demonstrated decreased cognitive performance only at the time of concussion. EEG data indicated that physiological recovery of brain function may extend well beyond the time course of clinical recovery and be related to clinical severity. Eisenberg, Andrea, Meehan, and Mannix (2013) followed consecutive emergency department patients between the ages of 11 and 22 presenting with concussion. Patients with a history of prior concussion experienced symptoms for a longer duration (24 days) than those with no prior concussion history (12 days). Median symptom duration was longer (28 days) for patients with a history of multiple concussions, as well as for those who had sustained a concussion in the past year (35 days). In a systematic review and meta-analysis of recovery time among high school and college athletes by Williams, Puetz, Giza, and Broglio (2015), high school athletes self-reported symptom recovery at 15 days compared to six days for college athletes. Neurocognitive recovery was similar between college and high school athletes, with a mean recovery time of five and seven days, respectively.

Other studies have attempted to identify demographic and symptom variables that predict the course of recovery from concussion. In the McCrea study cited above (McCrea et al., 2012), prolonged recover was associated with unconsciousness, posttraumatic amnesia, and more severe acute symptoms. In a comparison of 296 high school and college athletes, high school players generally demonstrated longer recovery time for cognitive performance compared to college players, suggesting a moderating effect of age on recovery (Covassin et al., 2012). In contrast, Meehan et al. (2013) found that symptom severity, and less reliably neurocognitive performance, were related to prolonged symptom duration, but sex, age, and loss of consciousness and amnesia at the time of injury were not related. Kontos et al. (2013) found that athletes with posttraumatic migraines were 7.3 times more likely to experience a protracted recovery than athletes without any headache, and 2.6 times more likely than a non-migraine headache group. Lau, Kontos, and Collins (2011) followed 107 male high school football players following concussion, and found that dizziness at the time of injury predicted protracted recovery, whereas other on-field signs and symptoms (e.g., confusion, loss of consciousness, amnesia, imbalance, visual problems, personality change, fatigue, sensitivity to light/noise, numbness, and vomiting) immediately following the concussion did not.

Thus, there is significant heterogeneity in the literature regarding both the expected time course of recovery from concussion, as well as demographic and other factors that predict the course of recovery. In general, it appears that younger athletes require more recovery time than older athletes, and symptom severity at the time of injury predicts longer recovery. Given the variability, an individualized approach in concussion management is warranted.

The Neuropsychological Evaluation

Neuropsychological evaluation always begins with a targeted clinical interview that provides the context for the psychometric testing that follows. Information about the presenting concern is obtained in detail. In the case of a concussion, factors that suggest the relative severity of the concussion are obtained, including whether or not the individual lost consciousness, and the duration of retrograde and posttraumatic amnesia. Retrograde amnesia refers to the inability to recall information that occurred from the point of the concussion backward, and post-traumatic amnesia refers to the inability to recall information from the concussion forward in time. Often, the athlete has (rightfully) presented to a physician or emergency department and other medical professionals prior to seeing a neuropsychologist, and it is important to obtain information about their course of treatment to that point (e.g., medications, therapies, and instructions regarding abstaining from activities). In addition to injury-specific information, it is critical to obtain a detailed premorbid history. It is vital to obtain information about prior concussions and other neurological events that might influence the course of recovery and the neuropsychological test results. Information about pre-existing learning disorders, Attention-Deficit/Hyperactivity Disorder (ADHD), and other conditions must be obtained to provide an estimated baseline (in the absence of an established pre-concussion baseline) from which to compare results that are obtained. Additionally, educational and occupational accomplishments (e.g., grades, standardized test scores, honors) also inform the estimation of premorbid abilities. Information about pre-existing psychiatric conditions is important to obtain, as depression and anxiety have been repeatedly demonstrated to influence an individual's appraisal of their own abilities at any point in time, and to influence the course of recovery (see section below on psychological contributors to symptom maintenance).

The selection of psychometrically sound neuropsychological tests is necessary in order to obtain accurate information about an individual's true level of functioning. A good neuropsychological test is reliable, valid, norm-referenced, and standardized. Reliability refers to a test yielding similar results upon repeated administrations, given similar circumstances. Factors such as practice effects (i.e., improved scores over repeated exposure to the test due to familiarity with the content) must be considered in choosing a test. The overall length of a test also affects reliability, with tests containing more items generally being more reliable than shorter tests. Validity refers to the property of a test measuring what it purports to measure. Using the example of a simple weight scale, a reliable scale would display the same weight every time, given that the same amount of weight in fact was placed upon it (though not necessarily the correct weight). A valid scale would accurately reflect the amount of weight that was placed upon it each time. Reliability is a necessary prerequisite for validity, but not vice versa. Thus, a test can be reliable without being valid, but a valid test by definition is also reliable.

One of the greatest threats to the validity of a neuropsychological test is the effort or motivation of the test-taker. For various reasons (e.g., litigation), the test-taker may be motivated to produce a score that is below their potential (i.e., feign or exaggerate deficits). In the case of an athlete, most often a hiatus from play due to a concussion would be a much-unwelcomed situation. As such, an athlete might be motivated to produce a very low baseline test score, so that they can meet or exceed that score when they are re-tested following a suspected concussion. For this reason, neuropsychological testing often includes validity checks, to ensure that the test-taker is responding in a forthright manner.

Norm-referencing refers to the administration of a test to a carefully selected control group to obtain expected performance levels in the absence of any neurological or other condition. Norm-referencing allows comparison of a patient's score to a standard, to determine the level of deficit that exists. The influence of demographic factors (e.g., age, sex, educational level) are measured, and, to the extent that such factors influence test scores, norms are stratified by levels of that variable. Standardization refers to the process of establishing strict guidelines for the administration of a test in order to ensure that the test is administered the same way every time. Standardization allows for the comparison of a patient's test score to the normative group. Many factors are involved in standardization, including the testing environment, instructions given prior to the test, and methods for measuring results. Factors such as a distracting environment, or variability in the manner in which the test is administered, can adversely affect the reliability and validity of the test.

Baseline and Post-Injury Computerized Cognitive Testing

Neuropsychological assessment can occur at various points in the pre- and post-injury process. In traditional neuropsychological assessment, normative information is utilized to determine one's level of performance compared to some expectation, due to the lack of information about their true premorbid level of functioning. In other words, most individuals do not present to a neuropsychologist with test results obtained before their injury or illness (i.e., a baseline). Given the relatively low probability of most neurologic insults, obtaining a baseline on every individual would be quite time-consuming and expensive. In the case of athletes, however, and particularly athletes in contact sports with a high probability of sustaining a concussion, obtaining a measure of their baseline performance is practical and valuable. Further, comparing one's own baseline to a post-concussion performance is superior to comparison to a normative sample, because the individual's baseline allows for an actual comparison to their premorbid abilities, rather than using an estimation. These individual baselines are particularly valuable in the case of an individual with premorbid conditions that adversely affect cognitive test performance, such as ADHD or a learning disorder.

For these reasons, athletes in sports with high incidences of concussion undergo baseline cognitive testing. Such testing most often involves the computerized administration of a relatively brief (typically 30 minutes or less) battery of tests measuring cognitive abilities known to be sensitive to the effects of concussion (e.g., attention, processing speed, memory). Given that the psychometric manifestations of a concussion are often subtle, it is critical to obtain as "clean" a baseline measure as possible. Given the demands of the athletic environment, such control can be challenging. For example, given the number of athletes that need to be tested at a particular school or sports organization, group testing is often conducted. This presents challenges in terms of providing a quiet, distraction-free testing environment. Variability in familiarity with computers can also introduce noise into the psychometric data. Given that most of the computerized programs are internet-based, it is possible to take the baseline test almost anywhere. Reputable companies (e.g., ImPACT Applications, Inc., a pioneer in baseline concussion testing), advise strongly against taking the test in an uncontrolled environment, such as in one's home. Also, the type of computer equipment used can influence test results. For example, ImPACT strongly recommends that an external pointing device (i.e., mouse) be used in responding to the test, rather than the touchpad that is often inherent to a laptop computer.

The interpretation of test results obtained from computerized concussion testing and the scope of use of that information are also important topics of discussion. Test companies have made both the test administration and interpretation of results quite user-friendly. In the case of the latter, reliable change thresholds are often highlighted to indicate a substantial change from baseline following a concussion. However, there is more to the interpretation of test scores than skimming the report for such highlighted scores. A neuropsychologist with advanced training in test theory, psychometrics, and brain-behavior relationships can analyze the output at a more sophisticated level to make informed decisions about return-to-play decisions.

The goal of computerized concussion testing for athletes is to determine when and if a player has returned to their pre-injury cognitive baseline and can return to sport participation. Test results are used in conjunction with other information (e.g., symptom endorsement, physical performance measures such as balance) to minimize the chance of an athlete sustaining another concussion before recovering from the first, with a potentially catastrophic outcome such as second impact syndrome (see Chapter 16). As is often stated by the test companies, the results are not designed to (and have not been validated to) *diagnose* a concussion, per se. Further, given the discussion above about reliability and test length, the results of computerized concussion testing should not be mistaken as equivalent to a comprehensive neuropsychological evaluation, which often involves four or more hours of psychometric testing.

The following is a vignette to illustrate the role of the neuropsychologist in interpreting computerized cognitive test data and participating in return-to-play decisions:

Joey is a 12-year-old football player who sustained a concussion in a game while making a tackle. He experienced alteration of mental status following the event, which was immediately identified by the coaching staff. Joey was immediately removed from the game, and he presented at a physician's office the next day when he was in fact diagnosed with a concussion. He experienced lingering concussion symptoms over the next few weeks, including headaches, dizziness, attention and memory problems, and irritability. Joey underwent baseline cognitive testing prior to the start of the season, and thus there was a basis of comparison for follow-up testing. He was administered three post-injury tests over the next month, which showed some improvement, but not to the point of returning to his baseline. This testing required waking up early to take the test at a concussion clinic that was overseeing his care. A few weeks later, Joey was given a fourth test, which showed significant decline in performance. At that point he was referred to a neuropsychologist. Upon his referral, it was verified that Joey had not sustained another injury, and there was no precipitous increase in his overall level of physical or cognitive activity that could account for the performance decline. Aware of the unlikelihood of a neurocognitive decline at this point in the recovery process, the neuropsychologist engaged in an extensive discussion with Joey, in which he shared his frustration over "being tested to death," having to wake up early to be tested, and not being allowed to return to play. He admitted that he became angry during the most recent test and did not try his best. With his assent, this information was shared with the treatment team in the spirit of advocacy for him. Another test was scheduled, in which he demonstrated return to his cognitive baseline, and he was gradually reintegrated into full participation.

Sideline Assessment of Concussion

The rapid and accurate identification of concussion in athletes during competition is critical for protecting them from second impact syndrome and potentially catastrophic outcomes. However, it is not practical to conduct a 30-minute computerized evaluation on every athlete who sustains a hard hit during the game. Thus, there is a need for tools that allow athletic trainers, psychologists, team physicians, and other professionals to quickly screen athletes during competition. To meet this need, brief paper-and-pencil assessments have been developed to screen athletes in just a few minutes. These instruments assess several domains sensitive to concussion, including concussion symptoms (e.g., dizziness, blurred vision), observable clinical signs (obvious disorientation, balance problems), as well as a formal, albeit brief, examination of orientation, memory, concentration, balance and coordination, and integrity of the neck. The neuropsychological measures on the instruments most often include questions about orientation to person, place, time, and situation; repetition of series of digits forward and backward; and learning and recall of a word list. In support of this type of cognitive testing, McCrea (2001) noted:

> standardized mental status testing can be a valuable tool to assist the sports medicine clinician in detecting the immediate effects of concussion on mental status, tracking resolution of immediate postconcussive mental status abnormalities, and making more informed decisions on return to play after injury.
>
> *(p. 274)*

One of the most commonly used instrument is the Sport Concussion Assessment Tool—Third Edition (SCAT3, 2013). The SCAT3 contains all of the aforementioned domains of assessment, highlighting the interdisciplinary approach that is necessary in concussion management.

Comprehensive Neuropsychological Evaluation Following Concussion

The clinical neuropsychologist is often called upon to answer questions beyond return-to-play readiness. Particularly in cases where symptoms persist beyond a few weeks, school, work, and general daily functioning are compromised. In such cases, a comprehensive neuropsychological evaluation is warranted to determine what objective areas of deficit are present, the overall emotional functioning of the individual, and what interventions are in place, either suggested by medical professionals or implemented independently by the patient, to cope with symptoms and facilitate recovery. Such an evaluation often lasts four or more hours, assessing the domains of global intellectual functioning, academic abilities, attention, executive functioning, language, sensorimotor processing and functioning, visuospatial skills, memory, and emotional functioning.

Once neuropsychological deficits (and areas of preserved functioning) are identified, recommendations can be made about potential intervention, as well as necessary accommodations in the classroom or workplace. Such interventions and accommodations can include cognitive rehabilitation therapy, the provision of extra time to complete assignments and job tasks, frequent and brief rest breaks, and a shortened work or school day. When informed by objective neurocognitive data, such recommendations can lay the foundations for effective intervention that increases the likelihood and speed of returning to one's premorbid level of functioning.

Psychological Factors Maintaining Post-Concussion Symptoms

There is longstanding scientific evidence that the subjective experience of cognitive deficits can occur following a concussion, even in the absence of objectively identifiable deficits on neuropsychological testing. This is not to suggest that all instances of prolonged post-concussion syndrome are without a neurological basis. Rather, a subset of cases can involve symptoms that appear to be maintained by factors other than those directly related to the neurological injury. Several studies have provided evidence suggesting no reliable association between mild traumatic brain injury and the development of post-concussion symptoms (e.g., Hanlon, Demery, Martinovich, & Kelly, 1999; Meares et al., 2011). In the work by Meares et al., premorbid anxiety and depressive disorders, as well as acute post-traumatic stress, were early markers for development of a post-concussion syndrome. Iverson and Lange (2011) conclude that:

> without question, a post-concussion syndrome can be worsened by psychological distress, social psychological factors (e.g., the nocebo effect, iatrogenesis, and misattributions), personality characteristics, and co-occurring conditions (e.g., chronic pain and insomnia).
>
> (p. 745)

Several studies (Ferguson, Mittenberg, Barone, & Schneider, 1999; Mittenberg, DiGiulio, Perrin, & Bass, 1992) have suggested that prolonged post-concussion syndrome results from an underestimation of pre-injury incidence of symptoms, and a re-attribution of these symptoms to the brain injury. Mittenberg and Strauman (2000) offer a framework that is useful for conceptualizing post-concussion syndrome. Their "expectation as etiology" theory is comprised of three components: (1) typical symptom expectancies are activated when mild traumatic brain injury occurs, and symptom expectancies bias selective attention to internal states; (2) normally occurring premorbid symptoms are attributed to mild traumatic brain injury, and selective attention to the inherent stress of the trauma subjectively magnifies these symptoms; and (3) symptom expectations are confirmed, and anxiety about the significance of symptoms maintains selective attention. This theory has implications for treatment of post-concussion syndrome (see the section on treatment in this chapter).

The Role of the Neuropsychologist on the Multi-Disciplinary Treatment Team

As was eluded to above in the introduction to this chapter, the neuropsychologist cannot fulfill all roles in the comprehensive management of concussion. A coordinated team is required to manage the medical, psychological, and practical aspects of recovering from a concussion. First a foremost, a coordinated team should include a physician with knowledge and expertise in concussion management. The physician is critical in assuring that the patient is stable and that the head injury is not life threatening. S/he also plays an important role in the ongoing medical management of recovery, including medications as appropriate. The neuropsychologist assists the physician in providing objective assessment of neurocognitive and psychological factors that are present, allowing for targeted treatment.

Various other health care professionals play a crucial role in concussion management, including providers with expertise in vision, vestibular functioning, and balance. Deficits in any of those areas can produce, or mimic, cognitive dysfunction. Coordinated assessment between the neuropsychologist and those professionals will allow for determination of the most efficacious mode(s) of treatment. Athletic trainers are often the "eyes and ears" of office-based medical professionals, able to provide timely information about an athlete's current level of functioning.

The clinical neuropsychologist also works closely with non-medical individuals involved in the athlete's daily life, such as teachers, coaches, and employers. Here, the neuropsychologist plays a critical role in informing those professionals of the concussion patient's current limitations, recommending accommodations as necessary, and helps to guide the athlete back to his/her premorbid activity level without placing them in further danger of re-injury, or risking academic or vocational errors that would be detrimental to their future.

Neuropsychological Intervention Following Concussion

Far from being an agent that merely provides assessment and diagnosis and refers the athlete on for treatment, the neuropsychologist serves a crucial role in the treatment and rehabilitation of concussions. By virtue of knowledge of brain-behavior relationships, the clinical neuropsychologist is well-suited to provide informed, effective rehabilitation interventions.

Neuroplasticity

Over the past few decades, much knowledge has been gained about the seemingly infinite ability of the brain to change over the lifespan, even in the context of neurological injury or illness. Through the principles of neuroplasticity, an injured brain can establish new connections, essentially re-wiring, and recovering function lost to an injury. Advances in neuroimaging have allowed access to the black box that is the brain, providing insight into the possibility for changes in connectivity. Neuroplasticity refers to the ability of the human brain to change in response to experience. Discovery of this phenomenon, in conjunction with the large and growing literature on its application to the treatment of neurological injuries such as concussion, has provided new hope for recovery of function not only in relatively uncomplicated concussion, but in more severe traumatic brain injuries as well. Such principles have also informed treatment interventions, providing a theoretical framework for concussion treatment.

Rest and Modulation of Activity Level

One of the cornerstones of concussion treatment has been the modulation of physical and cognitive activity post-injury. It has long been assumed that a period of rest is required following a concussion to facilitate cellular and metabolic recovery. Practitioners will often recommend taking time off from school or work immediately following a concussion, and minimizing or eliminating exposure to electronic devices. Consistent with this line of thinking, Brown et al. (2014) found that self-reported cognitive activity was positively associated with longer recovery from concussion. However, some studies suggest otherwise. For example, Grool et al. (2016) found that an early return to physical activity resulted in a lower risk of persistent post-concussion symptoms in children aged five to 18. Similarly, DiFazio et al. (2016) reviews research about the potential physical and psychological harm of prolonged activity restriction, citing the detrimental effects of removal from validating life activities and physical conditioning. The authors advocate for a model that promotes prompt reengagement in life activities as tolerated. Leddy, Baker, and Willer (2016) reviewed the recent literature on concussion recovery. They concluded that, contrary to conventional thinking that a patient with a concussion should rest until all symptoms have resolved, a more active treatment approach is warranted, including subthreshold aerobic exercise and cervical, vestibular, cognitive-behavioral, and vision therapies. They advocate for a thorough physical examination in the patient that articulates the nature of the post-concussion syndrome in that particular patient.

Anecdotally, this author has observed the harmful effects of total disengagement from life activities following a concussion:

> A young adult athlete sustained a minor concussion in a motor vehicle crash. There was no loss of consciousness, retrograde amnesia, or posttraumatic amnesia. In a effort to recover, the athlete, of his own volition, confined himself in his dark bedroom with no exposure to electronics for the better part of seven days. He emerged with a prolonged postconcussion syndrome that appeared to be maintained by psychological factors. Even the slightest contact to his head, such as lightly bumping it against a door, would produce significant symptoms and the perception that he had sustained another concussion

It has been the experience of this author that, aside from actual neurological injury, one of the most disruptive consequences of a sport-related concussion is the loss of one's routine and exposure to productive, goal-directed activity that comes with restriction from participation. Prior to a concussion, an athlete may be training for four or more hours per day, including travel time. If school or work are also part of their daily routine, they often move from one activity or role to another, with very little free time. One must be very organized to meet vocational and sport demands, arrive at commitments on time, obtain the necessary nutrition and sleep, etc. The time once spent engaged in athletic activity is often replaced by television or other electronic media, boredom, and possibly other bad habits (e.g., alcohol or other substance use). Effective treatment in those cases involves working with the athlete to establish a routine of productive activity that can be tolerated, but nonetheless provides challenge, structure, and a sense of accomplishment.

Cognitive Rehabilitation

Given that neuroplastic changes in the brain are possible even in the context of neurological injury, it can be inferred that rehabilitation of cognitive deficits following brain injury is possible. Cognitive rehabilitation interventions have long been employed with brain injuries of all severities to effect positive changes and restoration of function. In perhaps the most comprehensive and well-cited meta-analytic study on the topic, Cicerone and colleagues (2011) reviewed a total of 370 interventions in 65 class I or Ia studies and concluded that "there is substantial evidence to support interventions for attention, memory, social communication skills, executive function, and for comprehensive-holistic neuropsychological rehabilitation after TBI (pg. 519). Several of the findings were with sufficient support to warrant the recommendation level of a "practice standard." A practice standard is defined as:

> support from at least one well-designed class I study with an adequate sample, with support from class II or class III evidence, that directly addressed the effectiveness of the treatment in question, providing substantive evidence of effectiveness to support a recommendation that the treatment be specifically considered for people with acquired neurocognitive impairments and disability.
>
> *(p. 521)*

Recommendations that reached the threshold of a practice recommendation for traumatic brain injury included remediation of attention during postacute rehabilitation (including direct attention training and metacognitive training to promote development of compensatory strategies and foster generalization to real-world tasks); specific interventions for functional communication deficits, including pragmatic conversational skills, memory strategy training for mild memory impairments from TBI (including the use of internal strategies such as visual imagery and external compensation such as notebooks); metacognitive strategy training, such as self-monitoring and self-regulation for deficits in executive functioning after TBI, including impairments of emotional self-regulation, and as a component of interventions for deficits in attention, neglect, and memory; and comprehensive-holistic neuropsychologic rehabilitation during postacute rehabilitation to reduce cognitive and functional disability for persons with moderate or severe TBI.

Heart Rate Variability Biofeedback

Heart rate variability (HRV) training, discussed extensively in this volume, is an exciting area of potential intervention with sport-related concussion. Although not a mainstream neuropsychological intervention per se, HRV training exploits knowledge of brain-behavior relationships, which is a characteristic area of expertise for the neuropsychologist. The first step in demonstrating the effectiveness of HRV training in concussed individuals would be to establish that baseline difference in HRV parameters exist between concussed individual and normal controls. To this end, Bishop et al. (2017) measured heart rate and blood pressure parameters during rest and cognitive exertion (i.e., 10-second squat-stands) in concussed individuals and normal controls. Heart rate variability was significantly lower in the concussion group at rest, as well as during physical exertion. The authors interpreted these data as preliminary evidence for the dysregulation of autonomic function during the initial 72 hours post-concussion. Senthinathan, Mainwaring, and Hutchison (2017) demonstrated differences in HRV frequency domain parameters between concussed athletes and matched controls, both during the acute stages (i.e., symptomatic) and after returning to play. Paniccia et al. (2018) explored HRV parameters in concussed athletes between the ages of 13 and 18. They found higher HRV in older athletes overall, and lower HRV in younger athletes reporting more cognitive symptoms. Taken together, these studies provide good evidence for HRV disruption following sport-related concussion, establishing a rationale for interventions to normalize autonomic function.

There is a small but promising body of research on the potential for HRV biofeedback to help in ameliorating post-concussion symptoms. Lagos, Thompson, and Vaschillo (2013) presented preliminary data demonstrating the positive effect of a 10-week HRV biofeedback training on the improvement in mood disturbance, post-concussion symptoms, and headache severity. Robert and Alanna Condor (2014a, b) published studies reviewing the literature on HRV and concussion, including the potential neurocognitive benefit of HRV training in concussed athletes. Their studies provide a theoretical rationale for further exploration of HRV biofeedback as a treatment aspect of sport-related concussion.

Thus, there is convincing evidence for autonomic dysregulation in concussion, as evidenced by reduced variability and differences between patients and controls on other HRV parameters. Although few studies have systematically investigated the efficacy of HRV biofeedback training in concussion care, there is promise for such interventions due to the relative ease and non-invasiveness with which such training and practice can be initiated. Further research is needed to empirically investigate such interventions to increase awareness of their availability and determine their true value with concussed athletes.

Psychological Treatment for Prolonged Post-Concussion Syndrome

Given the literature on the tendency of post-concussion symptoms (PCS) to be maintained, by psychological and other non-injury factors, the development of psychological treatment interventions is an important component in the overall treatment arsenal. Several studies have examined the efficacy of single-session treatment interventions for PCS, as compared to a standard care group who receives only discharge instructions to return to the emergency room if physical symptoms (e.g., severe headaches) develop. Two studies (Minderhoud, Boelens, Huizenga, & Saan, 1980; Wade et al., 1998) found that a treatment group given written information and contact with a therapist had fewer PCS symptoms and reduced length of initial disability and absenteeism from work/school at six-month follow-up than a group receiving standard care. In a study by Gronwall (1986), a treatment group receiving printed material and reassurance were nine times less likely to complain of PCS symptoms after three months. Mittenberg, Zielinski, Fichera, and Rayls (1996) presented a treatment manual to patients and met with them to review the nature and incidence of expected symptoms, present a cognitive-behavioral model of symptom maintenance and treatment, teach techniques for reducing symptoms, and to provide instructions for gradual resumption of premorbid activities. This group, compared to a standard care group, showed a reduction in symptom frequency and severity, and produced earlier resolution of symptoms. Two studies have compared single-session treatments to control groups receiving a condition other than standard care. Alves, Macciocchi, and Barth (1993) demonstrated the superiority of a single-session group who received written information and reassurance that recovery was expected to be uncomplicated to both a standard care group and a group receiving only the written information. In a series of two studies, Paniak and colleagues (Paniak, Toller-Lobe, Nagy, & Durand, 1998; Paniak et al., 2000) compared a single session treatment group to a group that received a neuropsychological assessment, consultation with a physical therapist, and treatment-as-needed, initiated by the patient. No differences were found between these groups in symptom frequency at three and 12 months post-injury. The authors present these results as evidence of the equivalence of single-session treatments to more intensive interventions. This conclusion is suspect, though, as most patients in the treatment-as-needed group did not pursue this additional treatment, and as such therapeutic contact was not controlled.

More recently, Sayegh, Sanford, and Carson (2010) conducted a systematic review of psychological approaches to the treatment of post-concussion syndrome. From their analysis, they concluded that information, education, and reassurance alone may not be as beneficial as previously thought. They provide evidence of the effectiveness of cognitive-behavioral therapy (CBT) in the treatment of post-concussion syndrome. There was also somewhat limited evidence for the effectiveness of multi-faceted rehabilitation programs that include a psychotherapeutic element, or mindfulness-relaxation. Thus, there is empirical evidence for psychological interventions in the treatment of prolonged post-concussion syndrome. Given the complexity of concussion, an individualized approach is likely warranted, and additional research is needed to determine the parameters under which different interventions are effective.

Conclusions

Sport-related concussion, and concussions in general, are often "invisible injuries," at least to traditional neuroimaging. Accurate diagnosis depends on careful assessment of functioning in cognitive, emotional, and physical domains. The clinical neuropsychologist, by virtue of extensive education, training and experience in psychometrics, clinical neuroscience, and brain-behavior relationships, is uniquely suited to the task of cognitive assessment of an individual with concussion. The existing scientific literature on sport-related concussion presents a picture of significant variability, both in the cognitive and emotional sequelae of a concussion, as well as the projected time course of recovery. This makes logical sense given the diffuse nature of a concussion, the general non-specificity of concussion symptoms, and the individual variability in the structure of the brain and skull. Given the generally subtle, albeit clinically relevant, nature of cognitive deficits, precision is warranted in the assessment process. Tests with adequate reliability, validity, sensitivity, and specificity are required to provide an accurate clinical picture of the athlete at any given time. Baseline concussion testing is very helpful to provide the most precise basis of comparison between pre- and post-concussion functioning. Sideline cognitive testing instruments have been developed to quickly assess the potentially concussed athlete during games, in an effort to make sound decisions about return-to-play, attempting to avoid a potentially catastrophic second-impact syndrome. In instances where questions about an athlete's cognitive functioning go beyond return-to-play decisions (i.e., school or work functioning), a comprehensive neuropsychological evaluation may be warranted to more fully articulate their cognitive, emotional, and behavioral functioning. It is important to note that the clinical neuropsychologist does not act alone in the treatment of a concussed athlete. Ideally, a treatment team is established consisting of physicians, athletic trainers, psychologists, and specialists in vision, balance, and vestibular functioning. Participation from individuals with critical roles in the athlete's life is also important, such as educational professionals and employers.

The role of the clinical neuropsychologist extends beyond mere assessment of the athlete, and ideally includes participation in the treatment process. Employing current knowledge on neuroplasticity and the neurobiology of concussion, the neuropsychologist helps to modulate cognitive and physical activity in a such manner as to achieve maximal and timely recovery and return to premorbid level of functioning. Use of empirically validated cognitive rehabilitation interventions can help the athlete to recover cognitive functions that were compromised by the concussion. Advanced, emerging techniques such as heart rate variability biofeedback, though with only preliminary evidence of efficacy, provide promise for innovative and effective treatment modalities. Given the extensive literature on the contribution of psychological factors, the use of cognitive-behavioral therapy and other techniques can be very helpful in preventing or treating a prolonged post-concussion syndrome that is maintained by other than neurological factors. Ongoing research on the neuropsychology of concussion, broadly defined, is necessary to maximize the potential value that the clinical neuropsychologist can bring to the multi-disciplinary treatment of sport-related concussion.

References

Alves, W. M., Macciocchi, S. N., & Barth, J. T. (1993). Postconcussive symptoms after uncomplicated mild head injury. *Journal of Head Trauma Rehabilitation, 8*, 48–59.

American Psychological Association. Definition of a Clinical Neuropsychologist.

Bishop, S., Dech, R., Baker, T., Butz, M., Aravinthan, K., & Neary, J. P. (2017). Parasympathetic baroreflexes and heart rate variability during acute stage of sport concussion recovery. *Brain Injury, 31*, 247–259.

Brown, N. J., Mannix, R. C., O'Brien, M. J., Gostine, D., Collins, M. C., & Meehan, W. P. III (2014). Effect of cognitive activity level on duration of post-concussion symptoms. *Pediatrics, 133*, e299–e304.

Cicerone K. D, Langenbahn, D. M., Braden, C., Malec, J. F., Kalmar, K., Fraas, M., ... Ashman T. (2011). Evidence-based cognitive rehabilitation: Updated review of the literature from 2003 through 2008. *Archives of Physical Medicie and Rehabiltiation, 92*, 519–530.

Condor, R. L., & Condor, A. A. (2014a). Heart rate variability interventions for concussion and rehabilitation. *Frontiers in Psychology, 5*, 1–7.

Condor, R. L., & Condor, A. A. (2014b). Neuropsychological and psychological rehabilitation interventions in refractory sport-related post-concussion syndrome. *Brain Injury, 29*, 249–262.

Covassin, T., Elbin, R. J., Harris, W., Parker, T., & Kontos, A. (2012). The role of age and sex in symptoms, neurocognitive performance, and postural stability in athletes after concussion. *The American Journal of Sports Medicine, 40*, 1303–1312.

DiFazio, M., Silverberg, N. D., Kirkwood, M. W., Bernier, R., & Iverson, G. L. (2016). Prolonged activity restriction after concussion: Are we worsening outcomes? *Clinical Pediatrics, 55*, 443–451.

Eisenberg, M. A., Andrea, J., Meehan, W., & Mannix, R. (2013). Time interval between concussions and symptom duration. *Pediatrics, 132*, 8–17.

Ferguson, R. J., Mittenberg, W., Barone, D. F., & Schneider, B. (1999). Postconcussion syndrome following sports-related head injury: Expectation as etiology. *Neuropsychology, 13*, 582–589.

Gronwall, D. (1986). Rehabilitation programs for patients with mild head injury: Components, problems, and evaluation. *Journal of Head Trauma Rehabilitation, 1*, 53–63.

Grool, A. M., Aglipay, M., Momoli, F., Meehan, W. P. III, Freedman, S. B., Yeates, K. O., ... Barrowman, N. (2016). Association between early participation in physical activity following acute concussion and persistent postconcussion symptoms in children and adolescents. *Journal of the American Medical Association, 316*, 2504–2514.

Hanlon, R. E., Demery, J. A., Martinovich, Z., & Kelly, J. P. (1999). Effects of acute injury characteristics on neuropsychological status and vocational outcome following mild traumatic brain injury. *Brain Injury, 13*, 873–887.

Iverson G. L., & Lange R. T. (2011) Post-concussion syndrome. In M. R. Schoenberg & J. G. Scott (Eds.), *The little black book of neuropsychology*. Boston, MA: Springer.

Karr, J. E., Areshenkoff, C. N., & Garcia-Barrera, M. A. (2014). The neuropsychological outcomes of concussion: A systematic review of meta-analysis on the cognitive sequelae of mild traumatic brain injury. *Neuropsychology, 28*, 321–336.

Kontos, A. P., Elbin, R. J., Lau, B., Simensky, S., Freund, B., French, J., & Collins, M. W. (2013). Posttraumatic migraine as a predictor of recovery and cognitive impairment after sport-related concussion. *The American Journal of Sports Medicine, 41*, 1497–1504.

Lau, B. C., Kontos, A. P., & Collins, M. W. (2011). Which on-field signs/symptoms predict protracted recovery from sport-related concussion among high school football players? *The American Journal of Sports Medicine, 39*, 2311–2318.

Richard O. Temple

Lagos, L., Thompson, J., & Vaschillo, E. (2013). A preliminary study: Heart rate variability biofeedback for treatment of postconcussion syndrome. *Biofeedback, 41,* 136–143.

Leddy, J. J., Baker, J. G., & Willer, B. (2016). Active rehabilitation of concussion and post-concussion syndrome. *Physical Medicie Rehabilitation Clinics of North America, 27,* 437–454.

McCrea, M. M. (2001). Standardized mental status testing on the sideline after sport-related concussion. *Journal of Athletic Training, 36,* 274–279.

McCrea, M., Guskiewicz, K., Randolph, C., Barr, W. B., Hammeke, T. A., Marshall, S. W., ... Kelly, J. P. (2012). Incidence, clinical course, and predictors of prolonged recovery time following sport-related concussion in high school and college athletes. *Journal of the International Neuropsychological Society, 18,* 1–12.

Meares, S., Shores, E. A., Taylor, A. J., Batchelor, J., Bryant, R. A., Baguley, I. J., ... Marosszeky, J. E. (2011). The prospective course of postconcussion syndrome: The role of mild traumatic brain injury. *Neuropsychology, 25,* 454–465.

Meehan, W. P., Mannix, R. C., Stracciolini, A., Elbin, R. J., & Collins, M. C. (2013). Symptom severity predicts prolonged recovery after sport-related concussion, but age and amnesia do not. *The Journal of Pediatrics, 163,* 721–725.

Minderhoud, J. M., Boelens, M. E., Huizenga, J., & Saan, R. J. (1980). Treatment of minor head injuries. *Clinical Neurology and Neurosurgery, 82,* 127–140.

Mittenberg, W., DiGiulio, D. V., Perrin, S., & Bass, A. E. (1992). Symptoms following minor head injury: Expectation as aetiology. *Journal of Neurology, Neurosurgery, and Psychiatry, 41,* 611–616.

Mittenberg, W., & Strauman, S. (2000). Diagnosis of mild head injury and the postconcussion syndrome. *Journal of Head Trauma Rehabilitation, 15,* 783–791.

Mittenberg, W., Tremont, G., Zielinski, R. E., Fichera, S., & Rayls, K. R. (1996). Cognitive-behavioral prevention of postconcussion syndrome. *Archives of Clinical Neuropsychology, 11,* 139–145.

NAN Definition of a Clinical Neuropsychologist 2001: Official Position of the Natinal Academy of Neuropsychology.

Paniak, C., Toller-Lobe, G., Nagy, J., & Durand, A. (1998). A randomized trial of two treatments for mild traumatic brain injury. *Brain Injury, 12,* 1011–1023.

Paniak, C., Toller-Lobe, G., Reynolds, S., Melnyk, A., & Nagy, J. (2000). A randomized trial of two treatments for mild traumatic brain injury: One year follow-up. *Brain Injury, 14,* 219–236.

Paniccia, M., Verweel, L., Thomas, S., Taha, T., Keightley, M., Wilson, K.E., & Reed, N. (2018). Heart rate variability in healthy non-concussed youth athletes: Exploring the effect of age, sex, and concussion-like symptoms. *Frontiers in Neurology, 8,* 1–11.

Prichep, L. S., McCrea, M. M., Barr, W., Powell, M., & Chabot, R. J. (2013). Time course of clinical and electrophysiological recovery after sport-related concussion. *Journal of Head Trauma Rehabilitation, 28,* 266–273.

Sayegh, A. A., Sanford, D., & Carson, A. J. (2010). Psychological approaches to treatment of post-concussion syndrome: A systematic review. *Journal of Neurology, Neurosurgery, and Psychiatry, 81,* 1128–1134.

SCAT3. (2013). *British Journal of Sports Medicine, 47,* 259.

Senthinathan, A., Mainwaring, L. M., & Hutchison, M. (2017). Heart rate variability of athletes across concussion recovery milestones: A preliminary study. *Clinical Journal of Sports Medicine, 27,* 288–295.

Wade, D., King, N., Wenden, F., Crawford, S., & Caldwell, F. (1998). Routine follow-up after head injury: A second randomised controlled trial. *Journal of Neurology, Neurosurgery, & Psychiatry, 65,* 177–183.

Williams, R. M., Puetz, T. W., Giza, C. C., & Broglio, S. P. (2015). Concussion recovery time among high school and collegiate athletes: A systematic review and meta-analysis. *Sports Medicine, 45,* 893–903.

18

Beyond Physical Exercise

Designing Physical Activities for Cognitive Enhancement

David Moreau

Introduction

Human long-term memory is thought to be, for practical purposes, unlimited (Johnson & Hasher, 1987). We thus retain the capacity, throughout our lives, to accumulate knowledge without the risk of running out of storage space. By contrast, our ability to process and manipulate information decreases once we reach adulthood, with only subtle effects at first giving way to more dramatic changes eventually. In the scientific literature on intelligence, this difference is usually expressed with the distinction between crystallised and fluid intelligence, respectively (Cattell, 1963).

Consistent with the postulate of nearly infinite capacity, it is widely assumed that crystallised intelligence does not peak—that is, individuals keep gaining knowledge, skills, and experience well into older years. Therefore, apart from clinical conditions, intelligence can undoubtedly be enhanced via the acquisition of new skills and knowledge. What remains to be established, however, is the extent to which we can meaningfully influence fluid intelligence, so as to allow more efficient processing of information. This is a particularly important question given that fluid intelligence predicts performance in a wide range of settings, including professional and academic (Deary, Strand, Smith, & Fernandes, 2007). The malleability of cognitive abilities is also a critical area of investigation considering that fluid and crystallised intelligence are genetically determined in large part, with respective estimates of about 50% and 40% (Davies et al., 2011).

The notion that our cognitive abilities are strongly influenced by genetic factors does not imply however, that seeking improvement is a vain endeavour. *Strongly* here is not akin to *solely*, and there remains variance that is influenced by environmental—and possibly epigenetic—factors (Henikoff et al., 2016; Nikolova & Hariri, 2015). Consistent with this view, recent evidence suggests that the interaction between heritable traits and culture is more complex than initially postulated (Kan, Wicherts, Dolan, & van der Maas, 2013). As a result, the potential for enhancement has generated a lot of interest in different methods and techniques, ranging from pharmaceutical enhancers (i.e. nootropics) to brain stimulation and behavioural interventions. In this chapter, I will discuss the latter, with a particular focus on one of the most potent regimens, physical exercise (see for a review Moreau & Conway, 2013). Specifically, I will focus on how physical exercise interventions can be designed to promote cognitive growth. Behavioural interventions present important advantages over other approaches: they are usually safe, their underlying mechanisms are well understood, and they can be adapted to specific requirements.

As is the case for many research questions worth pursuing, definitive answers regarding the effectiveness of training programmes on cognition are elusive. In the computerised cognitive training literature, results have been mixed results thus far—several studies have suggested that fluid intelligence can be enhanced meaningfully via cognitive training (Astle, Barnes, Baker,

Colclough, & Woolrich, 2015; Au et al., 2014; Jaeggi, Buschkuehl, Jonides, & Perrig, 2008; Jaeggi, Buschkuehl, Jonides, & Shah, 2011; Jaeggi, Buschkuehl, Shah, & Jonides, 2014; Karbach, Strobach, & Schubert, 2014; Nouchi et al., 2013), while others have shown more scepticism (Redick et al., 2013; Shipstead, Redick, & Engle, 2012; Thompson et al., 2013). At the core of this disagreement lies the concept of transfer, or the extent to which a trained ability influences outcomes in ecological settings. Most would concur on the notion that improvements restricted to training are not the goal of cognitive interventions. This is because training-specific gains are by and large the norm rather than the exception – in typical settings, practice leads to enhanced performance. Professional musicians are well aware of that, as are elite athletes or students preparing for standardised tests. This justifies dedicated hours of practice, over years or even decades.

What is therefore targeted in cognitive training paradigms is enhancement *outside* training settings and demands, so as to potentially benefit numerous aspects of life. As alluded to earlier, and perhaps surprisingly, the most effective way to improve general cognitive abilities non-invasively is physical exercise. I explore the underlying processes of this remarkable effect in the next section.

Physical Exercise and Cognitive Enhancement

Physical exercise is known to be associated with numerous benefits, both in terms of physical and mental health. Low fitness indices are linked to decreases in incidence of a wide range of conditions, from stroke and cancer to diabetes and cardiovascular diseases (Blair, 1995). Sedentary habits are also correlated with higher risks for neurological conditions such as autism, schizophrenia, attention deficit/hyperactive disorder (ADHD), dementia and Alzheimer's disease, which all have been shown to benefit from exercise interventions (Penedo & Dahn, 2005).

Beyond neurological impairment, higher fitness is also associated with better executive function, an umbrella term relating to an array of important abilities such as planning, problem-solving, reasoning, and inhibiting (Colcombe & Kramer, 2003). Additional research has demonstrated that this association is not specific to executive tasks, and extend to a wider range of abilities in many domains of cognition (Moreau & Conway, 2013). Experimental designs have further confirmed that the link between physical exercise and cognition is causal: exercise interventions lead to cognitive improvements and enhanced performance both in academic settings and in the professional workplace (Castelli, Hillman, Buck, & Erwin, 2007; Coe, Pivarnik, Womack, Reeves, & Malina, 2006; Keeley & Fox, 2009). These findings also extend into studies with older populations, in which exercise typically elicits enhanced cognitive performance and quality of life (Cancela Carral & Ayán Pérez, 2007), as well as more stable mood and emotions (Blumenthal et al., 1991).

The underlying mechanisms mediating this association are now well understood. Physical exercise promotes neurogenesis—the creation of new neurons—(van Praag, Kempermann, & Gage, 1999; van Praag et al., 2002), neuronal survival (Vaynman, Ying, Yin, & Gomez-Pinilla, 2006), brain volume (Colcombe et al., 2006) and brain vascularisation (Black, Isaacs, Anderson, Alcantara, & Greenough, 1990). Chemical reactions in the brain are also altered by physical exercise, with changes in the concentration of hormones and neurotransmitters (Mora, Segovia, & del Arco, 2007). In particular, one of the key mediators of the relationship between physical exercise and cognitive enhancement is brain-derived neurotrophic factor (BDNF). Shortly after exercising, BDNF increases substantially in the hippocampus (Neeper, Gómez-Pinilla, Choi, & Cotman, 1995), a structure involved in learning, memory formation, and spatial navigation central to many aspects of cognitive function. In addition, enhanced concentrations of BDNF have been found in the spinal cord (Gómez-Pinilla, Ying, Opazo, Roy, & Edgerton, 2001), the cerebellum, and several cortical regions (Neeper, Gómez-Pinilla, Choi, & Cotman, 1996). These effects typically last at least several weeks (Berchtold, Kesslak, Pike, Adlard, & Cotman, 2001), and are thus thought to play a critical role in exercise-induced neural plasticity (Knaepen, Goekint, Heyman, & Meeusen, 2010).

Neurobiological changes also lead to alterations at the structural level. For example, fitness indices are associated with white matter integrity in children (Chaddock-Heyman et al., 2014), a finding corroborated by intervention designs (Krafft et al., 2014; Schaeffer et al., 2014). White matter tracts constitute the connections between neurons, and higher integrity is thought to enhance the processing and channelling of information throughout the brain. This line of research is based on diffusion tensor imaging (DTI), a technique that allows measuring the diffusion of water molecules along axonal pathways. Training influences the microstructural architecture of specific brain regions (Alexander, Lee, Lazar, & Field, 2007), and the diffusion of water is a proxy to measure these changes.

Functional changes in the brain are also associated with physical exercise. These differences are typically investigated with electroencephalography (EEG) or with functional magnetic resonance imaging (fMRI). Though the underlying rationales and assumptions of the two techniques are different, resulting in respective advantages and limitations that need to be considered depending upon the research question of interest, progress made via both techniques of investigation has been tremendous for the field in the past decades (Chaddock-Heyman et al., 2013; Davis et al., 2011; Hillman et al., 2014; Kamijo et al., 2011). A striking example comes from a study by Chaddock-Heyman and colleagues (2013), who reported decreases in neural activity in the right anterior prefrontal cortex while children were engaged in cognitive control tasks after a 1-year exercise intervention. Not only did children see alterations in neural activity with exercise, they also improved on behavioural measures of cognition, indicating that the underlying neural changes were beneficial to their cognitive abilities. Though the behavioural outcomes are typically consistent across studies, others have found increases in prefrontal activity following an exercise intervention (Davis et al., 2011). These results indicate that prefrontal activity is complex, and therefore requires further investigation with precise imaging techniques. Regardless, the benefits of physical exercise on cognition are well established (see for a review Moreau & Conway, 2013), and exciting questions have emerged as a result. For example, what type of intervention yields the best benefits? Related to this idea, do different regimens induce improvements in different cognitive functions? These and related questions represent promising avenues for future research, as they provide food for thought towards a better understanding of the fundamental process of enhancement, while also having obvious applications for diverse populations.

Increasing Cognitive Demands in Physical Activities

That physical exercise is the most effective way to elicit cognitive enhancement does not imply, however, that is should be used in isolation. It is possible that other forms of enhancement could induce gains that are additive and thus complement those elicited by physical exercise. This idea has been the basis for blended or combined regimens, where more than one method of enhancement is used, and has led to interventions pairing physical exercise with meditation (Astin et al., 2003), cognitive training (Curlik & Shors, 2013; Shatil, 2013), or transcranial direct current stimulation (tDCS, Ditye, Jacobson, Walsh, & Lavidor, 2012; Madhavan & Shah, 2012; Martin et al., 2013; Moreau, Wang, Tseng, & Juan, 2015).

If potential negative side effects are a concern with some of these approaches—for example, uncertainty over long-term effects in the case of tDCS (Davis, 2014), or unintended psychological stressors induced by mindfulness meditation (Lazarus, 1976; Shapiro, 1992)—behavioural interventions based on physical exercise induce remarkable health benefits in a very broad fashion. Effectiveness when multiple factors is particularly appealing considering recent concerns about opportunity costs related to computerised cognitive training regimens (Moreau & Conway, 2014). Many computerised programmes do not deliver on their promises, which is problematic given that training-specific skills improved as part of these regimens have limited relevance to ecological settings, in contrast with domains such as music, sports, or the arts. Indeed, if time and effort are to be invested in an activity solely intended to enhance brain function, it needs testing and validation.

Recently, several studies have questioned whether aerobic exercise, making up the vast majority of exercise interventions targeting cognitive enhancement, is indeed the most potent approach. Developments in the field of exercise physiology suggest that interventions based on short and intense bursts of exercise can induce physiological changes similar to those following aerobic exercise on a wide range of outcomes, including cardiovascular measures (Gayda, Ribeiro, Juneau, & Nigam, 2016), physical fitness and general health (Milanović, Sporiš, & Weston, 2015). HIT-induced improvements have in some instances surpassed those resulting from aerobic regimens (Rognmo, Hetland, Helgerud, Hoff, & Siørdahl, 2004). In line with the physiological literature, regimens based on resistance training have also shown sizeable effects on cognition (Best, Chiu, Liang Hsu, Nagamatsu, & Liu-Ambrose, 2015; Liu-Ambrose, Nagamatsu, Voss, Khan, & Handy, 2012), despite somewhat different mediating processes from those induced by aerobic exercise (Goekint et al., 2010).

Beyond mere physical exercise regimens, complex forms of motor training that combine high physical and cognitive demands further confirm the appeal of alternatives to traditional exercise-based cognitive training (Moreau, Morrison, & Conway, 2015). This type of regimens can elicit gains in measures of spatial ability and working memory capacity, together with health benefits (Moreau, Clerc, Mansy-Dannay, & Guerrien, 2012; Moreau et al., 2015; Moreau, 2015a). It should be noted that these effects are to be distinguished from short-term improvements immediately following acute bouts of exercise (Tomporowski, 2003), which typically dissipate after a few hours (Chang, Labban, Gapin, & Etnier, 2012).

Importantly, a large body of research on motor expertise supports the notion that the motor system exerts influence on cognitive abilities. For example, mental rotation problems that typically tap visual processes (Hyun & Luck, 2007) have been shown to recruit motor processes in elite athletes, resulting in better performance (Moreau, 2012). Interestingly, concurrent demands on the motor system impairs performance to a greater degree in elite athletes than novices, indicating that it is not the capacity to simultaneously manipulate motor content that increases with practice, but the propensity to involve motor processes in non-motor task (Moreau, 2012).

The underlying mechanisms of these differences are also well understood. It has been demonstrated consistently that mental manipulation of body parts (e.g. hands) implicitly induces motor simulation (Parsons, 1987a, 1987b, 1994; Sekiyama, 1982). As a result, measures that disrupt motor simulation, such as physically constraining movement, leads to decreased mental rotation performance (Ionta & Blanke, 2009; Ionta, Fourkas, Fiorio, & Aglioti, 2007). In contrast, the mental manipulation of abstract shapes (e.g. polygons) typically does not elicit motor activation (Jordan, Heinze, Lutz, Kanowski, & Jäncke, 2001; Kosslyn, DiGirolamo, Thompson, & Alpert, 1998), and thus restricting movement has little to no effect on performance (Moreau, 2013a). A radically different picture emerges when testing motor experts, however. When performing these mental rotation tasks with movement restriction, motor experts show impairment *both* with body parts and abstract shapes, as opposed to body parts only for controls (Moreau, 2013a). This finding suggests that motor experts recruit motor processes to perform tasks that are typically non-motor, and indicates that such strategies are not easily adaptable—more flexibility would allow recruitment of a different system (e.g. visual) to circumvent motor constraints (Moreau, 2015b). More generally, this phenomenon extends beyond mental rotation tasks, with similar results observed on working memory tasks (Moreau, 2013b).

This line of work, together with the idea of increasing cognitive demands via motor activities, stem from the motor simulation framework, which posits common neural mechanisms for motor simulation and execution (Jeannerod & Decety, 1995; Jeannerod, 2001). According to this view, overt actions shape motor simulation (de Lange, Roelofs, & Toni, 2008), and, transitively, cognitive tasks that can be supported or facilitated by motor simulation. Countless studies have confirmed this hypothesis, with observational or experimental evidence. Besides mental rotation and working memory (Amorim, Isableu, & Jarraya, 2006; Janczyk, Pfister, Crognale, & Kunde, 2012; Moreau,

2012, 2013b; Steggemann, Engbert, & Weigelt, 2011; Wraga, Thompson, Alpert, & Kosslyn, 2003), the interrelation between motor processes and other aspects of cognition have been largely documented, from language (Beilock, Lyons, Mattarella-Micke, Nusbaum, & Small, 2008) to problem solving (Broaders, Cook, Mitchell, & Goldin-Meadow, 2007), reasoning (Beilock & Goldin-Meadow, 2010; Cook, Mitchell, & Goldin-Meadow, 2008), and decision-making (Raab & Johnson, 2007). Overall, this body of work suggests that motor activities are a remarkably potent way to stimulate a vast array of cognitive abilities, with numerous possibilities and variations.

Implications for Education

Recent developments in the new-fangled field of educational neuroscience suggest prudence and caution when extrapolating laboratory findings to the classroom. Over the years, vernacular and concepts borrowed from neuroscience have spread remarkably well within education. Yet oftentimes, the new jargon adds very little, if anything, to discussions in education, sometimes blurring ideas to the detriment of clear understanding. Simple concepts become obscure. Children are reduced to brains capable of plastic changes, by opposition to so-called old views of a fixed brain. Nothing could be farther from the truth: that some brain regions retain plasticity across the lifespan has been known since the 1960s with the pioneer work of Joseph Altman (Altman, 1962) and James Hinds (Hinds, 1968). More strikingly perhaps, developmental plasticity was never really questioned, even prior to these seminal studies. As it turns out, manifestations of neuroplasticity presumably witnessed by teachers actually relate to changes in behaviour, or learning. The terminology might be new, but the rationale hardly is.

In contrast with the abuse of neurospeak in didactic settings, there are clear implications for the work bridging motor activities and cognition in the classroom. Experimental evidence has directly demonstrated the value of motor activities to enhance cognition, with encouraging results. Indeed, structured plays that incorporate cognitive demands within motor activities allow creating ecological situations that have the potential to elicit meaningful cognitive gains. As such, they represent an interesting avenue for teachers and educators, with great adaptability. The specific characteristics of this type of intervention matter less than the importance to get involved with any such programme; whether it is physical games (Tomporowski, Davis, Miller, & Naglieri, 2008), exergames (Staiano & Calvert, 2011), martial arts (Diamond & Lee, 2011), or designed sport (Moreau et al., 2015), the results have been extremely promising. Content can be adapted based on goals, feasibility and motivation, to offer interventions suitable to anyone.

Directly stemming from this idea, an important component inherent to programmes that target cognitive enhancement via physical activities is the range of possibilities they offer. Voluntary movement ranges from very simple, relying mostly on automated coordination, to extremely complex, requiring heightened and sustained attention. Due to complexity arising from the multiplicity of motor commands operating in synchrony, the latter often involves a progression through trial and error (Pritchett & Carey, 2014; Takiyama, Hirashima, & Nozaki, 2015). This represents a continuum educators can harness, adapt and tweak, to obtain the intended effects. Complex motor activities have the unique advantage of being more elaborate and diverse than the sum of their parts; in effect, situations are deliberately unconstrained so as to favour creative solutions. Product of this emergent property, challenging situations evolve in a unique way, directed but not constrained. The effects of these types of regimen on cognitive abilities have been remarkable (Moreau et al., 2015; Pesce et al., 2016; Tomporowski, Lambourne, & Okumura, 2011), to the point that they have become the preferred approach in numerous independent research groups (e.g. Curlik & Shors, 2013; Moreau et al., 2015; Tomporowski, McCullick, & Pesce, 2015).

Designing an intervention framework from a continuum also allows regimens to be adaptive, that is, propose individualised content to facilitate learning. Practice can thus be sustained at an optimum level of difficulty, to provide challenging but attainable goals. Adaptive training is a fundamental component of effective cognitive training (e.g. Zelinski et al., 2011), known in motor rehabilitation research as the "optimal challenge point" hypothesis (Guadagnoli & Lee, 2004). According to this view, skill learning is maximised when task difficulty is proportional to individual levels. Too easy, and individuals will stagnate and waste time. Too difficult, and they will not improve and might get frustrated. More generally, the idea stems from long-known mechanisms in motor learning, whereby demands of the environment slightly beyond an individual's capabilities yield the fastest learning rates (see for a review Schmidt & Wrisberg, 2008).

Further exploiting the blend of physical and cognitive demands, difficulty can also be nurtured in a different way. Concurrent physical and cognitive demands introduce competition for resources at various levels, especially related to physiological systems (Gómez-Pinilla, 2008). As exercise intensity increases, fewer resources (e.g. blood supply, oxygen, nutrients) are available for the brain to cope with cognitive demands, and maintaining adequate performance on a given task thus requires individuals to do more with less. This is consistent with the framework process of expertise acquisition—individuals typically recruit less cortical structures to perform a given task after learning (Wiesmann & Ishai, 2011). Concurrent exercise is therefore a positive stressor on the neural system, forcing efficiency. Cognitive tasks performed post-training without concurrent exercise often appear easier to most individuals, as the brain can then take advantage of plentiful resources and reclaim its place as the most energy-consuming organ (Tomasi, Wang, & Volkow, 2013).

Complex motor activities are also ideal to promote creativity, by setting the stage for an unlimited range of situations, without the need to plan and design each one of them *a priori*. Participants can modify existing situations, create new ones, and therefore produce unique conditions in which to solve problems and improve. Rich training environments that include variety and diversity are also critical factors to sustain motivation, which in turn may influence training outcomes. Loss of motivation is a common factor for dropping out of software-based cognitive regimens and aerobic exercise interventions, and physical exercise seems to be less effective when not voluntary, at least in rodents (Yuede et al., 2009).

However, great flexibility in an intervention program comes at a cost—the regimen is typically difficult to standardise, because the degrees of freedom are deliberately relaxed. In terms of validation, this is a major hurdle, because experiments require precise and constrained designs to facilitate reproducibility. With this limitation in mind, it is worth noting that constraining interventions too drastically prevents the very component targeted to develop, leading to an impoverished, simplified regimen. This approach might be suitable for laboratory-based testing, but it often reduces or annihilates the effects of interest, especially when the intervention under study is a complex blend.

How can these factors, seemingly antagonists, be reconciled? A promising solution lies in the combination of laboratory-based experiments to explore the basic processes of enhancement with large-scale ecological interventions that help quantify effect sizes in ecological settings. These two types of design can thus inform each other, and refine knowledge and applications. Such a combined approach also allows the study of cognitive malleability at different levels, from brain to behaviour. Each level of investigation can then inform others, leading to more scientifically sound interventions. This approach also facilitates theoretically driven hypotheses, thus reducing the rate of false positives and optimising the scientific enterprise as a whole. The trade-off between controlled laboratory experiments and ecological studies cannot be entirely circumvented, and has in fact bothered psychologists for decades (Brewer, 2000; Gibson, 1979). Yet combining findings from different research designs under a common framework will lead to better, more potent, interventions.

Concluding Remarks

Throughout this chapter, I have provided an overview of the vast amount of research dedicated to studying the link between physical exercise and cognition, and I have presented recent trends of research that advocate for complex physical activities, with potential for greater impact on cognitive abilities. These trends of research are promising, and are expected to provide ground for years of research to come.

Although the general feeling is one of optimism, there are still major challenges facing the field of cognitive enhancement. Among them, the personalisation of interventions holds a central place. Individuals differ in the extent to which they benefit from an intervention—some show impressive trends of improvement, while others do not seem to benefit at all, at least cognitively. Understanding the variability between individuals, as well as the dynamics of individual rates of improvement, is crucial to further our insight regarding the underlying mechanisms at play. Research at the intersection of psychology, neuroscience, physiology and genetics is particularly promising in this regard, providing footing for a more holistic approach of exercise-induced cognitive enhancement.

For practical concerns, acknowledging individual variability also allows training content needs to be adapted to specific demands, either based on expectations, or on inherent cognitive deficits. The potential of this type of approach has been underlined recently in the context of remediation for learning disorders (Moreau & Waldie, 2016); when cognitive deficits are identified in specific areas of cognition, training can be personalised so as to provide regimens optimised individually. Personalising regimens represents a promising but difficult endeavour—it is easy to fall intro the trap of modelling noise, via the personalisation of every single situation, when this approach might not be optimal.

Ultimately, understanding precisely mechanism of improvement requires solid theoretical grounds, still lacking at the moment. Researchers are only beginning to understand the dynamics of cognitive abilities induced by training—methods are progressively being refined, findings are better contextualised, and eventually these will call for an integrating framework. Only then can we envision accurate probabilistic estimates of training outcomes for a given individual, so as to maximise chances for a programme to be effective. This prospect holds remarkable promises, and constitutes a pivotal step for future research and applications.

References

Alexander, A. L., Lee, J. E., Lazar, M., & Field, A. S. (2007). Diffusion tensor imaging of the brain. *Neurotherapeutics : The Journal of the American Society for Experimental NeuroTherapeutics*, *4*(3), 316–329. doi:10.1016/j.nurt.2007.05.011

Altman, J. (1962). Are new neurons formed in the brains of adult mammals? *Science*, *135*, 1128–1129.

Amorim, M.-A., Isableu, B., & Jarraya, M. (2006). Embodied spatial transformations: "Body analogy" for the mental rotation of objects. *Journal of Experimental Psychology. General*, *135*(3), 327–347. doi:10.1037/0096-3445.135.3.327

Astin, J. A., Berman, B. M., Bausell, B., Lee, W.-L., Hochberg, M., & Forys, K. L. (2003). The efficacy of mindfulness meditation plus Qigong movement therapy in the treatment of fibromyalgia: A randomized controlled trial. *The Journal of Rheumatol*, *30*(10), 2257–2262.

Astle, D. E., Barnes, J. J., Baker, K., Colclough, G. L., & Woolrich, M. W. (2015). Cognitive training enhances intrinsic brain connectivity in childhood. *The Journal of Neuroscience : The Official Journal of the Society for Neuroscience*, *35*(16), 6277–6283. doi:10.1523/JNEUROSCI.4517-14.2015

Au, J., Sheehan, E., Tsai, N., Duncan, G. J., Buschkuehl, M., & Jaeggi, S. M. (2014). Improving fluid intelligence with training on working memory: A meta-analysis. *Psychonomic Bulletin & Review*. doi:10.3758/s13423-014-0699-x

Beilock, S. L., & Goldin-Meadow, S. (2010). Gesture changes thought by grounding it in action. *Psychological Science*, *21*(11), 1605–1610. doi:10.1177/0956797610385353

Beilock, S. L., Lyons, I. M., Mattarella-Micke, A., Nusbaum, H. C., & Small, S. L. (2008). Sports experience changes the neural processing of action language. *Proceedings of the National Academy of Sciences of the United States of America*, *105*(36), 13269–13273. doi:10.1073/pnas.0803424105

Berchtold, N. C., Kesslak, J. P., Pike, C. J., Adlard, P. A., & Cotman, C. W. (2001). Estrogen and exercise interact to regulate brain-derived neurotrophic factor mRNA and protein expression in the hippocampus. *The European Journal of Neuroscience*, *14*(12), 1992–2002.

Best, J. R., Chiu, B. K., Liang Hsu, C., Nagamatsu, L. S., & Liu-Ambrose, T. (2015). Long-term effects of resistance exercise training on cognition and brain volume in older women: Results from a randomized controlled trial. *Journal of the International Neuropsychological Society: JINS*, *21*(10), 745–756. doi:10.1017/S1355617715000673

Black, J. E., Isaacs, K. R., Anderson, B. J., Alcantara, A. A., & Greenough, W. T. (1990). Learning causes synaptogenesis, whereas motor activity causes angiogenesis, in cerebellar cortex of adult rats. *Proceedings of the National Academy of Sciences of the United States of America*, *87*(14), 5568–5572.

Blair, S. N. (1995). Changes in physical fitness and all-cause mortality. *JAMA*, *273*(14), 1093. doi:10.1001/jama.1995.03520380029031

Blumenthal, J. A., Emery, C. F., Madden, D. J., Schniebolk, S., Walsh-Riddle, M., George, L. K., … Coleman, R. E. (1991). Long-term effects of exercise on psychological functioning in older men and women. *Journal of Gerontology*, *46*(6), P352–P361.

Brewer, M. B. (2000). *Research design and issues of validity*. Cambridge: Cambridge University Press.

Broaders, S. C., Cook, S. W., Mitchell, Z., & Goldin-Meadow, S. (2007). Making children gesture brings out implicit knowledge and leads to learning. *Journal of Experimental Psychology. General*, *136*(4), 539–550. doi:10.1037/0096-3445.136.4.539

Cancela Carral, J. M., & Ayán Pérez, C. (2007). Effects of high-intensity combined training on women over 65. *Gerontology*, *53*(6), 340–346. doi:10.1159/000104098

Castelli, D. M., Hillman, C. H., Buck, S. M., & Erwin, H. E. (2007). Physical fitness and academic achievement in third- and fifth-grade students. *Journal of Sport & Exercise Psychology*, *29*(2), 239–252.

Cattell, R. B. (1963). Theory of fluid and crystallized intelligence: A critical experiment. *Journal of Educational Psychology*, *54*(1), 1–22. doi:10.1037/h0046743

Chaddock-Heyman, L., Erickson, K. I., Holtrop, J. L., Voss, M. W., Pontifex, M. B., Raine, L. B., … Kramer, A. F. (2014). Aerobic fitness is associated with greater white matter integrity in children. *Frontiers in Human Neuroscience*, *8*, 584. doi:10.3389/fnhum.2014.00584

Chaddock-Heyman, L., Erickson, K. I., Voss, M. W., Knecht, A. M., Pontifex, M. B., Castelli, D. M., … Kramer, A. F. (2013). The effects of physical activity on functional MRI activation associated with cognitive control in children: A randomized controlled intervention. *Frontiers in Human Neuroscience*, *7*, 72. doi:10.3389/fnhum.2013.00072

Chang, Y. K., Labban, J. D., Gapin, J. I., & Etnier, J. L. (2012). The effects of acute exercise on cognitive performance: A meta-analysis. *Brain Research*, *1453*, 87–101. doi:10.1016/j.brainres.2012.02.068

Coe, D. P., Pivarnik, J. M., Womack, C. J., Reeves, M. J., & Malina, R. M. (2006). Effect of physical education and activity levels on academic achievement in children. *Medicine and Science in Sports and Exercise*, *38*(8), 1515–1519. doi:10.1249/01.mss.0000227537.13175.1b

Colcombe, S. J., Erickson, K. I., Scalf, P. E., Kim, J. S., Prakash, R., McAuley, E., … Kramer, A. F. (2006). Aerobic exercise training increases brain volume in aging humans. *The Journals of Gerontology. Series A, Biological Sciences and Medical Sciences*, *61*(11), 1166–1170.

Colcombe, S. J., & Kramer, A. F. (2003). Fitness effects on the cognitive function of older adults: A meta-analytic study. *Psychological Science*, *14*(2), 125–130.

Cook, S. W., Mitchell, Z., & Goldin-Meadow, S. (2008). Gesturing makes learning last. *Cognition*, *106*(2), 1047–1058. doi:10.1016/j.cognition.2007.04.010

Curlik, D. M., & Shors, T. J. (2013). Training your brain: Do mental and physical (MAP) training enhance cognition through the process of neurogenesis in the hippocampus? *Neuropharmacology*, *64*, 506–514. doi:10.1016/j.neuropharm.2012.07.027

Davies, G., Tenesa, A., Payton, A., Yang, J., Harris, S. E., Liewald, D., … Deary, I. J. (2011). Genome-wide association studies establish that human intelligence is highly heritable and polygenic. *Molecular Psychiatry*, *16*(10), 996–1005. doi:10.1038/mp.2011.85

Davis, C. L., Tomporowski, P. D., McDowell, J. E., Austin, B. P., Miller, P. H., Yanasak, N. E., … Naglieri, J. A. (2011). Exercise improves executive function and achievement and alters brain activation in overweight children: A randomized, controlled trial. *Health Psychology : Official Journal of the Division of Health Psychology, American Psychological Association*, *30*(1), 91–98. doi:10.1037/a0021766

Davis, N. J. (2014). Transcranial stimulation of the developing brain: A plea for extreme caution. *Frontiers in Human Neuroscience*, *8*, 600. doi:10.3389/fnhum.2014.00600

de Lange, F. P., Roelofs, K., & Toni, I. (2008). Motor imagery: A window into the mechanisms and alterations of the motor system. *Cortex; a Journal Devoted to the Study of the Nervous System and Behavior*, *44*(5), 494–506. doi:10.1016/j.cortex.2007.09.002

Deary, I. J., Strand, S., Smith, P., & Fernandes, C. (2007). Intelligence and educational achievement. *Intelligence*, *35*(1), 13–21. doi:10.1016/j.intell.2006.02.001

Diamond, A., & Lee, K. (2011). Interventions shown to aid executive function development in children 4 to 12 years old. *Science (New York, NY)*, *333*(6045), 959–964. doi:10.1126/science.1204529

Ditye, T., Jacobson, L., Walsh, V., & Lavidor, M. (2012). Modulating behavioral inhibition by tDCS combined with cognitive training. *Experimental Brain Research*, *219*(3), 363–368. doi:10.1007/s00221-012-3098-4

Gayda, M., Ribeiro, P. A. B., Juneau, M., & Nigam, A. (2016). Comparison of different forms of exercise training in patients with cardiac disease: Where does high-intensity interval training fit? *The Canadian Journal of Cardiology*, *32*(4), 485–494. doi:10.1016/j.cjca.2016.01.017

Gibson, J. J. (1979). *The ecological approach to visual perception*. Boston, MA: Houghton Mifflin.

Goekint, M., De Pauw, K., Roelands, B., Njemini, R., Bautmans, I., Mets, T., & Meeusen, R. (2010). Strength training does not influence serum brain-derived neurotrophic factor. *European Journal of Applied Physiology*, *110*(2), 285–293. doi:10.1007/s00421-010-1461-3

Gómez-Pinilla, F. (2008). Brain foods: The effects of nutrients on brain function. *Nature Reviews. Neuroscience*, *9*(7), 568–578. doi:10.1038/nrn2421

Gómez-Pinilla, F., Ying, Z., Opazo, P., Roy, R. R., & Edgerton, V. R. (2001). Differential regulation by exercise of BDNF and NT-3 in rat spinal cord and skeletal muscle. *The European Journal of Neuroscience*, *13*(6), 1078–1084.

Guadagnoli, M. A., & Lee, T. D. (2004). Challenge point: A framework for conceptualizing the effects of various practice conditions in motor learning. *Journal of Motor Behavior*, *36*(2), 212–224. doi:10.3200/JMBR.36.2.212-224

Henikoff, S., Greally, J. M., Stern, C. D., Holliday, R., Pugh, J. E., Steffen, P. A., ... Hobert, O. (2016). Epigenetics, cellular memory and gene regulation. *Current Biology*, *26*(14), R644–R648. doi:10.1016/j.cub.2016.06.011

Hillman, C. H., Pontifex, M. B., Castelli, D. M., Khan, N. A., Raine, L. B., Scudder, M. R., ... Kamijo, K. (2014). Effects of the FITKids randomized controlled trial on executive control and brain function. *Pediatrics*, *134*(4), e1063–e1071. doi:10.1542/peds.2013-3219

Hinds, J. W. (1968). Autoradiographic study of histogenesis in the mouse olfactory bulb. II. Cell proliferation and migration. *The Journal of Comparative Neurology*, *134*(3), 305–321. doi:10.1002/cne.901340305

Hyun, J.-S., & Luck, S. J. (2007). Visual working memory as the substrate for mental rotation. *Psychonomic Bulletin & Review*, *14*(1), 154–158.

Ionta, S., & Blanke, O. (2009). Differential influence of hands posture on mental rotation of hands and feet in left and right handers. *Experimental Brain Research*, *195*(2), 207–217. doi:10.1007/s00221-009-1770-0

Ionta, S., Fourkas, A. D., Fiorio, M., & Aglioti, S. M. (2007). The influence of hands posture on mental rotation of hands and feet. *Experimental Brain Research*, *183*(1), 1–7. doi:10.1007/s00221-007-1020-2

Jaeggi, S. M., Buschkuehl, M., Jonides, J., & Perrig, W. J. (2008). Improving fluid intelligence with training on working memory. *Proceedings of the National Academy of Sciences of the United States of America*, *105*(19), 6829–6833. doi:10.1073/pnas.0801268105

Jaeggi, S. M., Buschkuehl, M., Jonides, J., & Shah, P. (2011). Short- and long-term benefits of cognitive training. *Proceedings of the National Academy of Sciences of the United States of America*, *108*(25), 10081–10086. doi:10.1073/pnas.1103228108

Jaeggi, S. M., Buschkuehl, M., Shah, P., & Jonides, J. (2014). The role of individual differences in cognitive training and transfer. *Memory & Cognition*, *42*(3), 464–480. doi:10.3758/s13421-013-0364-z

Janczyk, M., Pfister, R., Crognale, M. A., & Kunde, W. (2012). Effective rotations: Action effects determine the interplay of mental and manual rotations. *Journal of Experimental Psychology. General*, *141*(3), 489–501.

Jeannerod, M. (2001). Neural simulation of action: A unifying mechanism for motor cognition. *NeuroImage*, *14*(1 Pt 2), S103–S109. doi:10.1006/nimg.2001.0832

Jeannerod, M., & Decety, J. (1995). Mental motor imagery: A window into the representational stages of action. *Current Opinion in Neurobiology*, *5*(6), 727–732.

Johnson, M. K., & Hasher, L. (1987). Human learning and memory. *Annual Review of Psychology*, *38*, 631–668. doi:10.1146/annurev.ps.38.020187.003215

Jordan, K., Heinze, H.-J., Lutz, K., Kanowski, M., & Jäncke, L. (2001). Cortical activations during the mental rotation of different visual objects. *NeuroImage*, *13*(1), 143–152. doi:10.1006/nimg.2000.0677

Kamijo, K., Pontifex, M. B., O'Leary, K. C., Scudder, M. R., Wu, C.-T., Castelli, D. M., & Hillman, C. H. (2011). The effects of an afterschool physical activity program on working memory in preadolescent children. *Developmental Science*, *14*(5), 1046–1058. doi:10.1111/j.1467-7687.2011.01054.x

Kan, K.-J., Wicherts, J. M., Dolan, C. V, & van der Maas, H. L. J. (2013). On the nature and nurture of intelligence and specific cognitive abilities: The more heritable, the more culture dependent. *Psychological Science*, *24*(12), 2420–2428. doi:10.1177/0956797613493292

Karbach, J., Strobach, T., & Schubert, T. (2014). Adaptive working-memory training benefits reading, but not mathematics in middle childhood. *Child Neuropsychology: A Journal on Normal and Abnormal Development in Childhood and Adolescence*. doi:10.1080/09297049.2014.899336

Keeley, T. J. H., & Fox, K. R. (2009). The impact of physical activity and fitness on academic achievement and cognitive performance in children. *International Review of Sport and Exercise Psychology*, *2*(2), 198–214. doi:10.1080/17509840903233822

David Moreau

Knaepen, K., Goekint, M., Heyman, E. M., & Meeusen, R. (2010). Neuroplasticity - exercise-induced response of peripheral brain-derived neurotrophic factor: A systematic review of experimental studies in human subjects. *Sports Medicine (Auckland, NZ)*, *40*(9), 765–801. doi:10.2165/11534530-000000000-00000

Kosslyn, S. M., DiGirolamo, G. J., Thompson, W. L., & Alpert, N. M. (1998). Mental rotation of objects versus hands: Neural mechanisms revealed by positron emission tomography. *Psychophysiology*, *35*(2), 151–161.

Krafft, C. E., Schwarz, N. F., Chi, L., Weinberger, A. L., Schaeffer, D. J., Pierce, J. E., … McDowell, J. E. (2014). An 8-month randomized controlled exercise trial alters brain activation during cognitive tasks in overweight children. *Obesity (Silver Spring, MD)*, *22*(1), 232–242. doi:10.1002/oby.20518

Lazarus, A. A. (1976). Psychiatric problems precipitated by transcendental meditation. *Psychological Reports*, *39*(2), 601–602. doi:10.2466/pr0.1976.39.2.601

Liu-Ambrose, T., Nagamatsu, L. S., Voss, M. W., Khan, K. M., & Handy, T. C. (2012). Resistance training and functional plasticity of the aging brain: A 12-month randomized controlled trial. *Neurobiology of Aging*, *33*(8), 1690–1698. doi:10.1016/j.neurobiolaging.2011.05.010

Madhavan, S., & Shah, B. (2012). Enhancing motor skill learning with transcranial direct current stimulation – a concise review with applications to stroke. *Frontiers in Psychiatry*, *3*, 66. doi:10.3389/fpsyt.2012.00066

Martin, D. M., Liu, R., Alonzo, A., Green, M., Player, M. J., Sachdev, P., & Loo, C. K. (2013). Can transcranial direct current stimulation enhance outcomes from cognitive training? A randomized controlled trial in healthy participants. *The International Journal of Neuropsychopharmacology / Official Scientific Journal of the Collegium Internationale Neuropsychopharmacologicum (CINP)*, *16*(9), 1927–1936. doi:10.1017/S1461145713000539

Milanović, Z., Sporiš, G., & Weston, M. (2015). Effectiveness of high-intensity interval training (HIT) and continuous endurance training for VO2max improvements: A systematic review and meta-analysis of controlled trials. *Sports Medicine (Auckland, N.Z.)*, *45*(10), 1469–1481. doi:10.1007/s40279-015-0365-0

Mora, F., Segovia, G., & del Arco, A. (2007). Aging, plasticity and environmental enrichment: Structural changes and neurotransmitter dynamics in several areas of the brain. *Brain Research Reviews*, *55*(1), 78–88. doi:10.1016/j.brainresrev.2007.03.011

Moreau, D. (2012). The role of motor processes in three-dimensional mental rotation: Shaping cognitive processing via sensorimotor experience. *Learning and Individual Differences*, *22*(3), 354–359.

Moreau, D. (2013a). Constraining movement alters the recruitment of motor processes in mental rotation. *Experimental Brain Research*, *224*(3), 447–454.

Moreau, D. (2013b). Motor expertise modulates movement processing in working memory. *Acta Psychologica*, *142*(3), 356–361.

Moreau, D. (2015a). Brains and brawn: Complex motor activities to maximize cognitive enhancement. *Educational Psychology Review*, *27*(3), 475–482. doi:10.1007/s10648-015-9323-5

Moreau, D. (2015b). Unreflective actions? complex motor skill acquisition to enhance spatial cognition. *Phenomenology and the Cognitive Sciences*, *14*, 349–359. doi:10.1007/s11097-014-9376-9

Moreau, D., Clerc, J., Mansy-Dannay, A., & Guerrien, A. (2012). Enhancing spatial ability through sport practice: Evidence for an effect of motor training on mental rotation performance. *Journal of Individual Differences*, *33*(2), 83–88. doi:10.1027/1614-0001/a000075

Moreau, D., & Conway, A. R. A. (2013). Cognitive enhancement: A comparative review of computerized and athletic training programs. *International Review of Sport and Exercise Psychology*, *6*(1), 155–183. doi:10.1080/1750984X.2012.758763

Moreau, D., & Conway, A. R. A. (2014). The case for an ecological approach to cognitive training. *Trends in Cognitive Sciences*, *18*(7), 334–336. doi:10.1016/j.tics.2014.03.009

Moreau, D., Morrison, A. B., & Conway, A. R. A. (2015). An ecological approach to cognitive enhancement: Complex motor training. *Acta Psychologica*, *157*, 44–55. doi:10.1016/j.actpsy.2015.02.007

Moreau, D., & Waldie, K. E. (2016). Developmental learning disorders: From generic interventions to individualized remediation. *Frontiers in Psychology*, *6*, 2053. doi:10.3389/fpsyg.2015.02053

Moreau, D., Wang, C.-H., Tseng, P., & Juan, C.-H. (2015). Blending transcranial direct current stimulations and physical exercise to maximize cognitive improvement. *Frontiers in Psychology*, *6*, 678. doi:10.3389/fpsyg.2015.00678

Neeper, S. A., Gómez-Pinilla, F., Choi, J., & Cotman, C. (1995). Exercise and brain neurotrophins. *Nature*, *373*(6510), 109. doi:10.1038/373109a0

Neeper, S. A., Gómez-Pinilla, F., Choi, J., & Cotman, C. W. (1996). Physical activity increases mRNA for brain-derived neurotrophic factor and nerve growth factor in rat brain. *Brain Research*, *726*(1–2), 49–56.

Nikolova, Y. S., & Hariri, A. R. (2015). Can we observe epigenetic effects on human brain function? *Trends in Cognitive Sciences*, *19*(7), 366–373. doi:10.1016/j.tics.2015.05.003

Nouchi, R., Taki, Y., Takeuchi, H., Hashizume, H., Nozawa, T., Kambara, T., … Kawashima, R. (2013). Brain training game boosts executive functions, working memory and processing speed in the young adults: A randomized controlled trial. *PloS One*, *8*(2), e55518. doi:10.1371/journal.pone.0055518

Parsons, L. M. (1987a). Imagined spatial transformation of one's body. *Journal of Experimental Psychology. General*, *116*(2), 172–191. doi:10.1037/0096-3445.116.2.172

Parsons, L. M. (1987b). Imagined spatial transformations of one's hands and feet. *Cognitive Psychology*, *19*(2), 178–241. doi:10.1016/0010-0285(87)90011-9

Parsons, L. M. (1994). Temporal and kinematic properties of motor behavior reflected in mentally simulated action. *Journal of Experimental Psychology. Human Perception and Performance*, *20*(4), 709–730.

Penedo, F. J., & Dahn, J. R. (2005). Exercise and well-being: A review of mental and physical health benefits associated with physical activity. *Current Opinion in Psychiatry*, *18*(2), 189–193.

Pesce, C., Masci, I., Marchetti, R., Vazou, S., Sääkslahti, A., & Tomporowski, P. D. (2016). Deliberate play and preparation jointly benefit motor and cognitive development: Mediated and moderated effects. *Frontiers in Psychology*, *7*, 349. doi:10.3389/fpsyg.2016.00349

Pritchett, D. L., & Carey, M. R. (2014). A matter of trial and error for motor learning. *Trends in Neurosciences*, *37*(9), 465–466. doi:10.1016/j.tins.2014.08.001

Raab, M., & Johnson, J. G. (2007). Expertise-based differences in search and option-generation strategies. *Journal of Experimental Psychology. Applied*, *13*(3), 158–170. doi:10.1037/1076-898X.13.3.158

Redick, T. S., Shipstead, Z., Harrison, T. L., Hicks, K. L., Fried, D. E., Hambrick, D. Z., … Engle, R. W. (2013). No evidence of intelligence improvement after working memory training: A randomized, placebo-controlled study. *Journal of Experimental Psychology. General*, *142*(2), 359–379. doi:10.1037/a0029082

Rognmo, Ø., Hetland, E., Helgerud, J., Hoff, J., & Siørdahl, S. A. (2004). High intensity aerobic interval exercise is superior to moderate intensity exercise for increasing aerobic capacity in patients with coronary artery disease. *European Journal of Cardiovascular Prevention & Rehabilitation*, *11*(3), 216–222. doi:10.1097/01.hjr.0000131677.96762.0c

Schaeffer, D. J., Krafft, C. E., Schwarz, N. F., Chi, L., Rodrigue, A. L., Pierce, J. E., … McDowell, J. E. (2014). An 8-month exercise intervention alters frontotemporal white matter integrity in overweight children. *Psychophysiology*, *51*(8), 728–733. doi:10.1111/psyp.12227

Schmidt, R. A., & Wrisberg, C. A. (2008). *Motor learning and performance: A situation-based learning approach* (4th ed.). Champaign, IL: Human Kinetics.

Sekiyama, K. (1982). Kinesthetic aspects of mental representations in the identification of left and right hands. *Perception & Psychophysics*, *32*(2), 89–95.

Shapiro, D. H. (1992). Adverse effects of meditation: A preliminary investigation of long-term meditators. *International Journal of Psychosomatics : Official Publication of the International Psychosomatics Institute*, *39*(1–4), 62–67.

Shatil, E. (2013). Does combined cognitive training and physical activity training enhance cognitive abilities more than either alone? A four-condition randomized controlled trial among healthy older adults. *Frontiers in Aging Neuroscience*, *5*, 8. doi:10.3389/fnagi.2013.00008

Shipstead, Z., Redick, T. S., & Engle, R. W. (2012). Is working memory training effective? *Psychological Bulletin*, *138*(4), 628–654. doi:10.1037/a0027473

Staiano, A. E., & Calvert, S. L. (2011). Exergames for physical education courses: Physical, social, and cognitive benefits. *Child Development Perspectives*, *5*(2), 93–98. doi:10.1111/j.1750-8606.2011.00162.x

Steggemann, Y., Engbert, K., & Weigelt, M. (2011). Selective effects of motor expertise in mental body rotation tasks: Comparing object-based and perspective transformations. *Brain and Cognition*, *76*(1), 97–105. doi:10.1016/j.bandc.2011.02.013

Takiyama, K., Hirashima, M., & Nozaki, D. (2015). Prospective errors determine motor learning. *Nature Communications*, *6*, 5925. doi:10.1038/ncomms6925

Thompson, T. W., Waskom, M. L., Garel, K.-L. A., Cardenas-Iniguez, C., Reynolds, G. O., Winter, R., … Gabrieli, J. D. E. (2013). Failure of working memory training to enhance cognition or intelligence. *PloS One*, *8*(5), e63614. doi:10.1371/journal.pone.0063614

Tomasi, D., Wang, G.-J., & Volkow, N. D. (2013). Energetic cost of brain functional connectivity. *Proceedings of the National Academy of Sciences of the United States of America*, *110*(33), 13642–13647. doi:10.1073/pnas.1303346110

Tomporowski, P. D. (2003). Effects of acute bouts of exercise on cognition. *Acta Psychologica*, *112*(3), 297–324.

Tomporowski, P. D., Davis, C. L., Miller, P. H., & Naglieri, J. A. (2008). Exercise and children's intelligence, cognition, and academic achievement. *Educational Psychology Review*, *20*(2), 111–131. doi:10.1007/s10648-007-9057-0

Tomporowski, P. D., Lambourne, K., & Okumura, M. S. (2011). Physical activity interventions and children's mental function: An introduction and overview. *Preventive Medicine*, *52 Suppl 1*, S3–S9. doi:10.1016/j.ypmed.2011.01.028

Tomporowski, P. D., McCullick, B., & Pesce, C. (2015). *Enhancing children's cognition with physical activity games*. Champaign, IL: Human Kinetics.

van Praag, H., Kempermann, G., & Gage, F. H. (1999). Running increases cell proliferation and neurogenesis in the adult mouse dentate gyrus. *Nature Neuroscience*, *2*(3), 266–270. doi:10.1038/6368 van Praag, H., Schinder, A. F., Christie, B. R., Toni, N., Palmer, T. D., & Gage, F. H. (2002). Functional neurogenesis in the adult hippocampus. *Nature*, *415*(6875), 1030–1034. doi:10.1038/4151030a

Vaynman, S. S., Ying, Z., Yin, D., & Gomez-Pinilla, F. (2006). Exercise differentially regulates synaptic proteins associated to the function of BDNF. *Brain Research*, *1070*(1), 124–130. doi:10.1016/j.brainres.2005.11.062

Wiesmann, M., & Ishai, A. (2011). Expertise reduces neural cost but does not modulate repetition suppression. *Cognitive Neuroscience*, *2*(1), 57–65. doi:10.1080/17588928.2010.525628

Wraga, M., Thompson, W. L., Alpert, N. M., & Kosslyn, S. M. (2003). Implicit transfer of motor strategies in mental rotation. *Brain and Cognition*, *52*(2), 135–143.

Yuede, C. M., Zimmerman, S. D., Dong, H., Kling, M. J., Bero, A. W., Holtzman, D. M., … Csernansky, J. G. (2009). Effects of voluntary and forced exercise on plaque deposition, hippocampal volume, and behavior in the Tg2576 mouse model of Alzheimer's disease. *Neurobiology of Disease*, *35*(3), 426–432. doi:10.1016/j.nbd.2009.06.002

Zelinski, E. M., Spina, L. M., Yaffe, K., Ruff, R., Kennison, R. F., Mahncke, H. W., & Smith, G. E. (2011). Improvement in memory with plasticity-based adaptive cognitive training: Results of the 3-month follow-up. *Journal of the American Geriatrics Society*, *59*(2), 258–265. doi:10.1111/j.1532-5415.2010.03277.x

19

The Reticular-Activating Hypofrontality (RAH) Model

Arne Dietrich, Julien Dirani, and Zeead Yaghi

Introduction

This chapter summarizes the key points of a neurocognitive model of the effects of acute exercise on the brain. This model, which is known as the reticular-activating hypofrontality or RAH model, proposes a set of neural mechanisms for the cognitive and emotional changes that occur during exercise. To make sense of the varied data in the field, any attempt to provide a brain mechanism for the psychological effects of exercise has to make two categorical distinctions: (1) between chronic and acute exercise and (2) between executive functions and all other kinds of cognitive processes. While chronic exercise refers to exercise over long periods of time (e.g., weeks or months), acute exercise refers to exercise that is currently ongoing. As we will see, whether cognitive and emotional processes are facilitated or impaired with exercise depends on both factors, that is, what kind of mental process is measured and at what time point (during or after exercise) it is measured. Because the effects are orthogonal, any global statement about exercise and cognition is likely to be meaningless.

The available data shows that performance on cognitive tasks that require substantial executive processes are impaired during acute exercise (Audiffren et al., 2009; Davranche & McMorris, 2009; Del Giorno et al., 2010; Dietrich & Sparling, 2004; Mahoney et al., 2007; McMorris et al., 2009; Pontifex & Hillman, 2007). On the other hand, simpler reaction-time tasks show a facilitation effect during acute exercise; an effect that is true irrespective of the nature of the task or the type of exercise (Audiffren, 2009; Etnier et al., 1997; McMorris & Graydon, 2000; Tomporowski, 2003). However, this facilitation effect does not last into the post-exercise period (Audiffren et al., 2008; Brisswalter et al., 1997) or if exercise is maintained until exhaustion (Cian et al., 2000, 2001). Equally, executive functions might be facilitated when measured post-exercise (see Dietrich & Audiffren, 2011). Finally, exercise also has positive effects on emotions and well-being, which is true for acute as well as post-exercise assessments (Dietrich & McDaniel, 2004; Salmon, 2001; Scully et al., 1998).

The RAH model is an explanation for the psychological changes during a single bout of exercise. Exercise, however, also has long-term effects on mental function, such as the sparing of higher cognitive functions in aging (Colcombe & Kramer, 2003; Hillman, Erickson, & Kramer, 2008; Kramer, Erickson, & Colcombe, 2006). Such neuroprotective effects, the fruits of a life-long habit of exercising, must have different mechanisms underlying them. The durability of chronic effects cannot come from changes in neuronal activity patterns but require relatively permanent structural changes to the nervous system, such as angiogenesis (e.g., Swain et al., 2003), synaptogenesis (e.g., Chu & Jones, 2000), or neurogenesis (e.g., Cotman & Engesser-Cesar, 2002; van Praag et al., 1999). These molecular and cellular mechanisms are entirely outside the domain of the present model.

Basic Concepts of the RAH Model

A fundamental concept of the RAH model is the distinction between the implicit and the explicit system. While the explicit system is rule based and its content can be verbalized, the implicit system is skill or experience based and its content cannot be verbalized. That is, contrary to the content of the implicit system, the content of the explicit system is available to consciousness (Dienes & Perner, 1999, 2002; Reber, 1989; Schacter & Buckner, 1998; Squire, 1992; Willingham, 1998). The available literature shows that the brain circuitry that underlies the explicit system is heavily dependent on prefrontal regions, especially the dorsolateral prefrontal cortex (dlPFC), which is critical for working memory and executive attention (Baddeley, 1996; Cowan, 1995). Less is known about the specific circuitry of the implicit system, but the basal ganglia, cerebellum, and supplementary motor area (SMA) have been shown to be involved (Mishkin et al., 1984; Poldrack & Packard, 2003). It is generally agreed that both systems can be distinguished in terms of anatomy and function.

Another way to understand this difference is by seeing the explicit system as capable of representing knowledge at a higher-order level. As such, the explicit system has information about the information it contains (Keele et al., 2003). This omnidirectional availability makes the information accessible, via a global workspace, to other systems in the brain (Dehaene & Changeux, 2004). Information in the more primitive implicit system, however, is not available to consciousness, which means that it does not form higher-order representations and thus cannot engage in metacognitive processes (Cleeremans & Jiménez, 2002; Haider & Frensch, 2005; Karmiloff-Smith, 1992; Kihlstrom, 1996; MacDonald, 2008). This difference is best understood in terms of the flexibility-efficiency tradeoff. The complexity of the explicit system makes it cognitively flexible. But the tradeoff of such a complex system is inefficiency. The simplicity of the implicit system means that it is not burdened by higher-order processing and thus efficient and speedy in terms of motor execution. But it is exactly that simplicity that makes it also cognitively inflexible (Dietrich, 2004b; Radel et al., 2015).

This flexibility-efficiency tradeoff becomes obvious once we see it from an evolutionary perspective. Each system has evolved for a different purpose and these different purposes are mutually exclusive. Cognitive flexibility precludes efficiency and vice versa. One cannot have both in the same system. Once a system is complex in order to handle more cognitive flexibility, it is necessarily slow. But motor output in the real world has to happen in real time and for that one requires an efficient system that is not burdened by complexity (Dietrich, 2004a; Dietrich & Audiffren, 2011; Dienes & Perner, 1999, 2002; Reber, 1989). Since movement must occur in real time, a motor skill is most efficiently performed when controlled by the implicit system (Dietrich, 2004a, 2015).

The evolutionary benefit of a hypofrontality process during efficient motion is also highlighted by this tradeoff. Motion that is controlled by the explicit system, such as using your non-dominant hand to execute a tennis serve, is inefficient (DeCaro & Beilock, 2009; Ravizza, 1977; Wulf & Lewthwaite, 2009; Wulf & Prinz, 2001). In other words, thinking explicitly about a well-learned movement while executing it will lower its efficiency and accuracy. As a consequence, a motor skill is best done when the involvement of the explicit system is minimized. The adaptive role of a hypofrontality process, then, would be to minimize the involvement of complex prefrontal processes when they are not useful, that is, when time is of the essence. As any downhill skier can attest to, there is no point in engaging higher-order mental processes when you need to be quick. It is not difficult to understand why the notion of hypofrontality during physical exercise may seem counterintuitive at first. How can the downregulation of the prefrontal cortex be good for you? But from an evolutionary perspective, and in light of the opposing computational demands, the answer becomes immediately apparent.

In the next two sections, we will describe the basic neural and cognitive mechanisms that underlie these opponent processes of activation and deactivation. This yin-yang is known as the reticular-activating-hypofrontality or RAH model (Dietrich & Audiffren, 2011) to denote the idea that two specific brain mechanisms exist to accomplish this complex set of effects.

The first is an activation process. Physical activity leads to activation of arousal systems in the brainstem's reticular formation. There are several of those arousal systems that vary in terms of anatomy, neurotransmitter, and function (Robbins & Everitt, 1995, 2007). Together, they provide the energy required to maintain the exercise, including the activation of the endocrine and the autonomic nervous systems. In addition, they activate cortical regions that decrease reaction times for simpler perceptual and motor tasks.

The second is a deactivation process. The brain, in order to drive the bodily motion, is forced to make profound changes to the way it allocates its metabolic resources. This follows from three fundamental principles in neuroscience: (1) the brain has a finite energy supply; (2) bodily motion is an extremely demanding task for the brain, and (3) neural processing occurs on a competitive basis. This is to say, the brain cannot maintain activation in all its networks at once and activity in one structure must come at the expense of others (Gusnard & Raichle, 2001; Nybo & Secher, 2004; Woolsey et al., 1996). For exercise, the enormous demands on motor, sensory, and autonomic brain regions result in fewer resources available for activity in brain structures not directly involved in controlling the movements. So, as the brain sustains, during exercise, the massive and widespread neural activation that runs motor units, assimilates sensory inputs, and coordinates autonomic regulation, it must take metabolic resources, given their limited availability, away from neural structures whose functions are not critically needed at the time, which are first and foremost, according to the transient hypofrontality theory (THT), areas of the prefrontal cortex (Dietrich, 2006).

The Reticular-Activating Process

The reticular activating process is responsible for the facilitation of relatively simple and automatic processes during and shortly after exercise. It cannot explain the exercise-induced changes to explicit cognition, emotional processes, or changes to mental status. When seen from an evolutionary angle, this makes sense because the phylogenetically ancient arousal systems evolved to aid decision-making in the phylogenetically older implicit system in pressure situations. It did not evolve to affect the explicit system, which our ape ancestors did not have or to protect mental functions in old age, which our ape ancestors did not reach. This shows, at a minimum, that the extension of the reticular activating process to explain exercise-induced changes in explicit processing requires additional theoretical considerations.

As a neural mechanism for implicit, stimulus-driven task performance during exercise catecholaminergic arousal is well established and relatively uncontroversial. We thus keep this section concise, as the only new proposal it contains is that the reticular activating process should not be applied beyond implicit processing with respect to explaining the facilitating effects of acute exercise on cognition. We also keep short the discussion of the two cognitive-energetic models exercise scientists most commonly use to account for the data in the field (Kahneman, 1973; Sanders, 1983). That is, they remain relatively uncontroversial when applied to implicit processing. For explicit processing, however, they can no longer be used without accommodation. The reason for this lies in the same cause, the failure to come to terms with the consequences of the explicit/implicit distinction, especially for motion.

The reticular activating system consists of several distinct but interrelated arousal systems that are differentiated by anatomy (specific nuclei and their projections), neurotransmitter (norepinephrine, dopamine, and serotonin, mostly), and function (Robbins & Everitt, 2007).

Briefly, the noradrenergic system originates in the locus coeruleus of the pons and projects profusely to areas of the forebrain. It mediates alertness and appears to be involved in detecting sensory signals and maintaining discrimination processes under high levels of arousal and stress. Critically for exercise, increases in noradrenergic transmission improve the signal-to-noise ratio for signal detection.

The dopaminergic system originates from cell bodies located in the substantia nigra and the ventral tegmentum. It projects to (1) the dorsal and ventral striatum, which, in turn, modulate activity in a large network involving the motor thalamus, SMA, premotor area, and primary motor cortex; (2) several structures in the limbic system, such as the nucleus accumbens; and (3) cortical regions, particularly the prefrontal cortex. Together, these pathways activate or energize behavior and account for the vigor and frequency of behavioral outputs (Robbins & Everitt, 2007).

The serotonergic system originates from cell bodies located in the raphe nucleus and projects from there widely throughout the brain and spinal cord. This system appears to moderate the stimulating effects of catecholamine activity and thus promotes behavioral inhibition and cortical deactivation (Meeusen et al., 2006; Robbins & Everitt, 2007).

A large body of evidence shows that acute exercise activates all three of these monoamine systems (e.g., Meeusen & De Meirleir, 1995). As such, they have figured prominently in mechanistic explanations of the effects of exercise on mental processes. The link between exercise, arousal, central catecholamines and improvements in cognitive performance is based on the idea that exercise is an arousing stressor and today the arousing effects of exercise, on peripheral and central systems, are well documented. Acute exercise also activates both the sympathetic nervous system and the hypothalamo-pituitary-adrenal axis, which results in the release of catecholamines and indolamines, both centrally and peripherally (e.g., Meeusen & De Meirleir, 1995; Wittert, 2000). In conclusion, it is generally accepted that brain catecholamines are involved in the improvements of performance on procedural and relatively simple decisional tasks during exercise.

Cognitive psychology alone cannot explain the variability of mental performance during physical exercise (Hockey et al., 1986). Energetic considerations must supplement cognitive models in this case. Energetic psychology is more concerned with the intensive or energizing aspects of behavior as opposed to its directional or semantic aspects. Arousal and activation are concepts that were associated early on with energy mobilization or release within the organism (Duffy, 1962). Their relation to performance goes back even further, to the earliest days of experimental psychology and the famous U-shaped function (Yerkes & Dodson, 1908). Like the RAH model, the inverted-U model can account for some of the opposing effects of acute exercise on cognition. Given the idea that physical exercise is an arousing stressor (Cooper, 1973; Davey, 1973), one would expect an inverted-U function between exercise and cognition (Kahneman, 1973; Näätänen, 1973), but the empirical data has not lent support to this hypothesis (McMorris & Graydon, 2000; Tomporowski, 2003). Moreover, the inverted-U model is descriptive in nature; it does not contain, like the RAH model, an explanatory mechanism at either the neural or cognitive levels. As said, the most important shortcoming of it is, however, that it does not distinguish between explicit and implicit processing, which explains to a large extent why the cognitive data is so varied and inconclusive. In addition to arousal, it only considers task complexity and difficulty level.

Kahneman (1973) provided perhaps the first full cognitive-energetic model. This model regards the total amount of resources, which exist in a single, undifferentiated pool, as limited. The availability of resources depends on the level of arousal, which, in turn, is determined by two sources, task demand and several other sources, such as stimulus intensity, psychoactive drugs, anxiety, or, for that matter, exercise. The model postulates a so-called allocation policy mechanism that directs and supervises the allotment of resources, which, in turn, is determined by such factors as dispositions, intentions, or feedback from on-going activities. The level of arousal, then, corresponds to the amount of available resources and decrements in performance occur when task demands exceed the resource availability.

The Kahneman model assumes that there is a general, nonspecific pool of energetic resources that supports all cognitive functions. But such unitary concepts of arousal cannot explain the data, such as, for instance, the low correlations among different measures of arousal (Eysenck, 1982; Thayer, 1989) or the perfect time-sharing of two resource-demanding tasks (Wickens, 1984). In addition, the neural substrate underlying arousal, the reticular formation, is not, as already stated, a homogenous system, but consists of several highly differentiated systems. In response to such challenges, subsequent cognitive-energetic models of human performance shifted from a unidimensional conception of resources – one unique reservoir – to a multidimensional view that permits the operation of several different supply systems. In the model of Sanders (1983, 1998), probably the most commonly used by exercise scientists, there are three energetic mechanisms: arousal, activation, and effort. Each of these resource pools influences, at the cognitive level, a specific stage of information processing. Sanders linked arousal to sensory and perceptual processes, activation to the motor adjustment stage, and effort to response selection. An acute bout of exercise can increase the arousal and/or activation mechanism, which can modulate input (sensory processes) and/or output (motor processes), respectively.

Both cognitive-energetic models are all built on the assumption that there is only one, single cognitive system. This makes it impossible to explain the full range of psychological effects because exercise seems to affect the implicit and the explicit systems in opposing ways. This failure is not a problem with the models themselves, of course, as they predate this advance in cognitive psychology, but with the fact that none of these models were developed further in order to reflect this knowledge. This is curious insofar as this putative distinction between explicit and implicit processing is well known in exercise science.

As an example, consider effortless attention. Flow is a state in which superior performance is associated with a decrease in mental effort and attention (Bruya, 2009; Dietrich & Stoll, 2010). Flow, like other phenomena of effortless performance, is impossible to explain for traditional theories of attention and mental effort for the simple reason that they assume that better performance, even on a well-learned task, is associated with increased conscious effort allocated to that task. The effort mechanism, in both the Kahneman and Sanders models, also assumes that higher task demands require more effort, both objectively, in terms of caloric consumption by the brain, and subjectively, in terms of perceived, felt effort. In flow, however, the opposite is true. Here the mental effort decreases to the point of effortlessness, yet such automatic action is associated with improved performance. Flow is not a paradox at all if we uncouple explicit from implicit processes (Dietrich 2004a). In fact, improvements on well-learned, stimulus-driven tasks can only occur, according to the RAH model, if the explicit system, and thus effort, is decreased.

Another example is the impairment on executive tasks during exercise. Neither the Kahneman nor the Sanders model predicts such a selective effect on specific types of cognitive processes, which is likely a key reason why this phenomenon was not documented until a few years ago (Dietrich & Sparling, 2004). To clarify, both models do predict performance impairments. However, in the Kahneman model, performance is said to decline when exercise and the cognitive task compete for resources. In the Sanders model, decrements occur when that competition is over effort. Either concept, however, fails to explain why the negative effects of exercise are selective for explicit processing even if task difficulty and effort is controlled for. Finally, unlike the RAH model, the above cognitive-energetic models also fail to account for the effects of exercise on emotions.

The Sanders cognitive-energetic model is useful in localizing the facilitation effect physical exercise has on relatively simple cognitive processes. It identifies four stages: (1) a pre-processing stage influenced selectively by signal intensity; (2) a feature extraction stage influenced by signal quality; (3) a response selection stage influenced by stimulus-response compatibility; and, finally, (4) a motor adjustment stage influenced by the fore period duration. Using the additive factors methods of the discrete serial information processing model (Sternberg, 1998), one can pinpoint the processing stage exercise affects and the empirical data suggest that the facilitating effects of acute exercise on mean reaction time occur at the level of motor processes (Arcelin et al., 1998).

The sum of the evidence shows that the facilitating effects of exercise on stimulus-driven, bottom-up processing is modulated by arousal and activation, that is, the reticular activating process speeds up reaction times by enhancing early sensory as well as motor processes.

The Hypofrontality Process

The hypofrontality process has mental effects opposite to those induced by the reticular activating process. The process is anchored in the flexibility-efficiency tradeoff between the explicit and implicit system. From an evolutionary perspective, a hypofrontality process has to occur in a do-or-die situation involving physical motion; it simply is not adaptive to engage executive processes in such an event. With this in mind, we can now examine the neural mechanism that induces the hypofrontality process during exercise.

The general idea that exercise deactivates brain areas, and that such decreases in brain activity could explain some of the psychological data, was first mooted in the form of the transient hypofrontality theory (Dietrich, 2003, 2006). At first, this seemed counter-intuitive to many people because of a number of widely held but mistaken beliefs about the effects of exercise on brain health and, by extension, mental function. The most common were (are): (a) exercise increases blood supply to the brain and, therefore, oxygen and glucose uptake; (b) bodily motion is taxing for muscles but not (computationally) for brains; and (c) that improvements to mood and cognition must come from a boosting neural activity, a kind of activation-is-good fallacy (Dietrich, 2009). It simply did not make much sense to many people that all those creative ideas and positive feelings during exercise can come from a process that tends to deactivate the pinnacle of human evolution, the prefrontal cortex.

But, as said, the central idea behind the hypofrontality process is based on fundamental neuroscientific principles that are universally accepted by neuroscientists. In consequence, without additional metabolic resources, the brain is forced during exercise to make profound changes to the way it allocates its resources. In the case of exercise, the enormous demands on motor, sensory, and autonomic structures, powered by the reticular-activation process, result in fewer resources available for processes, cognitive or emotional, that are not involved directly in maintaining the motion (Dietrich, 2007).

A few crutches for the imagination may help to understand how computationally complex motor control really is and, as a result, how much resources the brain has to allocate to it. When taken together with the fact that the brain is not the recipient of additional resources – blood, oxygen, glucose, or otherwise – during exercise (see Astrand & Rodahl, 1986; Ide & Secher, 2000), one can grasp more easily the pivotal problem the brain must solve during exercise, especially when that exercise comes in a sustained manner involving large muscle groups, as it does in sports and exercise.

Consider first artificial intelligence, a field that has long understood motion as a gigantic computational problem. We still do not have robots remotely capable of returning a tennis serve. This is not because we cannot make the moveable equipment – arms, legs, joints, etc. – but because we cannot make the calculation for such super fast sensorimotor integration processes in real time. Motion is computationally, and thus metabolically, very costly indeed.

Another example is the brain's motor system. By simply listing the number of neural regions devoted to movement, one can get an idea of the complexity of moving the body around: primary motor cortex, secondary motor cortices (i.e., premotor and SMA), basal ganglia, the motor thalamus, cerebellum, red nucleus, substantia nigra, the massive pathway systems, and the motor neurons all along the spinal cord, among rather many others. This represents not just an enormous amount of brain volume but also a very high number, in percentage terms, of neurons. The cerebellum, for instance, has more neurons than any other structure in the brain, including the entire cerebral cortex. Movement also requires sensory processes and soon we are at yet another, nearly equally long list of brain structures that must be activated in order to process the relevant perceptual information during exercise. Add to this all the nuclei mediating autonomic regulation, such as in the hypothalamus, the reticular formation, and many nuclei in the medulla, and we can see how much the brain is activated for nothing other than the simple act of running (Dietrich, 2008). Given that the brain must balance its budget, there must be brain structures that pay for all this.

A detailed review of the existing evidence on exercise and cognitive function can be found elsewhere (Dietrich & Audiffren, 2011). In general, however, it can be stated that the weight of the animal and human literature permits the conclusion that the pattern of neural activity during aerobic exercise can be regarded as a state of generalized brain activation with the specific exclusion of the executive system in prefrontal and other cortical and limbic regions.

Acute exercise also has positive effects on emotions, especially depression, anxiety, and stress. Neither the reticular-activating process nor the cognitive-energetic models of Kahneman (1973) and Sanders (1983, 1998) can accommodate these data. Similarly, this change in mood states cannot be explained, as is sometimes done, by the activation of the opioid or serotonin systems (Dietrich & McDaniel, 2004). But the notion of a hypofrontality process suggest a possible neural mechanisms because evidence shows that some affective disorders, such as depression and several of the anxiety disorders, are accompanied by excessive activity in prefrontal and limbic regions (Baxter, 1990; Baxter et al., 1987; LeDoux, 1996; Mayberg, 1997; Mayberg et al., 1995). Treatment with serotonin reuptake inhibitors results in a normalization of this hypermetabolism in prefrontal regions (Mayberg et al., 1995). Interestingly, healthy subjects asked to think sad thoughts show a similar pattern of cortical activity (Damasio et al., 2000).

The concept of exercise-induced prefrontal downregulation suggests a brain mechanism by which exercise might be beneficial to mood. According to the THT, an exercising individual enters, sooner or later, a mental state marked by a transient decrease in prefrontal function. The massive neural activity caused by the large-scale bodily motion, coupled with the brain's finite metabolic resources, makes it impossible for the brain to sustain excessive neural activity in brain structures, such as the prefrontal cortex and the amygdala, that are not needed at the time. As the brain must run on safe mode the very structures that appear to compute the information engendering stress, anxiety, and negative thinking in the first place, we experience relief from life's worries (for details, see Dietrich, 2003, 2006).

In closing, it should be noted that the RAH model cannot provide a sound, mechanistic explanation for several other psychological changes that occur as a response to exercise, such as analgesia and sedation as well as the much rarer occurrences of euphoria and a state of bliss. The suppression of pain sensations, a sense of calm and well being, as well as the occasional experience of a euphoric state, especially in endurance athletes, has long been ascribed to endorphin release, but evidence for this possibility has only been supplied very recently (Boecker et al., 2008). In addition, there is also evidence that the endocannabinoid system is involved (Dietrich & McDaniel, 2004; Sparling et al., 2003). To what extent these mental phenomena are mediated by opioid and lipid neurotransmitters is not clear, but there is, at present, no solid, alternative explanation for them.

An Applied Example

What can the RAH model tell us about the brain activity of, say, a long-distance runner in the midst of a long run? Of course, one would not expect a few minutes of light jogging to have large-scale effects on a person's mental status. But a few hours of hard running can drastically alter cognitive performance. The question that arises then is how we get from A to B. What is the shape of the curve describing the progressive decline in cognitive function that must take place? Likewise, when – and why – is the initial improvement of automatic processing reversed into a impairment? And, where is the peak of that function?

Suppose a runner reaches a steady-state plateau just below the anaerobic threshold – a typical marathon pace. To keep things simple, suppose also that neither hydration nor glucose availability enters into the equation and that our runner possesses the muscular and cardiovascular fitness to run long enough to make matters interesting for the brain.

Almost immediately, our imaginary runner activates the various arousal systems in the brainstem. This activation supplies the energy needed for the relevant motor, sensory, and autonomic processes. This reticular activating process also stimulates cortical and subcortical regions that modulate relatively straightforward attention and decision-making processes. The limited data we have on this suggest that this facilitation effect seems to starts soon after movement starts, it is not dramatic enough to be noticed by the naked eye; that is, precise measurement is needed to detect it, and it can last for a considerable amount of time, certainly more than 40 minutes into the run.

The allocation of such a large part of the energetic resources has consequences for all brain structures that do not directly contribute to the on-going action. Within 5 to 10 minutes apparently, given the data (Kemppainen et al., 2005; Tashiro et al., 2001), some prefrontal and other cortical and limbic regions show decreased activity. As this hypofrontality process sets in, processing in the explicit system is held back by the shortage of resources. Since this sort of explicit processing is not needed – or desirable – in most cases, this effect, too, goes unnoticed by the naked eye; that is, a specific neuropsychological test is needed to detect this phenomenon. We do not know how strong this effect is but can assume that with continued running it can only get worse. The hypofunction of prefrontal areas then eliminates from phenomenology negative emotional processes, such as ruminating about the past or worrying about the future, that are caused by these very regions being hyperactive. As this excessive activity is checked by the on-going motion, our runner becomes calm and relaxed.

If we take a look at our runner's mental and brain state at 40 minutes, we cannot say that there is much drama. Aside from a bit of catecholaminergic arousal to quicken response latency and a bit of hypofrontality to take the edge off, effects which are both so weak that they escape most attempts of introspective detection, all that has noticeably changed is that our runner feels somewhat more peaceful and calm. Should our runner stop here, matters will never get critical and all bodily systems would return to normal.

Suppose our runner is sufficiently fit to push past 40 minutes. We have very little data to support claims about what happens from there on forward. For the explicit system, we can presuppose that the unrelenting metabolic taxation further takes its toll. This would, presumably, start at the highest-order brain structure, the prefrontal cortex, and continue down the functional hierarchy of the brain, one phenomenological subtraction at a time, leading to experiences of more profound distortions of thinking, such as ephemeral attention, the loss of the sense of self and agency, or feelings of timelessness (Dietrich, 2007). Note that such alterations cannot be explained by any other neuroscientific theory of exercise. These phenomena, however, readily conform, especially in terms of phenomenology, to a state of prefrontal hypofunction (Dietrich, 2003).

For implicit processing, the one thing we can say for sure is that somewhere, somehow, the initial facilitation also turns into a deficit (Cian et al., 2000, 2001; Grego et al., 2004). This is easily corroborated by commonsense; just think of your own cognitive capacity after an all-day hike to exhaustion. But it is far from clear what neural mechanism might lie behind this reversal of fortunes. There are several proposals for the so-called central fatigue hypothesis, which are neurobiological (Nybo & Secher, 2004) and psychological (Noakes et al., 2004) in nature. But the RAH model can also inform this body of work. For people so physically fit that they do not succumb to peripheral fatigue first – muscular or cardiovascular, that this – the brain's position, in terms of energetic resources, could become increasingly precarious with continued running. Inevitably, when somebody lives too long beyond his means, there will be, at some point, a rude awakening. Should this indeed be so, the brain would be forced, like a sinking ship, to throw overboard more and more neural networks until it reaches even those that drive the very motion itself. In the end, the failure to drive the relevant motor units might contribute to central fatigue.

References

Arcelin, R., Delignières, D., & Brisswalter, J. (1998). Selective effects of physical exercise on choice reaction processes. *Perceptual and Motor Skills, 87*, 175–185.

Astrand, P., & Rodahl, K. (1986). *Textbook of work physiology* (3rd ed.). New York, NY: McGraw Hill.

Audiffren, M. (2009). Acute exercise and psychological function: A cognitive-energetic approach. In T. McMorris, P. D. Tomporowski, & M. Audiffren (Eds.), *Exercise and Cognitive Function* (pp. 3–39). New York, NY: Wiley.

Audiffren, M., Tomporowski, P., & Zagrodnik, J. (2008). Acute aerobic exercise and information processing: Energizing motor processes doing a choice reaction time task. *Acta Psychologica, 129*, 410–419.

Audiffren, M., Tomporowski, P., & Zagrodnik, J. (2009). Acute aerobic exercise and information processing: Modulation of executive control in a random number generation task. *Acta Psychologica, 132*, 85–95.

Baddeley, A. (1996). Exploring the central executive. *Quarterly Journal of Experimental Psychology, 49A*, 5–28.

Baxter, L. R. (1990). Brain imaging as a tool in establishing a theory of brain pathology in obsessive-compulsive disorder. *Journal of Clinical Psychiatry, 51* (Suppl.), 22–25.

Baxter, L. R., Phelps, M. E., Mazziota, J. C., Guze, B. H., Schwartz, J. M., & Selin, C. E. (1987). Local cerebral glucose metabolic rates in obsessive-compulsive disorder: A comparison with rates in unipolar depression and normal controls. *Archives of General Psychiatry, 44*, 211–218.

Boecker, H., Sprenger, T., Spilker, M. E., Henriksen, G., Koppenhoefer, M., Wagner, K. J., Valet, M., Berthele, A., & Tolle, T. R. (2008). The runner's high: Opioidergic mechanisms in the human brain. *Cerebral Cortex, 18*, 2523–2531.

Brisswalter, J., Arcelin, R., Audiffren, M., & Delignieres, D. (1997). Influence of physical exercise on simple reaction time: Effects of physical fitness. *Perceptual and Motor Skills, 85*, 1019–1027.

Bruya, J. (2009). Effortlessness attention. In B. J. Bruya (Ed.), *Effortless attention: A new perspective in the cognitive science of attention and action* (pp. 1–28). Cambridge, MA: MIT Press.

Chu, C. J., & Jones, T. A. (2000). Experience-dependent structural plasticity in cortex heterotopic to focal sensorimotor cortical damage. *Experimental Neurology, 166*, 403–414.

Cian, C., Barraud, P. A., Melin, B., & Raphel, C. (2001). Effects of fluid ingestion on cognitive function after heat stress or exercise-induced dehydration. *International Journal of Psychophysiology, 42*, 243–251.

Cian, C., Koulmann, N., Barraud, P. A., Raphel, C., Jimenez, C., & Melin, B. (2000). Influences of variations in body hydration on cognitive function: Effects of hyperhydration, heat stress, and exercise-induced dehydration. *Journal of Psychophysiology, 14*, 29–36.

Cleeremans, A., & Jiménez, L. (2002). Implicit learning and consciousness: A graded, dynamic perspective. In R. M. French & A. Cleeremans (Eds.), *Implicit learning and consciousness* (pp. 1–40). London, UK: Psychology Press.

Colcombe, S., & Kramer, A. F. (2003). Fitness effects on the cognitive function of older adults: A meta-analytic study. *Psychological Science, 14*, 125–130.

Cooper, C. J. (1973). Anatomical and physiological mechanisms of arousal with specific reference to the effects of exercise. *Ergonomics, 16*, 601–609.

Cotman, C. W., & Engesser-Cesar, C. (2002). Exercise enhances and protects brain function. *Exercise and Sport Sciences Reviews, 30*, 75–79.

Cowan, N. (1995). *Attention and memory: An integrated framework.* Oxford Psychology Series, No 26. New York, NY: Oxford University Press.

Damasio, A. R., Graboweski, T. J., Bechera, A., Damasio, H., Ponto, L. L. B., Parvizi, J., & Hichwa, R. D. (2000). Subcortical and cortical brain activity during the feeling of self-generated emotions. *Nature Neuroscience, 3*, 1049–1056.

Davey, C. P. (1973). Physical exertion and mental performance. *Ergonomics, 16*, 595–599.

Davranche, K., & McMorris, T. (2009). Specific effects of acute moderate exercise on cognitive control. *Brain & Cognition, 69*, 565–570.

DeCaro, M.S., & Beilock, S. L. (2009). The benefits and perils of attentional control. In B. J. Bruya (Ed.), *Effortless attention: A new perspective in the cognitive science of attention and action* (pp. 51–74). Cambridge, MA: MIT Press.

Dehaene, S., & Changeux, J. P. (2004). Neural mechansims for access to consciousness. In M. S. Gazzaniga, (Ed.), *The Cognitive Neurosciences* (3rd ed., pp. 1145–1158). Cambridge, MA: MIT Press.

Del Giorno, J. M., Hall, E. E., O'Leary K. C., Bixby, W. R., & Miller, P. C. (2010). Cognitive function during acute exercise: A test of the transient hypofrontality theory. *Journal of Sport and Exercise Psychology, 32*, 312–323.

Dienes, Z., & Perner, J. (1999). A theory of implicit and explicit knowledge. *Behavioural and Brain Sciences, 5*, 735–808.

Dienes, Z., & Perner, J. (2002). A theory of the implicit nature of implicit learning. In R. M. French & A. Cleeremans (Eds.), *Implicit learning and consciousness* (pp. 68–92). New York, NY: Psychology Press.

Dietrich, A. (2003). Functional neuroanatomy of altered states of consciousness: The transient hypofrontality hypothesis. *Consciousness and Cognition, 12*, 231–256.

Dietrich, A. (2004a). Neurocognitive mechanisms underlying the experience of flow. *Consciousness and Cognition, 13*, 746–761.

Dietrich, A. (2004b). The cognitive neuroscience of creativity. *Psychonomic Bulletin and Review, 11*, 1011–1026.

Dietrich, A. (2006). Transient hypofrontality as a mechanism for the psychological effects of exercise. *Psychiatry Research, 145*, 79–83.

Dietrich, A. (2007). *Introduction to consciousness*. London, UK: Palgrave Macmillan.

Dietrich, A. (2008). Imaging the imagination: The trouble with motor imagery. *Methods, 45*, 319–324.

Dietrich, A. (2009). The cognitive neuroscience of exercise: The transient hypofrontality theory and its implications for cognition and emotion. In T. McMorris, P. D. Tomporowski, & M. Audiffren (Eds.), *Exercise and Cognitive Function* (pp. 69–90). New York, NY: Wiley.

Dietrich, A. (2015). *How creativity happens in the brain*. London, UK: Palgrave Macmillan.

Dietrich, A., & Audiffren, M. (2011). The reticular-activating hypofrontality (RAH) model of acute exercise. *Neuroscience & Biobehavioral Reviews, 35*, 1305–1325.

Dietrich, A., & McDaniel, W. F. (2004). Cannabinoids and exercise. *British Journal of Sports Medicine, 38*, 536–541.

Dietrich, A., & Sparling, P. B. (2004). Endurance exercise selectively impairs prefrontal-dependent cognition. *Brain and Cognition, 55*, 516–524.

Dietrich, A., & Stoll, O. (2010). Effortlessness attention, hypofrontality and perfectionism. In B. J. Bruya (Ed.), *Effortless attention: A new perspective in the cognitive science of attention and action* (pp. 159–178). Cambridge, MA: MIT Press.

Duffy, E. (1962). *Activation and behavior*. New York, NY: Wiley.

Etnier, J. L., Salazar, W., Landers, D. M., Petruzzello, S. J., Han, M., & Nowell, P. (1997). The influence of physical fitness and exercise upon cognitive functioning: A meta-analysis. *Journal of Sports & Exercise Psychology, 19*, 249–277.

Eysenck, M. W. (1982). *Attention and arousal*. Berlin: Springer-Verlag.

Grego, F., Vallier, J.-M., Collardeau, M., Bermon, S., Ferrari, P., Candito, M., Bayer, P., Magnié, M.-N., & Brisswalter, J. (2004). Effects of long duration exercise on cognitive function, blood glucose, and counterregulatory hormones in male cyclists. *Neuroscience Letters, 364*, 76–80.

Gusnard, D. A., & Raichle, M. E. (2001). Searching for a baseline: Functional imaging and the resting human brain. *Nature Review Neuroscience, 2*, 685–694.

Haider, H., & Frensch, P. A. (2005). The generation of conscious awareness in an incidental learning situation. *Psychological Research, 69*, 399–411.

Hillman, C. H., Erickson, K. I., & Kramer, A. F. (2008). Be smart, exercise your heart: Exercise effects on brain and cognition. *Nature Reviews Neuroscience, 9*, 58–65.

Hockey, G. R. J., Coles, M. G. H., & Gaillard, A. W. K. (1986). Energetical issues in research on human information processing. In G. R. J. Hockey, A. W. K. Gaillard, & M. G. H Coles. (Eds.), *Energetics and Human Information Processing* (pp. 3–21). Dordrecht, The Netherlands: Martinus Nijhoff Publishers.

Ide, K., & Secher, N. H. (2000). Cerebral blood flow and metabolism during exercise. *Progress in Neurobiology, 61*, 397–414.

Kahneman, D. (1973). *Attention and effort*. Englewood Cliffs, NJ: Prentice-Hall.

Karmiloff-Smith, A. (1992). Beyond modularity: A developmental perspective on cognitive science. Cambridge, MA: MIT Press.

Keele, S. W., Ivry, R., Mayr, U., Hazeltine, E., & Heuer, H. (2003). The cognitive and neural architecture of sequence representation. *Psychological Review, 110*, 316–339.

Kemppainen, J., Aalto, S., Fujimoto, T., Kalliokoski, K. K., Långsjö, J., Oikonen, V., Rinne, J., Nuutila, P., & Knuuti, J. (2005). High intensity exercise decreases global brain glucose uptake in humans. *Journal of Physiology, 568*, 323–332.

Kihlstrom, J. F. (1996). Perception without awareness of what is perceived, learning without awareness of what is learned. In M. Velmans (Ed.), *The science of consciousness: Psychological, neuropsychological and clinical reviews* (pp. 23–46). London, UK: Routledge.

Kramer, A. F., Erickson, K. I., & Colcombe, S. J. (2006). Exercise, cognition and the aging brain. *Journal of Applied Physiology, 101*, 1237–1242.

LeDoux, J. (1996). *The emotional brain*. New York, NY: Touchstone.

MacDonald, K. B. (2008). Effortful control, explicit processing, and the regulation of human evolved predispositions. *Psychological Review, 115*, 1012–1031.

Mahoney, C. R., Hirsch, E., Hasselquist, L., Lesher, L. L., & Lieberman, H. R. (2007). The effects of movement and physical exertion on soldier vigilance. *Aviation, Space, and Environmental Medicine*, *78*, B51–B57.

Mayberg, H. S. (1997). Limbic-cortical dysregulation: A proposed model of depression. *Journal of Neuropsychiatry and Clinical Neuroscience*, *9*, 471–481.

Mayberg, H. S., Mahurin, R. K., & Brannon, K. S. (1995). Parkinson's depression: Discrimination of mood-sensitive and mood insensitive cognitive deficits using fluoxetine and FDG PET. *Neurology*, *45*, A166.

McMorris, T., Davranche, K., Jones, G., Hall, B., Corbett, J., & Minter, C. (2009). Acute incremental exercise, performance of a central executive task, and sympathoadrenal system and hypothalamic-pituitary-adrenal axis activity. *International Journal of Psychophysiology*, *73*, 334–340.

McMorris, T., & Graydon, J. (2000). The effect of incremental exercise on cognitive performance. *International Journal of Sport Psychology*, *31*, 66–81.

Meeusen, R., & De Meirleir, K. (1995). Exercise and brain neurotransmission. *Sports Medicine*, *20*, 160–188.

Meeusen, R., Watson, P., Hasegawa, H., Roelands, B., & Piacentini, M., (2006). Central fatigue: The serotonin hypothesis and beyond. *Sports Medicine*, *36*, 881–909.

Mishkin, M., Malamut, B., & Bachevalier, J. (1984). Memory and habit: Two neural systems. In G. Lynch, J. J. McGaugh, & N. M. Weinberger (Eds.), *Neurobiology of learning and memory* (pp. 66–77). New York, NY: Guilford Press.

Näätänen, R. (1973). The inverted-U relationship between activation and performance: A critical review. In S. Kornblum (Ed.), *Attention and performance IV* (pp. 155–174). New York, NY: Academic Press.

Noakes, T. D., St Clair Gibson, A., & Lambert, E. V. (2004). From catastrophe to complexity: A novel model of integrative central neural regulation of effort and fatigue during exercise in humans. *British Journal of Sports Medicine*, *38*, 511–514.

Nybo, L., & Secher, N. H. (2004). Cerebral perturbations provoked by prolonged exercise. *Progress in Neurobiology*, *72*, 223–261.

Poldrack, R. A., & Packard, M. G. (2003). Competition among multiple memory systems: Converging evidence from animal and human brain studies. *Neuropsychologia*, *41*, 245–251.

Pontifex, M. B., & Hillman, C. H. (2007). Neuroelectric and behavioural indices of interference control during acute cycling. *Clinical Neurophysiology*, *118*, 570–580.

Radel, R., Davranche, K., Fournier, M., & Dietrich, A. (2015). The role of (dis)inhibition in creativity: Decreased inhibition improves idea generation. *Cognition*, *134*, 110–120.

Ravizza, K. (1977). Peak performances in sports. *Journal of Humanistic Psychology*, *4*, 35–40.

Reber, A. S. (1989). Implicit learning and tacit knowledge. *Journal of Experimental Psychology General*, *118*, 219–235.

Robbins, T. W., & Everitt, B. J. (1995). Arousal systems and attention. In M. S. Gazzaniga (Ed.), *The cognitive neurosciences* (pp. 703–720). Cambridge, MA: The MIT Press.

Robbins, T. W., & Everitt, B. J. (2007). A role for mesencephalic dopamine in activation: Commentary on Berridge (2006). *Psychopharmacology*, *191*, 433–437.

Salmon, P. (2001). Effects of physical exercise on anxiety, depression, and sensitivity to stress: A unifying theory. *Clinical Psychological Review*, *21*, 33–61.

Sanders, A. F. (1983). Towards a model of stress and human performance. *Acta Psychologica*, *53*, 61–97.

Sanders, A. F. (1998). *Elements of human performance: Reaction processes and attention in human skill*. Mahwah, NJ: Lawrence Erlbaum Associates.

Schacter, D. L., & Bruckner, R. L. (1998). On the relationship among priming, conscious recollection, and intentional retrieval: Evidence from neuroimaging research. *Neurobiology of Learning and Memory*, *70*, 284–303.

Scully, D., Kremer, J., Meade, M. M., Graham, R., & Dudgeon, K. (1998). Physical exercise and psychological well-being: A critical review. *British Journal of Sports Medicine*, *32*, 111–120.

Sparling, P. B., Giuffrida, A., Piomelli, D., Rosskopf, L., & Dietrich, A. (2003). Exercise activates the endocannabinoid system. *Neuroreport*, *14*, 2209–2211.

Squire, L. R. (1992). Memory and the hippocampus: A synthesis from findings with rats, monkeys and humans. *Psychological Review*, *99*, 195–231.

Sternberg, S. (1998). Discovering mental processing stages: The method of additive factors. In D. Scarborough, & S. Sternberg (Eds.), *An invitation to cognitive science, methods, models, and conceptual issues* (pp. 703–863). Cambridge, MA: MIT Press.

Swain, R. A., Harris, A. B., Wiener, E. C., Dutka, M. V., Morris, H. D., Theien, B. E., Konda, S., Engberg, K., Lauterbur, P. C., & Greenough, W. T. (2003). Prolonged exercise induces angiogenesis and increases cerebral blood volume in primary motor cortex of the rat. *Neuroscience*, *117*, 1037–1046.

Tashiro, M., Itoh, M., Fujimoto, T., Fujiwara, T., Ota, H., Kubota, K., Higuchi, M., Okamura, N., Ishi, K., Berecski, D., & Sasaki, H. (2001). 18F-FDG PET mapping of regional brain activity in runners. *Journal of Sports Medicine and Physical Fitness*, *41*, 11–17.

Thayer, R. E. (1989). *The biopsychology of mood and arousal*. New York, NY: Oxford Press.

Tomporowski, P. D. (2003). Effects of acute bouts of exercise on cognition. *Acta Psychologica, 112*, 297–324.

van Praag, H., Kempermann, G., & Gage, F. H. (1999). Running increases cell proliferation and neurogenesis in the adult mouse dentate gyrus. *Nature Neuroscience, 2*, 266–270.

Wickens, C. D. (1984). Processing resources in attention. In R. Parasuraman & D. R. Davies (Eds.), *Varieties of Attention* (pp. 63–102). Orlando, FL: Academic Press.

Willingham, D. G. (1998). A neuropsychological theory of motor skill learning. *Psychological Review, 105*, 558–584.

Wittert, G. (2000). The effect of exercise on the hypothalamo-pituitary-adrenal axis. In M. P. Warren & N. W. Constantini (Eds.), *Sports endocrinology* (pp. 43–55). Totowa, NJ: Humana Press.

Woolsey, T. A., Rovainen, C. M., Cox, S. B., Henegar, M. H., Liang, G. E., Liu, D., Moskalenko, Y. E., Sui, J. & Wei, L. (1996). Neuronal units linked to microvascular modules in cerebral cortex: Response elements for imaging the brain. *Cerebral Cortex, 6*, 647–660.

Wulf, G., & Lewthwaite, R. (2009). Effortless motor learning?: An external focus of attention enhances movement effectiveness and efficiency. In B. J. Bruya (Ed.), *Effortless attention: A new perspective in the cognitive science of attention and action* (pp. 74–102). Cambridge, MA: MIT Press.

Wulf, G., & Prinz, W. (2001). Directing attention to movement effects enhances learning: A review. *Psychonomic Bulletin & Review, 8*, 648–660.

Yerkes, R. M., & Dodson, J. D. (1908). The relation of strength of stimulus to the rapidity of habit formation. *Journal of Comparative and Neurology and Psychology, 18*, 459–482.

Section IV

Equipment, Instrumentation and Technology in Sport Neuroscience and Psychophysiology

20

Technology Product Options in Sport Neuroscience and Psychophysiology

Divya Jain and Ziba Atak

For sport neuroscience and psychophysiology researchers and practitioners, deciding what instrumentation to use can be challenging. To help keep up with the proliferation of neuropsychophysiological monitoring devices that range from basic consumer to advanced research grade systems, a select review of psychophysiological/neuroscience monitoring equipment that is available for purchase is presented. We have primarily featured systems that are used to monitor cardiac and brain activity. While the listed companies may manufacture a number of systems with differing capabilities, we only included one device per manufacturer that we deemed to be the most advanced and useful for the field of applied sport neuroscience and psychophysiology (applied practice & research). Instrumentation that is ambulatory and capable of wireless on-the playing-field recording is specified. Additional information on the presented systems can be obtained on the manufacturer's website or via e-mail.

In order assist researchers and practitioners in finding equipment that will suit their needs, we have rated instrumentation as follows:

***** Research grade, built-in analytics, real time data tracking, and automatic report generation
**** Research grade, built-in analytics but with third-party software for research-grade analytics
*** Research capable, with third party software for research analytics
** Consumer grade for basic monitoring and rudimentary research
* Consumer grade, with significant clinical/research limitations

We have also classified equipment/instrumentation systems by price:

***** USD 10000 and above
**** USD 7000–10000
*** USD 4000–7000
** USD 1000–3000
* Below USD 1000?

(for instrumentation where software comes with a monthly or yearly subscription, a notation has been made)

Limitations:

Exact prices and other details were not available for all devices mentioned.

The listing provided is selective, not exhaustive.

All information provided in this chapter was obtained from the manufacturer's website or via email correspondence. The authors have not tested most of the instruments listed in the review.

Device	Manufacturer	Website	Grade	Price	Description
Be Alert X24	Advanced Brain Monitoring	www.advancedbrainmonitoring.com	*****	Not available by editorial deadline	The B-Alert X24 is a two-channel EEG system, along with four optional channels for ECG, EMG, or EOG. A portable EEG device, its signals enable Power Spectral Density (PSD), validated Cognitive State Metrics1, and Cognitive Workload Metric2 computations in real-time or during offline analyses, as well as event-locked for single-trial or averaged Event-Related Potential (ERP) analyses. The B-Alert Series comes with both real time online as well as offline data and analytics. B-Alert Live is a visual EEG software solution that combines real-time and off-line processing and analysis tools. Using LabX, data can be analysed in three modes - Epoch by Epoch over time, Event Locked and LORETA/sLoreta.
Biocom HRM-02 USB Ear-Clip Pulse Wave Sensor	Biocom Technologies	www.biocomtech.com	*****	**	Comprised of an ear sensor that plugs into a computer via USB, the Biocom heart rate variability system offering both time as well as frequency domain HRV measures. While the Heart Rhythm Scanner PE is based on full short term HRV analysis during and after the session, the HRV Live! 1.0 offers continuous real-time short term HRV analysis.
Bodyguard 2	Firstbeat	www.firstbeat.com	*****	**	The Bodyguard 2 is designed for long term, 24-hour HRV monitoring with ECG electrodes. It records RR-intervals in 1 millisecond accuracy. In addition, the device has 3D acceleration sensor. The software included computes parameters including oxygen consumption, energy expenditure, excess post-exercise oxygen consumption (EPOC), respiration rate, stress level, recovery level, aerobic and anaerobic training effect, acute and chronic training load, and TRIMP in addition to time- and frequency domain parameters of HRV. The Firstbeat SPORTS Monitor is used for real-time monitoring of the training sessions and games, and to perform Quick Recovery Tests.
emWave Pro Plus	HeartMath	www.heartmath.com	*****	*	The emWave Pro Plus consists of an ear sensor along with USB module. It offers two HRV assessments: 1-minute deep breathing assessment with a visual breath pacer, and HRV assessments that range between 2 and 99 minutes. It captures both time and frequency domain measures.

Product	Manufacturer	URL	Rating	Cost	Description
EPOC +	Emotiv	www.emotiv.com/epoc	*****	* (yearly subscription additional)	Epoc + is a 14-channel wireless EEG, designed for contextualized research and Brain Computer Interface applications. The device offers 12 hours of continuous use and is compatible with Windows, OSX, Android and iOS. The EmotivPro is an integrated subscription-based software solution that provides real time display of data streams, including raw EEG, motion data, data packet acquisition and loss, and contact quality. It also allows to customize and view frequency data for live or recorded data with automatic FFT and power band graphs.
FlexComp System with BioGraph Infiniti Software- T7555M	Thought Technology	www.thoughttechnology.com/	*****	***	FlexComp System is a wired 10 high-speed channel system that can be used to record EEG, HRV, SEMG data. FlexComp offers real time monitoring or remote data storage modes and delivers instantaneous analysis of complex data. The FlexComp can be combined with specific software suites, including those for EEG, HRV, respiration with EKG or BVP Z-score biofeedback, peak performance and reaction time.
Freedom 7D	BrainMaster Technology	www.brainmaster.com/product/freedom-7d-gold-pkg-ii-braindx-z-scores/	*****	*****	Freedom 7D is a dry research grade wireless EEG headset with seven sensors positioned at choice of F3, F4, C3, C4, Pz, P3, and P4 locations of 10–20 International System.
I-330-C2+	J + J Engineering	www.jjengineering.com/	*****	**	The device includes four differential channels for EMG, ECG, EEG, and eight channels for temperature, skin resistance, and respiration, provide power, flexibility and functionality for a multitude of customized uses. The Windows software displays signals, provides feedback, collects data, prints reports, and exports database compatible files. Features include automatic testing of electrode impedance for connection quality, easy hookup with reusable gel free sensors, and fast channel sampling at 1024 SPS for high resolution spectral displays and precision filtering. The I-330-C2's 12 channel capability supports simultaneous monitoring of signals, such as: two-person monitoring for ECG, HRV, Respiration, Skin Resistance or Conductance, and Temperature; four EMG channels with spectral and raw signal displays, four Skin Resistance and Conductance, four Temperature; ECG, two EMG, two Respiration, two Skin Resistance, two Temperature; one, two, or four EEG channels, Respiration, SR, Temperature.

(Continued)

Device	Manufacturer	Website	Grade	Price	Description
MindWave Headset	Neurosky	www.neurosky.com	*****	*	A portable EEG headset, MindWave is designed to be used by developers. Research tools include NeuroView and NeuroSkyLab. NeuroView is designed for novice to intermediate researchers wishing to view and record EEG data in real time. This data can also be exported to other third-party applications for downstream data analysis and processing. Measurements can be taken in raw signal, neuroscience defined EEG power spectrum, eSense meter for Attention and eSense meter for Medication. The NeuroSkyLab on the other hand is targeted towards advanced EEG researchers who are familiar with the MATLAB environment, providing more customization and real time data viewing and analysis.
Mitsar Portable EEG System	Mitsar Medica	www.mitsar-medical.com	*****	Not available by editorial deadline	The Mitsar device is a Portable EEG System used essentially in clinical practice. The Mitsar-Porto uses a USB powered 25 channel amplifier. The supplied software package includes EEG acquisition, EEG analysis and report generation.
Muse: The brain sensing band	Muse	www.choosemuse.com	*****	*	Muse is a wireless EEG device containing 7 calibrated sensors-2 on the forehead, 2 behind the ears and 3 reference sensors. Compatible with Windows, Linux and iOS, Muse offers ran and quantization level EEG data, raw accelerometer data, raw gyroscope data, raw FFTs and band powers. It also corrects for artifacts associated with blinks and jaw clenches.
NEURO PRAX®	NeuroCare	www.neurocaregroup.com/ neuroconn-neuro-prax.html	*****	Not available by editorial deadline	The NEURO PRAX® series include full-band DC-EEG biofeedback and neurofeedback systems. The amplifiers detect EEG, EMG and EP ranging from very slow (up to 0.3 Hz) to very fast (up to 1200 Hz) frequencies. The systems are available with 32, 64 or 128 channels. It's software and hardware modules allow for online correction of artifacts caused by muscle and eye movements, topographical analyses, spectral and amplitude mapping, online averaging, bio- and neurofeedback. neuroCare technology fulfills technical requirements for applications in neuroscience research, including bio- and Neurofeedback/ QEEG/ fMRI-EEG/ EEG-tDCS/ EEG-tACS/ EEG-tRNS / TMS-EEG/ navigated EEG-TMS/ NIRS-EEG. It has been used in research involving ADHD, depression, rTMS and personalized medicine.

Product	Company	Website			Description
NeXus-32	Mind Media	www.mindmedia.com/en/products/nexus-32/	*****	Not available by editorial deadline	NeXus-32 is a lab-based device capable of measuring 32 physiological signals simultaneously. It has 24 inputs for unipolar EEG signals and up to four channels for EEG, EMG, ECG, respiration, temperature, skin conductance, SCP, EOG, Sp02, accelerometer and force. The BioTrace+ software allows for customized training application and audio-visual feedback options, extended analysis and reporting tools, artifact control and feedback controls for individual training. It also provides a dual monitor setup providing different screens to clients and researchers.
Neurobit Optima 4 unit	Neurobit Systems	www.neurobitsystems.com/neurobitoptima.htm	****	*	Neurobit Optima is a portable physiological data acquisition tool that can used to measure neurofeedback, EEG, sEMG, HRV, GSR, TEMP and can be used for scientific research. The device can be used with other third-party software for data processing.
Q-wiz suite	Pocket Neurobics	www.pocketneurobics.com/product/q-wiz-kit-complete/	****	**	Q-wiz suite supports EEG, ECG, EMG, SCG, HEG and pulse oximetry data acquisition. It has four channels. The device can be used with third party software such as BioExplorer and BioEra. It can connect to tablets and computers via USB or wireless. It comes with one set of electrodes, EEG cap, HEG headband. Finger sensor and wireless kit.
WaveRider Pro Hardware	Waverider	www.biof.com/onlinestore/waverider.asp	****	**	Waverider Pro has four channels to read brain, heart, and muscle signals. Outputs include music, tones, graphs, bars, and spectrogram as well as raw data and processed data. It is compatible with Windows and comes with WaveWare Software and accessories. WaveWare has export capabilities and stores raw data.
Polar V800 Sports Watch	Polar	www.polar.com/us-en/products/pro/V800	****	*	Polar V800 is a waterproof sports watch, integrated with GPS, allowing athletes to create and customize sport specific profiles. It comes with a chest strap and Polar H7 Bluetooth Smart Heart Rate Sensor. Data from the Polar Flow App can then be exported for HRV analysis using third party applications. Very artifact resistant.
SenzeBand	Neeuro	www.neeuro.com/senzeband/	***	*	Senzeband is a headband that measures EEG signals. It has six sensors–four individual channels and two reference sensors. Senzeband uses different levels of frequencies to measure the user's mental state. It has accelerometer to detect any head movements. It can track attention, focus, mental workload, and relaxation levels. Using Bluetooth, it is compatible with Android and iOS smartphones and tablets. Senzeband is extendable to be paired with Neeuro applications or customized applications through their SDK packages.

(*Continued*)

Device	Manufacturer	Website	Grade	Price	Description
Versus	Versus	www.getversuss.com	***	* (monthly subscription additional)	Versus is a five channel wireless EEG headset that connects to iPhones and iPads via Bluetooth. It accesses Fz, Cz, Pz, C3 and C4 and provides customized exercise protocols. It also includes NeuroPerformance Assessment – designed to identify strengths and weaknesses in mental acuity, concentration, problem solving, multitasking, resource management, decision making and sleep tendencies.
FocusBand	FocusBand	www.focusband.com/	**	*	FocusBand is a wearable headset that is used with a mobile app. It has 3 silver oxide sensors and 2 channel EEG system and measures brain frequency. It connects to your mobile device via Bluetooth and translates the data into easy to understand Avatar for visual and audio feedback. There are different apps for different uses such as FocusBand NeuroVision, FocusBand NeuroSkill, FocusBand Brain Training, FocusBand NeuroSelfCare etc.
GP Series	Physiocom	www.stressresilientmind.co.uk/biofeedback-neurofeedback-devices	**	*	The Physiocom GP series consists of multi-channel Biofeedback & Neurofeedback Amplifiers. Designed for consumers, they connect to a PC via USB. The parameters assessed include EMG, EEG, ECG for heart rate and heart rate variability (HRV), Pulse oximeter, skin temperature and breath detection.
L.I.F.E	Harmonic Energetic Technologies, Inc.	www.life-het.com/life/thesystem/	**	*****	The L.I.F.E. System is an electro-physiological Biofeedback device receiving signals through a 5-point harness system. This harness system contains eight LED's (Light Emitting Diodes) that provide a full spectrum of color used as feedback of stress and tension.
NeuroSystem 2/4	Zynex Neurodiagnostics	www.zynexneuro.com/neurosystem-24/	**	Not available by editorial deadline	The NeuroSystem 2/4 is an 6+ acquisition channel integrated instrumentation and software package for non-invasive biofeedback. It includes monitoring of PPG, sEMG, Temperature, Respiration and EDA Electrodermal Activity. Multiple report presentations are available to healthcare professions.
Health Tag	Spire	www.spire.io	**	*	Spire devices are long term HRV devices- they assess respiratory effort and are being expanded to include respiratory rate variability at 1-minute intervals, and cardiac information such as HR and HRV metrics. It consists of a consumer app, a clinical dashboard and an API. The former has reports on the stats screen and the latter two can be used to generate reports. It does not provide real time monitoring.

Device	Manufacturer	URL			Description
Tickr	Wahoo	www.wahoofitness.com/devices/heart-rate-monitors	**	*	Tickr is a waterproof activity tracker and heart rate monitor. Raw data from the device can be exported for HRV analytics.
Zephyr	Zephyr	www.zephyranywhere.com/resources/hxm	**	*	Zephyr Performance Systems include a heart rate sensor that can be attached to chest straps as well as compression and loose fit shirts. Data from the Zephyr BioModule device can be exported for heart rate variability analytics.
FitBit Versa	FitBit	www.fitbit.com/versa	*	*	FitBit Versa is a water-resistant activity tracker allows the users to track their heart rate and see trends, track sleeping, offers guided breathing sessions, and can be connected to mobile devices via Bluetooth.
Apple Watch Series 3	Apple	www.apple.com/apple-watch-series-3/	*	*	Apple Watch Series is a waterproof GPS wearable device that allows users to track heart rate while resting, walking, workout and recovery heart rate. It can be used with third party health apps.
IOM / LightStone Biofeedback System	Transparent Corp	www.transparentcorp.com/products/iom/index.php	*	Not available by editorial deadline	The IOM device measures both GSR (Skin Conductance) and heart rate utilizing three finger sensors and a USB plug. The IOM biofeedback system comes in a package with the Relaxing Rhythms software. Neuro-Programmer 3 (NP3) is capable of using the IOM biofeedback system to optimize brainwave entrainment as well.
Motiv Ring	Motiv	www.mymotiv.com/buy	*	*	Motiv ring monitors heart rate, resting heart rate, active minutes, steps and calories burned from the finger. It is waterproof and can also additionally track sleep duration. It Is It allows you to measure your distance and actively measure your heart rate.
NeurOptimal	NeurOptimal	www.neuroptimal.com	*	*****	NeurOptimal® is a neurofeedback system utilizing an original Dynamical Neurofeedback® algorithm. A consumer-based product, it has not been extensively used in medical or research settings.
Nokia Steel HR	Nokia	www.health.nokia.com/us/en/steel-hr	*	*	Nokia Steel Hr is a water-resistant heart rate and activity watch. Steel HR connects to Nokia Health Mate app and tracks health, sleep cycles, optimize workouts with continuous heart rate monitoring.
Samsung Gear Sport	Samsung	www.samsung.com/us/mobile/wearables/smartwatches/gear-sport-black-sm-r600nzkaxar/	*	*	Gear Sport watch is water resistant smart watch. It has GPS and can be connected to Samsung Pay and S Health and allows users to track heart rate.
TomTom Spark 3 Cardio + Music	TomTom	www.tomtom.com/en_us/sports/fitness-watches/	*	*	Spark 3 Cardio + Music comes with a built-in heart rate monitor. It measures heart rate in regular intervals. It has multiple sports modes, GPS tracking, and 24/7 activity tracking.
Vivoactive 3	Garmin	www.buy.garmin.com/en-US/US/p/571520	*	*	Vivoactive 3 is a smart watch which tracks fitness level with VO2 max and fitness age estimates, and wrist-based heart rate. It has 15 preloaded GPS and indoor sports apps.
Wild Divine – IomBLUE	Unyte	www.wilddivine.com/products/iom-blue	*	*	The IomBLUE is an ambulatory biofeedback device measuring HR, HRV and breathing. It transmits signals via an ear clip and is synced to Wild Divine Apps on iOS devices.

Index

Index

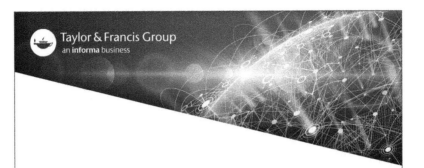

For Product Safety Concerns and Information please contact our EU
representative GPSR@taylorandfrancis.com
Taylor & Francis Verlag GmbH, Kaufingerstraße 24, 80331 München, Germany

www.ingramcontent.com/pod-product-compliance
Ingram Content Group UK Ltd.
Pitfield, Milton Keynes, MK11 3LW, UK
UKHW051834180425
457613UK00022B/1248